Alina Haider
16013

Illustrated Textbook of
Paediatrics
Fourth Edition

Commissioning Editor: *Pauline Graham*
Development Editor: *Sally Davies*
Project Manager: *Alan Nicholson*
Designer: *Stewart Larking*
Illustration Manager: *Gillian Richards*
Illustrator: *Cactus*

Illustrated Textbook of
Paediatrics
Fourth Edition

Edited by

Dr Tom Lissauer MB BChir FRCPCH
Honorary Consultant Paediatrician, Imperial College Healthcare Trust,
London, UK

Dr Graham Clayden MD FRCPCH FHEA
Honorary Reader in Paediatrics, Kings College London,
School of Medicine at Guy's, Kings and St Thomas' Hospitals,
London, UK

Foreword by

Professor Sir Alan Craft
Emeritus Professor of Child Health, Newcastle University,
Past President Royal College of Paediatrics and Child Health

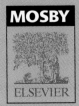

MOSBY

ELSEVIER

Edinburgh   London   New York   Oxford   Philadelphia   St Louis   Sydney   Toronto 2012

First edition 1997
Second edition 2001
Third edition 2007
Fourth edition 2012

ISBN 978 0 7234 3565 5
    Reprinted 2012
International ISBN 978 0 7234 3566 2
    Reprinted 2012

British Library Cataloguing in Publication Data
A catalogue record for this book is available from the British Library

Library of Congress Cataloging in Publication Data
A catalog record for this book is available from the Library of Congress

ELSEVIER your source for books, journals and multimedia in the health sciences
www.elsevierhealth.com

Working together to grow libraries in developing countries

www.elsevier.com | www.bookaid.org | www.sabre.org

ELSEVIER   BOOK AID International   Sabre Foundation

The publisher's policy is to use **paper manufactured from sustainable forests**

Printed in China

Contents

Foreword

When the late Frank A. Oski wrote the foreword for the first edition of this book in 1997, he gave it fulsome praise and predicted that it would become a 'standard by which all other medical textbooks will be judged'. He was a great man and a wonderful writer, so his prediction was no doubt welcomed by the authors, both well known for their contribution to undergraduate and postgraduate medical education and assessment.

I have a much easier task in writing the foreword for the fourth edition in 2011. The mere fact that there is a fourth edition is testimony in itself, but there is also the fact that this book has become the recommended paediatric textbook in countless medical schools throughout the world and has been translated into 8 languages. I have travelled the world over the last 15 years and wherever I have been in a paediatric department, the distinctive sunflower cover of 'Lissauer and Clayden' has been there with me. Whether it is Hong Kong, Malaysia, Oman or South Shields, it is there!

It is not surprising that it has won major awards for innovation and excellence at the British Medical Association and Royal Society of Medicine book awards. The book is well established and widely read for the simple reason that it is an excellent book. Medicine is now so complex and information so vast that students are no longer expected to know all there is to know about medicine. What they need are the core principles and guidance as to where to find out more. This book gives the core principles, but also provides a great deal more for the student who wishes to extend his or her knowledge. It is in a very accessible form and has a style and layout which facilitates learning. There are many diagrams, illustrations and case histories to bring the subject to life and to impart important messages. This new edition includes summaries to help revision and also provides access to online assessment tools.

It has been thoroughly updated with many new authors, each of whom is an expert in their own field, but who has been chosen because of their ability to impart the key principles in a non-specialist way. The text focuses on the key areas of paediatrics and new sections include child protection and global health.

There are now countless doctors throughout the world for whom this textbook has been their introduction to the fascinating and rewarding world of paediatrics.

For students, it is all they need to know and a bit more. For postgraduates, it provides the majority of information needed to get through postgraduate examinations and stimulates and guides the reader into the world of clinical paediatrics where practical experience can be gained, built on the sound foundation of the Lissauer and Clayden knowledge base.

The authors are to be congratulated on the continuing success of this book.

I can only echo what Frank Oski said in his preface to the first edition: 'I wish I had written this book'!

Professor Sir Alan Craft
Emeritus Professor of Child Health, Newcastle University
Past President Royal College of Paediatrics and Child Health

Acknowledgements

We would like to acknowledge the major contribution made to previous editions by the following contributors:

First edition:

Lynn Ball (Haematological disorders), Nigel Curtis (Paediatric emergencies, Infection and Immunity), Gill Du Mont (Skin), Tony Hulse (Growth and puberty; and Endocrine and metabolic disorders), Nigel Klein (Paediatric emergencies, Infection), Nicholas Madden (Genitalia), Angus Nicoll (Development, language, hearing and vision), Karen Simmer (Perinatal medicine, Neonatal medicine), Elizabeth Thompson (Genetics).

Second edition:

Paula Bolton-Maggs (Haematological disorders), Jon Couriel (Respiratory disorders), Ruth Gilbert (Evidence-based medicine), Dennis Gill (History and examination), Raanan Gillon (Ethics), Peter Hill (Emotions and behaviour), Nigel Klein (Infection and immunity), Simon Nadel (Paediatric emergencies), Barbara Phillips (Environment), Andrew Redington (Cardiac disorders), John Sills (Bones and joints), Rashmin Tamhne (The child in society), Michael Weindling (Perinatal medicine, Neonatal medicine).

Third edition:

Dr Ulrich Baumann (Liver disorders), Dr Mitch Blair (The child in society), Dr Tom Blyth (Allergy and immunity), Professor Ian Booth (Nutrition, Gastroenterology), Dr Michelle Cummins (Haematological disorders), Dr Iolo Doull (Respiratory disorders), Dr Saul Faust (Infection), Professor Elena Garralda (Emotions and behaviour), Dr Alison Giles (Paediatric Neurology), Professor George Haycock (Kidney and urinary tract), Dr Helen Jenkinson (Malignant disease), Professor Deirdre Kelly (Liver disorders), Dr Helen Kingston (Genetics), Professor Gideon Lack (Allergy and immunity), Mr Anthony Lander (Gastroenterology), Dr Vic Larcher (Care of the sick child – Ethics), Dr Hermione Lyall (Infection), Dr Ian Maconochie (Environment), Dr Maud Meates-Dennis (Care of the sick child – Evidence-based medicine), Dr Lesley Rees (Kidney and urinary tract), Dr Terry Segal (Adolescent medicine), Professor Jo Sibert (Environment), Professor Tauny Southwood (History and examination; Bones, joints and rheumatic disorders), Mr Mark Stringer (Genitalia), Dr Rob Tasker (Paediatric emergencies), Professor David Thomas (Genitalia), Dr Russell Viner (Adolescent medicine), Professor Andrew Whitelaw (Perinatal medicine; Neonatal medicine). We would also like to thank Dr Bernie Borgstein for advice on Paediatric Audiology, Professor Alistair Fielder and Ms Clare Roberts for advice on Paediatric Ophthalmology and Professor Ed Wraith for advice on Metabolic Disorders.

The contributors to this edition have extensively drawn on the material prepared for previous editions.

Preface

This textbook has been written for undergraduates. Our aim has been to provide the core information required by medical students for the 6–10 weeks assigned to paediatrics in the curriculum of most undergraduate medical schools. We are delighted that it has become so widely used not only in the UK but also in northern Europe, India, Pakistan, Australia, South Africa and other countries. We are also pleased that nurses, therapists and other health professionals who care for children have found the book helpful. It will also be of assistance to doctors preparing for postgraduate examinations such as the Diploma of Child Health (DCH) and Membership of the Royal College of Paediatrics and Child Health (MRCPCH).

The huge amount of positive feedback we have received on the first three editions from medical students, postgraduate doctors and their teachers in the UK and abroad has spurred us on to produce this new edition. We have updated the text and some sections, such as child protection and global health, have been rewritten to incorporate significant advances.

In order to make learning from this book easier, we have followed a lecture-note style using short sentences and lists of important features. Illustrations have been used to help in the recognition of important signs or clinical features and to make the book more attractive and interesting to use. Key learning points are identified and case histories chosen to demonstrate points within their clinical context. Summary boxes of important facts have been included to help with revision.

The male gender for children has been used throughout the book for stylistic simplicity.

We would like to thank all our contributors and Pauline Graham at Elsevier for their assistance in producing this new edition. Thanks also to Ann Goldman, Rachel and David and Sam Lissauer for their ideas and assistance, and for their understanding of the time taken away from the family in the preparation of this new edition.

We welcome any comments about the book.

Tom Lissauer and Graham Clayden

Contributors

Mrs Aruna Abhyankar
Consultant Paediatric Surgeon
University Hospital of Wales, Cardiff, UK
Ch. 19: Genitalia

Dr Shruti Agrawal
Consultant Paediatric Intensivist
St Mary's Hospital, Imperial College NHS Trust,
    London, UK
Ch. 6: Paediatric emergencies

Professor Stephen J Allen
Professor of Paediatrics and International
    Health
Swansea Medical School, Swansea, UK
Ch. 1: The child in society

Dr Cornelius Ani
Consultant Child and Adolescent Psychiatrist
    and Honorary Clinical Senior Lecturer
Academic Unit of Child and Adolescent
    Psychiatry, Imperial College London,
St Mary's Hospital, London, UK
Ch. 23: Emotions and behaviour

Dr Jonathan Bishop
Consultant in Paediatric Gastroenterology
Royal Hospital for Sick Children, Glasgow, UK
Ch. 12: Nutrition
Ch. 13: Gastroenterology
Ch. 20: Liver disorders

Dr Robert J Boyle
Clinical Senior Lecturer in Paediatrics
Imperial College London and Honorary
    Consultant Paediatric Allergist, St Mary's
    Hospital, London, UK
Ch. 15: Allergy

Dr Malcolm Brodlie
SpR in Paediatric Respiratory Medicine
Great North Children's Hospital, Newcastle
    Hospitals NHS Foundation Trust,
    Newcastle upon Tyne, UK
Ch. 16: Respiratory disorders

Dr Subarna Chakravorty
Clinical Research Fellow
Department of Haematology, Imperial College
    London, UK
Ch. 22: Haematological disorders

Professor Angus John Clarke
Professor and Honorary Consultant in Clinical
    Genetics
Institute of Medical Genetics, University
    Hospital of Wales, Cardiff, UK
Ch. 8: Genetics

Dr Graham Clayden
Honorary Reader in Paediatrics, Kings College
    London, School of Medicine at Guy's, Kings
    and St Thomas' Hospitals, London, UK
(Editor)

Dr Paul Dimitri
Consultant, Paediatric Endocrinology
    Sheffield Children's NHS Trust
Sheffield Children's Hospital, Sheffield, UK
Ch. 11: Growth and puberty
Ch. 25: Endocrine and metabolic disorders

Dr Rachel Dommett
Academic Clinical Lecturer
University of Bristol, School of Clinical
    Sciences, Bristol, UK
Ch. 21: Malignant disease

Professor Helen E Foster
Professor of Paediatric Rheumatology,
     Newcastle University and Honorary
     Consultant
Newcastle Hospitals NHS Foundation Trust,
     Newcastle upon Tyne, UK
Ch. 26: Musculoskeletal disorders

Dr Stephen Hodges
Consultant Paediatric Gastroenterologist
Newcastle Hospitals NHS Foundation Trust
Honorary Clinical Senior Lecturer Child Health
Newcastle University,
     Newcastle upon Tyne, UK
Ch. 12: Nutrition
Ch. 13: Gastroenterology
Ch. 20: Liver disorders

Dr Siobhan Jaques
Specialist Registrar in Paediatrics
Imperial College Healthcare Trust
London, UK
Ch. 2: History and examination

Dr Sharmila Jandial
Arthritis Research UK Research Fellow and
     Specialist Registrar in Paediatrics
Department of Paediatric Rheumatology,
     Newcastle Hospitals NHS Foundation Trust,
     Newcastle upon Tyne, UK
Ch. 26: Musculoskeletal disorders

Dr Larissa Kerecuk
Consultant Paediatric Nephrologist
Department of Paediatric Nephrology,
     Birmingham Children's Hospital
Birmingham, UK
Ch. 18: Kidney and urinary tract disorders

Dr Ike Lagunju
Consultant Paediatrician, Department of
     Paediatrics, University College Hospital,
Ibadan, Nigeria
Ch. 1: The child in society

Dr Tom Lissauer
Honorary Consultant Paediatrician
Imperial College Healthcare Trust, London, UK
(Editor)
Ch. 2: History and examination
Ch. 5: Care of the sick child
Ch. 9: Perinatal medicine
Ch. 10: Neonatal medicine

Dr Janet E McDonagh
Senior Lecturer in Paediatric and Adolescent
     Rheumatology and Clinical Lead for
     Adolescent Health
University of Birmingham, Institute of Child
     Health, Birmingham Children's Hospital
     NHS Foundation Trust, Birmingham, UK
Ch. 28: Adolescent medicine

Dr Michael C McKean
Consultant in Paediatric Respiratory Medicine
Great North Children's Hospital, Newcastle
     Hospitals NHS Foundation Trust,
     Newcastle upon Tyne, UK
Ch. 16: Respiratory disorders

Dr Richard W Newton
Consultant Paediatric Neurologist
Royal Manchester Children's Hospital,
     Manchester, UK
Ch. 27: Neurological disorders

Raúl Pardíñaz-Solís
Global Health Manager
Skillshare International, Leicester, UK
Ch. 1: The child in society

Dr Sanjay Patel
Clinical Research Fellow
Academic Department of Paediatrics,
     Paediatric Infectious Diseases, Imperial
     College London, London, UK
Ch. 2: History and examination

Dr Andrew Prendergast
Senior Lecturer in Paediatric Infection and
    Immunity
Wellcome Trust Intermediate Clinical Fellow
Honorary Consultant Paediatrican
Queen Mary and Westfield College, University
    of London, London, UK
Ch. 14: Infection and immunity

Professor Irene AG Roberts
Professor of Paediatric Haematology
Department of Haematology, Imperial College
    London, London, UK
Ch. 22: Haematological disorders

Dr Rebecca C Salter
Consultant in Paediatric Emergency Medicine
St Mary's Hospital, Imperial College Healthcare
    Trust, London, UK
Ch. 7: Accidents, poisoning and child protection

Dr Peter Sidebotham
Associate Professor of Child Health
University of Warwick, Coventry, UK
Ch. 1: The child in society

Dr Kathleen Sim
Academic Clinical Fellow
Paediatric Infectious Diseases, Imperial
    College London, St Mary's Hospital
    Campus, London, UK
Ch. 2: History and examination

Mr Gerard P S Siou
Consultant ENT and Head & Neck Surgeon
Freeman Hospital, Newcastle upon Tyne, UK
Ch. 16: Respiratory disorders

Dr Diane P L Smyth
Consultant in Paediatric Neurology and
    Neurodisability
St Mary's Hospital, Imperial College Healthcare
    Trust, London, UK
*Ch. 3: Normal child development, hearing and
    vision*
*Ch. 4: Developmental problems and the child
    with special needs*

Professor Michael Stevens
CLIC Professor of Paediatric Oncology
School of Clinical Sciences, University of
    Bristol, Bristol, UK
Ch. 21: Malignant disease

Dr Sharon E Taylor
Consultant Child and Adolescent Psychiatrist
Academic Unit of Child and Adolescent
    Psychiatry
Imperial College London and St Mary's
    Hospital, London, UK
Ch. 23: Emotions and behaviour

Dr Gareth Tudor-Williams
Reader and Honorary Consultant in Paediatric
    Infectious Diseases
Imperial College London and Imperial College
    Healthcare Trust, St Mary's Hospital,
    London, UK
Ch. 14: Infection and immunity

Dr Robert M R Tulloh
Consultant Paediatric Cardiologist
Bristol Royal Hospital for Children, Bristol, UK
Ch. 17: Cardiac disorders

Professor Julian L Verbov
Honorary Professor of Dermatology
University of Liverpool
Consultant Paediatric Dermatologist
Royal Liverpool Children's Hospital,
    Liverpool, UK
Ch. 24: Skin disorders

Dr Jerry K H Wales
Senior Lecturer in Paediatric Endocrinology
Academic Unit of Child Health, Sheffield
    Children's Hospital, Sheffield, UK
Ch. 11: Growth and puberty
Ch. 25: Endocrine and metabolic disorders

Professor Andrew R Wilkinson
Professor of Paediatrics & Perinatal Medicine
University of Oxford, Neonatal Unit, Women's
　　Centre, John Radcliffe Hospital, Oxford, UK
Ch. 9: Perinatal medicine
Ch. 10: Neonatal medicine

Dr Neil Wimalasundera
Consultant in Paediatric Neurodisability
The Wolfson Neurodisability Service, Great
　　Ormond Street Hospital, London, UK
*Ch. 3: Normal child development, hearing and
　　vision*
*Ch. 4: Developmental problems and the child
　　with special needs*

Contributors

1

The child in society

Most medical encounters with children involve an individual child presenting to a doctor with a symptom, such as diarrhoea. After taking a history, examining the child and performing any necessary investigations, the doctor arrives at a diagnosis or differential diagnosis and makes a management plan. This disease-oriented approach, which is the focus of most of this book, plays an important part in ensuring the immediate and long-term well-being of the child. Of course, the doctor also needs to understand the nature of the child's illness within the wider context of their world, which is the primary focus of this chapter. The context of any symptom will affect the:

- likely cause: if the diarrhoea is likely to be from a viral illness or from a contaminated water supply if in a developing country
- severity of the child's illness: the organism likely to be responsible and the child's nutritional status
- management options: who will take care of the child when ill; is pre-prepared oral rehydration therapy available; is hospital treatment possible and what facilities can it offer?

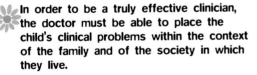 **In order to be a truly effective clinician, the doctor must be able to place the child's clinical problems within the context of the family and of the society in which they live.**

Important goals for a society are that its children and young people are healthy, safe, enjoy, achieve and make a positive contribution and achieve economic well-being (*Every Child Matters*, 2003 at: http://www.dcsf.gov.uk/everychildmatters). These are included in the UN Rights of the Child (see below). The way in which the environment impacts on a child achieving good health is exemplified by the contrast between the major child health problems in developed and developing countries. In developed countries these are a range of complex, often previously fatal, chronic disorders and behavioural, emotional or developmental problems. By contrast, in developing countries the

predominant problems are infection and malnutrition (Box 1.1).

The child's world

Children's health is profoundly influenced by their social, cultural and physical environment. This can be considered in terms of the child, the family and immediate social environment, the local social fabric and the national and international environment (Fig. 1.1). Our ability to intervene as clinicians needs to be seen within this context of complex interrelating influences on health.

The child

The child's world will be affected by gender, genes, physical health, temperament and development. The impact of the social environment varies markedly with age:

- Infant or toddler: life is mainly determined by the home environment
- Young child: by school and friends
- Teenager: also aware of and influenced by events nationally but also internationally, e.g. in music, sport, fashion or politics.

Immediate social environment

Family structure

Although the 'two biological parent family' remains the norm, there are many variations in family structure. In the UK, the family structure has changed markedly over the last 30 years (Fig. 1.2).

Single-parent households – One in four children now live in a single-parent household. Disadvantages of single parenthood include a higher level of unemployment, poor housing and financial hardship (Table 1.1). These social adversities may affect parenting resources, e.g. vigilance about safety, adequacy of nutrition,

Box 1.1 Contrast between main child health problems and associated factors in developed and developing countries

Developed countries – main child health problems	Problems in both developed and developing countries	Developing countries – main child health problems
• Severe, often previously fatal chronic disorders – malignant disease, cystic fibrosis • Provision of paediatric and neonatal intensive care, organ transplantation and other specialist services • Behavioural and emotional disorders – attention deficit hyperactivity disorder, anorexia nervosa • Neurodevelopmental disorders – language delay, reading difficulties, clumsiness, cerebral palsy • Excessive consumption – obesity • Drug and alcohol abuse, smoking, teenage pregnancies.	• Relative socioeconomic disadvantage among the 'have-nots' – lack of money, unemployment, inadequate housing and education • Lack of family cohesion • Healthcare – not available or poor quality or inequality of access	• High mortality rate for children, especially infants • Infection – respiratory tract, diarrhoea, malaria, tuberculosis, HIV • Malnutrition – marasmus, kwashiorkor, severe iron deficiency anaemia • Poor sanitation, water supply, food hygiene • Road traffic and other accidents • Developmental and learning problems of organic pathology – Down syndrome, congenital anomalies • High birth rate – large number of children requiring health care relative to population

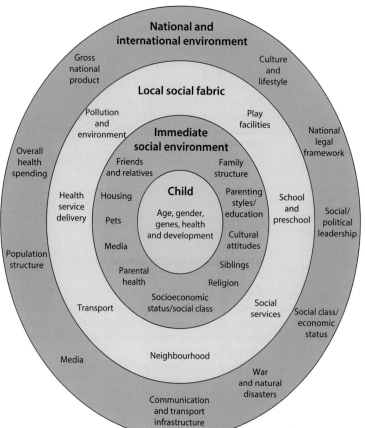

Figure 1.1 A child's world consists of overlapping, interconnected and expanding socioenvironmental layers, which influence children's health and development. (After Bronfenbrenner U. 1979. Contexts of child rearing – problems and prospects. *American Psychologist* 34:844–850.)

Table 1.1 Comparison between parents who are single or couples

	Lone-parent family	Couple family
Median weekly family income (£)	280	573
In lowest income quintile (%)	48	7
Living in social housing (%)	44	12
Parent with no educational qualification (%)	15	3
Child with school behaviour problems (%)	14	8

General Household Survey, Office for National Statistics, England 2008.

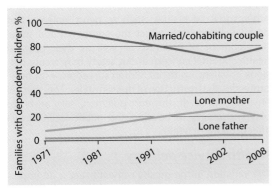

Figure 1.2 Changing structure of the family 1971–2008. (ONS, General Lifestyle Survey 2008).

take-up of preventive services, such as immunisation and regular screening, and ability to cope with an acutely sick child at home.

Reconstituted families – The increase in the number of parents who change partners and the accompanying rise in reconstituted families (1 in 10 children live in a stepfamily) mean that children are having to cope with a range of new and complex parental and sibling relationships. This may result in emotional, behavioural and social difficulties.

Looked after children – Approximately 3% of children under 16 years old in the UK live away from their family home. At any one time in England, over 60 000 children are cared for by Local Authorities. These 'looked after children' are known to have worse outcomes in terms of physical health, mental health, education and employment.

Asylum seekers – These are often placed in temporary housing and moved repeatedly into areas unfamiliar to them. In addition to the uncertainty as to whether or not they will be allowed to stay in the country, they face additional problems as a result of communication difficulties, poverty, fragmentation of families and racism. Many have lost family members and are uncertain about the safety of friends and family.

Parental employment – With many parents in employment, many young children are with childminders or at preschool nurseries. Parents are receiving conflicting opinions on the long-term consequences of caring for their young children at home in contrast to nursery care. Also, increasing attention is being paid to the quality of day-care facilities in terms of supervision of the children and improving the opportunities they provide for social interaction and learning.

Parenting styles

Children rely on their parents to provide love and nurture, stimulation and security, as well as catering for their physical needs of food, clothing and shelter. Parenting that is warm and receptive to the child, while imposing reasonable and consistent boundaries, will promote the development of an autonomous and self-reliant adult. This constitutes 'good enough' parenting as described by the paediatrician and psychotherapist, Donald Winnicott, and can reassure parents that perfection is not necessary. Some parents are excessively authoritarian or extremely permissive. Children's emotional development may be damaged by parents who neglect or abuse their children.

The child's temperament is also important, especially when there is a mismatch with parenting style, for example, a child with a very energetic temperament may be misperceived in a quiet family as having attention deficit hyperactivity disorder (ADHD).

Siblings and extended family

Siblings clearly have a marked influence on the family dynamics. How siblings affect each other appears to be determined by the emotional quality of their relationships with each other and also with other members of the family, including their parents. The arrival of a new baby may engender a feeling of insecurity in older brothers and sisters and result in attention-seeking behaviour. In contrast, children can benefit greatly from having siblings; and from having a close child companion, and can learn from and support each other. The role of grandparents and other family members varies widely and is influenced by the family's culture. In some, they are the main caregivers; in others, they provide valued practical and emotional support. However, in many families they now play only a peripheral role, exacerbated by geographical separation.

Cultural attitudes to child-rearing

The way in which children are brought up evolves within a community over generations, and is influenced by culture and religion, affecting both day-to-day issues to fundamental lifestyle choices. For example, in some societies children are given considerable self-autonomy, from deciding what food they want to eat, to their education and even to participating in major decisions about their medical care. By contrast, in other societies, children are largely excluded from decision-making. Other examples of marked differences between societies are the use of physical punishment to discipline children and the expected roles of males and females both as children and as adults.

Peers

Peers exert a major influence on children. Peer relationships and activities provide a 'sense of group belonging' and have potentially long-term benefits for the child. Conversely, they may exert negative pressure through inappropriate role modelling. Relationships can also go wrong, e.g. persistent bullying, which may result in or contribute to psychosomatic symptoms, misery and even, in extreme cases, suicide.

Socioeconomic status

Socioeconomic status is a key determinant of health and well-being of children. It is estimated that 2.8 million children in the UK are living in poverty (below 60% of the national median income after adjustment for housing costs). The proportion of children in poverty in different countries is shown in Figure 1.3. Health issues in the UK in which prevalence rates are increased by poverty include:

- low birthweight infants
- injuries
- hospital admissions
- asthma
- behavioural problems
- special educational needs
- child abuse.

Low socioeconomic status is often associated with multiple disadvantages, e.g. food of inadequate quantity or poor nutritional value, substandard housing or

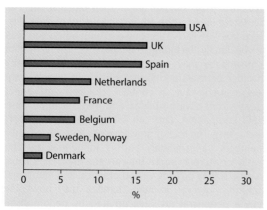

Figure 1.3 Percentage of children living in poverty. UNICEF definition is households with income below 50% of national median (UNICEF 2009). (Innocenti Research Centre. 2000. *British Medical Journal* 320:1621, reproduced with permission from the BMJ publishing group.)

homelessness, lack of 'good enough' parenting, parental education and health, and poor access to healthcare and educational facilities.

There are marked differences in living experiences between ethnic groups: 50% of Afro-Caribbean children live in single-parent households compared with 15% of white children and less than 10% of those from the Indian subcontinent. In 1992, in England and Wales, 12% of births were to mothers born outside the UK; in 2008 it was nearly 24%.

Local social fabric

Neighbourhood

Cohesive communities and amicable neighbourhoods are positive influences on children. Racial tension and other social adversities, such as gang violence and drugs, will adversely affect the emotional and social development of children, as well as their physical health. Parental concern about safety may create tensions in balancing their children's freedom with overprotection and restriction of their lifestyles. The physical environment itself, through pollution, safe areas for play and quality of housing and public facilities, will affect children's health.

Health service delivery

The variation in the quality of healthcare is an important component in preventing morbidity and mortality in children. Health services for children are increasingly provided within primary care. Some aspects of specialist paediatric care are also increasingly provided within the child's home, local community or local hospital through shared care arrangements and specialist community nursing and medical teams working within clinical networks. However, access to and the range of these services varies widely.

Schools

Schools provide a powerful influence on children's emotional and intellectual development and their subsequent lives. Differences in the quality of schools in different areas can accentuate inequalities already present in society. Schools provide enormous opportunities for influencing healthy behaviour through personal and social education and through the influence of peers and positive role models. They also provide opportunities for monitoring and promoting the health and well-being of vulnerable children.

 To educate a girl is to educate a whole family. And what is true of families is also true of communities and, ultimately, whole countries. Study after study has taught us that there is no tool for development more effective than the education of girls. No other policy is as likely to raise economic productivity, lower infant and maternal mortality, improve nutrition and promote health (Kofi Annan, Secretary General UN 2004).

Travel

The increasing ease of travel can broaden children's horizons and opportunities. Especially in rural areas, the ease and availability of transport allow greater access to medical care and other services. However, the increasing use of motor vehicles contributes to the large number of injuries sustained by children from road traffic accidents, mainly as pedestrians. It also decreases physical activity, as shown by the high proportion of children taken to school by car. Whereas 80% of children in the UK went to school by foot or bicycle in 1971, this has dropped to less than 10%.

National and international environment

Economic wealth

In general, there is an inverse relationship between a country's gross national product and income distribution and the quality of its children's health.

The lower the gross national income:

- the greater the proportion of the population who are children
- the higher the childhood mortality
- the higher the proportion of newborn infants with low birthweight
- the lower the immunisation rate.

However, even in countries with a high gross national product, many children live in financially deprived circumstances.

The dramatic reduction in childhood mortality in England over the last century is shown in Figure 1.4. It is primarily from improvements in living conditions such as improved sanitation and housing, and access to food and water. These have dramatically reduced

fatalities from infectious disease. More recent contributions to this reduction have been increased availability and uptake of immunisation and major medical improvements in perinatal and infant care.

In all countries difficult choices need to be made about the allocation of scarce resources. Should a developing country provide very expensive drugs and care for the small number of children with malignant disease or allocate its resources to preventive programmes for many children? In developed countries, difficult decisions also have to be faced in deciding the affordability of very expensive procedures, such as heart or liver transplantation, or neonatal intensive care for extremely premature infants and certain drugs, such as the genetically engineered enzyme replacement therapy for Gaucher disease or cytokine modulators ('biologics') and other immunotherapies. The public are becoming more engaged in these debates.

Media and technology

The media has a powerful influence on children. It can be positive and educational. However, the impact of television and computers and mobile technology can be negative owing to reduced opportunities for social interaction and active learning, lack of physical exercise and exposure to violence, sex and cultural stereotypes. The extent to which the aggressive tendencies of children may be exacerbated or encouraged by media exposure to violence is unclear.

The internet is enabling parents and children to become better informed about and gain support for their children's medical problems. This is especially beneficial for the many rare conditions encountered in paediatrics. A disadvantage is that it may result in the dissemination of information which is incorrect or biased, and may result in requests for inappropriate or untested investigations or treatment.

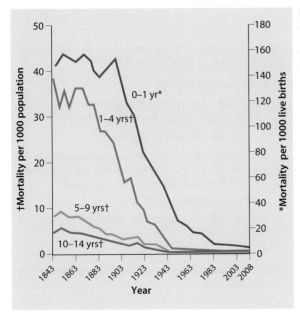

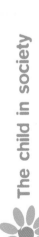

The child in society

Figure 1.4 Marked reduction in mortality of children aged 0–14 years between 1843 and 2008. In 1900, 15% of babies born in England died by 1 year of age and 23% by 14 years of age; in 2008 the figures were 0.46% and 0.64%, respectively.

War and natural disasters

Children are especially vulnerable when there is war, civil unrest or natural disasters (Box 1.2). Not only are they at greater risk from infectious diseases and malnutrition but also they may lose their care-givers and other members of their families and are likely to have been exposed to highly traumatic events.

Their lives will have been uprooted, socially and culturally, especially if they are forced to flee from their homes and become refugees.

Public health issues for young people

Important public health issues for the 11 million children and young people in the UK in which doctors play a role include:

Obesity – it is estimated that 6.5% of 9-year-olds and 15% of 15-year-olds are clinically obese (BMI >90th centile). Doctors can help promote healthy eating through supporting breast-feeding in infancy, advising parents and young people on healthy life-styles, monitoring growth parameters and the consequences of obesity, and through advocacy and support for local and national healthy lifestyle programmes.

Emotional and behavioural difficulties – 11% of boys and 8% of girls in this country suffer from a defined emotional or behavioural difficulty. In addition, these problems are often unrecognised and have significant ongoing impacts on children's overall well-being. Doctors can contribute to tackling these problems by being alert to and responding to the signs of mental health problems in childhood, and through promoting equitable distribution of resources to child and adolescent mental health services.

Disability – up to 5.4% have some form of disability and 7% have a long-standing illness that limits their activity. Doctors need to work closely with children and young people, families, local communities and other services to ensure that any individual child's needs are appropriately catered for. This may include outlining a child's health needs for a statement of special educational need, formulating an individual healthcare plan and advocating for the resources to implement this. Doctors can also provide education and social services with data on the numbers and levels of need within their own population.

Smoking, alcohol and drugs – a 2007 survey found that 6% of 11–15-year-olds smoke regularly; 10% had taken drugs in the past month and 20% had drunk alcohol in the past week. Doctors have been instrumental in campaigning for legislation to protect young people from targeted advertising and to raise awareness of the dangers of smoking, alcohol and drugs. There is some evidence that prevalence of all three behaviours are decreasing.

Doctors can also help children through advocacy about children's issues, by providing information to inform public debate. Examples of this are child protection, exploitation of children for labour or trafficking, the needs of refugee children and tobacco and alcohol advertising.

Children's rights

Children's rights are laid down in the United Nations Convention on the Rights of the Child, which has been ratified by all members of the United Nations, including the UK, but excepting the USA and Somalia (Box 1.3, Fig. 1.5). Unfortunately, the rights of many children are not met. Implications of the convention include the involvement of children in clinical decision-making and in issues of consent.

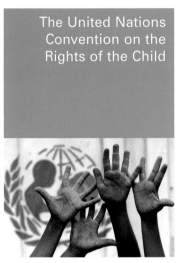

The United Nations
Convention on the
Rights of the Child

Figure 1.5 United Nations Convention On the Rights of the Child (1989). Reproduced with the permission of UNICEF.

Summary

Regarding child and young people's health

- For the individual child: depends on the child, the immediate social environment (family, parenting, peers, socioeconomic status), the local social fabric and the national and international environment
- The main problems in developed countries are chronic medical disorders, behavioural and emotional disorders, neurodevelopmental disorders, accidents, socioeconomic disadvantage, excessive consumption of food, drug and alcohol abuse, smoking and teenage pregnancies.

Global child health

Child mortality

Worldwide, each year, 8.8 million children under 5 years old die (Fig. 1.6). Infectious diseases, with undernutrition a major contributing factor, account for most deaths in children. Pneumonia and diarrhoea are the leading infectious causes of death. More than half of child deaths occurring after the neonatal period are due to just five preventable and treatable conditions: pneumonia, diarrhoea, malaria, measles and HIV.

Neonatal mortality (first 4 weeks of life) accounts for 41% of all under-5 deaths. Maternal health and care, especially at delivery, plays a crucial role. Preterm birth, infections and birth asphyxia are the leading causes of neonatal death; being underweight is an important contributing factor.

 Most child deaths in developing countries are preventable.

Where deaths occur

Not surprisingly, the mortality for infants and children living in poor countries is much higher than for those in rich countries. The lethal combination of poverty, HIV/AIDS and armed conflict underlies the very high under-5 mortality in some countries. In addition, many poor countries have warm, humid climates where tropical diseases such as malaria occur. However, even in these countries, much of the excess disease burden is due to illnesses such as respiratory infections and diarrhoea that occur at a much greater frequency and severity than in developed countries.

Although only about 48% of the world's estimated 629 million under-5s live in sub-Saharan Africa and

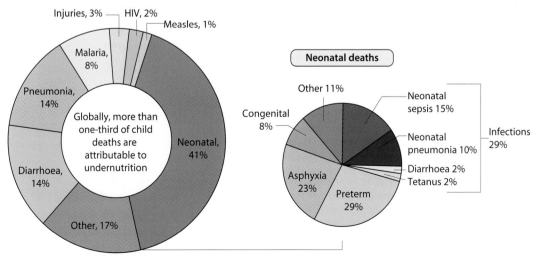

Figure 1.6 Causes of the 8.8 million deaths among children under 5 years old, 2008. (WHO and UNICEF 2010. http://www.childinfo.org. Reproduced with permission. Accessed January 2011).

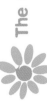

The child in society

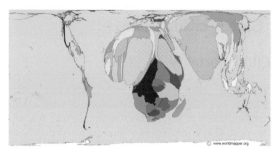

Figure 1.7 Territory size shows the proportion of all deaths of children aged 1–5 years. (http://www.worldmapper.org, 2002 data. Accessed January 2011).

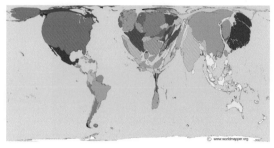

Figure 1.8 Territory size shows the proportion of doctors that work in that territory. (http://www.worldmapper.org, 2002 data. Accessed January 2011).

South Asia, 93% of child deaths occur in these two regions (Fig. 1.7). The difference in resources available is reflected in the difference in the number of healthcare professionals in different parts of the world. This is shown in diagrammatic form in Figure 1.8. Whereas the USA spends over $6000/person/year on health, the annual expenditure is only $25/person in the 49 lowest income countries. Put another way, the annual health budget available to the 1.2 billion people living in these countries is equivalent to that for the 6.5 million living in Arizona!

Over half of all child deaths occur in just five countries, which have high mortality rates and large populations: India, Nigeria, Democratic Republic of Congo (DRC), Pakistan and China. Nine countries have an under-5 years mortality rate of ≥180/1000 live births (Sierra Leone, Afghanistan, Chad, Equatorial Guinea, Guinea-Bissau, Mali, Burkina Faso, Nigeria, Burundi). This means that a child's chance of dying before age 5 years is 30-fold greater in these countries than in developed countries, where the under-5 years mortality rate is 6/1000 live births. The impact of poverty and limited health facilities on children is demonstrated by Case History 1.1.

Reducing child mortality

The international community has taken many steps to improve child health in poor countries. Some are listed in Box 1.4.

The launch of the Integrated Management of Childhood Illness (IMCI) in 1992 was a major advance (Fig. 1.10). It recognised that an integrated management approach to childhood illness is required, including nutrition and preventative care in families and communities. In health facilities, sick children are triaged according to the presence of specific danger signs and management is planned according to algorithms which can be followed by non-medical staff.

The major advance in global child health has been in the adoption of the Millennium Development Goals (MDGs), which has served as a major focus for the international community's commitment to reduce child mortality (Fig. 1.11). There are specific targets for each goal. For MDG 4 it is to reduce child mortality in children <5 years by two-thirds, between the years 2000

Case History

1.1 Burns to the face

This girl in West Africa sustained facial burns (Fig. 1.9). She fell into the open kitchen fire when she had a seizure. Although her epilepsy had initially responded well to phenobarbital, regular supplies were unavailable. Difficulty in finding affordable transport from the village to the health clinic delayed presentation by 4 days, by which time there was secondary infection and increased risk of cataract from conjunctival injury.

This simple example highlights the influence of environment on children's health. Her illness was readily treatable, her injuries were preventable with a fireguard, delayed treatment resulted in complications and only basic medical care was available at the clinic.

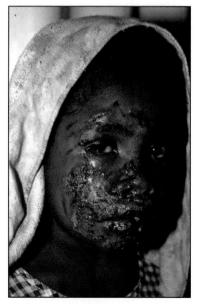

Figure 1.9 Facial burn in West Africa.

Box 1.4 Key international developments in maternal and child health

- 1946: UNICEF established from United Nations Emergency Fund
- 1948: WHO was formed
- 1974: Extended Programme of Immunisation (EPI) included diphtheria, pertussis, tetanus, polio, TB and measles
- 1978: Alma Ata. Primary Healthcare – Health for All
- 1980s: GOBI-FFF. Key primary care strategies: growth monitoring, oral rehydration therapy, breast-feeding, immunisation, family spacing, female education and food supplementation
- 1989: Convention on the Rights of the Child
- 1992: World Summit for Children – Child-to-Child strategy, Baby Friendly initiative, Integrated Management of Childhood Illness (IMCI)
- 2000: United Nations endorses Millennium Development Goals.

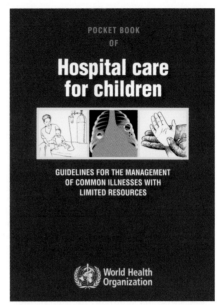

Figure 1.10 Integrated Management of Childhood Illness (IMCI) guidelines for countries with limited resources, WHO. Reproduced with permission.

The 8 Millennium Development Goals

Figure 1.11 Millennium Development Goals. (Available at: http://www.undp.rog/mdg. Accessed January 2011). UNDP Brazil. Reproduced with permission.

and 2015. Contributions are also made by MDGs to improve maternal health and reduce mortality from malaria by insecticide-treated bednets and appropriate anti-malarial drugs and from HIV and TB.

Some of the specific health measures targeted in maternal and child health are shown in Figure 1.12, together with the overall success in implementing them.

The health measures include:

- Contraception available
- One or more antenatal visits
- Skilled attendant at delivery
- Postnatal visit within 2 days
- Exclusive breast-feeding
- Case management of pneumonia
- Measles immunisation.

The aim is for 100% coverage.

Progress in reducing under-5-year-old mortality is being made (Fig. 1.13), although in many of the poorest countries it is slow and patchy, and considerable effort will be required to meet the MDG 4 target.

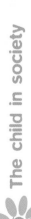

The child in society

9

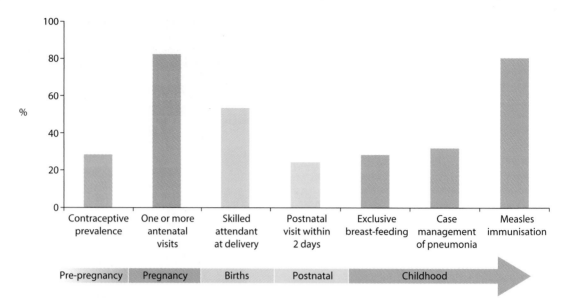

Figure 1.12 Coverage estimates for interventions across the continuum of care (2000–2006) (Countdown Coverage Writing Group; Countdown to 2015 Core Group, Bryce J, Daelmans B, Dwivedi A et al. 2008. Countdown to 2015 for maternal, newborn, and child survival: the 2008 report on tracking coverage of interventions. *Lancet* 371:1247–1258).

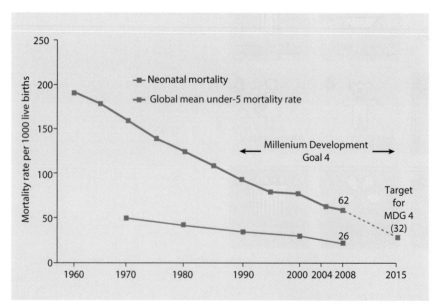

Figure 1.13 Global progress towards Millennium Development Goal 4 (MDG 4) for child survival (Adapted from Lawn J, Newborn survival in low resource settings – are we delivering? *BJOG* 116 (Suppl 1):49–59, 2009. updated 2010 for data to 2008).

Conclusion

Children are vulnerable members of society. They rely on their parents and society to care for them and provide an environment where they can grow both physically and emotionally to reach their full potential. Their health is dependent on a nurturing environment and good health services. Where these are deficient, whether in developed or developing countries, children suffer, but in developing countries they not infrequently lead to death. A global child health perspective empowers the student or child health professional to contribute to the global health workforce, join in international education and research and, most importantly, serve as an effective advocate for the world's children.

Further reading

Blair M, Stewart-Brown S, Waterston T, et al: *Child Public Health*, ed 2, Oxford, 2010, Oxford University Press.

Countdown Coverage Writing Group, Countdown to 2015 Core Group, Bryce J, Daelmans B, Dwivedi A, et al: Countdown to 2015 for maternal, newborn, and child survival: the 2008 report on tracking coverage of interventions. *Lancet* 371:1247–1258, 2008.

Crisp N: *Turning the World Upside Down: the Search for Global Health in the 21st Century*, London, 2010, Royal Society of Medicine Press Ltd.

World Health Organization: *Pocket Book of Hospital Care for Children*. Guidelines for the Management of Common Illnesses with Limited Resources, Geneva, 2005, WHO.

Websites (Accessed May 2011)

The Lancet Global Health Collection. Available at: http://www.thelancet.com/collections/global-health.collexcode=110.

UNICEF. Childinfo. Available at: http://www.childinfo.org.

UNICEF. Countdown to 2015. Available at: http://www.countdown2015mnch.org.

UNICEF. State of the World's Children annual reports. Available at: http://www.unicef.org/sowc.

UNDP. Millennium Development Goals. Available at: http://www.undp.org/mdg.

The child in society

History and examination

The cornerstone of clinical practice continues to be history-taking and clinical examination. Good doctors will continue to be admired for their ability to distil the important information from the history, for their clinical skills, for their attitude towards patients and for their knowledge of diseases, disorders and behaviour problems.

Parents are acutely interested in and anxious about their children. They will quickly recognise doctors who demonstrate interest, empathy and concern. They will seek out doctors who possess the appropriate skills and attitudes towards their children.

In approaching clinical history and examination of children, it is helpful to visualise some common clinical scenarios in which children are seen by doctors:

- An acute illness, e.g. respiratory tract infection, meningitis, appendicitis
- A chronic problem, e.g. failure to thrive, chronic cough
- A newborn infant with a congenital malformation or abnormality, e.g. developmental dysplasia of the hip, Down syndrome
- Suspected delay in development, e.g. slow to walk, talk or acquire skills
- Behaviour problems, e.g. temper tantrums, hyperactivity, eating disorders.

The aims and objectives are to:

- establish the relevant facts of the history; this is always the most fruitful source of diagnostic information
- elicit all relevant clinical findings
- collate the findings from the history and examination
- formulate a working diagnosis or differential diagnosis on the basis of logical deduction
- assemble a problem list and management plan.

The above can be summarised by the acronym HELP:

H = history
E = examination
L = logical deduction
P = plan of management.

Key points in paediatric history and examination are:

- the child's age – a key feature in the history and examination (Fig. 2.1) as it determines:
  - the nature and presentation of illnesses, developmental or behaviour problems
  - the way in which the history-taking (Fig. 2.2) and examination are conducted
  - the way in which any subsequent management is organised
- the parents, who are astute observers of their children. Never ignore or dismiss what they say.

Taking a history

Introduction

- Make sure you have read any referral letter and scanned the notes *before* the start of the interview.
- Observe the child at play in the waiting area and observe their appearance, behaviour and gait as they come into the clinic room. The continued observation of the child during the whole interview may provide important clues to the diagnosis and management.
- When you welcome the child, parents and siblings, check that you know the child's first name and gender. Ask how the child prefers to be addressed.

Paediatrics is a specialty governed by age

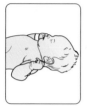
Infant

| Neonate (<4 weeks) Infant (<1 year) |

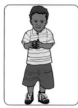
Toddler

| Approx 1–2 years |

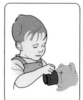
Preschool

| Young child (2–5 years) |

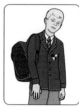
School-age

| Older child |

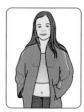
Teenager

| Adolescent |

Figure 2.1 The illnesses and problems children encounter are highly age-dependent. The child's age will determine the questions you ask on history-taking; how you conduct the examination; the diagnosis or differential diagnosis and your management plan.

 Paediatrics stretches from newborn infants to adolescents. Whenever you consider a paediatric problem, whether medical, developmental or behavioural, first ask, 'What is the child's age?'

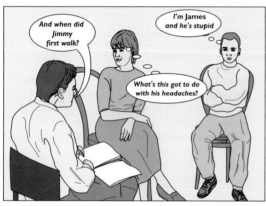

Figure 2.2 The history must be adapted to the child's age. The age when a child first walks is highly relevant when taking the history of a toddler but irrelevant for a teenager with headaches.

- Introduce yourself.
- Determine the relationship of the adults to the child.
- Establish eye contact and rapport with the family. Infants and some toddlers are most secure in parents' arms or laps. Young children may need some time to get to know you.
- Ensure that the interview environment is as welcoming and unthreatening as possible. Avoid having desks or beds between you and the family, but keep a comfortable distance.
- Have toys available. Observe how the child separates, plays and interacts with any siblings present.

- Do not forget to address questions to the child, when appropriate.
- There will be occasions when the parents will not want the child present or when the child should be seen alone. This is usually to avoid embarrassing older children or teenagers or to impart sensitive information. This must be handled tactfully, often by negotiating to talk separately to each in turn.

Presenting symptoms

Full details are required of the presenting symptoms. Let the parents and child recount the presenting complaints in their own words and at their own pace. Note the parent's words about the presenting complaint: onset, duration, previous episodes, what relieves/aggravates them, time course of the problem, if getting worse and any associated symptoms. Has the child's or the family's lifestyle been affected? What has the family done about it?

Make sure you know:

- What prompted referral to a doctor
- What the parents think or fear is the matter.

The scope and detail of further history-taking are determined by the nature and severity of the presenting complaint and the child's age. While the comprehensive assessment listed here is sometimes required, usually a selective approach is more appropriate (Fig. 2.3). This is not an excuse for a short, slipshod history, but instead allows one to focus on the areas where a thorough, detailed history is required.

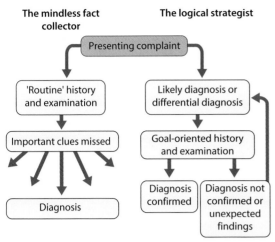

The mindless fact collector | The logical strategist

Figure 2.3 The history and examination should be goal-oriented, based on the presenting complaint. Comprehensive history-taking is best reserved for training or for complex, multi-system disorders. (Adapted from Hutson JM, Beasley SW. 1988. *The Surgical Examination of Children*. Heinemann Medical Books, London.)

General enquiry

Check:

- General health – how active and lively?
- Normal growth
- Pubertal development (if appropriate)
- Feeding/drinking/appetite
- Any recent change in behaviour or personality.

Systems review

Selected, as appropriate:

- General rashes, fever (if measured)
- Respiratory – cough, wheeze, breathing problems
- ENT – throat infections, snoring, noisy breathing (stridor)
- Cardiovascular – heart murmur, cyanosis, exercise tolerance
- Gastrointestinal – vomiting, diarrhoea/constipation, abdominal pain
- Genitourinary – dysuria, frequency, wetting, toilet-trained
- Neurological – seizures, headaches, abnormal movements
- Musculoskeletal – disturbance of gait, limb pain or swelling, other functional abnormalities.

Make sure that you and the parent or child mean the same thing when describing a problem.

Past medical history

Check:

- Maternal obstetric problems, delivery, prolonged rupture of membranes, group B streptococcus status, maternal pyrexia (pertinent if neonate)
- Birthweight and gestation
- Perinatal problems, whether admitted to special care baby unit, jaundice, etc.
- Immunisations (ideally from the personal child health record)
- Past illnesses, hospital admissions and operations, accidents and injuries.

Medication

Check:

- Past and present medications
- Known allergies.

Family history

Families share houses, genes and diseases!

- Have any members of the family or friends had similar problems or any serious disorder?

Any neonatal/childhood deaths?

- Draw a family tree. If there is a positive family history, extend family pedigree over several generations.
- Is there consanguinity?

Social history

Check:

- Relevant information about the family and its community – parental occupation, economic status, housing, relationships, parental smoking, marital stresses.
- Is the child happy at home? What are the child's preferred play or leisure activities?
- Is the child happy at nursery/school?
- Is there a social worker involved?

This 'social snapshot' is crucial, since many childhood illnesses or conditions are permeated by adult problems, for example:

- alcohol and drug abuse
- long-term unemployment/poverty
- poor, damp, cramped housing
- parental psychiatric disorders
- unstable partnership.

Development

Check:

- Parental worries about vision, hearing, development
- Key developmental milestones (Fig. 2.4)
- Previous child health surveillance developmental checks
- Bladder and bowel control
- Child's temperament, behaviour
- Sleeping problems
- Concerns and progress at nursery/school.

Look through the personal child health record.

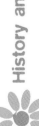

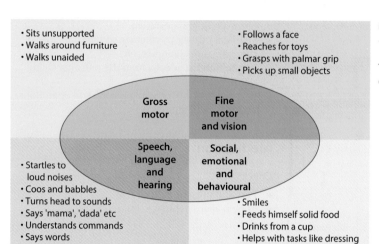

• Sits unsupported
• Walks around furniture
• Walks unaided

Gross motor

• Follows a face
• Reaches for toys
• Grasps with palmar grip
• Picks up small objects

Fine motor and vision

Speech, language and hearing

• Startles to loud noises
• Coos and babbles
• Turns head to sounds
• Says 'mama', 'dada' etc
• Understands commands
• Says words
• Talks in sentences

Social, emotional and behavioural

• Smiles
• Feeds himself solid food
• Drinks from a cup
• Helps with tasks like dressing
• Toilet-trained

Figure 2.4 Some key developmental milestones in infants and young children. These are considered in detail in Chapter 3.

An approach to examining children

Obtaining the child's cooperation

- Make friends with the child.
- Be confident but gentle.
- Avoid dominating the child.
- Short mock examinations, e.g. auscultating a teddy or the mother's hand, may allay a young child's fears.
- When first examining a young child, start at a non-threatening area, such as a hand or knee.
- Explain what you are about to do and what you want the child to do, in language he can understand. As the examination is essential, not optional, it is best not to ask his permission, as it may well be refused!
- A smiling, talking doctor appears less threatening, but this should not be overdone as it can interfere with one's relationship with the parents.
- Leave unpleasant procedures until last.

Adapting to the child's age

Adapt the examination to suit the child's age. While it may be difficult to examine some toddlers and young children fully, it is usually possible with resourcefulness and imagination on the doctor's part.

- Babies in the first few months are best examined on an examination couch with a parent next to them.
- A toddler is best initially examined on his mother's lap or occasionally over a parent's shoulder.
- Parents are reassuring for the child and helpful in facilitating the examination if guided as to what to do (Fig. 2.5).
- Preschool children may initially be examined while they are playing.
- Older children and teenagers are often concerned about privacy. Teenage girls should normally be

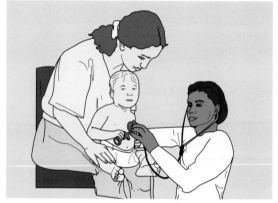

Figure 2.5 Distracting a toddler with a toy allows auscultation of the heart.

examined in the presence of their mother, or a nurse or suitable chaperone. Be aware of cultural sensitivities in different ethnic groups.

Undressing children

Be sensitive to children's modesty. The area to be examined must be inspected fully but this is best done in stages, re-dressing the child when each stage has been completed. It is easiest and kindest to ask the child or parent to do the undressing.

Warm, clean hands

Hands must be washed before (and after) examining a child. Warm smile, warm hands and a warm stethoscope all help.

Developmental skills

A good overview of developmental skills can be obtained by watching the child play. A few simple toys, such as some bricks, a car, doll, ball, pencil and paper, pegboard, miniature toys and a picture book, are all that is required, as they can be adapted for any age. If developmental assessment (see Ch. 3) is the focus of the examination, it is advisable to assess this before the physical examination, as cooperation may then be lost.

Examination

Initial observations

Careful observation is usually the key to success in examining children. Look before touching the child. Inspection will provide information on:

- severity of illness
- growth and nutrition
- behaviour and social responsiveness
- level of hygiene and care.

Severity of illness

Is the child sick or well? If sick, how sick? For the acutely ill infant or child, perform the '60-second rapid assessment':

- Airway and Breathing – respiration rate and effort, presence of stridor or wheeze, cyanosis
- Circulation – heart rate, pulse volume, peripheral temperature, capillary refill time
- Disability – level of consciousness.

The care of the seriously ill child is described in Chapter 6.

Measurements

As abnormal growth may be the first manifestation of illness in children, always measure and plot growth on centile charts for:

- weight, noting previous measurements from personal child health record
- length (in infants, if indicated) or height in older children
- head circumference in infants.

Also, as appropriate:

- temperature
- blood pressure
- peak expiratory flow rate.

General appearance

The face, head, neck and hands are examined. The general morphological appearance may suggest a chromosomal or dysmorphic syndrome. In infants, palpate the fontanelle and sutures.

Respiratory system

Cyanosis

Central cyanosis is best observed on the tongue.

Clubbing of the fingers and/or toes

Clubbing (Fig. 2.6a) is usually associated with chronic suppurative lung disease, e.g. cystic fibrosis, or cyanotic congenital heart disease. It is occasionally seen in inflammatory bowel disease or cirrhosis.

Tachypnoea

Rate of respiration is age-dependent (Table 2.1).

Dyspnoea

Laboured breathing. Increased respiratory rate (may be the only sign of increased work of breathing).
Increased work of breathing is judged by:

- nasal flaring
- expiratory grunting – to increase positive end-expiratory pressure
- use of accessory muscles, especially sternomastoids
- retraction (recession) of the chest wall, from use of suprasternal, intercostal and subcostal muscles
- difficulty speaking (or feeding).

Chest shape

- Hyperexpansion or barrel shape (Fig. 2.6b), e.g. asthma
- *Pectus excavatum* (hollow chest) or *pectus carinatum* (pigeon chest)
- Harrison's sulcus (indrawing of the chest wall from diaphragmatic tug), e.g. from poorly controlled asthma
- Asymmetry of chest movements.

Palpation

- Chest expansion: this is 3–5 cm in school-aged children. Measure maximal chest expansion with a tape measure. Check for symmetry.
- Trachea: checking that it is central is seldom helpful and is disliked by children. To be done selectively.
- Location of apex beat to detect mediastinal shift.

Percussion

- Needs to be done gently, comparing like with like, using middle fingers.
- Seldom informative in infants.
- Localised dullness: collapse, consolidation, fluid.

Auscultation (ears and stethoscope)

- Note quality and symmetry of breath sounds and any added sounds
- Harsh breath sounds from the upper airways are readily transmitted to the upper chest in infants
- Hoarse voice – abnormality of the vocal cords
- Stridor – harsh, low-pitched, mainly inspiratory sound from upper airways obstruction

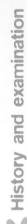

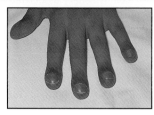

Figure 2.6a Clubbing of the fingers. There is increased curvature, loss of nail angle and fluctuation. This child had cystic fibrosis.

Table 2.1 Respiratory rate in children (breaths/min)

Age	Normal	Tachypnoea
Neonate	30–50	>60
Infants	20–30	>50
Young children	20–30	>40
Older children	15–20	>30

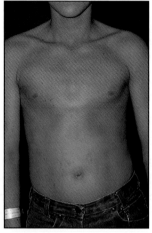

Figure 2.6b Hyperexpanded chest from chronic obstructive airways disease. This boy had severe asthma.

Table 2.2 Chest signs of some common chest disorders of children

	Chest movement	Percussion	Auscultation
Bronchiolitis	Laboured breathing Hyperinflated chest Chest recession	Hyper-resonant	Fine crackles in all zones Wheezes may/may not be present
Pneumonia	Reduced on affected side Rapid, shallow breaths	Dull	Bronchial breathing Crackles
Asthma	Reduced but hyperinflated Use of accessory muscles Chest wall retraction	Hyper-resonant	Wheeze

 Infants with pneumonia may not have any abnormal signs on auscultation.

 Sputum is rarely produced by children, as they swallow it. The main exception is suppurative lung disease from cystic fibrosis.

- Breath sounds – normal are vesicular; bronchial breathing is higher-pitched and the length of inspiration and expiration equal
- Wheeze – high-pitched, expiratory sound from distal airway obstruction (Table 2.2)
- Crackles – discontinuous 'moist' sounds from the opening of bronchioles (Table 2.2).

Cardiovascular system

Cyanosis

Observe the tongue for central cyanosis.

Clubbing of fingers or toes

Check if present.

Pulse

Check:

- Rate (Table 2.3)
- Rhythm – sinus arrhythmia (variation of pulse rate with respiration) is normal
- Volume – small in circulatory insufficiency or aortic stenosis; increased in high-output states (stress, anaemia); collapsing in patent ductus arteriosus, aortic regurgitation.

Inspection

Look for:

- respiratory distress
- precordial bulge – caused by cardiac enlargement

Table 2.3 Normal resting pulse rate in children

Age	Beats/min
<1 year	110–160
2–5 years	95–140
5–12 years	80–120
>12 years	60–100

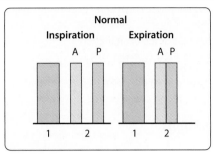

Figure 2.7 The splitting of the second heart sound is easily heard in children.

 Features of heart failure in infants:
- **Poor feeding/failure to thrive**
- **Sweating**
- **Tachypnoea**
- **Tachycardia**
- **Gallop rhythm**
- **Cardiomegaly**
- **Hepatomegaly.**

 Features suggesting that a murmur is significant:
- **Conducted all over the precordium**
- **Loud**
- **Thrill (equals grade 4–6 murmur)**
- **Any diastolic murmur**
- **Accompanied by other abnormal cardiac signs.**

- ventricular impulse – visible if thin, hyperdynamic circulation or left ventricular hypertrophy
- operative scars – mostly sternotomy or left lateral thoracotomy.

Palpation

Thrill = palpable murmur.

Apex (4th–5th intercostal space, mid-clavicular line):

- not palpable in some normal infants, plump children or dextrocardia
- heave from left ventricular hypertrophy.

Right ventricular heave at lower left sternal edge – right ventricular hypertrophy.

Percussion

Cardiac border percussion is rarely helpful in children.

Auscultation

Listen for heart sounds and murmurs.

Heart sounds

- Splitting of second sound is usually easily heard and is normal (Fig. 2.7).
- Fixed splitting of second heart sound in atrial septal defects.
- Third heart sound in mitral area is normal in young children.

Murmurs

- Timing – systolic/diastolic/continuous
- Duration – mid-systolic (ejection)/pansystolic

- Loudness – systolic murmurs graded:
  - 1–2: soft, difficult to hear
  - 3: easily audible, no thrill
  - 4–6: loud with thrill
- Site of maximal intensity – mitral/pulmonary/aortic/tricuspid areas
- Radiation:
  - to neck in aortic stenosis
  - to back in coarctation of the aorta or pulmonary stenosis.

Draw your findings (see Ch. 17 on cardiac disorders).

Hepatomegaly

Important sign of heart failure in infants. An infant's liver is normally palpable 1–2 cm below the costal margin.

Femoral pulses

In coarctation of the aorta:

- Decreased volume or may be impalpable in infants
- Brachiofemoral delay in older children.

Blood pressure (see later in chapter)

 Heart disease is more common in children with other congenital abnormalities or syndromes, e.g. Down and Turner syndromes.

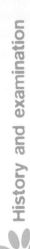

Abdomen

Abdominal examination is performed in three major clinical settings:

- The routine part of the examination
- An 'acute abdomen' – ?cause (see Ch.13, Gastroenterology)
- Recurrent abdominal pain/distension/constipation mass.

Associated signs

Examine:

- The eyes for signs of jaundice and anaemia
- The tongue for coating and central cyanosis
- The fingers for clubbing.

Inspection

The abdomen is protuberant in normal toddlers and young children. The abdominal wall muscles must be relaxed for palpation.

Generalised abdominal distension is most often explained by the five 'F's:

- Fat
- Fluid (ascites – uncommon in children, most often from nephrotic syndrome)
- Faeces (constipation)
- Flatus (malabsorption, intestinal obstruction)
- Fetus (not to be forgotten after puberty).

Occasionally, it is caused by a grossly enlarged liver and/or spleen or muscle hypotonia.

Causes of localised abdominal distension are:

- Upper abdomen – gastric dilatation from pyloric stenosis, hepato/splenomegaly
- Lower abdomen – distended bladder, masses.

Other signs:

- Dilated veins in liver disease, abdominal striae
- Operative scars (draw a diagram)
- Peristalsis – from pyloric stenosis, intestinal obstruction.

Are the buttocks normally rounded, or wasted as in malabsorption, e.g. coeliac disease or malnutrition?

Palpation

- Use warm hands, explain, relax the child and keep the parent close at hand. First ask if it hurts.
- Palpate in a systematic fashion – liver, spleen, kidneys, bladder, through four abdominal quadrants.
- Ask about tenderness. Watch the child's face for grimacing as you palpate. A young child may become more cooperative if you palpate first with their hand or by putting your hand on top of theirs.

Tenderness

- *Location* – localised in appendicitis, hepatitis, pyelonephritis; generalised in mesenteric adenitis, peritonitis

- *Guarding* – often unimpressive on direct palpation in children. Pain on coughing, on moving about/walking/bumps during car journey suggests peritoneal irritation. Back bent on walking may be from psoas inflammation in appendicitis. By incorporating play into examination, more subtle guarding can be elicited. For example, a child will not be able to jump on the spot if they have localised guarding.

Hepatomegaly (Table 2.4, Fig. 2.8)

- Palpate from right iliac fossa
- Locate edge with tips or side of finger
- Edge may be soft or firm
- Unable to get above it
- Moves with respiration
- Measure (in cm) extension below costal margin in mid-clavicular line.

Percuss downwards from the right lung to exclude pseudohepatomegaly due to lung hyperinflation.

Liver tenderness is likely to be due to inflammation from hepatitis.

Splenomegaly (Table 2.5)

- Palpate from right iliac fossa
- Edge is usually soft
- Unable to get above it
- Notch occasionally palpable if markedly enlarged
- Moves on respiration (ask the child to take a deep breath)
- Measure size below costal margin (in cm) in mid-clavicular line.

If uncertain whether it is palpable:

- Use bimanual approach to spleen
- Turn child onto right side.

A palpable spleen is at least twice its normal size!

Kidneys

These are not usually palpable beyond the neonatal period unless enlarged or the abdominal muscles are hypotonic.

On examination:

- Palpate by balloting bimanually
- They move on respiration
- One can get above them.

Tenderness implies inflammation.

Abnormal masses

- *Wilms' tumour* – renal mass, sometimes visible, does not cross midline
- *Neuroblastoma* – irregular firm mass, may cross midline; the child is usually very unwell
- *Faecal masses* – mobile, non-tender, indentable
- *Intussusception* – acutely unwell, mass may be palpable, most often in right upper quadrant.

Table 2.4 Causes of hepatomegaly

Infection	Congenital, infectious mononucleosis, hepatitis, malaria, parasitic infection
Haematological	Sickle cell anaemia, thalassaemia
Liver disease	Chronic active hepatitis, portal hypertension, polycystic disease
Malignancy	Leukaemia, lymphoma, neuroblastoma, Wilms' tumour, hepatoblastoma
Metabolic	Glycogen and lipid storage disorders, mucopolysaccharidoses
Cardiovascular	Heart failure
Apparent	Chest hyperexpansion from bronchiolitis or asthma

 On examining the abdomen:
- **Inspect first, palpate later**
- **Superficial palpation first, deep palpation later**
- **Guarding is unimpressive in children**
- **Silent abdomen – serious!**
- **Immobile abdomen – serious!**

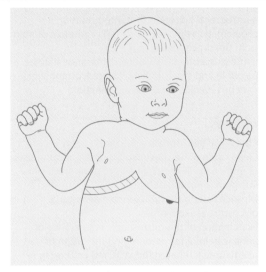
Figure 2.8 Normal findings. The liver edge is 1–2 cm below the costal margin in infants and young children. The spleen may be 1–2 cm below the costal margin in infants.

Table 2.5 Causes of splenomegaly

Infection	Viral, bacterial, protozoal (malaria, leishmaniasis), parasites, infective endocarditis
Haematological	Haemolytic anaemia
Malignancy	Leukaemia, lymphoma
Other	Portal hypertension, systemic juvenile idiopathic arthritis (Still's disease)

Percussion

- *Liver* – dullness delineates upper and lower border. Record span
- *Spleen* – dullness delineates lower border
- *Ascites* – shifting dullness. Percuss from most resonant spot to most dull spot.

Auscultation

Not very useful in 'routine' examination, but important in 'acute abdomen':

- Increased bowel sounds – intestinal obstruction, acute diarrhoea
- Reduced or absent bowel sounds – paralytic ileus, peritonitis.

Genital area

The genital area is examined routinely in young children, but in older children and teenagers this is done only if relevant, e.g. vaginal discharge. Is there an inguinal hernia or a perineal rash?

In *males*:

- Is the penis of normal size?
- Is the scrotum well developed?
- Are the testes palpable? With one hand over the inguinal region, palpate with the other hand. Record if the testis is descended, retractile or impalpable.
- Is there any scrotal swelling (hydrocele or hernia)?

In *females*:

- Do the external genitalia look normal?

Does the anus look normal? Any evidence of a fissure?

Rectal examination

- This should not be performed routinely, and only for specific reasons
- Unpleasant and disliked by children
- Its usefulness in the 'acute abdomen' (e.g. appendicitis) is debatable in children, as they have

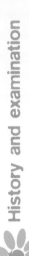

a thin abdominal wall and so tenderness and masses can be identified on palpation of the abdomen. Some surgeons advocate it to identify a retrocaecal appendix, but interpretation is problematic as most children will complain of pain from the procedure.

- If intussusception is suspected, the mass may be palpable and stools looking like redcurrant jelly may be revealed on rectal examination.

Urinalysis

- Checked if appropriate
- Clean catch urine specimen preferred and the use of urine bags in the diagnosis of urine tract infection is not advisable
- Dipstick testing for proteinuria, haematuria, glycosuria, leukocyturia
- Examination of the microscopic appearance of urine is helpful for determining the origin of haematuria (crenated red cells, red cell casts).

✿ **Lung hyperexpansion in bronchiolitis or asthma may displace the liver and spleen downwards, mimicking hepato/splenomegaly**

Neurology/neurodevelopment

Brief neurological screen

A quick neurological and developmental overview should be performed in all children. When doing this:

- Use common sense to avoid unnecessary examination
- Adapt it to the child's age
- Take into consideration the parent's account of developmental milestones.

Watch the child play, draw or write. Are the manipulative skills normal? Can he walk, run, climb, hop, skip, dance? Are the child's language skills and speech satisfactory? Are the social interactions appropriate? Does vision and hearing appear to be normal?

In infants, assess primarily by observation:

- Observe posture and movements of the limbs.
- When picking the infant up, note their tone. The limbs and body may feel normal, floppy or stiff. Head control may be poor, with abnormal head lag on pulling to sitting.

Most children are neurologically intact and do not require formal neurological examination of reflexes, tone, etc. More detailed neurological assessment is performed only if indicated. Specific neurological concerns or problems in development or behaviour require detailed assessment.

More detailed neurological examination

If the child has a neurological problem, a detailed and systematic neurological examination is required.

Patterns of movement

Observe walking and running: normal walking is with a heel–toe gait. Assessment can be incorporated into playing a game, for example: 'pretend you are on a tightrope, how fast can you run?' A toe–heel pattern of walking (toe-walkers) although often idiopathic, may suggest pyramidal tract (corticospinal) dysfunction, a foot drop (common or superficial peroneal nerve lesion), or tight tendo-achilles due to a neuromuscular disease. Children with myopathy may also develop tight Achilles tendon due to weakness. If you are unsure whether a gait is heel–toe or toe–heel, look at the pattern of shoe wear.

A broad-based gait may be due to an immature gait (normal in a toddler) or secondary to a cerebellar disorder. Proximal muscle weakness around the hip girdle can cause a waddling gait. Corticospinal tract lesions give a dynamic pattern of movement involving shoulder adduction, forearm pronation, elbow and wrist flexion with burying of the thumb, whereas internal hip rotation and flexion at the hip and knee and plantar flexion at the ankle give a characteristic circumduction pattern of lower limb movement. If subtle, these are more evident with asking the child to adopt an unusual pattern of walking, e.g. to walk on his heels or toes or with feet inverted. Extrapyramidal lesions give fluctuating tone, with difficulty in initiating or involuntary movements. Look for asymmetry (see Fig. 4.4).

Observe standing from lying down supine. Children up to 3 years of age will turn prone in order to stand because of poor pelvic muscle fixation; beyond this age, it suggests neuromuscular weakness (e.g. Duchenne muscular dystrophy) or low tone, which could be due to a central (brain) cause. The need to turn prone to rise or, later, as weakness progresses, to push off the ground with straightened arms and then climb up the legs is known as Gowers sign (see Fig. 27.6).

Coordination

Assess this by:

- asking the child to build one brick upon another or using a peg-board, and do up and undo buttons, draw, copy patterns, write
- asking the child to hold his arms out straight and close his eyes, and then observing for drift or tremor (this is really looking for asymmetry, position sense, and neglect of one side with visual cues removed)
- finger–nose testing (use teddy's nose to reach out and touch if necessary)
- rapid alternating movements of hands and fingers
- touching tip of each finger in turn with thumb
- asking the child to walk heel–toe, jump and hop.

Subtle asymmetries in gait may be revealed by Fogg's test – children are asked to walk on their heels, the outside and then the inside of their feet. Watch for the pattern of abnormal movement in the upper limbs. Observe them running.

Inspection of limbs

Muscle bulk

- Wasting may be secondary to cerebral palsy, meningomyelocele, muscle disorder or from previous poliomyelitis.
- Increased bulk of calf muscles may indicate Duchenne muscular dystrophy, or myotonic conditions.

Muscle tone

Tone, in limbs

- Best assessed by taking the weight of the whole limb and then bending and extending it around a single joint. Testing is easiest at the knee and ankle joints. Assess the resistance to passive movement as well as the range of movement.
- Increased tone (spasticity) in adductors and internal rotators of the hips, clonus at the ankles or increased tone on pronation of the forearms at rest is usually the result of pyramidal dysfunction. This can be differentiated from the lead-pipe rigidity seen in extrapyramidal conditions, which, if accompanied by a tremor may be termed 'cog-wheel' rigidity.
- The posture of the limbs may give a clue as to the underlying tone, e.g. scissoring of the legs, pronated forearms, fisting, extended legs suggests increased tone (see Figs 4.3 and 4.4). Sitting in a frog-like posture of the legs suggests hypotonia (see Fig. 8.2a), while abnormal posturing and extension suggests fluctuating tone (dystonia).

Truncal tone

- In extra-pyramidal tract disorders, the trunk and head tend to arch backwards (extensor posturing).
- In muscle disease and some central brain disorders, the trunk may be hypotonic (Fig. 2.9a and Fig. 27.8). The child feels floppy to handle and cannot support the trunk in sitting.

Head lag

- This is best tested by pulling the child up by the arms from the supine position (Fig. 2.9b).

Power

Difficult to test in babies. Watch for antigravity movements and note motor function. Both will tell you a lot about power. From 6 months onwards, watch the pattern of mobility and gait. Watch the child standing up from lying and climbing stairs. From the age of 4 years, power can be tested formally against gravity and resistance, first testing proximal muscle and then distal muscle power and comparing sides.

Reflexes

Test with the child in a relaxed position and explain what you are about to do before approaching with a tendon hammer, or demonstrate on parent or toy first. Brisk reflexes may reflect anxiety in the child or a pyramidal disorder. Absent reflexes may be due to a neuromuscular problem or a lesion within the spinal cord, but may also be due to inexpert examination technique. Children will reinforce reflexes if asked.

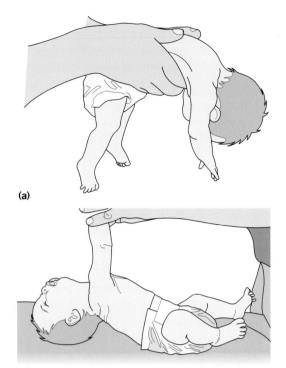

(a)

(b)

Figure 2.9 A hypotonic infant. **(a)** When held prone, the infant flops like a rag doll. **(b)** Marked head lag on traction of the arms.

Plantar responses

In children the responses are often equivocal and unpopular as it is unpleasant. They are unreliable under 1 year of age. Upgoing plantar responses provide additional evidence of pyramidal dysfunction.

Sensation

Testing the ability to withdraw to tickle is usually adequate as a screening test. If loss of sensation is likely, e.g. meningomyelocele or spinal lesion (transverse myelitis, etc.), more detailed sensory testing is performed as in adults. In spinal and cauda equina lesions there may be a palpable bladder or absent perineal sensation.

Cranial nerves

Before about 4 years old you need some ingenuity to test for abnormal or asymmetric signs – make it a game; ask them to mimic you:

I	Need not be tested in routine practice. Can be done by recognising the smell of a hidden mint sweet.
II	Visual acuity – determined according to age. Direct and consensual pupillary response tested to light and accommodation. Visual fields can be tested if the child is old enough to cooperate.

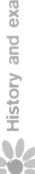

III, IV, VI	Full eye movement through horizontal and vertical planes. Is there a squint? Nystagmus – avoid extreme lateral gaze, as it can induce nystagmus in normal children.
V	Clench teeth and waggle jaw from side to side against resistance.
VII	Close eyes tight, smile and show teeth.
VIII	Hearing – ask parents, although unilateral deafness could be missed this way. If in doubt, needs formal assessment in a suitable environment.
IX	Levator palati – saying 'aagh'. Look for deviation of uvula.
X	Recurrent laryngeal nerve – listen for hoarseness or stridor.
XI	Trapezius and sternomastoid power – shrug shoulders and turn head against resistance.
XII	Put out tongue and look for any atrophy or deviation.

Bones and joints

A rapid screen to identify disorders of the musculoskeletal is pGALS (paediatric Gait, Arms, Legs, Spine; Fig. 2.10). If an abnormality is found, a more detailed regional examination of the affected joint as well as the joint above and below should be performed (Fig. 2.11).

Neck

Thyroid

- Inspect – swelling uncommon in childhood; occasionally at puberty
- Palpate from behind and front for swelling, nodule, thrill
- Auscultate if enlarged
- Look for signs of hypo/hyperthyroidism.

Lymph nodes

Examine systematically – occipital, cervical, axillary, inguinal. Note size, number, consistency of any glands felt:

- Small, discrete, pea-sized, mobile nodes in the neck, groin and axilla – common in normal children, especially if thin
- Small, multiple nodes in the neck – common after upper respiratory tract infections (viral/bacterial)
- Multiple lymph nodes of variable size in children with extensive atopic eczema – frequent finding, no action required
- Large, hot, tender, sometimes fluctuant node, usually in neck – infected/abscess
- Variable size and shape:
  - infections: viral, e.g. infectious mononucleosis, or TB
  - rare causes: malignant disease (usually non-tender), Kawasaki disease, cat-scratch.

Blood pressure

Indications

Must be closely monitored if critically ill, if there is renal or cardiac disease or diabetes mellitus, or if receiving drug therapy which may cause hypertension, e.g. corticosteroids (Box 2.1). Not measured often enough in children.

Technique

When measured with a sphygmomanometer:

- Show the child that there is a balloon in the cuff and demonstrate how it is blown up.
- Use largest cuff which fits comfortably, covering at least two-thirds of the upper arm.
- The child must be relaxed and not crying.
- Systolic pressure is the easiest to determine in young children and clinically the most useful.
- Diastolic pressure is when the sounds disappear. May not be possible to discern in young children. Systolic pressure used in clinical practice.

Measurement

Must be interpreted according to a centile chart (see Fig. A.3, in the Appendix). Blood pressure is increased by tall stature and obesity. Charts relating blood pressure to height are available and preferable; however, for convenience, charts relating blood pressure to age are often used. An abnormally high reading must be repeated, with the child relaxed, on at least three separate occasions.

Eyes

Examination

Inspect eyes, pupils, iris and sclerae. Are eye movements full and symmetrical? Is nystagmus detectable? If so, may have ocular or cerebellar cause, or testing may be too lateral to the child. Are the pupils round (absence of posterior synechiae), equal, central and reactive to light? Is there a squint? (see Ch. 4).

Epicanthic folds are common in Asian ethnic groups.

Ophthalmoscopy

- In infants, the red reflex is seen from a distance of 20–30 cm. Absence of red reflex occurs in corneal clouding, cataract, retinoblastoma.
- Fundoscopy – difficult. Requires experience and cooperation. In infants, mydriatics are needed and an ophthalmological opinion may be required. Retinopathy of prematurity and retinopathy of

Box 2.1 Measuring blood pressure in children

- Sphygmomanometer (Fig. 2.12)
  - stethoscope in older children
  - Doppler ultrasound in infants
- Oscillometric (e.g. Dynamapp) – unreliable in infants and young children
- Invasive – direct measurement from an arterial catheter is preferable if critically ill.

pGALS – musculoskeletal screening for school-aged children

(Differences from adult GALS highlighted in bold)

Screening questions
· **Do you (or your child) have any pain or stiffness in your joints, muscles or your back?**
· **Do you (or your child) have any difficulty getting yourself dressed without any help?**
· **Do you (or your child) have any difficulty going up and down stairs?**

POSTURE AND GAIT   ARMS

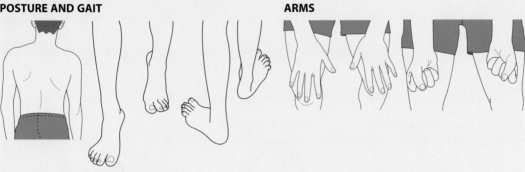

Observe standing (from front, back and sides)

Observe walking **'Walk on your tip-toes, walk on your heels'**

'Put your hands out straight in front of you'

'Turn your hands over and make a fist'

ARMS

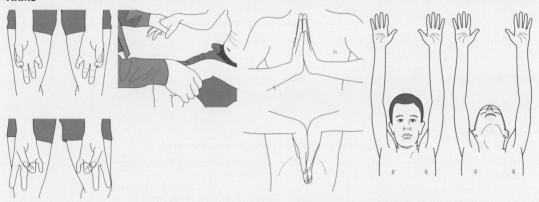

'Pinch your index finger and thumb together'

'Touch the tips of your fingers with your thumb'

Squeeze the metacarpo-phalangeal joints for tenderness

'Put your hands together palm to palm'

'Put your hands back to back'

'Reach up and touch the sky'

'Look at the ceiling'

Figure 2.10 pGALS (paediatric Gait, Arms, Legs, Spine) musculoskeletal screening for school-aged children (Foster HE et al., Musculoskeletal screening examination (pGALS) for school-aged children based on the adult GALS screen. Arthritis Rheum 2006; 55(5):709-16 and see http://www.arthritisresearchuk.org/videos/pgals.aspx to view video of the examination)

Continued

History and examination

pGALS – musculoskeletal screening for school-aged children—cont'd

(Differences from adult GALS highlighted in bold)

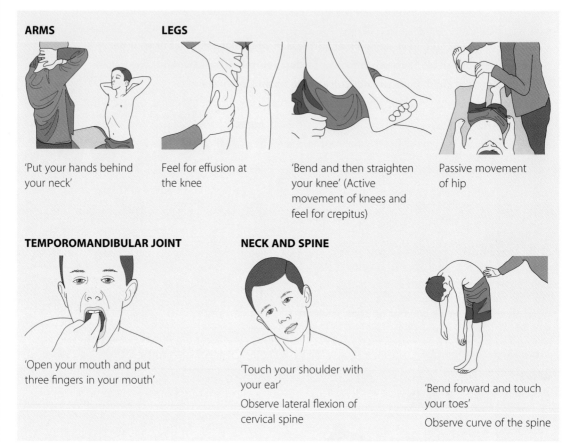

ARMS

'Put your hands behind your neck'

LEGS

Feel for effusion at the knee

'Bend and then straighten your knee' (Active movement of knees and feel for crepitus)

Passive movement of hip

TEMPOROMANDIBULAR JOINT

'Open your mouth and put three fingers in your mouth'

NECK AND SPINE

'Touch your shoulder with your ear'

Observe lateral flexion of cervical spine

'Bend forward and touch your toes'

Observe curve of the spine

Figure 2.10, cont'd

Regional musculoskeletal assessment

Look:
- For signs of discomfort
- Skin abnormalities – rashes, scars, bruising, colour, nail abnormalities
- Limb alignment, leg length, muscle bulk and evidence of asymmetry
- Bony deformity, soft tissue, joint swelling or muscle changes

Feel:
- Each joint, long bones and neighbouring soft tissues:
- Palpate along bones and joint line for tenderness
- Feel for warmth *(infection or inflammation)*
- Delineate bony or soft tissue swellings
- Check for joint effusion, most readily at the knee

Move:
- For each joint, ask to move the joint first (active movement).
  Observe for discomfort, symmetry and range of movement.
- Passively move the joint, noting range of any restriction of movement (compare sides but note bilateral changes)
- Lateral and rotational movements may be as important as flexion and extension.

Function:
- For lower limb joints – check gait
- For small joints such as hands - check grip

Figure 2.11 A regional musculoskeletal assessment. (See Foster HE and Brogan P. *Oxford Handbook of Paediatric Rheumatology*, Oxford, 2011, Oxford University Press and http://www.arc.org.uk/arthinfo/medpubs/6321/6321. asp)

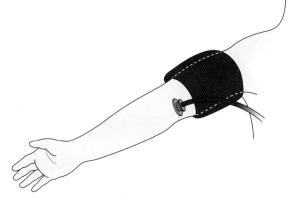

Cuff >2/3 upper arm.
(Smaller cuffs give artificially
high readings)

Age	Upper limit of normal systolic blood pressure
1–5 years	110 mmHg
6–10 years	120 mmHg

Figure 2.12 Measurement of blood pressure.

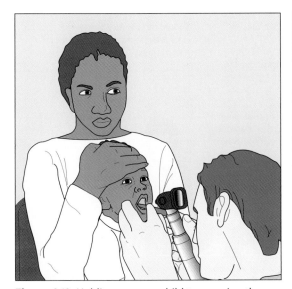

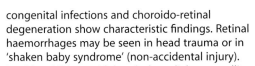

Figure 2.13 Holding a young child to examine the throat. The mother has one hand on the head and the other across the child's arms.

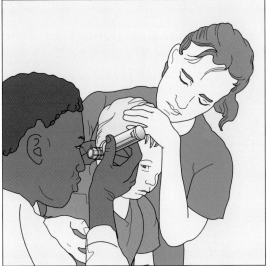

Figure 2.14 Holding a young child correctly is essential for successful examination of the ear with an auroscope. The mother has one hand on the child's head and the other hand holding the upper arm.

congenital infections and choroido-retinal degeneration show characteristic findings. Retinal haemorrhages may be seen in head trauma or in 'shaken baby syndrome' (non-accidental injury).

- In older children with headaches, diabetes mellitus or hypertension, optic fundi should be examined. Mydriatics are not usually needed.

Ears and throat

Examination is usually left until last, as it can be unpleasant. Explain what you are going to do. Show the parent how to hold and gently restrain a younger child to ensure success and avoid possible injury (Figs 2.13 and 2.14).

Throat

Try quickly to get a look at the tonsils, uvula, pharynx and posterior palate. Older children (5 years +) will open their mouths as wide as possible without a spatula. A spatula is required for young children. Look for redness, swelling, pus or palatal petechiae. Also check the teeth for dental caries and other gross abnormalities.

Ears

Examine ear canals and drums gently, trying not to hurt the child. Look for anatomical landmarks on the ear drum and for swelling, redness, perforation, dullness, fluid.

Communicating with children

Throughout the consultation, make sure that your communication with the child is appropriate for the child's age and stage of development (Table 2.6).

Table 2.6 The reasons for talking with children

Why talk to children when you can get the information from the parent? The reasons are:
- To establish rapport
- To obtain the child's own views about their problems
- To know how the child feels about their health and life
- To reduce anxiety and fear and to improve compliance with assessment and treatment
- To determine the presence of associated emotional or psychiatric problems

	Preschool child (2–5 years)	School-age child (6–11 years)	Adolescent (12–18 years)
Thought processes	When I close my eyes, Mum goes away (world viewed differently, from own perspective)

I am asleep, so everyone is asleep (centre of their world)

When I fell, the floor hurt me (objects are alive)

My toy elephant is crying because the other elephants won't play with him (involvement in pretend play) | I have been invited to Katie and Jane's parties - maybe I could go for some time to each (able to start solving concrete problems)

Am I going to be chosen for the school choir? (develops worries about the future)

Mum gets really upset when Dad gets drunk, but Dad does not care (able to see another person's point of view and take on more than one perspective) | I can handle things without Mum's help (seeking autonomy and separation)

Should our country be at war? (develops concern about social issues) 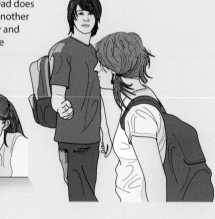 |
| **Effect on the way we talk to them** | Use short, concrete questions within their immediate experience.

To avoid yes/no answers use a choice of options, e.g. when you go to nursery, what do you like to do – draw or dress up or something else?

Use toys or puppets while interviewing, e.g. to represent different people in the child's life | Use familiar examples of experience of others to explore the child's feelings and behaviour, e.g. when a boy was bullying another boy at school, he came to see me so we could talk about how he controls his temper. Do you ever get angry and bully others?

You can get at their hopes and dreams by asking them, 'If I was a magician and could give you three wishes, what would they be?' | Should be given an opportunity to be seen alone as they may have problems and difficulties not known to the parents and that the adolescent does not want to share with them

Upsetting thoughts can be explored in some adolescents using metaphors |

Summary

In taking a history and performing a clinical examination:

- The child's age is a key feature – it will determine the nature of the problem, how the consultation is conducted, the likely diagnosis and its management.
- The interview environment should be welcoming – with suitable toys for young children.
- Most information is usually obtained from a focused history and observation, rather than detailed examination although examination is also important.
- Check growth, including charts in personal child health record, and development.
- With young children – be confident but gentle, do not ask their permission to examine them or they may say 'no', and leave unpleasant procedures (ears and throat) until last.
- Involve children with the consultation, as appropriate to their age.

Remember child protection when taking a history or examining a child where there are unusual findings.

Summary and management plan

At the end of the history and examination:

- Summarise the key problems (in physical, emotional, social and family terms, if relevant).
- List the diagnoses or differential diagnoses. Draw up a management plan to address the problems, both short and long term. This could be reassurance, a period of observation, performing investigations or therapeutic intervention.
- Provide explanation to the parents and to the child, if old enough. Consider providing further information, either written or on the internet.
- If relevant, discuss what to tell other members of the family.
- Consider which other professionals should be informed.
- Write a brief summary in the child's personal child health record.
- Ensure your notes are dated and signed.

Further reading

Gill D, O'Brien N: *Paediatric Clinical Examination Made Easy*, ed 5, Edinburgh, 2007, Churchill Livingstone.

Normal child development, hearing and vision

Children acquire functional skills throughout childhood. The term 'child development' is used to describe the skills acquired by children between birth and about 5 years of age, during which there are rapid gains in mobility, speech and language, communication and independence skills. During school age, evidence of developmental progression is predominantly through cognitive development and abstract thinking, although there is also some further maturation of early developmental skills.

Normal development in the first few years of life is monitored:

- by parents, who are provided with guidance about normal development in their child's personal child health record and in a book *Birth to Five*, given to all parents in the UK
- at regular child health surveillance checks
- whenever a young child is seen by a healthcare professional, when a brief opportunistic overview is made.

The main objective of assessing a young child's development is the early detection of delayed or abnormal development in order to:

- help children achieve their maximum potential
- provide treatment or therapy promptly (particularly important for impairment of hearing and vision)
- act as an entry point for the care and management of the child with special needs.

This chapter covers normal development. Delayed or abnormal development and the child with special needs are considered in Chapter 4.

Influence of heredity and environment

A child's development represents the interaction of heredity and the environment on the developing brain. Heredity determines the potential of the child, while the environment influences the extent to which that potential is achieved. For optimal development, the environment has to meet the child's physical and psychological needs (Fig. 3.1). These vary with age and stage of development:

- Infants are totally physically dependent on their parents and require a limited number of carers to meet their psychological needs.
- Primary school-age children can meet some of their physical needs and cope with many social relationships.
- Adolescents are able to meet most of their physical needs while experiencing increasingly complex emotional needs.

Fields of development

There are four fields of developmental skills to consider whenever a young child is seen (Fig. 3.2):

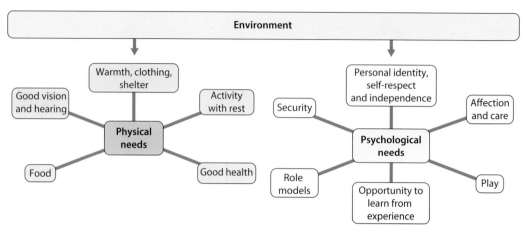

Figure 3.1 Development can be impaired if the environment fails to meet the child's physical or psychological needs.

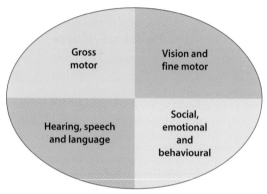

Figure 3.2 The four functional areas of child development and their core features.

- Gross motor
- Vision and fine motor
- Hearing, speech and language
- Social, emotional and behavioural.

Gross motor skills are the most obvious initial area of developmental progress. As fine motor skills require good vision, these are grouped together; similarly, normal speech and language development depends on reasonable hearing and so these are also considered together. Social, emotional and behavioural skills are a spectrum of psychological development.

The acquisition of developmental abilities for each skill field follows a remarkably constant pattern between children, but may vary in rate. It is like a sequential story. Thus, the normal pattern for acquisition of skills:

- is sequentially constant
- should always be considered longitudinally, relating each stage to what has gone before and what lies ahead
- varies in rate between children.

A deficiency in any one skill area can have an impact on other areas. For instance, a hearing impairment may affect a child's language, social and communication skills and behaviour. As a child grows, additional skills become important, such as attention and concentration and how an individual child manages to integrate their skills.

Developmental milestones

Chronological age, physical growth and developmental skills usually evolve hand in hand. Just as there are normal ranges for changes in body size with age, so there are ranges over which new skills are acquired. Important developmental stages are called developmental milestones.

When considering developmental milestones:

- The *median age* is the age when half of a standard population of children achieve that level; it serves as a guide to when stages of development are likely to be reached but does not tell us if the child's skills are outside the normal range.
- *Limit ages* are the age by which they should have been achieved. Limit ages are usually 2 standard deviations (SD) from the mean. They are more useful as a guide to whether a child's development is normal than the median ages. Failure to meet them gives guidance for action regarding more detailed assessment, investigation or intervention.

Median and limit ages

The difference between median and limit ages is shown by considering the age range for the developmental milestone of walking unsupported. The percentage of children who take their first steps unsupported is:

- 25% by 11 months
- 50% by 12 months
- 75% by 13 months
- 90% by 15 months
- 97.5% by 18 months.

The median age is 12 months and is a guide to the common pattern to expect, although the age range is wide. The limit age is 18 months (2 SDs from the mean).

Of those not achieving the limit age, many will be normal late walkers, but a proportion will have an underlying problem, such as cerebral palsy, a primary muscle disorder or global developmental delay. A few may be understimulated from social deprivation. Hence, any child who is not walking by 18 months should be assessed and examined. Thus, 18 months can be set as a 'limit age' for children not walking. Setting the limit age earlier may allow earlier identification of problems, but will also increase the number of children labelled as 'delayed' who are in fact normal.

Variation in the pattern of development

There is variation in the pattern of development between children. Taking motor development as an example, normal motor development is the progression from immobility to walking, but not all children do so in the same way. While most achieve mobility by crawling (83%), some bottom-shuffle and others crawl with their abdomen on the floor, so-called commando crawling (creeping) (Fig. 3.3). A very few just stand up and walk. The locomotor pattern (crawling, creeping, shuffling, just standing up) determines the age of sitting, standing and walking.

The limit age of 18 months for walking applies predominantly to children who have had crawling as their early mobility pattern. Children who bottom-shuffle or commando crawl tend to walk later than crawlers, so that within those not walking at 18 months there will be some children who demonstrate a locomotor variant pattern, with their developmental progress still being normal. For example, of children who become mobile by bottom-shuffling, 50% will walk independently by 18 months and 97.5% by 27 months of age, with even later ages for those who initially commando crawl.

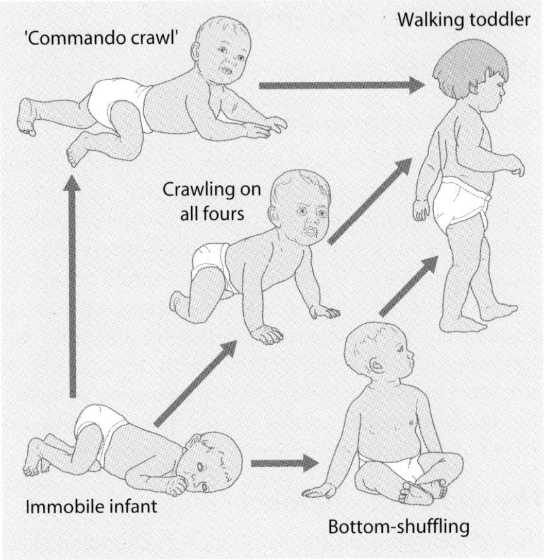

Adjusting for prematurity

If a child has been born preterm, this should be allowed for when assessing developmental age by calculating it from the expected date of delivery. Thus the anticipated developmental skills of a 9-month-old baby (chronological age) born 3 months early at 28 weeks' gestation are more like those of a 6-month-old baby (corrected age). Correction is not required after about 2 years of age when the number of weeks early the child was born no longer represents a significant proportion of the child's life.

Is development normal?

When evaluating a child's developmental progress and considering whether it is normal or not:

- Concentrate on each field of development (gross motor; vision and fine motor; hearing, speech and language; social, emotional and behavioural) separately.
- Consider the developmental pattern by thinking longitudinally and separately about each

Figure 3.3 Early locomotor patterns. Most children crawl on all fours prior to walking, but some 'bottom-shuffle' and others 'commando crawl' (creep). Bottom-shuffling often runs in families. The late walking that often goes with this locomotor variant needs to be differentiated from an abnormality such as cerebral palsy.

'Commando crawl'

Walking toddler

Crawling on all fours

Immobile infant

Bottom-shuffling

> **Summary**
>
> **Assessing child development**
>
> When assessing a young child's development:
> - Consider the four fields of developmental skills: gross motor; vision and fine motor; hearing, speech and language; social, emotional, behavioural
> - The acquisition of developmental abilities follows a similar pattern between children, but may vary in rate, and still be normal.
>
> Terms used are:
> - Developmental milestones: the acquisition of important developmental skills
> - Median age – when half the population acquire a skill; serves as a guide to normal pattern of development
> - Limit age – when a skill should have been acquired; further assessment is indicated if not achieved.
>
> When evaluating a child's development, consider:
> - the sequence of developmental progress
> - the stage the child has reached for each skill field
> - if progress is similar in each skill field
> - how the child's developmental achievements relate to age.

developmental field. Ask about the sequence of skills achieved as well as those skills to be anticipated shortly.

- Determine the level the child has reached for each skill field.
- Now relate the progress of each developmental field to the others. Is the child progressing at a similar rate through each skill field, or does one or more field of development lag behind the others?
- Then relate the child's developmental achievements to age (chronological or corrected).

This will enable you to decide if the child's developmental progress is normal or delayed. Normal development implies steady progress in all four developmental fields with acquisition of skills occurring before limit ages are reached. If there is developmental delay, does it affect all four developmental fields (global delay), or one or more developmental field only (specific developmental delay)? As children grow older and acquire further skills, it becomes easier to make a more accurate assessment of their abilities and developmental status.

Pattern of child development

This is shown pictorially for each field of development, including key developmental milestones and limit ages:

- Gross motor development (Fig. 3.4 and Table 3.1)
- Vision and fine motor (Fig. 3.5)
- Hearing, speech and language (Fig. 3.6)
- Social, emotional and behavioural (Fig. 3.7).

In order to screen a young child's development, it is necessary to know only a limited number of key developmental milestones and their limit ages.

Cognitive development

Cognition refers to higher mental function. This evolves with age. In infancy, thought processes are centred around immediate experiences. The thought processes of preschool children (which have been called preoperational thought by Piaget, who described children's intellectual development) tend to be that:

- they are the centre of the world
- inanimate objects are alive and have feelings and motives
- events have a magical element
- everything has a purpose. Toys and other objects are used in imaginative play as aids to thought, to help make sense of experience and social relationships.

In middle-school children, the dominant mode of thought is practical and orderly, tied to immediate circumstances and specific experiences. This has been called operational thought.

It is only in the mid-teens that an adult style of abstract thought (formal operational thought) begins to develop, with the ability for abstract

Table 3.1 The primitive reflexes present at birth gradually disappear as postural reflexes develop, which are essential for independent sitting and walking

Primitive reflexes	Postural reflexes
Moro – sudden extension of the head causes symmetrical extension, then flexion of the arms	**Labyrinthine righting** – head moves in opposite direction to which the body is tilted
Grasp – flexion of fingers when an object is placed in the palm	**Postural support** – when held upright, legs take weight and may push up (bounce)
Rooting – head turns to the stimulus when touched near the mouth	**Lateral propping** – in sitting, the arm extends on the side to which the child falls as a saving mechanism
Stepping response – stepping movements when held vertically and dorsum of feet touch a surface	**Parachute** – when suspended face down, the arms extend as though to save themself
Asymmetrical tonic neck reflex – lying supine, the infant adopts an outstretched arm to the side to which the head is turned	

reasoning, testing hypotheses and manipulating abstract concepts.

Analysing developmental progress

Detailed assessment

So far, emphasis has been mainly on thinking about developmental progress in a longitudinal way, taking each skill field and its progression separately, and then relating the progress in each to the others and to chronological age. This is the fundamental concept of learning how to think about developmental assessment of children. Detailed questioning and observation is required to assess children with developmental problems but is unnecessary when screening developmental progress in normal clinical practice, when a short-cut approach can be adopted.

The short-cut approach

This concentrates on the most actively changing skills for the child's age. The age at which developmental progress accelerates differs in each of the developmental fields. Figure 3.8 demonstrates the age when there is the most rapid emergence of skills in each developmental field. This means there is for:

- gross motor development: an explosion of skills during the first year of life

Gross motor development (median ages)

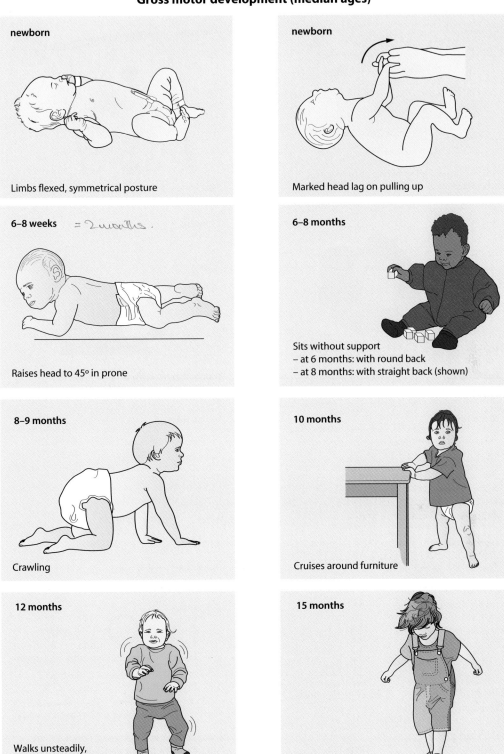

newborn

Limbs flexed, symmetrical posture

newborn

Marked head lag on pulling up

6–8 weeks = 2 months.

Raises head to 45° in prone

6–8 months

Sits without support
– at 6 months: with round back
– at 8 months: with straight back (shown)

8–9 months

Crawling

10 months

Cruises around furniture

12 months

Walks unsteadily,
broad gait, hands apart

15 months

Walks steadily

Figure 3.4 Gross motor development (median ages).

Vision and fine motor (median ages)

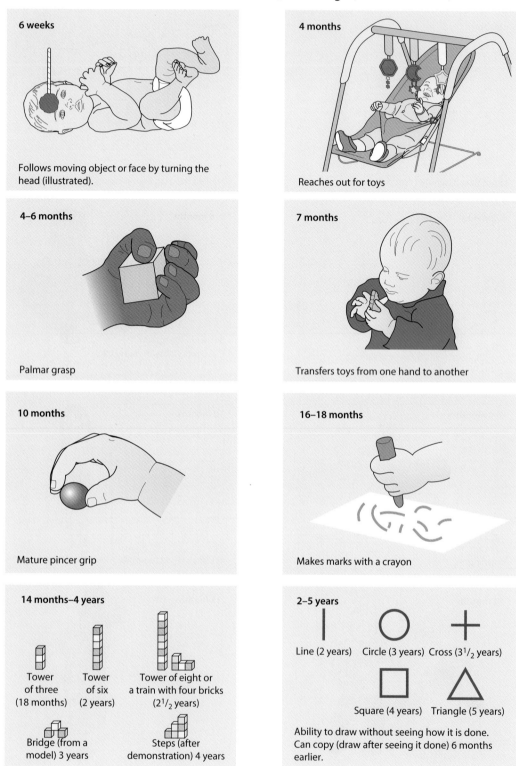

6 weeks

Follows moving object or face by turning the head (illustrated).

4 months

Reaches out for toys

4–6 months

Palmar grasp

7 months

Transfers toys from one hand to another

10 months

Mature pincer grip

16–18 months

Makes marks with a crayon

14 months–4 years

Tower of three (18 months)

Tower of six (2 years)

Tower of eight or a train with four bricks (2½ years)

Bridge (from a model) 3 years

Steps (after demonstration) 4 years

2–5 years

Line (2 years)   Circle (3 years)   Cross (3½ years)

Square (4 years)   Triangle (5 years)

Ability to draw without seeing how it is done. Can copy (draw after seeing it done) 6 months earlier.

Figure 3.5 Vision and fine motor skills (median ages).

Hearing, speech and language (median ages)

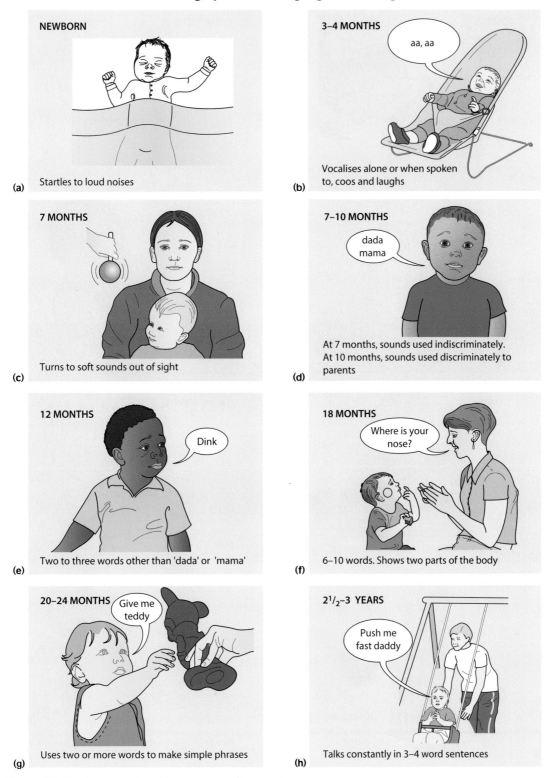

(a) NEWBORN — Startles to loud noises

(b) 3–4 MONTHS — "aa, aa" — Vocalises alone or when spoken to, coos and laughs

(c) 7 MONTHS — Turns to soft sounds out of sight

(d) 7–10 MONTHS — "dada mama" — At 7 months, sounds used indiscriminately. At 10 months, sounds used discriminately to parents

(e) 12 MONTHS — "Dink" — Two to three words other than 'dada' or 'mama'

(f) 18 MONTHS — "Where is your nose?" — 6–10 words. Shows two parts of the body

(g) 20–24 MONTHS — "Give me teddy" — Uses two or more words to make simple phrases

(h) 2½–3 YEARS — "Push me fast daddy" — Talks constantly in 3–4 word sentences

Figure 3.6 Hearing, speech and language (median ages).

Social, emotional and behavioural development (median ages)

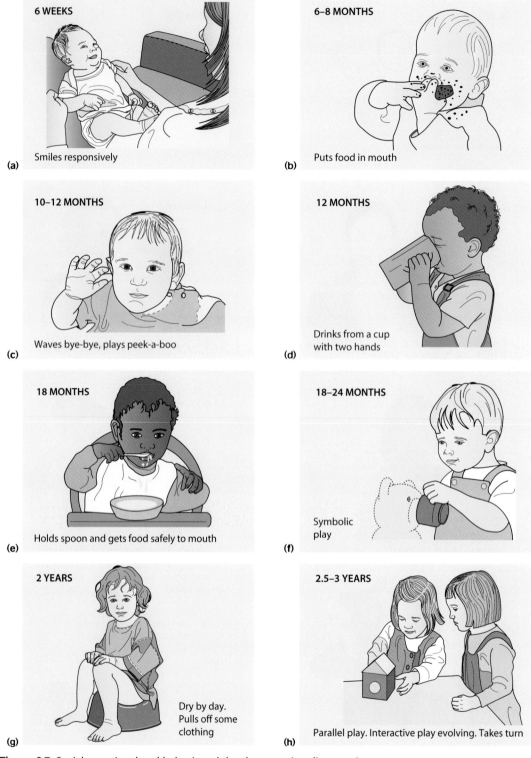

Figure 3.7 Social, emotional and behavioural development (median ages).

Fields of development with limit ages

Gross motor development

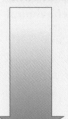

- Acquisition of tone and head control
- Primitive reflexes disappear
- Sitting
- Locomotor patterns
- Standing, walking, running
- Hopping, jumping, peddling

Gross motor	Limit ages	
Head control	4 months	
Sits unsupported	9 months	
Stands independently	12 months	
Walks independently	18 months	

Vision and fine motor development

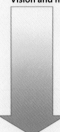

- Visual alertness, fixing and following
- Grasp reflex, hand regard
- Voluntary grasping, pincer, points
- Handles objects with both hands, transfers from hand to hand
- Writing, cutting, dressing

Vision and fine motor	Limit ages	
Fixes and follows visually	3 months	
Reaches for objects	6 months	
Transfers	9 months	
Pincer grip	12 months	

Hearing, speech and language development

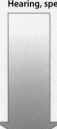

- Sound recognition, vocalisation
- Babbling
- Single words, understands simple requests
- Joining words, phrases
- Simple and complex conversation

Hearing, speech and language	Limit ages	
Polysyllabic babble	7 months	
Consonant babble	10 months	
Saying 6 words with meaning	18 months	
Joins words	2 years	
3-word sentences	2.5 years	

Social, emotional, behaviour development

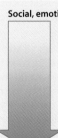

- Smiling, socially responsive
- Separation anxiety
- Self-help skills, feeding, dressing, toileting
- Peer group relationships
- Symbolic play
- Social/communication behaviour

Social behaviour	Limit ages	
Smiles	8 weeks	
Fear of strangers	10 months	
Feeds self/spoon	18 months	
Symbolic play	2–2.5 years	
Interactive play	3–3.5 years	

Normal child development, hearing and vision

Summary

Developmental milestones by median age

Age	Gross motor	Vision and fine motor	Hearing, speech and language	Social, emotional and behavioural
Newborn	Flexed posture	Fixes and follows face	Stills to voice Startles to loud noise	Smiles – by 6 weeks
7 months	Sits without support	Transfers objects from hand to hand	Turns to voice Polysyllabic babble	Finger feeds Fears strangers
1 year	Stands independently	Pincer grip (10 months) Points	1–2 words Understands name	Drinks from cup Waves
15-18 months	Walks independently	Immature grip of pencil Random scribble	6–10 words Points to four body parts	Feeds self with spoon Beginning to help with dressing
2½ years	Runs and jumps	Draws	3–4 word sentences Understands two joined commands	Parallel play Clean and dry

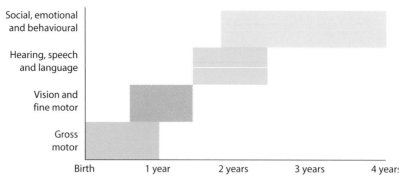

Figure 3.8 Diagram highlighting the ages when there is the most rapid emergence of skills in each developmental field.

- vision and fine motor development: more evident acquisition of skills from 1 year onwards
- hearing, speech and language: a big expansion of skills from 18 months
- social, emotional and behavioural development: expansion in skills is most obvious from 2.5 years.

Understanding the time when acceleration in each skill field becomes more obvious and knowing the child's age helps guide the direction of initial developmental questioning. Thus for a child aged:

- <18 months – it is likely to be most useful to begin questions around gross motor abilities, acquisition of vision and hearing skills, followed by questions about hand skills.
- 18 months to 2.5 years – initial developmental questioning is likely to be most usefully directed at acquisition of speech and language and fine motor (hand) skills with only later and brief questioning

about gross motor skills (as it is likely the child would have presented earlier if these were of concern).
- 2.5 to 3.5 years – initial questions are best focused around speech and language and social, emotional and behaviour development.

Developmental questioning needs to cover all areas of developmental progression but this more focused way of taking a developmental history allows a useful short-cut approach. It directs the assessment to current abilities instead of concentrating on parents trying to remember the age when their child acquired developmental milestones some time in the past.

Observation during questioning

Of equal importance to taking the developmental history is the examiner's ability to observe the child throughout any visit. Not only will this provide an almost immediate guide to where to begin questioning but also it will offer the opportunity for a rapid overview of the child's abilities, behaviour, peer group and parent–child relationships, all of which will go towards determining the overall picture about the child and his developmental abilities.

Equipment for developmental testing

Simple basic equipment is all that is needed for most developmental assessments. Equipment is aimed at bringing out the child's skills using play. Cubes, a ball, picture book, doll and miniature toys such as a tea-set, crayons and paper allow a quick but useful screen of mobility, hand skills, play, speech and language. These items allow the child to relax by having fun at the same time as facilitating observer assessment of his skills.

Developmental screening and assessment

Developmental screening (checks of whole populations of children at set ages by trained professionals) is a formal process within the child health surveillance and promotion programme. It is also an essential role of all health professionals to screen a young child's developmental progress opportunistically at every health contact, e.g. by the general practitioner for a sore throat, in the Accident and Emergency department for a fall or on admission to a paediatric ward. In this way, every child contact is optimised to check that development is progressing normally.

There are a number of problems inherent in developmental screening:

- It is a subjective clinical opinion, and therefore has its limitations
- A single observation of development may be limited by the child being tired, hungry, shy or simply not wishing to take part
- While much of the focus of early developmental progress in infants is centred on motor development, this is a poor predictor of problems in cognitive function and later school performance. Development of speech and language is a better predictor of cognitive function but is less easy to assess rapidly and may come at a time of less contact with health professionals.

The reliability of screening tests can be improved by adding a questionnaire completed by parents beforehand. Screening is being increasingly targeted towards children at high risk or when there are parental concerns.

Developmental assessment is the detailed analysis of particular areas of development and follows concern after screening that a child's developmental progress may be abnormal in some way. It is part of the diagnostic process and includes investigation, therapy and advice on how to optimise the child's progress. Developmental assessment is by referral to a specialist service and this may be the developmental paediatrician, therapy disciplines, or the local multidisciplinary child development service, which will include a paediatrician.

A range of tests have been developed to screen or to assess development in a formal reproducible manner. Screening tests include the Schedule of Growing Skills and the Denver Developmental Screening Test. Standardised tests that assess the development of infants and young children include the Griffiths and the Bailey Infant Development Scales. They are used, for example, in follow-up studies of preterm infants. There are also standardised tests concentrating on assessing specific aspects of development (e.g. the Reynell language scale, the Gross Motor Function Measure (GMFM) and the Autism Diagnostic Interview). All but the screening tests are time-consuming and require training for reliable results.

Cognitive function (higher mental function) can be assessed objectively with formal IQ tests by clinical or educational psychologists. However, IQ tests:

- may be affected by cultural background and linguistic skills
- do not test all skill areas
- do not necessarily reflect an individual child's ultimate potential
- may be compromised by individual disabilities, such as a motor disorder as in cerebral palsy.

'Verbal' intelligence tests, especially those for younger children, reflect general intellectual skills, particularly relating to language. 'Performance' or 'non-verbal' intelligence tests assess abilities independent of language. Verbal and performance intelligence testing allows formulation of a verbal IQ (VIQ) and performance IQ (PIQ), which together give an overall IQ figure.

Summary

Pattern of child development

When analysing a young child's developmental progress:
- Consider the child's age and then focus your questions on the areas of likely current developmental progress
- Offer the child suitable toys to find out about skills through play
- Observe how the child uses the toys and interacts with people.

Summary

Developmental screening and assessment

- *Developmental screening* – checks of whole populations or groups of children at set ages by trained professionals
- *Developmental assessment* – detailed analysis of overall development or specific areas of development.

Children with disabilities may have problems with speech or hand skills that may compromise testing, so that results in these situations have to be interpreted with care.

Cognitive (higher mental function) assessment of school-age children using IQ and other tests is carried out by clinical or educational psychologists.

Child health surveillance

In the UK, the healthy child programme (HCP) was introduced in 2009 (previously the child health promotion programme). It spans from pregnancy to 19 years old, but the main emphasis is on ages 0–5 years.

It offers families a programme of:

- Screening tests – early detection
- Immunisation – disease prevention
- Developmental reviews – including a specific screening at 2 years, an age when less obvious areas of developmental concern may arise with language skills
- Health promotion – information and guidance to support parenting and healthy choices.

There is a 'universal' programme, and a 'progressive' programme for families thought to be more at risk. Those in the progressive programme include infants or children with health or developmental problems, children at increased risk of obesity or families considered to be at higher risk, e.g. at-risk first-time mothers; parents with learning difficulties, drug or alcohol abuse or serious mental illness, insensitive (i.e. intrusive or passive) parenting interactions or domestic violence. These families receive additional intervention according to need. The programme is a compromise between the desire to detect problems and provide early intervention for all, while avoiding an excessive number of assessments. The way the healthy child programme

(HCP) is organised is shown in Table 3.2. At each review, a check is made for specific physical abnormalities and on the child's overall development, health and growth. Selected health promotion topics are considered. There is an emphasis on parental opinion for vision, hearing, speech and language, as parents are usually excellent at the early detection of these problems. Details of each review are entered into the child's personal child health record kept by parents and brought whenever the child is seen by a health professional.

The HCP is carried out in primary care, usually by health visitors. If problems are identified, an action plan is made for the child, which could involve advice and monitoring progress or referral to the general practitioner or specialist.

> **Summary**
>
> **The child health surveillance and promotion programme**
>
> - is provided in primary care
> - includes immunisation, health promotion and developmental screening
> - emphasises the role of parents in the early detection of developmental problems.

Hearing

During the later stages of pregnancy, the fetus responds to sound. At birth, a baby startles to sound, but there is a marked preference for voices. The ability to locate and turn towards sounds comes later in the first year. A checklist for parents of normal hearing responses during infancy is shown in Box 3.1.

Box 3.1 Hearing checklist for parents

Shortly after birth	Startles and blinks at a sudden noise, e.g. slamming of door
By 1 month	Notices sudden prolonged sounds, e.g. a vacuum cleaner, and pauses and listens when they begin
By 4 months	Quietens or smiles to the sound of your voice even when he cannot see you. He may also turn his head or eyes towards you if you come up from behind and speak to him from the side
By 7 months	Turns immediately to your voice across the room or to very quiet noises made on each side, so long as he is not too occupied with other things
By 9 months	Listens attentively to familiar everyday sounds and searches for very quiet sounds made out of sight. Should also show pleasure in babbling loudly and tunefully
By 12 months	Shows some response to his own name and to other familiar words. May respond when you say 'no' and 'bye-bye', even when he cannot see any accompanying gesture

If you suspect that your baby is not hearing normally, seek advice from your health visitor or doctor.

Used with permission from Dr Barry McCormick, Children's Hearing Assessment Centre, Nottingham, UK.

Table 3.2 The healthy child programme (HCP) provided by integrated local services, usually led by a health visitor

Age and checked by whom	Screening	General examination and immunisation	Health promotion
Antenatal (by 12th week of pregnancy) Midwife, GP or obstetrician	Antenatal screening for fetal conditions (see NICE guidelines for antenatal care)	Maternal health, fetal growth, maternal immunisation (rubella)	Universal: smoking and alcohol intake, mental health, breast-feeding
Newborn–72 h Usually hospital doctor; may be trained midwife, neonatal nurse practitioner or GP	Screening on examination includes eyes (red reflex), developmental dysplasia of the hip (DDH), testes in boys. Newborn Hearing Screening Programme. Bilirubin check by 48 h if jaundiced	Normal newborn examination: general examination, weight and head circumference plotted on centile graph, BCG offered (repeated at 1, 2, 12 months) if at risk. Hepatitis B vaccine if indicated (mother HepBsAg positive). Vitamin K	Universal: feeding, personal child health record and *Birth to Five* book, promoting sensitive parenting, prevention of sudden infant death syndrome
5–8 days (ideally Day 5) Midwife	Blood spot test for biochemical and haematological screening		
New baby review (by 14 days) Home visit by midwife or health visitor	Assess child and family health needs, including parental mental health needs	Examine baby for nutritional status and prolonged jaundice	Infant feeding, promote sensitive parenting, advice on promoting development, home safety
6–8 weeks General practitioner	Physical examination: cardiac abnormalities (heart murmurs and femoral pulses), DDH, testicular descent in boys, red reflex of fundus, matters of parental concern	Full physical examination, weight, head circumference and plot growth centiles. Vision/hearing – any parental concern? 1st immunisation – DTaP/IPV, Hib, PCV	Nutrition, immunisations, recognition of illness, avoid passive smoking, crying and sleep problems, maternal mental health
3 months Child health clinic	General review of progress, address parental concerns such as growth	2nd immunisation – DTaP/IPV/Hib, MenC	Support families by providing access to parenting and child health information
4 months Child health clinic	General review of progress	Third immunisation – DTaP/IPV/Hib, PCV MenC	Weaning on to solids around 6 months
7–9 months Health visiting team	Systematic assessment of the child's physical, emotional and social development and family needs	If parental concern – hearing, vision, development, growth	Distribution of books,[a] accident prevention: choking, scalds and burns, safety gates, nutrition and dental care, skin care (sunburn)
12–13 months Child health clinic	General review of progress	Immunisation – Hib, MenC, PCV, MMR	Dental health
2–2½ year review Health visiting team coordinate this key review	Nutrition, active play, personal, social and emotional development, speech, language and communication	Review immunisation status and physical status according to parental concerns	Obesity prevention, injury prevention, advice on how to seek medical help
3–5 years (preschool) Heath visiting team	General review of progress	3-4 years immunisation – MMR, DTaP/IPV	Health promotion and supporting parents
By 5 years (to be completed soon after school entry) School nurse	Orthoptist: screen all children for visual impairment (4–5 years). School nurse: hearing screening (audiometry), growth	Review immunisation status. Measure height and weight, plot centiles[b]. Physical examination if parental concern	Health promotion and supporting parents
5–11 years School nurse	Share information about preschool background, assessment of emotional health, psychological well-being and mental health	Nursing care provided according to needs	Promote healthy weight, support for parents and carers
11–16 years School nurse	Health review at school transition at 10–11 and 15–16 years by questionnaires, engaging primary care in mid-teens, emotional health, psychological well-being and mental health	Immunisation (13–16 years) – Td/IPV. Human papilloma virus (HPV) in girls. If at risk – BCG, Hep B, influenza	Sexual health, promote healthy weight
16–19 years (Further Education) School nurse, GP	Share information from school with adult services, emotional health, psychological well-being and mental health	Review immunisation status	Sexual health, encourage physical activity, support for parents and carers

Adapted from: The Healthy Child Programme 2009, Department of Health, London, UK.
DTaP/IPV: Diphtheria, tetanus, pertussis, polio immunization; Hib: *Haemophilus B influenzae*; PCV: Pneumococcal; MenC: Meningitis C; Td/IPV: Diphtheria, tetanus, polio; MMR: Measles, Mumps and Rubella.
[a]Bookstart – national programme to encourage parents and carers to enjoy books with their children from an early age.
[b]The national child measurement programme – height and weight of all reception and year 6 children.

Normal child development, hearing and vision

Hearing tests

Newborn

Early detection and treatment of hearing impairment improves the outcome for speech and language and behaviour. In order to detect hearing impairment in the newborn period, hearing can be tested by:

- Evoked otoacoustic emission (EOAE) (Fig. 3.9a) – an earphone produces a sound which evokes an echo or emission from the ear if cochlear function is normal.
- Auditory brainstem response (ABR) audiometry (Fig. 3.9b) – computer analysis of EEG waveforms evoked in response to a series of auditory stimuli.

Universal neonatal hearing screening has been introduced in many countries. In the UK, initial screening is performed using different combinations of EOAE testing or ABR audiometry. If a normal response cannot be obtained, the child is referred to an audiologist.

Distraction testing

This was the mainstay of hearing screening but has been replaced by universal neonatal screening. It is now only used as a screening test for infants who have not had newborn screening or as a diagnostic test. It is performed at 7–9 months of age (Fig. 3.10). The test relies on the baby locating and turning appropriately towards sounds. High- and low-frequency sounds are presented out of the infant's field of vision. Testing is unreliable if not carried out by properly trained staff, since it can be difficult to identify hearing-impaired infants as they are particularly adept at using non-auditory cues.

Visual reinforcement audiometry

This is particularly useful to assess impairment in infants between 10 and 18 months, although it can be used between the age of 6 months and 3 years. Hearing thresholds are established using visual rewards (illumination of toys) to reinforce the child's head turn to stimuli of different frequencies. Localisation of the stimuli is not necessary and insert earphones may be used to obtain ear-specific information, thus making it more useful than free field tests such as distraction and performance testing (Fig. 3.11).

Performance and speech discrimination testing

Performance testing using high- and low-frequency stimuli and speech discrimination testing using miniature toys can be used for children with suspected hearing loss at 18 months to 4 years of age (Fig. 3.12).

Audiometry

Threshold audiometry using headphones, where the child responds to a pure tone stimulus, can be used to detect and assess the severity of hearing loss in children from 4 years old.

Parental concern

At all ages, parental concern about hearing warrants further assessment.

Summary

Hearing

- Early detection and treatment of hearing impairment improves the outcome of speech and language, and behaviour.
- Newborn hearing screening is performed for the early identification of hearing impairment.
- If there is parental concern about hearing, further assessment is warranted.

Vision

A newborn infant's vision is limited; the visual acuity is only about 6/200 (can see at 6 metres what a normally sighted adult can see at 200 metres). The peripheral retina is well developed but the fovea is immature and the optic nerve unmyelinated. Well-focused images on the retina are required for the acquisition of visual acuity and any obstruction to this, e.g. from a cataract, will interfere with the normal development of the optic pathways and visual cortex unless corrected early in life.

Many newborn infants can fix and follow horizontally a face or coloured ball or the image of a target of concentric black and white circles. Most squint transiently, particularly when the baby tries to look at near objects and the eyes over-converge.

By about 6 weeks of age, both eyes should move together when following a light source. By 12 weeks, no squint should be present. Babies slowly develop the ability to focus at different distances. Visual acuity also improves: from 6/60 at 3 months to being able to poke at 1 cm objects at 8 months and at 1 mm objects (e.g. 'hundreds and thousands' cake sprinkles) at 15 months. Adult levels are reached by 3–4 years of age, when the child can match pictures or letters at 6/6 using both eyes together.

Summary

Vision

- Term newborn infants can fix and follow horizontally and prefer to watch faces.
- Visual acuity is poor in the newborn but increases to adult levels by 4 years of age.
- Vision screening is performed at school entry or in preschool children.

Hearing screening of newborn infants

(a) Evoked otoacoustic emission (EOAE)

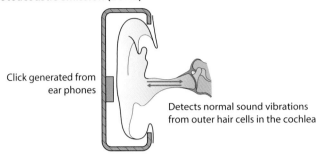

Click generated from ear phones

Detects normal sound vibrations from outer hair cells in the cochlea

Advantages:
- Simple and quick to perform, though is affected by ambient noise

Disadvantages:
- Misses auditory neuropathy as function of auditory nerve or brain not tested
- Relatively high false-positive rate in first 24 hours after birth as vernix or amniotic fluid are still in ear canal
- Not a test of hearing but a test of cochlear function

(b) Automated auditory brainstem response (AABR)

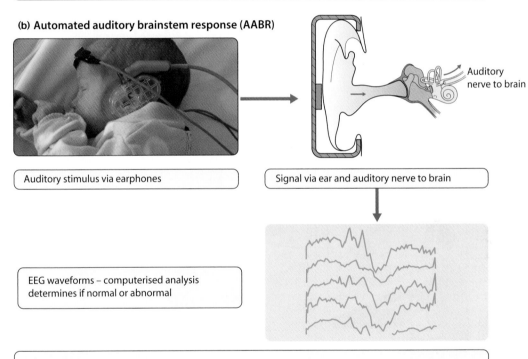

Auditory nerve to brain

Auditory stimulus via earphones

Signal via ear and auditory nerve to brain

EEG waveforms – computerised analysis determines if normal or abnormal

Advantages:
- Screens hearing pathway from ear to brainstem
- Low false-positive rate

Disadvantages:
- Affected by movement, so infants need to be asleep or very quiet, so time consuming
- Complex computerised equipment, but is mobile
- Requires electrodes applied to infant's head, which parents may dislike

Figure 3.9 Universal neonatal hearing screening is usually performed using **(a)** otoacoustic emission testing or **(b)** auditory brainstem response audiometry.

Normal child development, hearing and vision

Normal child development, hearing and vision

3

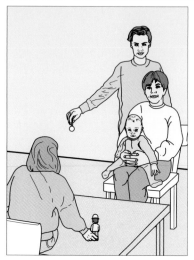

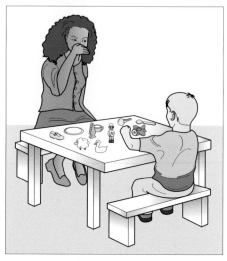

Figure 3.10 Distraction hearing test. The test is hard to perform reliably as babies with hearing difficulties learn to compensate by using shadows, smells and guesswork to locate the presenter. The test must be done by well-trained professionals.

Figure 3.12 Speech discrimination testing using miniature toys to detect hearing loss in children between 18 months and 4 years of age.

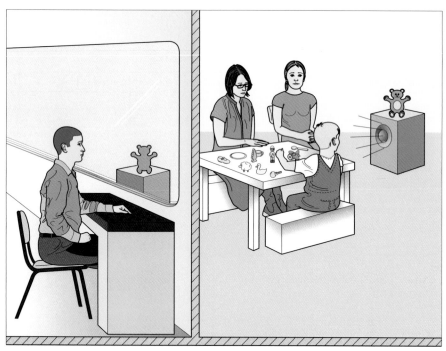

Figure 3.11 Visual reinforcement audiometry. While an assistant plays with the child, sounds of a specific frequency are emitted from a speaker. When the child turns to it, the tester lights up a toy by the speaker to reinforce the sound with a visual reward. This test is particularly useful at 10–18 months.

Vision testing

The assessment of vision at different ages is shown in Table 3.3. All children in the UK are screened for visual acuity and squint at school entry. In some parts of the UK, screening is carried out in preschool children at 4–5 years.

Table 3.3 Testing vision at different ages

Age	Test
Birth	Face fixation and following
6–8 weeks	Fix and follow bright toy, optokinetic nystagmus
6 months	Reaches well for toys, preferential looking tests
2½ years	Can identify or match pictures of reducing size (Kay pictures)
4 years	Can identify or match letters in linear optotype book (Crowded LogMAR)
6 years onwards	Can identify or match letters on a LogMAR chart

Note: Using single letters/pictures instead of lines underestimates amblyopia severity (see Ch. 4).

Further reading

Meggitt C: *Child Development*, Oxford, 2007, Heinemann.

Website (accessed May 2011)

Department of Health: *Birth to Five*, 2009. Available at www.nhs.uk/birthtofive.

Normal child development, hearing and vision

4

Developmental problems and the child with special needs

Any child whose development is delayed or disordered needs assessment to determine the cause and management. Neurodevelopmental problems present at all ages, with an increasing number now recognised antenatally (Table 4.1). Many are identified in the neonatal period because of abnormal neurology or dysmorphic features. During infancy and early childhood, problems often present at an age when a specific area of development is most rapid and prominent, i.e. motor problems during the first 18 months of age, speech and language problems between 18 months and 3 years and social and communication disorders between 2 and 4 years. Abnormal development may be caused not only by neurodevelopmental problems (Table 4.2) but also by ill health or if the child's physical or psychological needs are not met.

When performing a clinical examination on a young child with a developmental problem:

- Ask the parent what their child can and cannot do. Start at a level below what a child is likely to be able to do to retain confidence of the parent and child.
- *Observe* the child from the first moment seen.
- Make it fun. Your examination should be perceived as a game by the child, although they may not always follow your rules.
- Toys to use are cubes, a ball, car, doll, pencil, paper, pegboard, miniature toys, picture book. Adapt their use to the child.

- Formulate a developmental picture in terms of gross motor; vision and fine motor; hearing, speech and language; and social, emotional and behaviour. As you become more confident you will screen all these skills simultaneously.
- At the end of developmental screening you should be able to describe what a child is able to do and what the child cannot do, if the abilities are within normal limits for age and, if not, which developmental fields are outside the normal range.
- Clinical signs to look for that may aid diagnosis or guide investigation are:

  - patterns of growth: height, weight, head circumference with centile plotting
  - dysmorphic features: face, limbs, body proportions, cardiac, genitalia
  - skin: neurocutaneous stigmata, injuries, cleanliness
  - central nervous system examination: abnormal posture/symmetry, wasting, power and tone, deep tendon reflexes, clonus, plantar responses, sensory examination, cranial nerves
  - cardiovascular examination: abnormalities are associated with many dysmorphic syndromes
  - visual function and ocular abnormalities
  - hearing: by questioning parents about hearing and language development and checking if neonatal hearing screening was done

Table 4.1 Features that may suggest neurodevelopmental concerns by age

Prenatal	Positive family history, e.g. affected siblings or family members; ethnicity, e.g. Tay–Sachs disease in Jewish parents
	Antenatal screening tests, e.g. ultrasound including nuchal thickness and triple blood test for conditions such as Down syndrome, neural tube defects (spina bifida) and hydrocephalus. Amniocentesis for chromosomal disorders
Perinatal	Following birth asphyxia/neonatal encephalopathy
	Preterm infants with intraventricular haemorrhage/periventricular leucomalacia, post-haemorrhagic hydrocephalus
	Dysmorphic features
	Abnormal neurological behaviour – tone, feeding, movement, seizures, visual inattention
Infancy	Global developmental delay
	Delayed or asymmetric motor development
	Vision or hearing concerns by parent or after screening
	Neurocutaneous/dysmorphic features
Preschool	Speech and language delay
	Abnormal gait, clumsy motor skills
	Poor social communication skills
School age	Problems with balance and coordination
	Learning difficulties
	Attention control
	Hyperactivity
	Specific learning difficulties, e.g. dyslexia, dyspraxia
	Social communication difficulties
Any age	Acquired brain injury, e.g. after meningitis, head injury
	Loss of skills

— patterns of mobility, dexterity, hand dominance, communication and social skills, general behaviour

— cognition.

Many examination findings can be predicted from *observation* of functional skills.

Many parental concerns about their child's development are found to be variations of the norm, in which case the parents should be reassured. If in doubt, observe the child's progress over a period of time.

Abnormal development – key concepts

The terminology can be confusing, but:

- *Delay* – implies slow acquisition of all skills (global delay) or of one particular field or area of skill (specific delay), particularly in relation to developmental problems in the 0–5 years age group

- *Learning difficulty* – used in relation to children of school age and may be cognitive, physical, both or relate to specific functional skills
- *Disorder* – maldevelopment of a skill.

The following are agreed definitions:

- *Impairment* – loss or abnormality of physiological function or anatomical structure
- *Disability* – any restriction or lack of ability due to the impairment
- *Disadvantage* – this results from the disability, and limits or prevents fulfilment of a normal role. It is situationally specific; a child with a learning disability may for example be a good skier or enjoy swimming.

The term 'handicap' is now discouraged as it can imply a person deserves pity. Difficulty and disability are often used interchangeably, but difficulty is used particularly in an educational context.

The *pattern* of abnormal development (global or specific) can be categorised as (Fig. 4.1):

Table 4.2 Conditions which cause abnormal development and learning difficulty

Prenatal	
Genetic	Chromosome/DNA disorders, e.g. Down syndrome, fragile X syndrome, chromosome microdeletions or duplications
	Cerebral dysgenesis, e.g. microcephaly, absent corpus callosum, hydrocephalus, neuronal migration disorder
Vascular	Occlusions, haemorrhage
Metabolic	Hypothyroidism, phenylketonuria
Teratogenic	Alcohol and drug abuse
Congenital infection	Rubella, cytomegalovirus, toxoplasmosis, HIV
Neurocutaneous syndromes	Tuberous sclerosis, neurofibromatosis
Perinatal	
Extreme prematurity	Intraventricular haemorrhage/periventricular leucomalacia
Birth asphyxia	Hypoxic-ischaemic encephalopathy
Metabolic	Symptomatic hypoglycaemia, hyperbilirubinaemia
Postnatal	
Infection	Meningitis, encephalitis
Anoxia	Suffocation, near drowning, seizures
Trauma	Head injury – accidental or non-accidental
Metabolic	Hypoglycaemia, inborn errors of metabolism
Vascular	Stroke
Other	
Unknown (about 25%)	

The site and severity of brain damage influences the clinical outcome, i.e. whether specific or global developmental delay, learning and/or physical disability.

- slow but steady
- plateau effect
- showing regression.

The *severity* can be categorised as:

- mild
- moderate
- severe
- profound.

Other features of developmental delay are:

- The gap between normal and abnormal development becomes greater with increasing age and therefore becomes more apparent over time (Fig. 4.2).
- It may be the presentation of a wide variety of underlying conditions (Table 4.2).
- The site and severity of brain damage influences the clinical outcome, i.e. whether there will be specific or global developmental delay, learning and/or physical disability.
- It may be genetic, with important implications for the family.
- There is a wide age band across which it can be normal to achieve a developmental skill. Limit ages denote beyond the normal range.

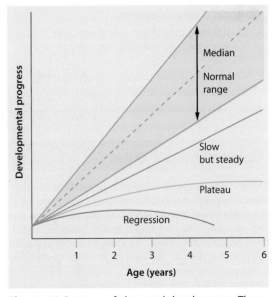

Figure 4.1 Patterns of abnormal development. These may be slow but steady, plateau or regression.

51

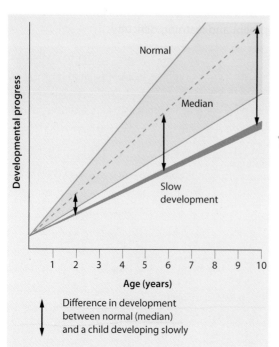

Developmental progress

Normal

Median

Slow development

Age (years)

Difference in development between normal (median) and a child developing slowly

Figure 4.2 For children with abnormal development, the gap between their abilities and what is normal widens with age.

The choice of investigations to identify the cause is influenced by the child's age, the history and clinical findings (Table 4.3). In some children, no cause can be identified even after extensive investigation.

Summary

Abnormal development

- Incorporates global and specific delay or disorder, learning difficulty, impairment and disability
- Varies in pattern of progression and severity
- Becomes more apparent with age.

Developmental delay

Global developmental delay (also called early developmental impairment) implies delay in acquisition of all skill fields (gross motor, vision and fine motor, hearing and speech, and language and cognition, social/emotional and behaviour). It usually becomes apparent in the first 2 years of life. Global developmental delay is likely to be associated with cognitive difficulties, although these may only become apparent several years later. The presence of global developmental delay should always generate investigation into a possible cause such as those listed in Table 4.2. When children become older and the clinical picture is clearer, it is more appropriate to describe the individual

difficulties such as learning disability, motor disorder and communication difficulty, rather than using the term global developmental delay.

Specific developmental impairment is when one field of development or skill area is more delayed than others. It may also be developing in a disordered way.

🌼 **Global developmental delay usually presents in the first 2 years of life.**

Abnormal motor development

This may present as delay in acquisition of motor skills, e.g. head control, rolling, sitting, standing, walking or as problems with balance, an abnormal gait, asymmetry of hand use, involuntary movements or rarely loss of motor skills. Concern about motor development usually presents between 3 months and 2 years of age when acquisition of motor skills is occurring most rapidly. Examination may reveal underlying abnormal motor signs.

Causes of abnormal motor development include:

- central motor deficit e.g. cerebral palsy
- congenital myopathy/primary muscle disease
- spinal cord lesions, e.g. spina bifida
- global developmental delay, as in many syndromes or of unidentified cause.

As hand dominance is not acquired until 1–2 years or later, asymmetry of motor skills during the first year of life is always abnormal and may suggest an underlying hemiplegia.

Late walking (>18 months old) may be caused by any of the above but also needs to be differentiated from children who display the normal locomotor variants of bottom-shuffling or commando crawling (see Ch. 3), where walking occurs later than with crawlers.

Concern about abnormal motor development needs assessment by a neurodevelopmental paediatrician and physiotherapist. Ongoing physiotherapy input and subsequent involvement of an occupational therapist is likely to be needed.

Cerebral palsy (CP)

Cerebral palsy may be defined as an abnormality of movement and posture, causing activity limitation attributed to non-progressive disturbances that occurred in the developing fetal or infant brain. The motor disorders of CP are often accompanied by disturbances of cognition, communication, perception, sensation, behaviour and seizure disorder and secondary musculoskeletal problems. Although the lesion is non-progressive, the clinical manifestations emerge over time, reflecting the balance between normal and abnormal cerebral maturation. Cerebral palsy is the most common cause of motor impairment in children, affecting about 2 per 1000 live births. The term is usually used for brain injuries occurring up to the age of 2 years. After this age, it is more appropriate to use acquired brain injury as the diagnosis. Although the

Table 4.3 Investigations or assessment to consider for developmental delay

Cytogenetic	Chromosome karyotype[a]
	Fragile X analysis[a]
	DNA FISH analysis, e.g. for chromosome 7, 15, 22 deletions, CGH microarray (comparative genomic hybridisation), telomere screen
Metabolic	Thyroid function tests, liver function tests, bone chemistry, urea and electrolytes, plasma amino acids[a]
	Creatine kinase, blood lactate, VLCFA (very long chain fatty acids), ammonia, blood gases, white cell (lysosomal) enzymes, urine amino and organic acids, urine mucopolysaccharides (GAG) and oligosaccharide screen, urine reducing substances, lead levels, urate, ferritin, biotinidase
	Maternal amino acids for raised phenylalanine
Infection	Congenital infection screen
Imaging	Cranial ultrasound in newborn
	CT and MRI brain scans
	Skeletal survey, bone age
Neurophysiology	EEG (for seizures and can be specific for some progressive neurological disorders and syndromes)
	Nerve conduction studies, EMG, VEP (visual evoked potentials), ERG (electroretinogram)
Histopathology/ histochemistry	Nerve and muscle biopsy
Other	Hearing[a]
	Vision[a]
	Clinical genetics
	Cognitive assessment
	Therapy assessment – physiotherapy, occupational therapy and speech and language therapy
	Child psychiatry
	Dietician
	Nursery/school reports

[a]Basic screening tests.

underlying cause is static, the resulting motor disorder may evolve, giving the impression of deterioration. The diagnosis for each child should formulate: the distribution of the motor disorder, the movement type, the cause and any associated impairment.

Causes

About 80% of cerebral palsy is antenatal in origin due to vascular occlusion, cortical migration disorders or structural maldevelopment of the brain during gestation. Some of these problems are linked to gene deletions. Other antenatal causes are genetic syndromes and congenital infection.

Only about 10% of cases are thought to be due to hypoxic-ischaemic injury during delivery and this proportion has remained relatively constant over the last decade. About 10% are postnatal in origin.

Preterm infants are especially vulnerable to brain damage from periventricular leucomalacia (PVL) secondary to ischaemia and/or severe intraventricular haemorrhage. The rise in survival of extremely preterm infants has been accompanied by an increase in survivors with cerebral palsy, although the number of such children is relatively small.

Postnatal causes are meningitis/encephalitis/encephalopathy, head trauma from accidental or non-accidental injury, symptomatic hypoglycaemia, hydrocephalus and hyperbilirubinaemia.

MRI brain scans may assist in identifying the cause of the cerebral palsy but a scan is not necessary to make the diagnosis.

Clinical presentation

Many children who develop cerebral palsy will have been identified as being at risk in the neonatal period. Early features of cerebral palsy are as follows:

- Abnormal limb and/or trunk posture and tone in infancy with delayed motor milestones (Fig. 4.3); may be accompanied by slowing of head growth
- Feeding difficulties, with oromotor incoordination, slow feeding, gagging and vomiting
- Abnormal gait once walking is achieved
- Asymmetric hand function before 12 months of age.

In CP, primitive reflexes, which facilitate the emergence of normal patterns of movement and which need to disappear for motor development to progress, may persist and become obligatory (see Ch. 3).

The diagnosis is made by clinical examination, with particular attention to assessment of posture and the pattern of tone in the limbs and trunk, hand function and gait. There are three main clinical subtypes: spastic (90%), dyskinetic (6%) and ataxic (4%). A mixed pattern may occur. Functional ability is described using the Gross Motor Function Classification System (Table 4.4).

Spastic cerebral palsy

In this type, there is damage to the upper motor neurone (pyramidal or corticospinal tract) pathway. Limb tone is persistently increased (spasticity) with associated brisk deep tendon reflexes and extensor plantar responses. The tone in spasticity is velocity dependent, so the faster the muscle is stretched the greater the resistance it will have. This elicits a dynamic catch which is the hallmark of spasticity. The increased limb tone may suddenly yield under pressure in a 'clasp knife' fashion. Limb involvement is increasingly described as unilateral or bilateral to acknowledge asymmetrical signs. Spasticity tends to present early and may even be seen in the neonatal period. Sometimes there is initial hypotonia, particularly of the head and trunk. There are three main types of spastic cerebral palsy:

- *Hemiplegia* – unilateral involvement of the arm and leg (Fig. 4.4). The arm is usually affected more than the leg, with the face spared. Affected children often present at 4–12 months of age with

fisting of the affected hand, a flexed arm, a pronated forearm, asymmetric reaching or hand function. Subsequently a tiptoe walk (toe–heel gait) on the affected side may become evident. Affected limbs may initially be flaccid and hypotonic, but increased tone soon emerges as the predominant sign. The past medical history may be normal, with an unremarkable birth history with no evidence of hypoxic-ischaemic encephalopathy. In some, the condition is caused by neonatal stroke. Larger brain lesions (strokes) may cause a hemianopia (loss of half of visual field) of the same side as the affected limbs

- *Quadriplegia* – all four limbs are affected, often severely. The trunk is involved with a tendency to opisothonus (extensor posturing), poor head control and low central tone (Fig. 4.5). This more severe cerebral palsy is often associated with seizures, microcephaly and moderate or severe intellectual impairment. There may have been a history of perinatal hypoxic-ischaemic encephalopathy.
- *Diplegia* – all four limbs, but the legs are affected to a much greater degree than the arms, so that hand function may appear to be relatively normal. Motor difficulties in the arms are most apparent with functional use of the hands. Walking is abnormal. Diplegia is one of the patterns associated with preterm birth due to periventricular brain damage.

Dyskinetic cerebral palsy

Dyskinesia refers to movements which are involuntary, uncontrolled, occasionally stereotyped, and often more evident with active movement or stress. Muscle tone is variable and primitive motor reflex patterns predominate. May be described as:

- Chorea – irregular, sudden and brief non-repetitive movements
- Athetosis – slow writhing movements occurring more distally such as fanning of the fingers
- Dystonia – simultaneous contraction of agonist and antagonist muscles of the trunk and proximal muscles often giving a twisting appearance.

Intellect may be relatively unimpaired. Affected children often present with floppiness, poor trunk control and delayed motor development in infancy. Abnormal movements may only appear towards the end of the first year of life. The signs are due to damage or dysfunction in the basal ganglia or their associated pathways (extrapyramidal). In the past the commonest cause was hyperbilirubinaemia (kernicterus) due to rhesus disease of the newborn but it is now hypoxic-ischaemic encephalopathy at term.

Ataxic (hypotonic) cerebral palsy

Most are genetically determined. When due to acquired brain injury (cerebellum or its connections), the signs occur on the same side as the lesion but are usually relatively symmetrical. There is early trunk and limb hypotonia, poor balance and delayed motor development. Incoordinate movements, intention tremor and an ataxic gait may be evident later.

Table 4.4 Gross Motor Function Classification System (GMFCS)

Level I	Walks without limitations
Level II	Walks with limitations
Level III	Walks using a handheld mobility device
Level IV	Self-mobility with limitations; may use powered mobility
Level V	Transported in a manual wheelchair

See http://www.canchild.ca/en/measures/gmfcs.asp for further details (accessed January 2011).

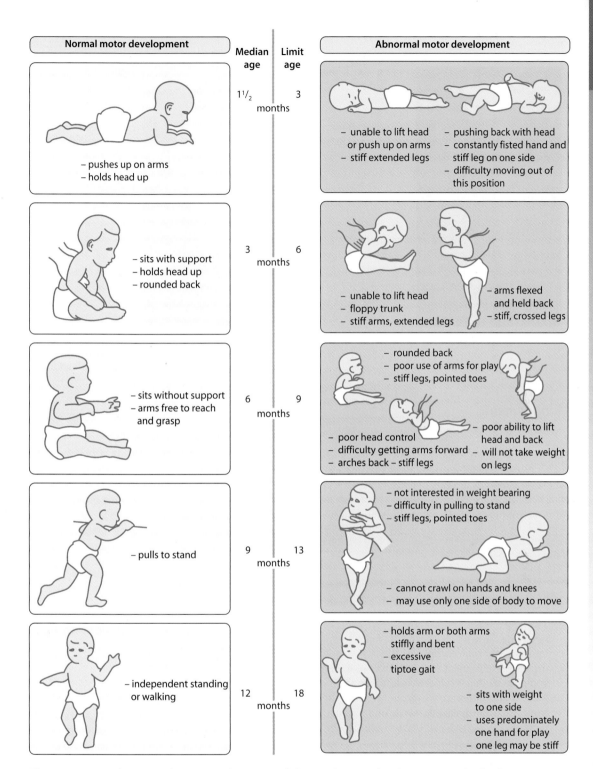

Normal motor development	Median age	Limit age	Abnormal motor development

Normal motor development

– pushes up on arms
– holds head up

– sits with support
– holds head up
– rounded back

– sits without support
– arms free to reach and grasp

– pulls to stand

– independent standing or walking

Median age / Limit age

1½ months / 3 months

3 months / 6 months

6 months / 9 months

9 months / 13 months

12 months / 18 months

Abnormal motor development

– unable to lift head or push up on arms
– stiff extended legs

– pushing back with head
– constantly fisted hand and stiff leg on one side
– difficulty moving out of this position

– unable to lift head
– floppy trunk
– stiff arms, extended legs

– arms flexed and held back
– stiff, crossed legs

– rounded back
– poor use of arms for play
– stiff legs, pointed toes

– poor head control
– difficulty getting arms forward
– arches back – stiff legs

– poor ability to lift head and back
– will not take weight on legs

– not interested in weight bearing
– difficulty in pulling to stand
– stiff legs, pointed toes

– cannot crawl on hands and knees
– may use only one side of body to move

– holds arm or both arms stiffly and bent
– excessive tiptoe gait

– sits with weight to one side
– uses predominately one hand for play
– one leg may be stiff

Figure 4.3 Normal motor milestones and patterns of abnormal motor development. Cerebral palsy (hemiplegia or quadriplegia) is the commonest cause of developmental problems. (Adapted from Pathways Awareness Foundation, 123 North Wacker Drive, Chicago, IL. Tel. (+1) 800 326 8154; see also http://www.pathwaysawareness.org. Accessed May 2011.)

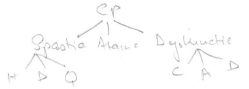

Developmental problems and the child with special needs

55

Cerebral palsy

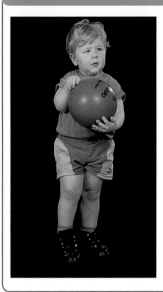

Figure 4.4 A child with a right spastic hemiplegia. His right arm is hyperpronated, flexed, hand fisted.

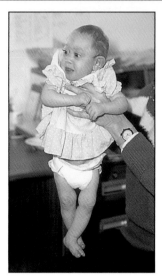

Figure 4.5 A child with spastic quadriplegia showing scissoring of the legs from excessive adduction of the hips, pronated forearms and 'fisted' hands.

Management

Parents should be given details of the diagnosis as early as possible, but prognosis is difficult during infancy until the severity and pattern of evolving signs and the child's developmental progress have become clearer over several months or years of life. Children with cerebral palsy are likely to have a wide range of associated medical, psychological and social problems, making it essential to adopt a multidisciplinary approach to assessment and management, as described later in this chapter.

> **Summary**
>
> **Cerebral palsy**
> * has many causes. Only about 10% follow hypoxic-ischaemic encephalopathy
> * usually presents in infancy with abnormal tone and posture, delayed motor milestones and feeding difficulties
> * may be spastic, dyskinetic, ataxic or a mixed pattern.

Abnormal speech and language development

A child may have a deficit in either receptive or expressive speech and language, or both. The deficit may be a delay or a disorder.

Speech and language *delay* may be due to:

* hearing loss
* global developmental delay
* difficulty in speech production from an anatomical deficit, e.g. cleft palate, or oromotor incoordination, e.g. cerebral palsy
* environmental deprivation/lack of opportunity for social interaction
* normal variant/familial pattern.

Speech and language *disorders* include disorders of:

* language comprehension
* language expression – inability or difficulty in producing speech whilst knowing what is needing to be said
* phonation and speech production such as stammering (dysfluency), dysarthria or verbal dyspraxia
* pragmatics (difference between sentence meaning and speaker's meaning), construction of sentences, semantics, grammar
* social/communication skills (autistic spectrum disorder).

Speech and language problems are usually first suspected by parents or primary healthcare professionals. A hearing test and assessment by a speech and language therapist are the initial steps. In early years, there is considerable overlap between language and cognitive (intellectual) development. Involvement of a neurodevelopmental paediatrician and paediatric audiological physician is indicated. Speech and language therapy may be provided on a continuous, burst or review basis. The speech therapist may promote alternative methods of communication such as signing (with Makaton or the Picture Exchange Communication System, PECS). Special schooling (usually language units attached to a mainstream primary school) are available but only appropriate for a very few. Many children with early speech and language problems will need learning support at school entry.

There are many tests of language development. These include:

- The Symbolic Toy test, which assesses very early language development.
- The Reynell test for receptive and expressive language, used for preschool children.

Abnormal development of social/communication skills (autistic spectrum disorders)

Children who fail to acquire normal social and communication skills may have an autistic spectrum disorder. The prevalence of autistic spectrum disorder is 3–6/1000 live births. It is more common in boys. Presentation is usually between 2 and 4 years of age when language and social skills normally rapidly expand. The child presents with a triad of difficulties and associated co-morbidities (Box 4.1).

Where only some of the behaviours are present, the child may be described as having autistic features but not the full spectrum.

Asperger syndrome refers to a child with the social impairments of an autistic spectrum disorder but at the milder end, and near-normal speech development. Such children still have major difficulties with the give-and-take of ordinary social encounters, a stilted way of speaking and narrow, strange interests which they do not share with others, and are often clumsy. In reality autistic spectrum disorders are a continuum of behavioural states ranging from the severe form of autism with or without severe learning difficulties to the milder Asperger syndrome, to autistic features occurring secondary to other clinical problems. Autism is diagnosed by observation of behaviour, including the use of formal standardised tests. It may arise as the result of different organic processes but in many cases no specific cause can be identified. There is probably multiple aetiology with a genetic component in at least some. The condition is not the result of emotional trauma or deviant parenting. There is no evidence for a suggested link with the MMR vaccine.

Management

The condition has lifelong consequences of varying degree for the child's social/communication and learning skills. Parents need a great deal of support. They often feel initial guilt that they did not recognise the problem earlier. A wide range of interventions have been promoted over the last 10 years but with little evidence except for applied behavioural analysis (ABA), a behaviour modification approach that helps to reduce ritualistic behaviour, develop language, social skills and play and to generalise use of all these skills. It is currently the most widely accepted treatment approach but requires 25–30 h of individual therapy each week, so is costly and time-consuming. An appropriate educational placement needs to be sought; some schools incorporate this approach. Less than 10% of children with autism are able to function independently as adults.

Box 4.1 Features of autistic spectrum disorders

Impaired social interaction:

- does not seek comfort, share pleasure, form close friendships
- prefers own company, no interest or ability in interacting with peers (play or emotions)
- gaze avoidance
- lack of joint attention
- socially and emotionally inappropriate behaviour
- does not appreciate that others have thoughts and feelings
- lack of appreciation of social cues

Speech and language disorder:

- delayed development, may be severe
- limited use of gestures and facial expression
- formal pedantic language, monotonous voice
- impaired comprehension with over-literal interpretation of speech
- echoes questions, repeats instructions, refers to self as 'you'
- can have superficially good expressive speech

Imposition of routines with ritualistic and repetitive behaviour:

- on self and others, with violent temper tantrums if disrupted
- unusual stereotypical movements such as hand flapping and tiptoe gait
- concrete play
- poverty of imagination in play and general activities
- peculiar interests and repetitive adherence
- restriction in behaviour repertoire

Co-morbidities:

- general learning and attention difficulties (about two-thirds)
- seizures (about one-quarter, often not until adolescence).

Autistic spectrum disorder
- **Presents at 2–4 years with impaired social interaction, speech and language disorder and imposition of routines with ritualistic and repetitive behaviour**
- **Usually managed by behaviour modification such as applied behavioural analysis (ABA).**

Slow acquisition of cognitive skills/general learning difficulty

The term 'learning difficulty or disability' (reflecting cognitive learning difficulties) is now preferred to 'mental retardation' or 'mental handicap'. Medical and educational classification of Intelligence Quotients can be different, with medical models having lower ranges. The educational levels below are useful for general use.

Children with borderline and mild (IQ 70–80) learning difficulties are usually supported by additional helpers (learning support assistants, LSAs) in mainstream schools, whereas children with moderate (IQ 50–70), severe (IQ 35–50) and profound (IQ < 35) learning difficulties are likely to need the resources of special schools.

Severe or profound learning difficulties are usually apparent from infancy as marked global developmental delay, whereas moderate learning difficulties emerge only as delay in speech and language becomes apparent. Mild learning difficulties may only become apparent when the child starts school or much later.

A child with profound learning difficulties will have no significant language and be completely dependent for all of his needs. A child with severe learning difficulties is likely to be able to learn minimal self-care skills and acquire simple speech and language. Both will need high or total supervision and support throughout life.

The prevalence of severe learning difficulty is about 3–4 per 1000 children. Most have an organic cause irrespective of social class, in contrast to moderate learning difficulty (30 per 1000 children) in which children of parents from lower socioeconomic classes are over-represented.

Common causes of developmental delay and learning difficulty are listed in Table 4.3.

Specific learning difficulty

Specific learning difficulty implies the skill described is more delayed than would be expected for the child's level of cognitive ability.

Developmental coordination disorder (DCD) or dyspraxia

Developmental coordination disorder (dyspraxia) is a disorder of motor planning and/or execution with no significant findings on standard neurological examination. It is a disorder of the higher cortical processes and there may be associated problems of perception (how the child interprets what he sees and hears), use of language and putting thoughts together.

The difficulties may impact on educational progress and self-esteem and suggest the child has greater academic difficulties than may be the case. Features include problems with:

- handwriting, which is typically awkward, messy, slow, irregular and poorly spaced
- dressing (buttons, laces, clothes)
- cutting up food
- poorly established laterality
- copying and drawing
- messy eating from difficulty in coordinating biting, chewing and swallowing (oromotor dyspraxia). Dribbling of saliva is common.

Assessment and advice is primarily from an occupational therapist or when necessary a speech and language therapist (oromotor skills/speech). A visual assessment may also be helpful. Dyspraxia in its milder form often goes undetected during the first few years of life as the child achieves gross motor milestones at the normal times. With therapy (emphasis on sensory integration, sequencing and executive planning) and maturity, the condition should improve.

Dyslexia

Dyslexia is a disorder of reading skills disproportionate to the child's IQ. The term is often used when the child's reading age is more than 2 years behind his chronological age. Assessment needs to include vision and hearing and involves an educational psychologist.

Dyscalculia, dysgraphia

These are disorders in the development of calculation or writing skills.

Disorder of executive functions

Executive functions are a collection of cognitive processes that are responsible for activities such as planning and organisation, self-regulation, cognitive flexibility, problem solving and abstract reasoning. They are very necessary to function in and interact with one's social environment. Deficits in executive function can occur as a consequence of acquired brain injury such as those following infection, stroke or trauma. Executive dysfunction may manifest as poor concentration, forgetfulness, volatile mood, overeating and poor social skills.

Associated co-morbidities of specific learning disorders

These are:

- Attention deficit disorder
- Hyperactivity
- Poor sensory integration skills (touch, balance)
- Depression, conduct disorders.

Management of specific learning disorders

Assessment may include vision and hearing and assessment by an occupational therapist, physiotherapist, speech and language therapist and educational psychologist. Co-morbidities need to be identified. Treatment is aimed at improving skill acquisition, with educational and information technology support as appropriate.

Problems with concentration and attention

Attention deficit disorder (ADD) and attention deficit hyperactivity disorder (ADHD) are considered in Chapter 23.

Hearing impairment

Any concern about hearing impairment should be taken seriously. Any child with delayed language or speech, learning difficulties or behavioural problems should have their hearing tested, as a mild hearing loss may be the underlying cause without parents or other carers realising it. Hearing loss may be:

- sensorineural – caused by a lesion in the cochlea or auditory nerve and is usually present at birth
- conductive – from abnormalities of the ear canal or the middle ear, most often from otitis media with effusion.

The causes, natural history and management of hearing loss are listed in Table 4.5. Hearing tests are described in Chapter 3. The typical audiogram in sensorineural and conductive hearing loss is shown in Figure 4.6.

Sensorineural hearing loss

This type of hearing loss is uncommon (1 in 1000 of all live births; 1 in 100 in extremely low birthweight infants). It is usually present at birth or develops in the first few months of life. It is irreversible and can be of any severity, including profound.

The child with severe bilateral sensorineural hearing impairment will need early amplification with hearing aids for optimal speech and language development.

Hearing aid use requires close supervision, beginning in the home together with the parents and continuing into school. Children often resist wearing hearing aids because background noise can be amplified unpleasantly. Cochlear implants may be required where hearing aids give insufficient amplification (Fig. 4.7).

Many children with moderate hearing impairment can be educated within the mainstream school system or in partial hearing units attached to mainstream schools. Children with hearing impairment should be placed in the front of the classroom so that they can readily see the teacher. Gesture, visual context and lip movement will also allow children to develop language concepts. Speech may be delayed, but with appropriate therapy can be of good quality. Modified and simplified signing such as Makaton can be helpful for children who are both hearing-impaired and learning-disabled. Specialist teaching and support in preschool and school years is provided by peripatetic teachers for children with hearing impairment. Those with profound hearing impairment may need to attend a school for children who are deaf.

Conductive hearing loss

Conductive hearing loss from middle ear disease is usually mild or moderate but may be severe. It is much more common than sensorineural hearing loss. In association with upper respiratory tract infections, many children have episodes of hearing loss which are usually self-limiting. In some cases of chronic otitis media with effusion, the hearing loss may last many months or years. In most affected children, there are no identifiable risk factors present but children with Down syndrome, cleft palate and atopy are particularly prone to hearing loss from middle ear disease.

Table 4.5 Causes and management of hearing loss

	Sensorineural	Conductive
Causes	Genetic (the majority)	Otitis media with effusion (glue ear)

	Antenatal and perinatal:
	  Congenital infection
	  Preterm
	  Hypoxic-ischaemic encephalopathy
	  Hyperbilirubinaemia
		Eustachian tube dysfunction:
		  Down syndrome
		  Cleft palate
		  Pierre Robin sequence
		  Mid-facial hypoplasia

	Postnatal:
	  Meningitis/encephalitis
	  Head injury
	  Drugs, e.g. aminoglycosides, furosemide (frusemide)
	  Neurodegenerative disorders
		Wax (only rarely a cause of hearing loss)

Hearing loss	May be profound (>95 dB hearing loss)	Maximum of 60 dB hearing loss
Natural history	Does not improve and may progress	Intermittent or resolves
Management	Amplification or cochlear implant if necessary	Conservative, amplification or surgery

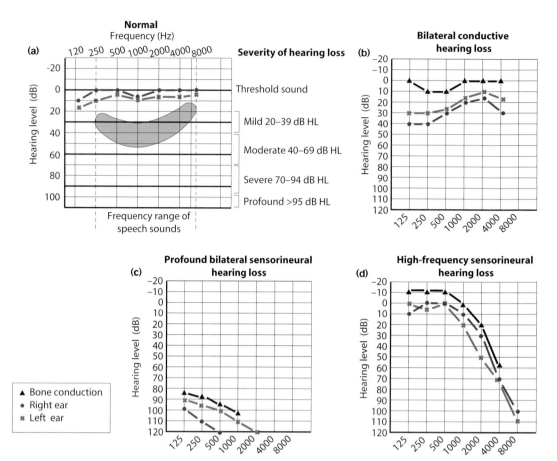

Figure 4.6 (a) Audiogram showing normal hearing and the loudness of normal speech (blue area). The consonants are high-frequency sounds, the vowels are low-frequency sounds. (b) Audiogram showing bilateral conductive hearing loss. There is a 30–40 dB hearing loss in both the right and left ears. (c) Audiogram showing bilateral profound sensorineural hearing loss. (d) Audiogram showing bilateral high-frequency sensorineural hearing loss.

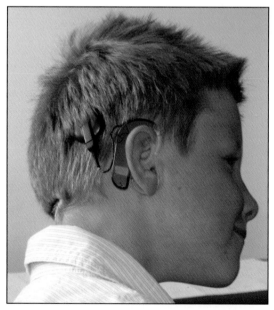

Figure 4.7 Cochlear implant. There is a microphone to detect sound, a speech processor and a transmitter and receiver/stimulator. They convert speech into electric impulses which are conveyed to the auditory nerve, bypassing the ear. It provides a deaf person with a representation of sounds.

Summary

Hearing loss

Sensorineural hearing loss:
- is usually present at birth and is irreversible
- for severe hearing impairment, early amplification with hearing aids or cochlear implants is needed for optimal speech and language development
- assistance from peripatetic teachers for children with hearing impairment is required.

Conductive hearing loss:
- is usually due to middle ear disease, often otitis media with effusion
- is usually mild or moderate and transient
- if it does not resolve, insertion of tympanostomy tubes (grommets) with or without the removal of adenoids will need to be considered.

Impedance audiometry tests, which measure the air pressure within the middle ear and the compliance of the tympanic membrane, determine if the middle ear is functioning normally. If the condition does not improve spontaneously, medical treatment (decongestant or a long course of antibiotics or treatment of nasal allergy) can be given. If that fails, surgery is considered, with insertion of tympanostomy tubes (grommets) with or without the removal of adenoids. Hearing aids are used in cases where problems recur after surgery.

The decision whether to intervene surgically should be based on the degree of functional disability rather than on absolute hearing loss.

 Any child with poor or delayed speech or language must have their hearing assessed.

Abnormalities of vision

Normal visual development and tests of vision are described in Chapter 3.

Visual impairment may present in infancy with:

- loss of red reflex from a cataract
- a white reflex in the pupil, which may be due to retinoblastoma, cataract or retinopathy of prematurity (ROP).
- not smiling responsively by 6 weeks post-term
- lack of eye contact with parents
- visual inattention
- random eye movements
- nystagmus
- squint
- photophobia.

Squint (strabismus)

In this common condition there is misalignment of the visual axes. The history may be helpful as squints are often intermittent. The parents are usually correct if they report deviation of the eyes. There may be a history of squint in the family. Newborn babies usually have transient misalignments up to 3 months of age. In some infants and young children, marked epicanthic folds may give an appearance of a squint. Any infant with a squint should have red reflexes checked and those persisting beyond 3 months of age should be referred for a specialist ophthalmological opinion. A squint is usually caused by failure to develop binocular vision due to refractive errors, but cataracts, retinoblastoma and other intraocular causes must be excluded.

Squints are commonly divided into:

- *Concomitant* (non-paralytic, common) – usually due to a refractive error in one or both eyes, which is often treated by correction with glasses but may require surgery. These squints are particularly common in children with neurodevelopmental delay. The squinting eye most often turns inwards (convergent), but there can be outward (divergent) or, rarely, vertical deviation.
- *Paralytic* (rare) – varies with gaze direction due to paralysis of the motor nerves. This can be sinister because of the possibility of an underlying space-occupying lesion such as a brain tumour.

Corneal light reflex test

For the non-specialist, the light reflex test is used to detect squints (Fig. 4.8). It is easiest to use a pen-torch held at a distance to produce reflections on both corneas simultaneously. The light reflection should appear in the same position in the two pupils. If it does not, a squint is present. However, a minor squint may be difficult to detect.

Cover test

When a squint is present and the fixing eye is covered, the squinting eye moves to take up fixation (Fig. 4.9). The child's interest can be attracted with a toy or light. The test should be performed with the object near (33 cm) and distant (at least 6 m), as certain squints are present only at one distance. Occlusion

Squints

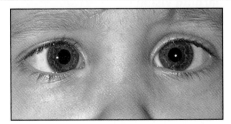

Figure 4.8 Corneal light reflex (reflection) test to detect a squint. The reflection is in a different position in the two eyes because of a small convergent squint of the right eye.

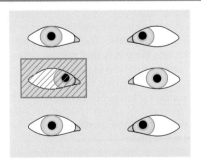

Figure 4.9 The cover test is used to identify a squint. If the fixing eye is covered, the squinting eye moves to take up fixation. This diagram shows a left convergent squint.

Box 4.2 Causes of visual impairment

Genetic	Antenatal and perinatal	Postnatal
Cataract	Congenital infection	Trauma
Albinism	Retinopathy of prematurity	Infection
Retinal dystrophy	Hypoxic-ischaemic encephalopathy	Juvenile idiopathic arthritis
Retinoblastoma	Cerebral abnormality/damage	
	Optic nerve hypoplasia	

should be with a card or plastic occluder. These tests are difficult to perform and reliable results are best obtained by an orthoptist or ophthalmologist.

Refractive errors

Hypermetropia (long sight)

This is the most common refractive error in young children. High degrees or asymmetric hypermetropia should be corrected early to avoid irreversible damage to vision (amblyopia). This is more likely if accompanied by a squint but may occur without.

Myopia (short sight)

This is relatively uncommon in young children and is less likely to cause amblyopia unless it is severe or only one eye is affected.

Astigmatism (abnormal corneal curvature)

High levels of astigmatism may cause amblyopia.

Amblyopia

This is a potentially permanent loss of visual acuity in an eye that has not received a clear image. It affects 2–3% of children. In most cases, it affects one eye; rarely, both are involved. Any interference with visual development may cause amblyopia, such as refractive errors, squint or visual deprivation, e.g. ptosis or cataract. Treatment is by relieving deprivation and correction of any refractive error with glasses, together with patching of the 'good' eye for specific periods of the day to force the 'lazy' eye to work and therefore develop better vision. It is continued until the vision in the 'lazy' eye no longer improves. The longer treatment is delayed, the less likely it is that normal vision will be obtained. Early treatment is essential, as after 7 years of age improvement is unlikely. Considerable encouragement and support often needs to be given to both the child and parents, as young children usually dislike having their eye patched, particularly if vision in the unpatched eye is poor.

Severe visual impairment

This affects 1 in 1000 live births in the UK but is higher in developing countries. A family history of severe visual impairment, developmental delay or extreme prematurity places the infant at an increased risk. The main causes are listed in Box 4.2. In developed countries, about 50% of severe visual impairment is genetic; in developing countries acquired causes such as infection are more prevalent. When visual impairment is of cortical origin, resulting from cerebral damage, examination of the eye, including the pupillary responses, may be normal.

Although few causes of severe visual impairment can be cured, early detection is important, as certain elements may require treatment and much can be done to help the child and parents. Parents of a partially sighted or severely visually impaired child need appropriate advice on how to provide non-visual stimulation using speech and touch, on providing a safe home environment and on how to build the child's confidence. In the UK, advice is usually provided by peripatetic teachers for children with visual impairment. The teachers provide input at both preschool and school ages. Partially sighted children may be able to attend a mainstream school but require special assistance with low vision aids, which include filtered lenses, high-powered magnifiers and small telescopic devices and computers. Severely visually impaired children may need special schooling. Some will need to be taught Braille to enable them to read. While many severely visually impaired children have a visual disability alone, at least half have additional neurodevelopmental problems.

Summary

Regarding vision

- Abnormal eye movements in a newborn infant or not smiling responsively by 6 weeks post-term – can the infant see?
- Any infant with a squint (fixed or otherwise) after 3 months of age – refer for an ophthalmological opinion.
- Concomitant squint – common, usually due to a refractive error in one or both eyes.
- Paralytic squint – rare, due to paralysis of the motor nerves; if rapid onset, consider space-occupying lesion.
- Testing for squints – corneal light reflex (reflection) test for the non-specialist, cover test for the specialist.

Multidisciplinary child development services

Although children with a wide range of conditions have additional needs, the term 'special needs' is usually used for children with developmental problems and disabilities. In order to optimise their assessment and care on an ongoing basis, child development services have been developed nationally on a geographic area as a secondary care service.

A child development service (CDS):

- is multidisciplinary with predominantly health professionals (paediatrician, physiotherapist, occupational therapist, speech and language therapist, clinical psychologist, specialist health visitor, dietician) in the team but often also includes a social worker (Fig. 4.10)
- is multi-agency (Fig. 4.11) and may include health, social services, education, volunteers, voluntary agencies, parent support groups
- aims to provide a coordinated service with good inter-agency liaison to meet the functional needs of the child
- predominantly sees preschool children with moderate or severe difficulties but may have resources to support children with milder problems
- may provide multidisciplinary support and monitor children up to school-leaving age (16–19 years)
- maintains a register of children with disabilities and special needs (this may be held by Social

Hearing
Conductive or sensorineural hearing impairment

Vision
Squint
Impaired visual acuity
Visual field deficits

Orthopaedic
Hip subluxation/dislocation
Fixed joint contractures
Dynamic muscle contractures
Painful muscle spasm
Spinal deformity
Osteoporosis/fractures

Specialist health visitor
Helps coordinate multidisciplinary and multi-agency care
Advice on development of play or local authority schemes
e.g. Portage

Dietician
Advice on feeding and nutrition

Social worker/ Social services
Advice on benefits: disability, mobility, housing, respite care, voluntary support agencies
Day nursery placements
Advocate for child and family
Register of children with special needs

Psychologist (clinical and educational)
Cognitive testing
Behaviour management
Educational advice

Gastrointestinal
Gastro-oesophageal reflux
Oromotor incoordination
Aspiration of food or saliva
Constipation

Urogenital
Urinary tract infection
Delay in establishing continence
Unstable bladder
Vesico-ureteric reflux
Neuropathic bowel and bladder

Common medical problems

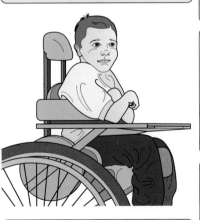

Child Development Services

Paediatrician
Assessment, investigation and diagnosis
Continuing medical management
Coordination of input from therapists and other agencies – health, social services, education

Respiratory
Respiratory infections
Aspiration pneumonia
Chronic lung disease
Sleep apnoea

Neurological
Epilepsy
Microcephaly/ hydrocephalus
Cerebral palsy

Nutrition
Poor weight gain
Failure to thrive

Behaviour
Organic or reactive
Sibling behaviour
Parental distress

Speech and language therapist
Feeding
Language development
Speech development
AAC (augmentative and alternative communication) aids e.g. Makaton sign language, Bliss symbol boards, voice synthesisers

Occupational therapist
Eye–hand coordination
ADL (activities of daily living) – feeding, washing, toileting, dressing, writing
Seating
Housing adaptations

Physiotherapist
Balance and mobility
Postural maintenance
Prevention of joint contractures, spinal deformity
Mobility aids, orthoses

Figure 4.10 Common medical conditions and the many professionals in the child development services involved in the care of children with developmental problems.

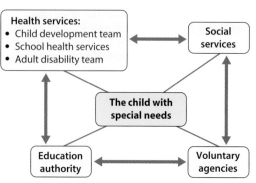

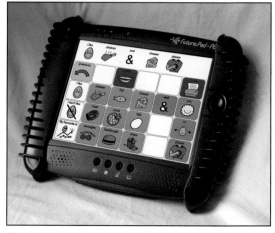

Figure 4.11 Children with special needs are supported by the integrated input of health and social services, local education authorities and voluntary agencies.

Figure 4.12 An example of a touch screen speaking communication aid to assist children who may have speaking and movement difficulties.

Services, but there is an increasing trend to single multi-agency Special Needs registers)

- is community or hospital based but has emphasis on children's needs within the community (home, nursery, school), regardless of its location
- often has a nominated key worker for a child, to facilitate parents getting access to information and services their child may need.

Child development services in the UK now usually use the Common Assessment Framework (CAF) to allow multidisciplinary sharing of information.

Emphasis is on:

- diagnosis
- assessment of functional skills
- provision of therapy
- regular review
- a coordinated approach to care (multidisciplinary, multi-agency).

Functional skills kept under review include:

- mobility
- hand function
- vision
- hearing
- speech, language and communication, including social/communication skills
- behaviour, social and emotional skills
- self-help skills, including continence
- learning.

Many children with special needs have medical problems (Fig. 4.10) which require investigation, treatment and review. Good inter-professional communication is vital for well-coordinated care. This is assisted by all professionals keeping entries in the child's personal child health record up to date.

In addition to locally organised child development services, specialist neurodisability services are required for:

- Rehabilitation following acquired brain injury
- Surgery for cerebral palsy, scoliosis
- Gait analysis
- Spasticity management, including botulinum toxin injections to muscles

- Epilepsy unresponsive to two or more anticonvulsants or where there is severe cognitive and behavioural regression related to epilepsy
- Complex communication disorders, diagnosis and therapeutic intervention
- Mixed complex learning problems, often with neuropsychiatric co-morbid symptoms
- Provision of communication aids (Fig. 4.12).
- Sensory impairments, e.g. cochlear implants
- Services for severe visual and hearing impairment
- Specialised seating/wheelchairs and orthoses (Fig. 4.13).
- Management of movement disorders, e.g. continuous infusion of intrathecal baclofen and deep brain stimulation to basal ganglia.

Needs are likely to change over time with key stages being at transition to school and adult services. A care plan should be developed at each stage and needs to be shared with the child and family and then regularly reviewed. Involvement with specialist services may be of variable frequency throughout childhood. Collaboration across services is vital in promoting a service tailored around the child and family.

Summary

Children with developmental problems and disabilities

- are looked after by local multidisciplinary child development services
- often have complex medical needs
- need regular review, as needs change with time affecting a child's activity and participation
- require coordination of care between the family and the many professionals involved, as well as close liaison with education and social services.

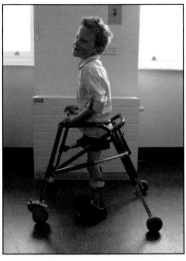

(a)

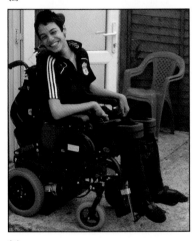

(b)

Figure 4.13 (a) A boy with spastic cerebral palsy is able to walk with the help of a frame. **(b)** Motorised wheelchair which enables this young person with cerebral palsy to be mobile.

'notification', usually by the paediatrician if preschool or by an education professional if at school. Notification is a statutory requirement if a health professional identifies that a child may have special educational needs.

The 2000 Code of Practice suggests that pupils' needs may fall within four broad areas:

- Cognition and learning
- Communication and interaction
- Behaviour, emotional and social development
- Sensory and/or physical needs.

Where a child is identified as having special educational needs, a special educational needs' coordinator (SENCO) within the teaching staff is responsible for formulating an individual education plan (IEP) for the child within the school or nursery or for seeking help from external services, e.g. educational psychology.

Extra educational provision in school is commonly provided at three levels: *School action* is the first internal level of extra support; *School action plus* may involve external support services, such as a behaviour specialist or teacher for the visually impaired. If a child's needs are more significant, the LEA is asked to conduct a statutory assessment of a child's educational needs. This may lead to a Statement of Special Educational Needs, which is a document identifying the extra help the child needs and is reviewed annually. Parents can also request such an assessment. The statementing process may start before school age in preparation for a child who is expected to have SEN, such as children with Down syndrome or severe cerebral palsy.

Although children are integrated into mainstream school where practicable, special schools or units are usually more suitable for children with severe learning difficulties and sometimes for those with severe physical, sensory, communication or behaviour problems. Many special educational placements will have a need for therapy input (physiotherapy, occupational and speech/language therapy) as well as specialised teaching resources. Support for the behavioural needs of a child may come from a clinical or educational psychologist.

Education

In England and Wales, several Education Acts and the 2000 Code of Practice have made provision for children with special educational needs to receive educational input appropriate to their requirements. This includes their right to integration into mainstream education whenever possible. Education authorities have a duty to identify children whose special educational needs will require additional resources.

Initial recognition that a child may have special educational needs (SEN) may occur at the preschool stage in children with specific or global developmental delay or with specific disabilities, or may only become evident when the child is of school age. Early identification and initiating appropriate help maximises the child's opportunity to progress. The local education authority (LEA) is informed of these children by a process called

Transition of care to adult services

In the UK, adult disability services are in general still poorly developed by comparison to those provided for children. Young adults with severe learning and physical disabilities are supported by Adult Learning Disability Teams, but there is only limited national provision for those with mild or moderate learning disabilities or with a predominantly physical disability. Major issues for young adults with disabilities include social challenges: namely, care, housing, mobility, finance, leisure, employment, and genetic and sexual counselling. Health information must be properly transferred from child to adult health services if reinvestigation of already well-clarified conditions is to be avoided.

The rights of disabled children

Irrespective of their disability, the aspirations and rights of children, as affirmed by the United Nations Convention on the Rights of the Child, need to be respected (see Ch. 1). Technological advances to improve mobility, communication and emotional expression are helping enable people with disability to better achieve their full potential, rather than being held back by their disability. However, this requires skilled assistance and adequate resources. Prominent public figures who function effectively despite disabilities help to make the public appreciate what can be achieved and serve as an inspiration to those with disabilities. The World Health Organization's model of the international classification of functioning, disability and health (ICF) stresses the important outcomes of activity and participation. Any interventions for people with disability either on an individual level or in society as a whole should aim to improve these outcomes.

Further reading

Common Assessment Framework. 2006. Government directive as part of Every Child Matters 2003.

Department for Education and Science: *Together From the Start: Practical Guidance for Professionals Working with Disabled Children and Their Families,* London, 2002, DfES.

Department of Health: *National Service Framework for Children, Young People and Maternity Services: Disabled Children and Young People and those with Complex Health Needs,* London, 2003, DoH.

Hall D, Elliman D: *Health for all Children,* ed 4, Oxford, 2003, Oxford University Press.

Hall D, Williams J, Elliman D: *The Child Surveillance Handbook,* ed 3, Oxford, 2009, Radcliffe Medical Press.

Meggitt C: *Child Development. An Illustrated Guide,* ed 2, Oxford, 2006, Heinemann Educational.

UK Government Campaign. 2006. Every Disabled Child Matters.

World Health Organization: Model of the International Classification of Functioning, Disability and Health (ICF), Geneva, 2001, WHO.

Website (Accessed May 2011)

National Autistic Society (national recommendations for management of autistic spectrum disorder 2003 and national plan for autism). Available at: http://www.autism.org.uk.

Care of the sick child

Most sick children are cared for by their parents at home. Medical management is initially given by general practitioners or, in some countries, primary care paediatricians. Most hospital admissions are at secondary care level. A smaller number of children will require tertiary care in a specialist centre, e.g. paediatric intensive care unit, cardiac or oncology unit. Most specialist centres now share care within clinical networks, with the centre linked to a number of surrounding hospitals. For very rare and complex treatments, e.g. organ transplantation and craniofacial surgery, there are a few national centres (Fig. 5.1).

rapidly, and parents require rapid access to a general practitioner or other healthcare professionals working in primary care, who in turn require ready access to secondary care. Advice may also be obtained from a health professional by telephone, e.g. via NHS Direct, via the internet with NHS Direct Online or by NHS Direct cable TV services. Although an individual general practitioner will care for relatively few children with serious chronic illnesses (e.g. cystic fibrosis, diabetes mellitus) or disability (e.g. cerebral palsy), each affected child and family are likely to require considerable input from the whole of the primary care team.

Primary care

The majority of acute illness in children is mild and transient (e.g. upper respiratory tract infection, gastroenteritis) or readily treatable (e.g. urinary tract infection). Although serious conditions are uncommon (Fig. 5.2), they must be identified promptly. The condition of sick children, especially infants, may deteriorate

Hospital care

Accident and Emergency

Approximately 3 million children (1 in 4) attend an Accident and Emergency (A&E) department each year in England and Wales. The services which should be provided for children are shown in Box 5.1. The number

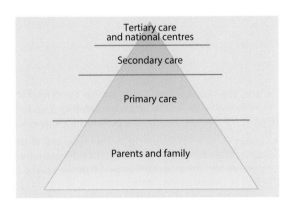

Figure 5.1 Schematic representation of the 'clinical iceberg' of the provision of care for sick children. (Adapted from Audit Commission, Children First, 1993.)

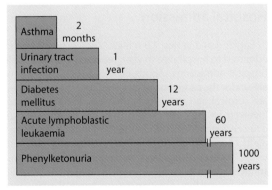

Figure 5.2 Number of years a general practitioner needs to work before encountering a child newly presenting with these conditions.

Box 5.1 Services which should be available for children attending an Accident and Emergency (A&E) department

Environment	Staff	Medical care
Separate waiting area, play facilities, child friendly treatment and recovery areas	Medical and nursing staff trained and experienced in the care and treatment of children	Resuscitation and other equipment for children. Priority for prompt treatment
Access for parents to examination, X-ray and anaesthetic rooms	Non-paediatric staff trained in communicating with children and families	Rapid transfer if inpatient admission is needed.
		Child protection policies in place
	Effective communication with other health professionals	Procedures and counselling in place following the sudden death of a child

Adapted from *Welfare of Children in Hospital*, HMSO, London, 1991.

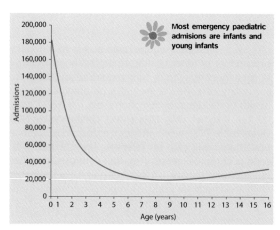

Most emergency paediatric admissions are infants and young infants

Figure 5.3 Hospital inpatient admission for children and young people aged 0–16 years in England. (Adapted from *Trends in Children and Young People's Care: Emergency Admission Statistics, 1996/97–2006/07, England*. Department of Health, London.)

Table 5.1 Reason for emergency admission of children <15 years old to hospital

System	Specific disorders
Respiratory 25%	Respiratory infections 20%
	Asthma 3%
Injuries and poisoning 17%	Head injury 5%
	Poisoning 1%
Gastroenterological 13%	Gastroenteritis 5%
Infection 6%	Viral infection 5%
Urogenital 3%	Urinary tract infection 2%
Neurological 2%	Seizures 1%
Endocrine and metabolic 2%	Diabetes mellitus 1%
Skin 2%	
Muskuloskeletal 2%	
Other 28%	

Data based on 58 061 admissions, 2009–2010. ISD, Scotland.

of departments able to meet these expectations is increasing, often by creating a dedicated children's A&E department.

Hospital admission

In England and Wales, 1.9 million, i.e. 1 in 6 children is admitted to hospital each year, representing 16% of all hospital admissions. About 60% of acute admissions are under the care of paediatricians, and the remainder are surgical patients (although a paediatrician is also involved in their care while they are in hospital, to oversee any medical requirements) (Fig. 5.3). Most paediatric admissions are of infants and young children under 5 years of age and are emergencies, whereas surgical admissions peak at 5 years of age, one-third of which are elective. The reasons for medical admission are shown in Table 5.1.

Although primary and community health services for children have improved markedly over the last

decade, the hospital admission rate has continued to rise, although it may now be plateauing (Fig. 5.4). The reasons for this are unclear, but probably include:

- Lower threshold for admission: there appears to be an increased expectation of hospital admission by parents and medical staff worried that the child's clinical condition may deteriorate
- Repeated hospital admission of children with complex conditions who would have died in the past but are now surviving, e.g. very low birthweight infants from neonatal intensive care units, children with cancer or organ failure.

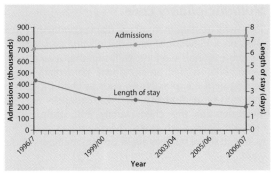

Figure 5.4 There has been an increase in the number of children and young people (0–19 years) admitted to hospital. This is because of a marked increase in the number of paediatric admissions, whereas surgical admissions have declined slightly. However, the average length of stay continues to fall. (Adapted from *Trends in Children and Young People's Care: Emergency Admission Statistics, 1996/97–2006/07, England.* Department of Health, London.)

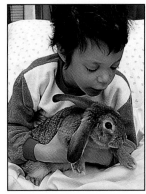

Figure 5.5 Providing terminal care in a child's home. Although this child required a subcutaneous morphine infusion to control her pain from malignant disease, she was able to remain at home and enjoyed playing with her pet rabbit. (By kind permission of her parents and Dr Ann Goldman.)

Strenuous efforts are made to reduce the rate and length of hospitalisation (Fig. 5.4):

- Speciality of ambulatory paediatrics has been developed; it encompasses specialist paediatricians providing hospital care for immediate medical problems outside inpatient paediatric wards
- Dedicated children's short stay beds within or alongside the A&E department are increasingly available to allow children to be treated or observed for a number of hours and discharged home directly, avoiding the need for admission to the ward
- Day-case surgery has been instituted for many operations which used to require overnight stay.
- Day units are used for complex investigations and procedures instead of inpatient wards
- Shared care may be provided between hospitals and primary care, with paediatricians and other healthcare professionals seeing children at home or in primary care settings
- Homecare teams aim to provide care in the child's home and thereby reduce hospital attendance, admission and length of stay. Most teams comprise community paediatric nurses, but some include doctors, and either cover all aspects of paediatric care within a geographical area or are for a specific condition, e.g. cystic fibrosis or malignancy, usually centred around a tertiary referral centre. The problems managed at home by such teams include:
  - Changing postoperative wound dressings or managing burns
  - Day-to-day management and support for the family for chronic illnesses, e.g. diabetes mellitus, asthma and eczema
  - Specialist care, e.g. home oxygen therapy, intravenous infusions via a central venous catheter (e.g. antibiotics or chemotherapy) or peritoneal dialysis

  - Symptom and pain control and emotional support of terminally ill children (Fig. 5.5)
- Children's hospices provide respite or terminal care for children with life-threatening conditions, including malignancy disease, neurodegenerative, metabolic and other disorders.
- Some teams provide a 'hospital at home' service for children who are acutely ill, in order to avoid hospitalisation.

 Hospital admission of children:

- Hospital admission of children should be avoided whenever possible.
- Most medical admissions are infants and young children; surgical admissions occur throughout childhood.

Children in hospital

Children should only be admitted to hospital if their care cannot be provided safely at home. Removing young children from their familiar environment to a strange ward is stressful and frightening for the child, parents and family. Ill or injured children may regress in their behaviour, acting younger than their actual age. It also disrupts family routines, not only of the child in hospital but also of siblings who still need to be looked after at home and transported to and from nursery or school.

Family-centred care

Care in hospital should be child- and family-centred. Parents and siblings should be involved in the child's care, which should be appropriate for the child's

Care of the sick child

physical and emotional maturity and needs. A holistic approach should be adopted towards the child and his family rather than simply focusing on the medical condition. Young children may interpret the pain experienced in hospital and separation from their home or parents as punishment. In general, the distress arising from separating children from their mothers is greatest in young children, and increases the longer the length of stay and the more frequently the child is admitted. Parents of infants and young children should be encouraged to stay with their child overnight and continue to provide the care and support they would give at home. Parents know best about their child's usual behaviour and habits and due attention must be paid to their worries or comments. Many parents rapidly learn some of the nursing skills, e.g. tube feeding, required by their child. Good communication is needed between staff and parents to arrive at a mutually agreed plan of responsibilities for looking after the child. This will avoid parents either feeling pressurised to accept responsibilities they are not confident about or feeling brushed aside and undervalued by staff. Parents should be able to stay overnight with their child.

Child-orientated environment

Children should be cared for within a children's ward. Adolescents should be with others of their own age and not forced to accept ward arrangements designed for babies or adults. Education and facilities for play should be provided.

Information and psychosocial support

Detailed information should be provided, given personally and preferably also written and available in appropriate ethnic languages. Staff should be sensitive to the family's individual needs according to their social, educational, cultural and religious background. Play specialists should be part of the ward team because they can help children understand their illness and its treatment through play. Emotional and psychological support should be available. For elective admissions, children and their families should be offered an advance visit and have details of proposed treatment and management explained at an appropriate level.

Skilled staff

Children in hospital should be cared for by specially trained medical, nursing and support staff. Every child admitted to hospital should be supervised by a children's physician or surgeon. Children constitute only a relatively small proportion of the workload in acute surgical specialities, so surgeons and anaesthetists should treat a sufficient number of children to maintain their skills. There should be a 'named nurse' responsible for planning and coordinating care by other nurses to ensure that families receive all the information they need and provide a link with staff involved in discharge planning and post-discharge arrangements.

Multidisciplinary care

Successful management of paediatric conditions often relies on a network of multidisciplinary care, with all the professionals working well together as a coordinated team. If this breaks down, particularly when dealing with complex issues such as child protection and long-term disability, the consequences may be disastrous for the child, family and professionals involved. Child psychiatrists, the community paediatric team and social services are important members of the team.

Tertiary care

As the number of children requiring tertiary care is relatively small, it is concentrated in specialist centres. Increasingly, the centre is linked to several district general hospitals to form a clinical network. These centres have the advantage of having a wide range of specialists, not only medical staff but also nursing and other healthcare professionals, and diagnostic and other services. A disadvantage is that they are often some distance from the child's home and hospital stay may be prolonged, e.g. following a bone marrow transplant. Accommodation for parents should be provided. Shared care arrangements between tertiary centres and local hospitals are designed to minimise the need for the child to travel to the specialist centre, but depend on excellent communication to be effective and valued by the family. For example, a child with leukaemia would attend a tertiary centre for the initial diagnostic assessment and treatment, and subsequently for specialised treatment and periodic review, but much of the maintenance therapy would be provided by the local hospital together with monitoring of their health and regular blood and other tests performed by a specialist nurse at home.

Summary

Children in hospital should be provided with:

- Family-centred care: holistic approach to family, parent able to stay and provide parental care
- Child-oriented environment: appropriate for child's age, together with education and play facilities
- Information and psychosocial support: verbal and written information for both parents and child
- The opportunity for children and families to express their views and fears and be listened to
- Skilled staff: specially trained to care for children
- Multidisciplinary care
- Access to tertiary care: with shared care arrangements with local hospital and primary care.

Pain

It is easy to ignore or underestimate pain in children. Pain should ideally be anticipated and prevented.

Acute pain

This may be caused by:

- Tissue damage, e.g. burns or trauma
- Specific disease process, e.g. sickle cell crisis
- Medical intervention, i.e. investigations or procedures
- Surgery.

Chronic pain

In children, chronic severe pain sometimes occurs as a result of disease such as malignant disease or juvenile idiopathic arthritis. Intermittent pain of mild or moderate severity, e.g. headache or recurrent abdominal pain, is more common.

Older children can describe the nature and severity of the pain they are experiencing. In younger children, assessing pain is more difficult. Observation and parental impression are commonly used and a number of self-assessment tools have been designed for children over 3 years old (Fig. 5.6).

Management

The approaches to pain management are listed in Box 5.2. This should allow pain to be prevented or kept to a minimum. Age-appropriate explanation should be given when possible and the approach be reassuring; however, it is imperative not to lie to children, otherwise they will lose trust in what they are told in the future. Distraction techniques such as blowing bubbles, telling stories, holding family toys or playing computer games, as well as the involvement of trained play specialists, can be highly successful in ameliorating pain in children. Some children develop particular preferences for a particular venepuncture site or distraction technique, and this should be accommodated as far as possible.

For minor medical procedures, e.g. venepuncture or inserting an intravenous cannula, pain can be alleviated by explanation and the use of a topical anaesthetic. Additional and appropriate use of inhalation agents such as nitrous oxide (laughing gas) or the adjunctive use of mild sedation alongside pain relief, e.g. intranasal midazolam, can be helpful for more painful procedures such as suturing a wound. For more invasive procedures, e.g. bronchoscopy, a general anaesthetic should be given.

Postoperative pain can be markedly reduced by local infiltration of the wound, nerve blocks and postoperative analgesics. For severe pain, there was reluctance in the past to use morphine in children for fear of depressing breathing. This should not occur when morphine is given in appropriate dosage under nursing supervision to children with a normal respiratory drive. Intravenous morphine can be given using a patient-controlled delivery system in older children or a nurse-controlled system in young children.

 Pain should be anticipated and prevented rather than treated.

Box 5.2 Approaches to pain management

Explanation and information

- Psychological, by the parent, doctor, nurse or play specialist
- Behavioural
- Distraction
- Hypnosis

Medical

- Local: anaesthetic cream, local anaesthetic infiltration, nerve blocks, warmth or cold, physiotherapy, transcutaneous electrical nerve stimulation (TENS)
- Analgesics:
  - Mild – paracetamol, NSAIDs
  - Moderate – codeine, NSAIDs
  - Strong – morphine
- Sedatives and anaesthetic agents:
  - Intranasal midazolam, nitrous oxide, general anaesthetic
- Anti-epileptic and antidepressant drugs for neuropathic pain

Consider the route for analgesics – oral if possible, otherwise intravenous, subcutaneous or rectal.
(NSAIDs, non-steroidal anti-inflammatory drugs).

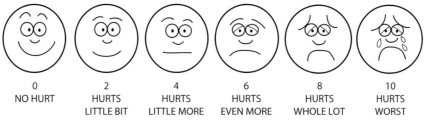

| 0 | 2 | 4 | 6 | 8 | 10 |
| NO HURT | HURTS LITTLE BIT | HURTS LITTLE MORE | HURTS EVEN MORE | HURTS WHOLE LOT | HURTS WORST |

Figure 5.6 An example of a scoring system for pain assessment in children. Wong Baker Faces scale. (From Wong DL et al. 2001. *Wong's Essentials of Pediatric Nursing,* St Louis, MO. Copyright Mosby. Reprinted with permission).

Prescribing medicines for children

There are marked differences in the absorption, distribution and elimination of drugs between children and adults.

Absorption

In the neonate and infant, oral formulations of drugs are given as liquids. However, their intake cannot be guaranteed and absorption is unpredictable as it is affected by gastric emptying and acidity, gut motility and the effects of milk in the stomach. In acutely ill neonates and infants, drugs are given intravenously to ensure reliable and adequate blood and tissue concentrations. Intramuscular injections should be avoided if at all possible as there is little muscle bulk available for injection, absorption is variable and they are painful. Rectal administration can be used for some drugs; absorption is more reliable, but this route is not popular in the UK. Significant systemic absorption can occur across the skin, particularly in pre-term infants. Occasionally this can be used therapeutically, but is a potential cause of toxicity, e.g. alcohol and iodine absorption from cleansing solutions applied to the skin for procedures.

Young children find it difficult to take tablets and a liquid formulation is required. Most are glucose-free. Persuading children to take medicines is often a problem, especially if the preparation has an unpleasant taste; experience and imagination help to overcome their reluctance. Adherence (compliance) is improved when medicines are only required once or twice a day and if regimens are kept simple.

Distribution

Water comprises a larger percentage of the body in the neonate (80%) than in older children and adults (55%). Drugs which distribute within the extracellular fluid will require a larger dose relative to body weight in infants than in adults. As extracellular fluid correlates with body surface area, this is used when accurate drug dosage is required, e.g. cytotoxic agents. For drugs with a high margin of safety, drug dosages are expressed per kilogram body weight or based on age, with the assumption that the child is of average size. Weight-based dosages should not simply be extrapolated to older children, as the dosage will be excessively large.

In the first few months of life, the plasma protein is low. More of a drug may be unbound and pharmacologically active. In jaundiced babies, bilirubin may compete with some drugs, e.g. sulphonamides, for albumin binding sites, making such drugs unsuitable for use in this situation.

Elimination

In neonates, drug biotransformation is reduced, as microsomal enzymes in the liver are immature. This leads to a prolonged half-life of drugs metabolised in the liver, e.g. theophylline. Renal excretion is reduced by the low glomerular filtration rate, which increases the half-life of some drugs, e.g. vancomycin. Measuring the plasma drug concentration is necessary under these circumstances.

Summary

Regarding medicines for children

- Oral formulations need to be given as liquids in infants and young children
- Medicines are usually prescribed per kilogram of body weight, but check the maximum dose
- Intramuscular drugs should be avoided if at all possible
- Intravenous drug dosages can easily be miscalculated as they vary widely in children because of their different size, and drugs often need to be diluted; all dosages and dilutions must be checked independently by two trained members of staff
- To improve compliance, use formulations requiring the least number of times to be taken per day
- Always check drug dosage in the BNF (*British National Formulary*) for children.

Breaking bad news

Doctors often face the difficult task of imparting bad news to parents and children. In paediatric practice, it may be because there is:

- a serious congenital abnormality at birth, e.g. chromosomal disorder
- the diagnosis of a disabling condition, e.g. cerebral palsy, neurodegenerative disorder, gross intracranial abnormality seen at ultrasound in pre-term infants
- a serious illness, e.g. meningitis or malignant disease, or an accident, e.g. head injury
- sudden death of a child, e.g. sudden infant death syndrome (SIDS).

Initial interview

The manner in which the initial interview is conducted is very important. It may have a profound influence on the parents' ability to cope with the problem and their subsequent relationship with health professionals. Parents often continue to recall and recount, for many years, details of the initial interview when they were informed that their child had a serious problem. Parents of children with life-threatening illnesses have said that what they valued most was open, sympathetic, direct and uninterrupted discussion in private that allowed sufficient time for doctors to repeat and clarify information and for them to ask questions (Box 5.3).

Discharge from hospital

Children should be discharged from hospital as soon as clinically and socially appropriate. Although there is increasing pressure to reduce the length of hospital stay to a minimum, this must not allow discharge planning to be neglected. Before discharge from hospital, parents and children should be informed of:

- The reason for admission and any implications for the future

Box 5.3 How parents wish to be told the diagnosis of a life-threatening illness

Setting

- In private
- Uninterrupted
- Unhurried
- Both parents (or friend/relative) present if possible
- Senior doctor
- Nurse or social worker present

Establish contact

- Find out what the family knows or suspects
- Respect the family's vulnerability
- Use the child's name
- Do not avoid looking at them
- Be direct, open, sympathetic

Provide information

- Flexibility is essential
- Do not protect from bad news, but pace giving it
- Name the illness
- Describe symptoms relevant to child's condition
- Discuss aetiology – parents will usually want to know
- Anticipate and answer questions. Do not avoid difficult issues because parents have not thought to ask

Explain long-term prognosis

- If the child is likely to die, listen to concerns about time, place and nature of death
- Outline the support/treatment available

Address feelings

- Be prepared to tolerate reactions of shock, especially anger or weeping
- Acknowledge uncertainty
- How is it likely to affect the family?
- What and how to tell other children, relatives and friends?

Concluding the interview

- Elicit what parents have understood
- Clarify and repeat
- Acknowledge that it may be difficult for parents to absorb all the information
- Mention sources of support
- If possible, give parents contact telephone number
- Give address of self-help group

Follow-up

- Offer early follow-up
- Suggest to families that they write down questions in preparation for the next appointment
- Ensure adequate communication of content of interview to:
  - other members of staff
  - general practitioner and health visitor
  - other professionals, e.g. a referring paediatrician.

Adapted from Woolley H, Stein A, Forrest GC et al. 1989. Imparting the diagnosis of life-threatening illness in children. *British Medical Journal* 298:1623–1626.

- Details of medication and other treatment
- Any clinical features which should prompt them to seek medical advice, and how this should be obtained
- The existence of any voluntary self-help groups if appropriate
- Problems or questions likely to be asked by other family members or in the community. These should be anticipated by the doctor and discussed. What do the nursery or school, baby-sitters or friends need to know? What about sports, etc?

In addition:

- Suitability of home circumstances needs to be assessed, particularly when the home requires adaptation for special needs
- Social support may need to be arranged, especially in relation to child protection
- Medical information should be added to the child's personal child health record
- Consider which professionals should be informed about the admission and what information it is relevant for them to receive. This must be done before or at the time of discharge. The aim is to provide a seamless service of care, treatment and support, with the family and all the professionals fully informed (Fig. 5.7). This can be facilitated for children with a chronic illness or disability by having a key worker to coordinate their care.

Ethics

Situations arise in paediatric practice in which the course of action that should be followed is unclear. Knowledge of the ethical theories and principles which underpin medical practice is helpful in understanding the issues involved. It is important to justify decisions to investigate or treat in accordance with these principles, and in language that is clear to all concerned.

Definitions of the principles of medical ethics

- *Non-maleficence* – do no harm (psychological and/or physical)
- *Beneficence* – positive obligation to do good (these two principles have been part of medical ethics since the Hippocratic Oath)

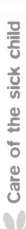

73

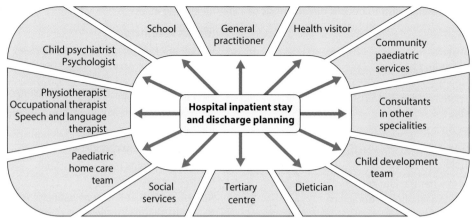

Figure 5.7 Some of the professionals who may need to be informed on admission or discharge about a child admitted to hospital.

- *Justice* – fairness for all, equity and equality of care
- *Respect for autonomy* – respect for individuals' rights to make informed and thought-out decisions for themselves in accordance with their capabilities
- *Truth-telling and confidentiality* – important aspects of autonomy that support trust, essential in the doctor–patient relationship
- *Duty* – the moral obligation to act irrespective of the consequences in accordance with moral laws which are universal, apply equally to all and which respect persons as autonomous beings
- *Utility* – the obligation to do the greatest good for the greatest number
- *Rights* – justifiable moral claims, e.g. the right to life, respect, education, which impose moral obligations upon others.

Application of ethical principles to paediatrics

Non-maleficence

Children are more vulnerable to harm. This includes their suffering from fear of procedures, which they may be too young to express verbally. Doctors may do harm from lack of skill or knowledge, especially if they do not treat children frequently.

Beneficence

The child's interest is paramount. In the UK, this is enshrined in the Children Act 1989 and the UN Convention on the Rights of the Child. This may sometimes conflict with parental autonomy, such as the emergency treatment of a child where the parent is not immediately available or when details are given to social workers in suspected child abuse.

Justice

This involves ensuring a comprehensive child health service, including the prevention of illness, and equal access to healthcare, even when poverty, language barriers and parental disability are present.

Autonomy

Children have restricted but developing rights in law. Parents are trusted to make decisions on their child's behalf because they will usually act in the child's best interests, but there may be circumstances, e.g. child abuse, in which this is not the case.

Truth-telling

It is more difficult with children than adults to be sure that they understand what is happening to them. For example, it is easy to reassure children falsely that procedures will not hurt; when they find this is untrue, trust will be lost for future occasions.

Consent

Valid consent is required for all medical interventions other than emergencies or when urgent intervention is necessary to prevent serious risk of present or future harm. It provides the ethical and legal authority for action which would otherwise be a common assault or interfere with the right of individuals to decide what should be done to them (autonomous choice). To be valid, consent must be sufficiently informed, and freely given by a person who is competent to do so. Clinicians have a duty to provide sufficient information to enable a reasonable person to make the decision and must answer all questions honestly. Information has to be given in language that is clear and understandable. In UK law, the legal age of consent to medical treatment is 16 years. The right of children below this age to give consent depends on their competence rather than their age. They may consent to medical examination and treatment provided they can demonstrate that they have the maturity and judgement to understand and appraise the nature and implications of the proposed treatment, including the risks and alternative courses of action. This is known as Gillick competence.

When a child lacks the maturity and judgement to give consent, this capacity is given to a person having parental responsibility – usually a natural parent, or to a court. In practice, problems occur only when there is disagreement between the child and the parents and clinicians over treatment, e.g. contraception for under 16-year-olds.

When a girl less than 16 years of age requests contraception without parental knowledge, a professional can provide it if satisfied that she cannot be persuaded to inform her parents, that she is likely to have sex with or without contraception and that receiving contraception is in her best interests. These are known as the Fraser guidelines.

Despite including children's views in consent, legal judgements have not supported children who refuse treatment parents and clinicians feel to be in their best interests, especially if its purpose is to save life or prevent serious harm, e.g. heart transplantation for acute cardiomyopathy in an intelligent 15-year-old patient. Where disputes cannot be resolved by negotiation or mediation, or there is doubt over the legality of what is proposed, legal advice should be sought. Whatever the outcome, children should have their views heard and be given reasons as to why they are being over-ridden.

Confidentiality

Children are owed the same duty of confidentiality as adults, irrespective of their legal capacity. In general, personal information about them should not be shared without their consent or agreement unless it is necessary for their health or to protect them from serious harm, e.g. in actual or suspected child abuse.

Best interests

It is a general ethical and legal maxim that the best interests of the child are paramount. Doctors therefore have a duty to save life, restore health and prevent disease by treatments that confer maximum benefit and minimal harm and which respect the autonomy of the child as far as possible. Parents have the ethical and legal duty to make decisions on behalf of their child, provided that they act in their best interests. Disputes may arise over what constitutes best interests and who should decide about them; they may require legal intervention, especially when the withholding or withdrawing of life-sustaining treatment is involved. Courts have generally been supportive of the position that in some circumstances the burden to the child of providing life-sustaining treatment outweighs its benefits.

Case Histories 5.1 and 5.2 demonstrate some of the ethical problems encountered in paediatrics.

The ethics of research in paediatrics

Research involving children is important in promoting children's health and well-being and may provide an evidence base for practice. Children differ from adults in their anatomy, physiology, disease patterns and responses to therapy but many drugs in current use have not been tested on them. However, children are perhaps more vulnerable to the harm which may be produced by research and should be protected against it.

Distinction is often made between therapeutic research, where there is an intention to benefit the individual subject, and non-therapeutic research, which carries a wider societal benefit but without intent to benefit individuals. Research that fails to benefit individuals may be ethical provided that it involves an acceptable level of risk.

Where a child suffers from a particular disease, e.g. acute lymphoblastic leukaemia, randomised clinical trials may be used to compare treatment regimens. The ethical justification for such trials is that there is no good reason to believe that one of the treatments would be better than the other – 'therapeutic equipoise' – and that the standard treatment used for comparative purposes is the best currently available.

The situation is different when an investigation, e.g. blood test, X-ray or intervention, is proposed for normal

Case History

5.2 Acute lymphatic leukaemia, truth-telling and stopping treatment

Jane, aged 10 years, has acute lymphoblastic leukaemia which was diagnosed 4 years ago. She has relapsed, with early involvement of the central nervous system. She is well known to the staff of her local children's ward as she has had four relapses of her leukaemia and a previous bone marrow transplant. It is the opinion of her paediatric consultant that no further medical treatment is likely to be curative. Jane asks one of the junior paediatric doctors why her parents had been so upset following a recent discussion with the consultant, at which she had not been present. The parents had made it very clear to all the staff that they did not want their child to be informed of the poor prognosis, nor would they tell her why she was not having further chemotherapy.

The parents have heard of a new drug which is claimed, in some reports on the internet, to help such children. However, it is very expensive, there is evidence that it does not cross the blood–brain barrier and the doctors consider it highly unlikely to be of benefit. The parents insist on a trial of the drug.

Ethical issues to consider are:

- *Autonomy* – the parents claim the right to control the information reaching their child on the grounds that it is in her best interests as judged by them.
- *Truth-telling* – the staff feel that it would be wrong to reassure her falsely.
- *Non-maleficence* – the parents wish to avoid the shock of the news and the loss of hope in their daughter.
- *Beneficence* – the staff wish to support the child effectively, which would be difficult if she were to be isolated by ignorance of what is upsetting her family and carers.
- *Justice* – should scarce resources be used on this new drug? Because her parents are desperate, should Jane be given a drug which, in the specialist's opinion, will not benefit her?
- *Best interests* – what are Jane's best interests and who should decide them? What weight should be given to Jane's own views based on her experience of her illness?

In such situations, further discussion between the parents and staff whom they trust is usually the key to resolving the situation. The parents will need to understand the mutual benefits of adopting as open a pattern of communication as possible. They may be helped by a member of staff being present or helping them talk or listen to the child, who will usually understand more than the parents suspect.

Parents almost always wish to do the best for their child. Detailed explanation is likely to help them see that the child's best interests may not be to seek further cure but to accept a change of focus towards palliative care. A second opinion from an independent specialist may be helpful, as may a specific ethical review. If, despite all efforts to reach agreement, the parents reject the doctor's advice, it is fairest to let a court of law decide whether or not to accept the parents' demands.

---

children as part of a control group in a trial or for the purpose of establishing a normal range. Both can be ethically justified provided that the procedure in question carries no more risk than generally encountered and accepted in everyday life.

Whatever the nature of the research a number of criteria must be met:

- Appropriate research should be first carried out in adults or older children.
- The project should have a sound scientific basis and be well designed.
- The researchers should be competent to carry it out in the time specified.
- Sufficient information should be given in a form comprehensible to the child and family to enable them to give valid consent to participation, e.g. by provision of information sheets in an appropriate form and language or by the use of independent translators.
- Parents must have the option to withdraw their child from the research at any stage without prejudice.
- The project must be reviewed and approved by an independent scientific and ethical process (Research Ethics Committee).

Summary

Ethics in paediatrics

- Both clinicians and parents aim to do what is in their child's best interests
- Conflicting views can usually be resolved by good communication
- If not resolved – help may be sought from further, wider communication, or a second, truly independent opinion, or sometimes from hospital ethical committees; or may go to court.
- Older children who understand the issues and have strong views as to what should or should not be done to them – there is increasing ethical and legal support for them to exercise as much autonomy as they are capable of.

Evidence-based paediatrics

Clinicians have always sought to make decisions in the best interests of their patients. However, such decisions have often been made intuitively, given as clinical opinion, which is difficult to generalise, scrutinise or challenge. Evidence-based practice provides a systematic approach to enable clinicians to efficiently use the best available evidence, usually from research, to help them solve their clinical problems. The difference between this approach and old-style clinical practice is that clinicians need to know how to turn their clinical problems into questions that can be answered by the research literature, to search the literature efficiently, and to analyse the evidence, using epidemiological and biostatistical rules (Figs 5.8, 5.9). Sometimes, the best available evidence will be a high-quality systematic review of randomised controlled trials, which are directly applicable to a particular patient. For other questions, lack of more valid studies may mean that one has to base one's decision on previous experience with a small number of similar patients. The important factor is that, for any decision, clinicians know the strength of the evidence, and therefore the degree of uncertainty. As this approach requires clinicians to be explicit about the evidence they use, others involved in the decisions (patients, parents, managers and other clinicians) can debate and judge the evidence for themselves.

Why practise evidence-based paediatrics?

There are many examples from the past where, through lack of evidence, clinicians have harmed children, e.g.

- *Blindness from retinopathy of prematurity*. In the 1950s, following anecdotal reports, many neonatal units started nursing all premature infants in additional ambient oxygen, irrespective of need. This reduced mortality, but as no properly conducted trials were performed of this new therapy, it took several years for it to be realised that it was also responsible for many thousands of babies becoming blind from retinopathy of prematurity.
- *Advice that babies should sleep lying on their front (prone), which increases the risk of sudden infant death syndrome (SIDS)*. Medical advice given during the 1970s and 1980s, to put babies to sleep prone, appears to have been based on physiological studies in preterm babies, which showed better oxygenation when nursed prone. Furthermore, autopsies on some infants who died of SIDS showed milk in the trachea, which was assumed to have been aspirated and this was thought to be more likely if they were lying on their back. However, an accumulation of more valid evidence from cohort and case–control studies showed that placing term infants prone was associated with an *increased* risk of SIDS.

Evidence-based medicine allows clinicians to be explicit about the probability (or risk) of important outcomes. For example, in discussing with parents the prognosis of a child who has had a febrile seizure, one can state that 'the risk of developing epilepsy is 1 in 100', instead of using vague terms, such as 'he/she is unlikely to develop epilepsy'.

Explicit analysis of evidence has also become more important with the increasing delivery of healthcare by teams rather than individuals. Each team member needs to understand the rationale for decisions and the probability of different outcomes in order to make their own clinical decisions and to provide consistent information to patients and parents.

To what extent is paediatric practice based on sound evidence?

There are two paediatric specialities in which there is a considerable body of reliable, high-quality evidence underpinning clinical practice, namely paediatric oncology and, to a lesser extent, neonatology. Management protocols of virtually all children with cancer are part of multicentre trials designed to identify which treatment gives the best possible results. The trials are national or, increasingly, international, and include short- and long-term follow-up. Examples of the range of evidence available in paediatrics are given in Box 5.4. In general, the evidence base for paediatrics is poorer than in adult medicine. Reasons for this include:

- The relatively small number of children with significant illness requiring investigation and treatment. To overcome this, multicentre trials are required, which are more difficult to organise and expensive.
- Additional ethical limitations
  - Subjecting children to additional investigations or giving a new treatment is severely limited by the inability of the child to give consent. Some parents are concerned that participating in a trial could mean that their child could receive treatment that turns out to be inferior to the standard treatment and could have unknown side-effects.
  - There is concern over the ability of parents to give truly informed consent immediately after the acute onset of serious illness, e.g. the birth of a preterm infant, meningococcal septicaemia or meningitis.
- There is limited investment by the pharmaceutical industry in drug trials, as drug use in children is insufficient to justify the cost and ethical difficulties of conducting trials. As a result, approximately 50% of drug treatments in children are unlicensed ('off label').

The consequence is that there is less of a culture of randomised controlled trials in paediatrics compared with adult medicine.

For evidence-based practice to become more widespread, clinicians must recognise the need to ask

Care of the sick child

77

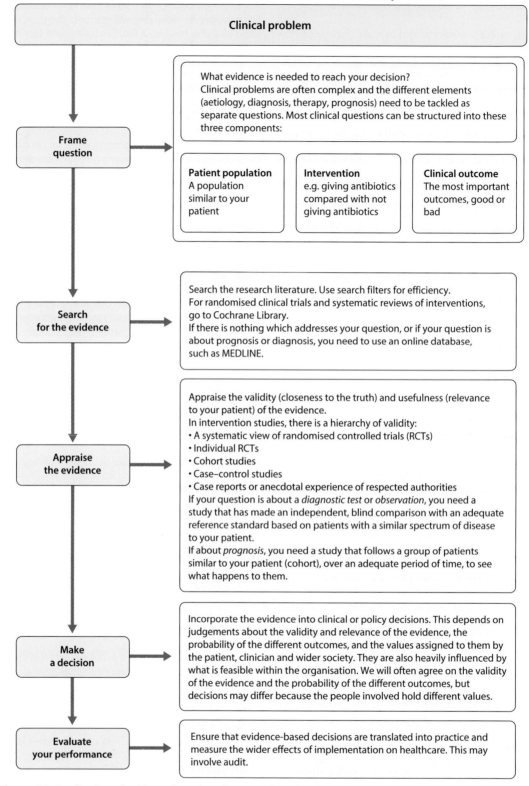

Application of evidence-based medicine to clinical problems

Clinical problem

Frame question

What evidence is needed to reach your decision?
Clinical problems are often complex and the different elements (aetiology, diagnosis, therapy, prognosis) need to be tackled as separate questions. Most clinical questions can be structured into these three components:

Patient population
A population similar to your patient

Intervention
e.g. giving antibiotics compared with not giving antibiotics

Clinical outcome
The most important outcomes, good or bad

Search for the evidence

Search the research literature. Use search filters for efficiency.
For randomised clinical trials and systematic reviews of interventions, go to Cochrane Library.
If there is nothing which addresses your question, or if your question is about prognosis or diagnosis, you need to use an online database, such as MEDLINE.

Appraise the evidence

Appraise the validity (closeness to the truth) and usefulness (relevance to your patient) of the evidence.
In intervention studies, there is a hierarchy of validity:
• A systematic view of randomised controlled trials (RCTs)
• Individual RCTs
• Cohort studies
• Case–control studies
• Case reports or anecdotal experience of respected authorities
If your question is about a *diagnostic test* or *observation*, you need a study that has made an independent, blind comparison with an adequate reference standard based on patients with a similar spectrum of disease to your patient.
If about *prognosis*, you need a study that follows a group of patients similar to your patient (cohort), over an adequate period of time, to see what happens to them.

Make a decision

Incorporate the evidence into clinical or policy decisions. This depends on judgements about the validity and relevance of the evidence, the probability of the different outcomes, and the values assigned to them by the patient, clinician and wider society. They are also heavily influenced by what is feasible within the organisation. We will often agree on the validity of the evidence and the probability of the different outcomes, but decisions may differ because the people involved hold different values.

Evaluate your performance

Ensure that evidence-based decisions are translated into practice and measure the wider effects of implementation on healthcare. This may involve audit.

Figure 5.8 Application of evidence-based medicine to clinical problems.

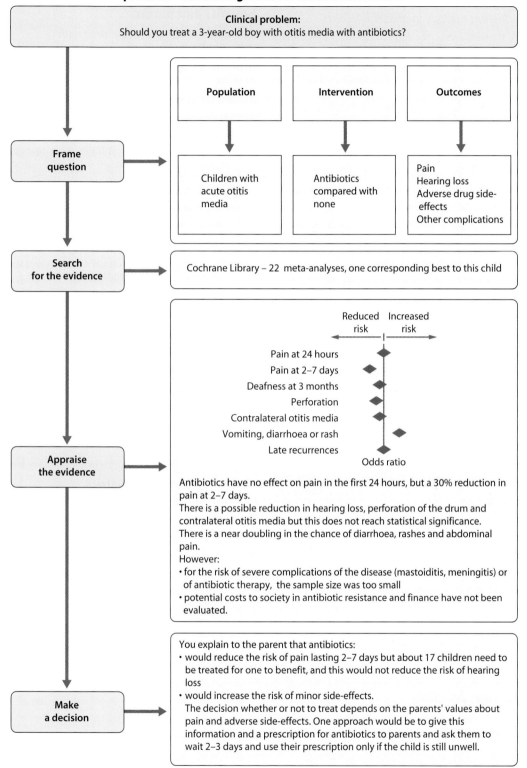

Example of evidence-based practice in solving a clinical problem – the management of acute otitis media

Clinical problem:
Should you treat a 3-year-old boy with otitis media with antibiotics?

Frame question

Population	Intervention	Outcomes
Children with acute otitis media	Antibiotics compared with none	Pain Hearing loss Adverse drug side-effects Other complications

Search for the evidence

Cochrane Library – 22 meta-analyses, one corresponding best to this child

Appraise the evidence

Reduced risk ← | → Increased risk

Pain at 24 hours
Pain at 2–7 days
Deafness at 3 months
Perforation
Contralateral otitis media
Vomiting, diarrhoea or rash
Late recurrences

Odds ratio

Antibiotics have no effect on pain in the first 24 hours, but a 30% reduction in pain at 2–7 days.
There is a possible reduction in hearing loss, perforation of the drum and contralateral otitis media but this does not reach statistical significance.
There is a near doubling in the chance of diarrhoea, rashes and abdominal pain.
However:
• for the risk of severe complications of the disease (mastoiditis, meningitis) or of antibiotic therapy, the sample size was too small
• potential costs to society in antibiotic resistance and finance have not been evaluated.

Make a decision

You explain to the parent that antibiotics:
• would reduce the risk of pain lasting 2–7 days but about 17 children need to be treated for one to benefit, and this would not reduce the risk of hearing loss
• would increase the risk of minor side-effects.
The decision whether or not to treat depends on the parents' values about pain and adverse side-effects. One approach would be to give this information and a prescription for antibiotics to parents and ask them to wait 2–3 days and use their prescription only if the child is still unwell.

Figure 5.9 An example of an evidence-based medicine approach to a clinical problem – the treatment of acute otitis media with antibiotics. (Sanders S, Glasziou PP, Del Mar C et al. (2004 last updated 2008). Antibiotics for acute otitis media in children. *Cochrane Database of Systematic Reviews* (1) CD000219).

Care of the sick child

Box 5.4 Examples of the range of evidence available in paediatrics

1. Clear evidence of benefit

Surfactant therapy in pre-term infants

The meta-analysis (see Fig. 10.12) from a Cochrane systematic review shows that mortality is reduced by 40% in preterm infants with respiratory distress syndrome (RDS) treated with surfactant compared with placebo.

This evidence was rapidly produced and introduced into practice as:

- Respiratory distress syndrome is a common cause of death and morbidity in a neonatal intensive care unit
- There is a clearly understood disease mechanism for respiratory distress syndrome, i.e. surfactant deficiency
- The effect of surfactant treatment was immediately obvious at the cot-side – ventilator settings usually have to be reduced shortly after administration
- Potential benefits and side-effects could be clearly defined and identified
- Neonatologists are a relatively small group of doctors who meet regularly – national and international studies could be organised and their results quickly disseminated
- There was financial support and involvement from the pharmaceutical industry.

2. Clear evidence, but need to balance benefits and harms

Antibiotic treatment for children with otitis media

As shown in Figure 5.9, there is a balance of risk and benefits.

3. No clear evidence

Bulk-forming laxatives for constipation

Bulk-forming laxatives, such as methylcellulose or ispaghula husk, are used in children with constipation. However, this is not based on clear evidence. There are no systematic reviews and no randomised controlled studies of these agents in children.

Some possible reasons for the lack of evidence on the use of these laxatives in this common condition are:

- constipation is not a life-threatening disorder
- the causes are multifactorial and the disease mechanism is not clearly defined
- there is a belief that there are likely to be few side-effects to the use of bulk-forming laxatives and clinicians are prepared to prescribe them without clear evidence
- there is limited support for studies from the pharmaceutical industry
- the research agenda is not driven by such clinical problems.

questions, particularly about procedures or interventions which are common practice. However, evidence-based medicine is not cookbook medicine. Incontrovertible evidence is rare, and clinical decisions complex, which is why clinical care is provided by clinicians and not technicians. Evidence-based healthcare cannot change this, but is an essential tool to help clinicians make rational, informed decisions together with their patients. In addition, evidence-based paediatrics provides a way for clinicians to articulate their priorities for research and thereby set a research agenda which is relevant to service needs.

Summary

Evidence-based paediatrics

- requires clinical problems to be framed into questions, to search the literature and then appraise the evidence in order to make a decision
- is less well developed than in adult medicine
- should be adopted whenever possible; however, clinical decisions are complex and the evidence base usually informs rather than determines clinical decision-making.

Further reading

Websites (Accessed May 2011)

CEBM (Centre for Evidence-Based Care, Oxford)
Available at: http://www.cebm.net

Every Child Matters – national framework for services for children and young people. Available at: www.education.gov.uk

http://www.tripdatabase.com

http://clinicalevidence.bmj.com/ceweb

http://www.cochrane.org

Paediatric emergencies

There are few situations that provoke greater anxiety than being called to see a child who is seriously ill. This chapter outlines a basic approach to the emergency management of seriously ill children.

The seriously ill child

The rapid clinical assessment of the seriously ill child will identify if there is potential respiratory, circulatory or neurological failure. This should take less than 1 minute. Normal vital signs are shown in Figure 6.1 and how a rapid assessment is performed is shown in Figure 6.2.

Resuscitation is given immediately, if necessary, followed by secondary assessment and other emergency treatment.

The seriously ill child may present with shock, respiratory distress, as a drowsy/unconscious or fitting child or with a surgical emergency. Their causes are listed in Figure 6.4. In children, the key to successful outcome is the early recognition and active management of conditions that are life-threatening and potentially reversible.

 Doctors should be able to provide life support for children of all ages, from newborn to adolescents.

Summary

Regarding the seriously ill child

- Prevention of cardiopulmonary arrest is by early recognition and treatment of respiratory distress, respiratory or circulatory failure.

Cardiopulmonary resuscitation

In adults, cardiopulmonary arrest is often cardiac in origin, secondary to ischaemic heart disease. In contrast, children usually have healthy hearts but experience hypoxia from respiratory or neurological failure or shock. If this occurs, irrespective of the cause, basic life support must be started immediately.

Vital signs

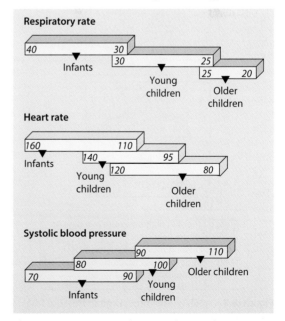

Figure 6.1 Variation in the normal range for respiratory rate, heart rate and systolic blood pressure with age.

Assessment of the seriously ill child

The rapid clinical assessment: **ABCDE** Should take < 1 min **Airway and Breathing** **Look, listen and feel for:** Airway obstruction or respiratory distress Work of breathing (respiratory effort) Respiratory rate Stridor, wheeze Auscultation for air entry Cyanosis **Circulation** **Feel and assess:** Heart rate Pulse volume Capillary refill time (Fig 6.3) Blood pressure **Disability** **Observe and note:** Level of consciousness (Box 6.1) Posture – hypotonia, decorticate, decerebrate Pupil size and reactivity **Exposure**	**Resuscitation (if necessary)** **Includes Basic/Advanced life support** **Consider:** Jaw and neck positioning Oxygen Suction and foreign body removal Supporting breathing Chest compression Monitoring pulse oximetry and heart rate

Secondary assessment

History from:
- parents
- witnesses
- general practitioner
- paramedical staff
- police

Examination including:
- evidence of trauma
- rash, e.g. meningococcal
- smell, e.g. ketones, alcohol
- scars, e.g. underlying congenital heart disease
- MedicAlert bracelet

Investigations
- blood glucose

Other emergency interventions

Figure 6.2 Assessment of the seriously ill child.

Capillary refill time

Press on the skin of the sternum or a digit at the level of the heart
Apply blanching pressure for 5 seconds
Measure time for blush to return
Prolonged capillary refill if >2 seconds

Figure 6.3 Capillary refill time. Digital pressure for 5 seconds. Normal <2 seconds.

❋ **Capillary refill time is affected by body exposure to a cold environment.**

Box 6.1 AVPU rapid assessment of level of consciousness – more detailed evaluation is with the Glasgow Coma Scale (see Table 6.2)

A	ALERT
V	Responds to VOICE
P	Responds to PAIN
U	UNRESPONSIVE

A score of P means that the child's airway is at risk and will need to be maintained by a manoeuvre or adjunct.

Basic life support

See Figure 6.5.

Advanced life support (Fig. 6.6)

Children who have been resuscitated successfully should be transferred to a paediatric high-dependency or intensive care unit.

The seriously injured child

Management of the seriously injured child must take account of potential injury to the cervical spine and other bones and internal injuries (Fig. 6.7).

Presentation and causes of serious illness in children

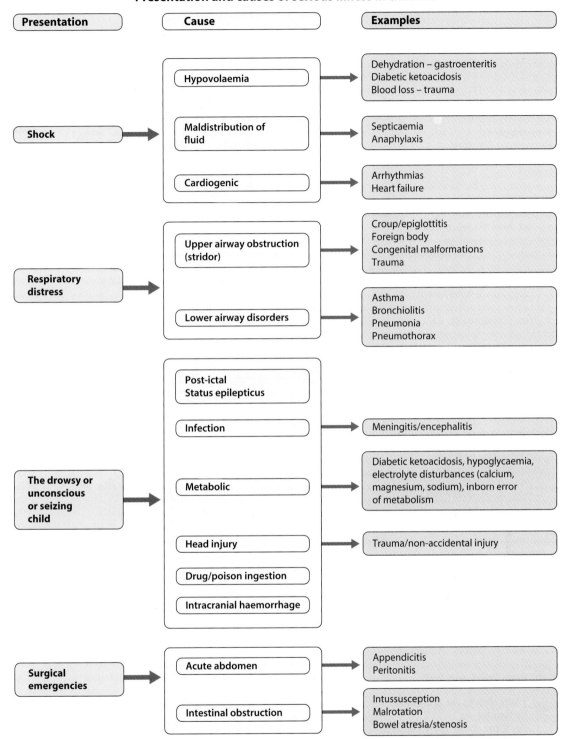

Presentation	Cause	Examples

Shock
- Hypovolaemia → Dehydration – gastroenteritis / Diabetic ketoacidosis / Blood loss – trauma
- Maldistribution of fluid → Septicaemia / Anaphylaxis
- Cardiogenic → Arrhythmias / Heart failure

Respiratory distress
- Upper airway obstruction (stridor) → Croup/epiglottitis / Foreign body / Congenital malformations / Trauma
- Lower airway disorders → Asthma / Bronchiolitis / Pneumonia / Pneumothorax

The drowsy or unconscious or seizing child
- Post-ictal / Status epilepticus
- Infection → Meningitis/encephalitis
- Metabolic → Diabetic ketoacidosis, hypoglycaemia, electrolyte disturbances (calcium, magnesium, sodium), inborn error of metabolism
- Head injury → Trauma/non-accidental injury
- Drug/poison ingestion
- Intracranial haemorrhage

Surgical emergencies
- Acute abdomen → Appendicitis / Peritonitis
- Intestinal obstruction → Intussusception / Malrotation / Bowel atresia/stenosis

Figure 6.4 The main modes of presentation of serious illness in children and their causes.

Paediatric emergencies

83

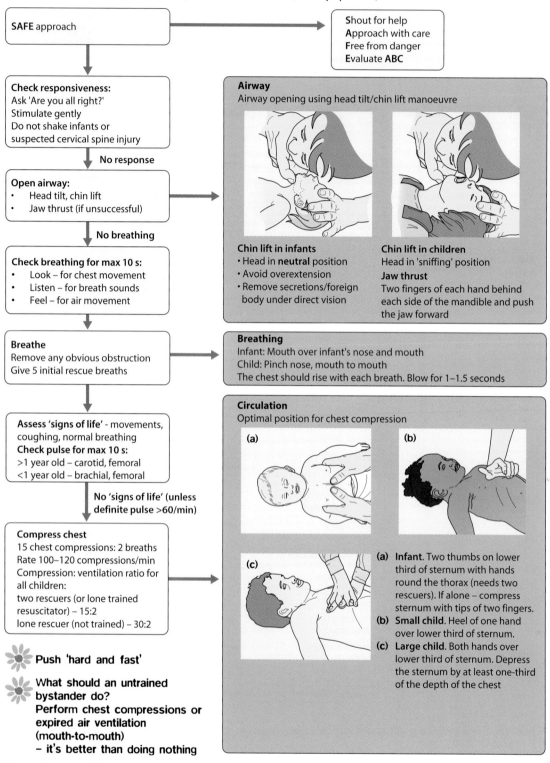

Basic life support
(Trained resuscitator, no equipment)

SAFE approach → **S**hout for help
Approach with care
Free from danger
Evaluate **ABC**

Check responsiveness:
Ask 'Are you all right?'
Stimulate gently
Do not shake infants or
suspected cervical spine injury

No response

Open airway:
- Head tilt, chin lift
- Jaw thrust (if unsuccessful)

No breathing

Check breathing for max 10 s:
- Look – for chest movement
- Listen – for breath sounds
- Feel – for air movement

Breathe
Remove any obvious obstruction
Give 5 initial rescue breaths

Assess 'signs of life' - movements,
coughing, normal breathing
Check pulse for max 10 s:
>1 year old – carotid, femoral
<1 year old – brachial, femoral

*No 'signs of life' (unless
definite pulse >60/min)*

Compress chest
15 chest compressions: 2 breaths
Rate 100–120 compressions/min
Compression: ventilation ratio for
all children:
two rescuers (or lone trained
resuscitator) – 15:2
lone rescuer (not trained) – 30:2

❀ **Push 'hard and fast'**

❀ **What should an untrained
bystander do?**
**Perform chest compressions or
expired air ventilation
(mouth-to-mouth)
– it's better than doing nothing**

Airway
Airway opening using head tilt/chin lift manoeuvre

Chin lift in infants
• Head in **neutral** position
• Avoid overextension
• Remove secretions/foreign
  body under direct vision

Chin lift in children
Head in 'sniffing' position
Jaw thrust
Two fingers of each hand behind
each side of the mandible and push
the jaw forward

Breathing
Infant: Mouth over infant's nose and mouth
Child: Pinch nose, mouth to mouth
The chest should rise with each breath. Blow for 1–1.5 seconds

Circulation
Optimal position for chest compression

(a)
(b)
(c)

(a) **Infant.** Two thumbs on lower
third of sternum with hands
round the thorax (needs two
rescuers). If alone – compress
sternum with tips of two fingers.
(b) **Small child.** Heel of one hand
over lower third of sternum.
(c) **Large child.** Both hands over
lower third of sternum. Depress
the sternum by at least one-third
of the depth of the chest

Figure 6.5 Basic life support. (Adapted from Resuscitation Council (UK). 2010. Resuscitation Guidelines.)

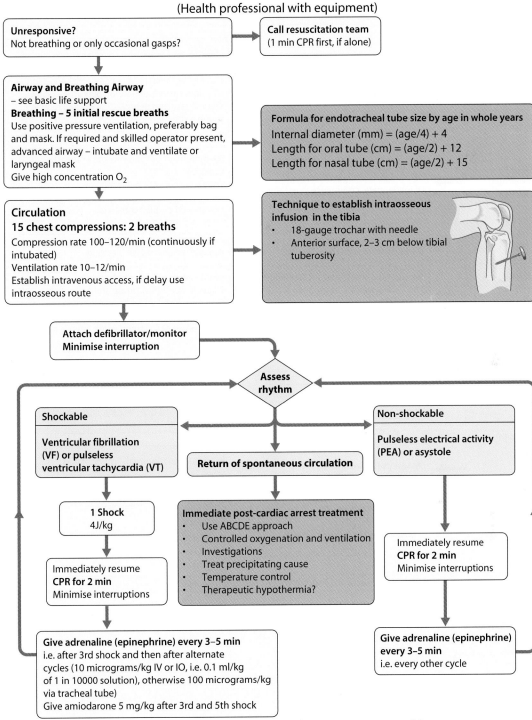

Advanced life support
(Health professional with equipment)

| Unresponsive? |
| Not breathing or only occasional gasps? |

→

| Call resuscitation team |
| (1 min CPR first, if alone) |

Airway and Breathing Airway
– see basic life support
Breathing – 5 initial rescue breaths
Use positive pressure ventilation, preferably bag and mask. If required and skilled operator present, advanced airway – intubate and ventilate or laryngeal mask
Give high concentration O_2

→

Formula for endotracheal tube size by age in whole years
Internal diameter (mm) = (age/4) + 4
Length for oral tube (cm) = (age/2) + 12
Length for nasal tube (cm) = (age/2) + 15

Circulation
15 chest compressions: 2 breaths
Compression rate 100–120/min (continuously if intubated)
Ventilation rate 10–12/min
Establish intravenous access, if delay use intraosseous route

→

Technique to establish intraosseous infusion in the tibia
• 18-gauge trochar with needle
• Anterior surface, 2–3 cm below tibial tuberosity

Attach defibrillator/monitor
Minimise interruption

Assess rhythm

Shockable

Ventricular fibrillation (VF) or pulseless ventricular tachycardia (VT)

Return of spontaneous circulation

Non-shockable

Pulseless electrical activity (PEA) or asystole

1 Shock
4J/kg

Immediate post-cardiac arrest treatment
• Use ABCDE approach
• Controlled oxygenation and ventilation
• Investigations
• Treat precipitating cause
• Temperature control
• Therapeutic hypothermia?

Immediately resume
CPR for 2 min
Minimise interruptions

Immediately resume
CPR for 2 min
Minimise interruptions

Give adrenaline (epinephrine) every 3–5 min
i.e. after 3rd shock and then after alternate cycles (10 micrograms/kg IV or IO, i.e. 0.1 ml/kg of 1 in 10000 solution), otherwise 100 micrograms/kg via tracheal tube)
Give amiodarone 5 mg/kg after 3rd and 5th shock

Give adrenaline (epinephrine) every 3–5 min
i.e. every other cycle

During CPR
• Ensure high-quality CPR: rate, depth, recoil
• Plan actions before interrupting CPR
• Give oxygen
• Vascular access (intravenous, intraosseous)
• Give adrenaline (epinephrine) every 3–5 min
• Consider advanced airway and capnography (end-tidal CO_2 monitoring)
• Continuous chest compressions when advanced airway in place
• Correct reversible causes

Reversible causes
• Hypoxia
• Hypovolaemia
• Hypo-/hyperkalaemia/metabolic
• Hypothermia
• Tension pneumothorax
• Toxins
• Tamponade – cardiac
• Thromboembolism

Figure 6.6 Advanced life support. (Adapted from Resuscitation Council (UK). 2010. Resuscitation Guidelines.)

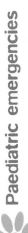

Paediatric emergencies

Management of the seriously injured child

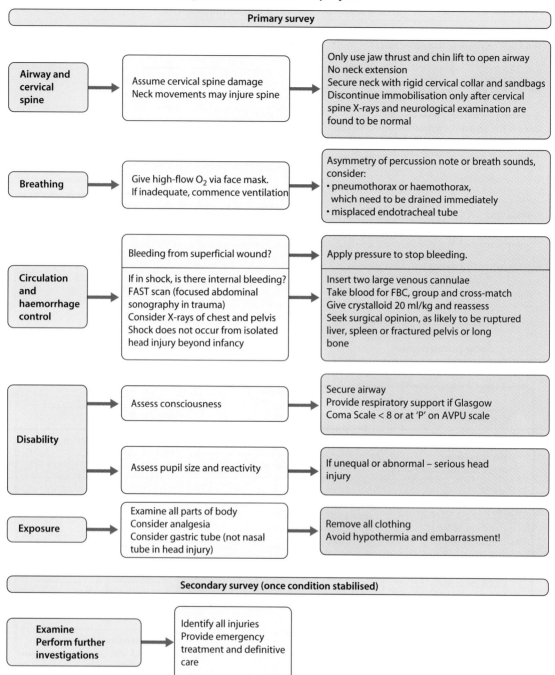

Primary survey

Airway and cervical spine → Assume cervical spine damage
Neck movements may injure spine → Only use jaw thrust and chin lift to open airway
No neck extension
Secure neck with rigid cervical collar and sandbags
Discontinue immobilisation only after cervical spine X-rays and neurological examination are found to be normal

Breathing → Give high-flow O₂ via face mask.
If inadequate, commence ventilation → Asymmetry of percussion note or breath sounds, consider:
• pneumothorax or haemothorax, which need to be drained immediately
• misplaced endotracheal tube

Circulation and haemorrhage control →
Bleeding from superficial wound? → Apply pressure to stop bleeding.

If in shock, is there internal bleeding?
FAST scan (focused abdominal sonography in trauma)
Consider X-rays of chest and pelvis
Shock does not occur from isolated head injury beyond infancy → Insert two large venous cannulae
Take blood for FBC, group and cross-match
Give crystalloid 20 ml/kg and reassess
Seek surgical opinion, as likely to be ruptured liver, spleen or fractured pelvis or long bone

Disability →
Assess consciousness → Secure airway
Provide respiratory support if Glasgow Coma Scale < 8 or at 'P' on AVPU scale

Assess pupil size and reactivity → If unequal or abnormal – serious head injury

Exposure → Examine all parts of body
Consider analgesia
Consider gastric tube (not nasal tube in head injury) → Remove all clothing
Avoid hypothermia and embarrassment!

Secondary survey (once condition stabilised)

Examine
Perform further investigations → Identify all injuries
Provide emergency treatment and definitive care

Figure 6.7 Management of the seriously injured child.

Shock

Shock is present when the circulation is inadequate to meet the demands of the tissues. Critically ill children are often in shock, usually because of hypovolaemia due to fluid loss or maldistribution of fluid, as occurs in sepsis or intestinal obstruction.

Why are children so susceptible to fluid loss?

Children normally require a much higher fluid intake per kilogram of body weight than adults (Table 6.1). This is because they have a higher surface area to volume ratio and a higher basal

Table 6.1 Fluid intake at different ages

Body weight	Fluid requirement/24 h	Volume/kg per hour (approximate)
First 10 kg	100 ml/kg	4 ml/kg
Second 10 kg	50 ml/kg	2 ml/kg
Subsequent kg	20 ml/kg	1 ml/kg
Examples of calculations		
Infant (7 kg)	700 ml	28 ml/h
Child (18 kg)	1000 + 400 = 1400 ml	40 + 16 = 56 ml/h
Adolescent (42 kg)	1000 + 500 + 440 = 1940 ml	40 + 20 + 22 = 82 ml/h

Box 6.2 Clinical signs of shock

Early (compensated)	Late (decompensated)
Tachypnoea	Acidotic (Kussmaul) breathing
Tachycardia	Bradycardia
Decreased skin turgor	Confusion/depressed cerebral state
Sunken eyes and fontanelle	
Delayed capillary refill (>2 s)	Blue peripheries
Mottled, pale, cold skin	Absent urine output
Core–peripheral temperature gap (>4°C)	Hypotension
Decreased urinary output	

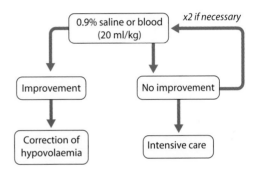

Figure 6.8 Initial fluid resuscitation in shock.

metabolic rate. Children may therefore become dehydrated if:

- they are unable to take oral fluids
- there are additional fluid losses due to fever, diarrhoea or increased insensible losses (e.g. due to increased sweating or tachypnoea)
- there is loss of the normal fluid-retaining mechanisms, e.g. burns, the permeable skin of premature infants, increased urinary losses or capillary leak.

Clinical features

The clinical features of shock are manifestations of compensatory physiological mechanisms to maintain the circulation and the direct effects of poor perfusion of tissues and organs (Box 6.2).

In early, compensated shock, the blood pressure is maintained by increased heart and respiratory rate, redistribution of blood from venous reserve volume and diversion of blood flow from non-essential tissues such as the skin in the peripheries, which become cold, to the vital organs like brain and heart. In shock due to dehydration, there is usually >10% loss of body weight (see Ch. 13) and a profound metabolic acidosis which

is compounded by failure to feed and drink while severely ill. After acute blood loss or redistribution of blood volume because of infection, low blood pressure is a late feature. It signifies that compensatory responses are failing.

In late or uncompensated shock, compensatory mechanisms fail, blood pressure falls and lactic acidosis increases. It is important to recognise early compensated shock, as this is reversible, in contrast to uncompensated shock, which may be irreversible.

Management priorities

Fluid resuscitation

Rapid restoration of the intravascular circulating volume is the priority (Fig. 6.8). This will usually be with 0.9% saline, or blood if following trauma.

Subsequent management

If there is no improvement following fluid resuscitation or there is progression of shock and respiratory failure, a paediatric intensive care unit should be involved and transfer arranged as the child may need:

- tracheal intubation and mechanical ventilation
- invasive monitoring of blood pressure
- inotropic support
- correction of haematological, biochemical and metabolic derangements
- support for renal or liver failure.

Septicaemia

Bacteria may cause a focal infection or proliferate in the bloodstream, leading to septicaemia. In septicaemia, the host response includes the release of inflammatory cytokines and activation of endothelial cells, which may lead to septic shock. The commonest cause of septic shock in childhood is meningococcal infection, which may or may not be accompanied by meningitis. Fortunately, its incidence in the UK has fallen markedly since immunisation was introduced against meningococcal C, but other strains are still prevalent. *Pneumococcus* is the commonest organism causing bacteraemia, but it is unusual for it to cause septic shock. In neonates, the commonest causes of septicaemia are group B streptococcus or Gram-negative organisms acquired from the birth canal.

Clinical features

See Box 6.3

Management priorities

Children with septic shock need to be rapidly stabilised and may require transfer to a paediatric intensive care unit.

Antibiotics

Choice depends on the child's age and any predisposition to infection.

Fluids

Significant hypovolaemia is often present, owing to fluid maldistribution, which occurs due to the release of vasoactive mediators by host inflammatory and endothelial cells. There is loss of intravascular proteins and fluid which may occur due to the development of 'capillary leak' caused by endothelial cell dysfunction. Circulating plasma volume is lost into the interstitial fluid. Central venous pressure monitoring and urinary catheterisation may be required to guide the assessment of fluid balance. Capillary leak into the lungs causes pulmonary oedema, which may lead to respiratory failure, necessitating mechanical ventilation.

Circulatory support

Myocardial dysfunction occurs as inflammatory cytokines and circulating toxins depress myocardial contractility. Inotropic support may be required.

Disseminated intravascular coagulation (DIC)

Abnormal blood clotting causes widespread microvascular thrombosis and consumption of clotting factors. If bleeding occurs, clotting derangement should be corrected with fresh frozen plasma and platelet transfusions.

Steroids

There is no evidence that steroids are of benefit in septic shock.

> **Summary**
>
> **Septicaemia**
> - The most common cause of septic shock in children is meningococcal disease
> - May occur without meningitis
> - Early antibiotic therapy and fluid resuscitation are life-saving
> - May need admission to paediatric intensive care for multi-organ failure.

Coma

In coma, there is disturbance of the functioning of the cerebral hemispheres and/or the reticular activating system of the brainstem. The level of awareness may range from excessive drowsiness to unconsciousness.

Box 6.3 Clinical features of septicaemia

History	Examination
Fever	Fever
Poor feeding	Tachycardia, tachypnoea, low blood pressure
Miserable, irritable, lethargy	
History of focal infection, e.g. meningitis, osteomyelitis, gastroenteritis, cellulitis	Purpuric rash (meningococcal septicaemia) (Fig. 6.9).
	Shock
Predisposing conditions, e.g. sickle cell disease, immunodeficiency	Multi-organ failure

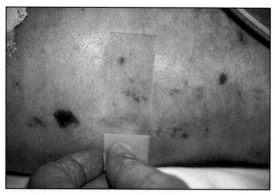

Figure 6.9 The glass test for meningococcal purpura. Parents are advised to suspect meningococcal disease if their child is febrile and has a rash that does not blanch when pressed under a glass. (Courtesy of Dr Parviz Habibi.)

Table 6.2 Glasgow Coma Scale, incorporating Children's Coma Scale

	Glasgow Coma Scale (4–15 years)	**Children's Coma Scale (<4 years)**	
	Response	Response	Score
Eyes	Open spontaneously	Open spontaneously	4
	Verbal command	React to speech	3
	Pain	React to pain	2
	No response	No response	1
Best motor response			
Verbal command	Obeys	Spontaneous or obeys verbal command	6
Painful stimulus	Localises pain	Localises pain	5
	Withdraws	Withdraws	4
	Abnormal flexion	Abnormal flexion (decorticate posture)	3
	Extension	Abnormal extension (decerebrate posture)	2
	No response	No response	1
Best verbal response	Oriented and converses	Smiles, orientated to sounds, follows objects, interacts	5
	Disoriented and converses	Fewer than usual words, spontaneous irritable cry	4
	Inappropriate words	Cries only to pain	3
	Incomprehensible sounds	Moans to pain	2
	No response	No response to pain	1

A score of <8 out of 15 means that the child's airway is at risk and will need to be maintained by a manoeuvre or adjunct.

It is assessed rapidly by using AVPU (**A**lert, responds to **V**oice, responds to **P**ain, **U**nresponsive) or the Glasgow Coma Scale (Table 6.2).

The immediate assessment of a child in coma is shown in Figures 6.10 and 6.11. The causes, clinical features and investigations of coma are listed in Table 6.3. In contrast to adults, most children have a diffuse metabolic insult rather than a structural lesion.

The history, examination and investigation of coma are directed towards the cause. Early treatment of treatable causes, especially hypoglycaemia and infection, is paramount. Raised intracranial pressure is treated with:

- the head positioned midline
- the head end of the bed tilted by 20–30°
- isotonic fluids at 60% maintenance
- intubation and ventilation if Glasgow Coma Score <9
- mannitol or 3% saline as osmotic diuretics
- maintaining normothermia and high normal blood pressure.

An intracranial mass lesion may require neurosurgical intervention.

Status epilepticus

This is a seizure lasting 30 minutes or longer, or when successive seizures occur so frequently that the patient does not recover consciousness between them. After immediate primary assessment and resuscitation, the priority is to stop the seizure as quickly as possible (Fig. 6.12).

Anaphylaxis

Anaphylaxis is rapid in onset and may be fatal. It has an incidence of one episode every 20 000 person years, and about 1 in 1000 cases are fatal. In children, 85% of anaphylaxis is caused by food allergy; most are IgE-mediated reactions with significant respiratory or cardiovascular compromise. Other causes include insect stings, drugs, latex, exercise, inhalant allergens and idiopathic. While most paediatric anaphylaxis occurs in children <5 years, when food allergy is most prevalent, the majority of fatal paediatric anaphylaxis occurs in adolescents with allergy to nuts; asthma is an additional risk factor. The acute management of anaphylaxis relies

Paediatric emergencies

89

Initial assessment and management of coma

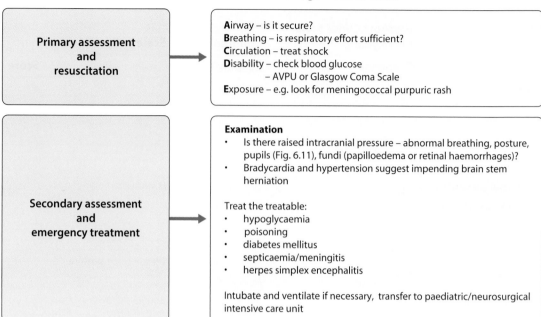

Primary assessment and resuscitation

Airway – is it secure?
Breathing – is respiratory effort sufficient?
Circulation – treat shock
Disability – check blood glucose
            – AVPU or Glasgow Coma Scale
Exposure – e.g. look for meningococcal purpuric rash

Secondary assessment and emergency treatment

Examination
•   Is there raised intracranial pressure – abnormal breathing, posture, pupils (Fig. 6.11), fundi (papilloedema or retinal haemorrhages)?
•   Bradycardia and hypertension suggest impending brain stem herniation

Treat the treatable:
•   hypoglycaemia
•   poisoning
•   diabetes mellitus
•   septicaemia/meningitis
•   herpes simplex encephalitis

Intubate and ventilate if necessary, transfer to paediatric/neurosurgical intensive care unit

Figure 6.10 Initial assessment and management of coma.

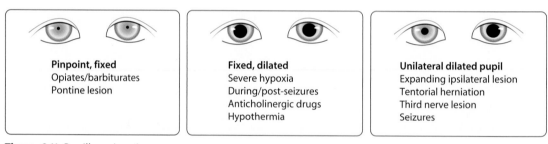

Pinpoint, fixed
Opiates/barbiturates
Pontine lesion

Fixed, dilated
Severe hypoxia
During/post-seizures
Anticholinergic drugs
Hypothermia

Unilateral dilated pupil
Expanding ipsilateral lesion
Tentorial herniation
Third nerve lesion
Seizures

Figure 6.11 Pupillary signs in coma.

on early administration of adrenaline (epinephrine) (Fig. 6.13). Long-term management involves detailed strategies and training for allergen avoidance, a written management plan with instructions for the treatment of allergic reactions and the provision of adrenaline (epinephrine) auto-injector(s). In some cases, such as insect sting anaphylaxis, allergen immunotherapy may be effective in preventing future episodes. The experience of an anaphylactic reaction can have a significant psychological impact on the child and family.

Summary

Anaphylaxis in children/adolescents

•   Reaction is mainly to foods – 1 in 1000 episodes is fatal
•   Risk factors for fatal outcome include adolescent age group, coexistent asthma and nut allergy
•   Acute management is early administration of intramuscular adrenaline (epinephrine).

Apparent life-threatening events (ALTE)

These occur in infants and are a combination of apnoea, colour change, alteration in muscle tone, choking or gagging, which are frightening to the observer. They are most common in infants less than 10 weeks old and may occur on multiple occasions. They may be the presentation of a potentially serious disorder, although often no cause is identified.

Management requires a detailed history and thorough examination to identify problems with the baby or in caregiving. The infant should be admitted to hospital. Causes and investigations to be considered are listed in Box 6.4. Multi-channel overnight monitoring is usually indicated.

In most, the episode is brief, with rapid recovery, and the baby is well clinically. Baseline investigations and overnight monitoring of oxygen saturation, respiration and ECG are found to be normal. The parents should be taught resuscitation and will find it helpful to receive follow-up from a specialist paediatric nurse and paediatrician.

Table 6.3 Causes, history and examination and investigation of coma

Cause	History and examination	Diagnostic investigations
Infection Meningitis or meningoencephalitis	Fever Irritability, lethargy, drowsiness Poor feeding, vomiting Rash, e.g. meningococcal purpura Seizures Neck stiffness and pain; bulging fontanelle Overseas travel	Full blood count Culture of blood, urine, infected sites, CSF (unless contraindicated) for bacteria and viruses Acute-phase reactant Rapid bacterial antigen/PCR tests for organisms
Status epilepticus or post-ictal	Past history of seizures Neurocutaneous lesions on the skin Developmental delay Ongoing seizure activity, e.g. abnormal eye movements Focal neurological signs	Blood glucose Electrolytes – sodium, potassium, calcium, magnesium Drug levels if on anticonvulsants EEG CT scan
Trauma – accidental/non-accidental	History of road traffic accident, fall, etc. Bruising, haemorrhage Fractures – cervical spine, etc. Focal neurology Retinal haemorrhages	Radiological – plain X-rays or CT/MRI scans
Intracranial tumour or haemorrhage/infarct/abscess	Symptoms or signs of raised intracranial pressure Focal neurological signs, e.g. squint	Cranial CT/MRI scan Haemorrhage – coagulation screen, screen for procoagulant disorders (protein C/S deficiency)
Metabolic		
1. **Diabetes mellitus**	Previously diagnosed diabetes mellitus Diabetic ketoacidosis	Blood glucose, plasma electrolytes Urine for glucose and ketones Blood gas analysis
2. **Hypoglycaemia**	Any acutely ill child Known diabetes mellitus Sudden onset of coma	Low blood glucose
3. **Inborn errors of metabolism**	Previous history of loss of consciousness Sudden collapse Consanguinity, death or illness of siblings Developmental delay Hepatomegaly	Blood glucose Blood gas analysis Blood ammonia, lactate Urine amino and organic acids Plasma amino acids
4. **Hepatic failure**	Jaundice Abnormal bleeding	Abnormal liver function tests Prolonged prothrombin time
5. **Acute renal failure**	Oliguria, hypertension	Abnormal creatinine
Poisoning	Accidental – poison usually identified Deliberate – tablets may be found, also illicit drugs and alcohol	Toxicology screen Plasma level for paracetamol and salicylates
Shock	Septicaemia Dehydration Cardiac failure	Full blood count and cultures Urea, electrolytes, blood gas
Hypertension	Symptoms and signs of raised intracranial pressure Fundoscopy – hypertensive changes	Left ventricular hypertrophy on ECG or echocardiography Creatinine and electrolytes
Respiratory failure	Respiratory failure	Chest X-ray Arterial blood gas – hypoxia, hypercarbia

Paediatric emergencies

91

Management protocol for status epilepticus

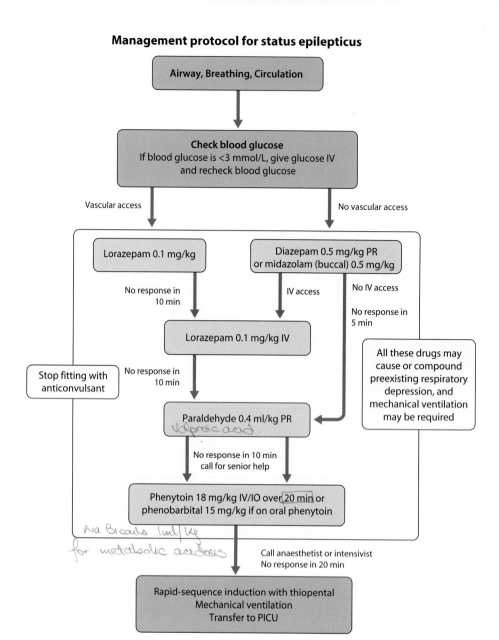

Figure 6.12 Management protocol for status epilepticus. (Adapted from Advanced Life Support Group. 2005. *Advanced Paediatric Life Support. The Practical Approach*, 4th edn. Blackwell BMJ Books, London.)

Detailed specialist investigation and assessment will be required if clinical, biochemical or physiological abnormalities are identified.

The death of a child

The risk of death is four times greater during infancy than at any other age in childhood. In many, a serious condition will have been diagnosed before or after birth, such as a congenital abnormality or complications of prematurity. Deaths which occur suddenly and unexpectedly in infancy are known as sudden unexpected death in infancy (SUDI). In some, a previously undiagnosed congenital abnormality, e.g. congenital heart disease, will be found at autopsy. Rarely, an inherited metabolic disorder is identified, in particular the fatty acid oxidation defect medium-chain acyl-CoA dehydrogenase deficiency (MCAD), which can very rarely result in sudden death in infants, but is increasingly identified in the UK from routine biochemical screening (Guthrie test). After 1 month of age, in most instances of sudden death in a previously well infant, no cause is identified and the death is classified as sudden infant death syndrome (SIDS). The vast majority of such deaths, even when occurring more than once in the same family, are due to natural causes. Rarely, the death may be due to suffocation or other forms of non-accidental injury.

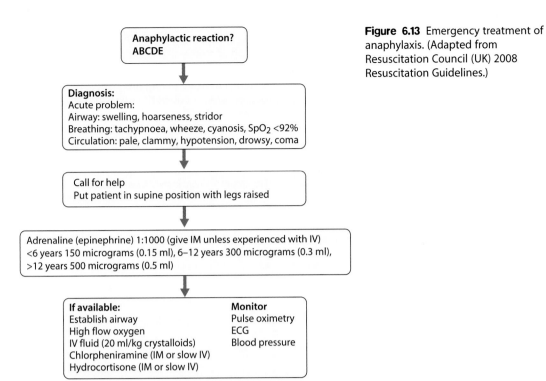

Figure 6.13 Emergency treatment of anaphylaxis. (Adapted from Resuscitation Council (UK) 2008 Resuscitation Guidelines.)

Anaphylactic reaction?
ABCDE

↓

Diagnosis:
Acute problem:
Airway: swelling, hoarseness, stridor
Breathing: tachypnoea, wheeze, cyanosis, SpO_2 <92%
Circulation: pale, clammy, hypotension, drowsy, coma

↓

Call for help
Put patient in supine position with legs raised

↓

Adrenaline (epinephrine) 1:1000 (give IM unless experienced with IV)
<6 years 150 micrograms (0.15 ml), 6–12 years 300 micrograms (0.3 ml),
>12 years 500 micrograms (0.5 ml)

↓

If available:
Establish airway
High flow oxygen
IV fluid (20 ml/kg crystalloids)
Chlorpheniramine (IM or slow IV)
Hydrocortisone (IM or slow IV)

Monitor
Pulse oximetry
ECG
Blood pressure

Box 6.4 Causes and investigations to be considered in apparent life-threatening events

Causes

- Infections – respiratory syncytial virus (RSV), pertussis
- Seizures
- Gastro-oesophageal reflux (present in one-third of normal infants)
- Upper airways obstruction – natural or imposed
- No cause identified

Uncommon causes

- Cardiac arrhythmia
- Breath-holding
- Anaemia
- Heavy wrapping/heat stress
- Central hypoventilation syndrome
- Cyanotic spells from intrapulmonary shunting

Investigations to be considered

- Blood glucose (as soon as possible)
- Blood gas (as soon as possible)
- Oxygen saturation monitoring
- Cardiorespiratory monitoring
- EEG
- Oesophageal pH monitoring
- Barium swallow
- Full blood count
- Urea and electrolytes, liver function tests
- Lactate
- Urine (collect and freeze first sample)
  - metabolic studies
  - microscopy and culture
  - toxicology
- ECG – for QT_c conduction pathway abnormality
- Chest X-ray
- Lumbar puncture.

Sudden infant death syndrome

This is defined as the sudden and unexpected death of an infant or young child for which no adequate cause is found after a thorough postmortem examination. There is marked variation in the incidence of SIDS in different countries, suggesting that environmental factors are important (Box 6.5). SIDS occurs most commonly at 2–4 months of age (Fig. 6.14). The risk for subsequent children is slightly increased.

In the UK, the incidence of SIDS has fallen dramatically during the last 20 years (Fig. 6.15), coinciding with a national 'Back to Sleep' campaign (Fig. 6.16). This advocates that:

- Infants should be put to sleep on their back (not their front or side)
- Overheating by heavy wrapping and high room temperature should be avoided
- Infants should be placed in the 'feet to foot' position

Box 6.5 Factors associated with SIDS

The infant

- Age 1–6 months, peak at 12 weeks
- Low birthweight and preterm (but 60% are normal birthweight term infants)
- Sex (boys 60%)
- Multiple births

The parents

- Low income[a]
- Poor or overcrowded housing
- Maternal age (mother aged <20 years has three times the risk of a mother aged 25–29 years, but 80% of affected mothers are >20 years old)[a]

- Single unsupported mother (twice the rate of supported mothers)
- High maternal parity[a]
- Maternal smoking during pregnancy (1–9 cigarettes/day doubles the risk: >20/day increases the risk five-fold)[a]
- Parental smoking after baby's birth

The environment

- The infant sleeps lying prone
- The infant is overheated from high room temperature and too may clothes and covers, particularly when ill.

[a]Three of these four factors are present in over 40% of SIDS but only 8% of control families.
Based on data from Fleming P, Blair P, Bacon C et al. 2000. *Sudden Unexpected Deaths in Infancy.* The Stationery Office, London.

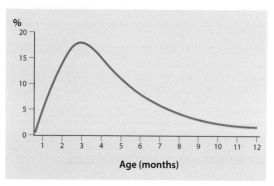

Figure 6.14 Age distribution of SIDS. (Based on data from Fleming P, Blair P, Bacon C et al. 2000. *Sudden Unexpected Deaths in Infancy.* The Stationery Office, London, with permission.)

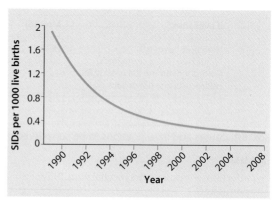

Figure 6.15 Decline in the number of deaths from SIDS in the UK from 1.9/1000 live births in 1989 to 0.31 in 2008.

Prevention of sudden infant death syndrome

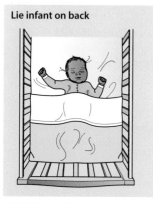

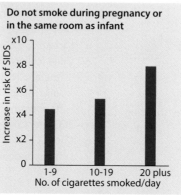

Figure 6.16 Key features of the 'Back to Sleep' campaign.

Management of the sudden unexpected death of an infant

Resuscitation → Infant found dead at home – take to Accident and Emergency Department
Initiate resuscitation unless inappropriate

Care of parents → Should be cared for by specific member of staff
History should be obtained

Baby pronounced dead → Detailed clinical examination by consultant
Remove endotracheal tube and intraosseous needles but retain venous lines
Retain child's clothes and any bedding and nappy for police
Investigations performed:
- Nasopharyngeal aspirate for virology and bacteriology
- Blood for toxicology, metabolic screen (on Guthrie card), chromosomes if dysmorphic
- Blood culture
- Urine (catheter specimen) – for biochemistry, toxicology and freeze immediately
- Lumbar puncture – CSF for virology and routine culture, if clinically indicated
SUDI paediatrician, coroner, police and primary care team and other healthcare professionals informed

Breaking the news to the parents → Performed by the paediatrician. Explain that the police and coroner will be involved, a postmortem is required, tissue blocks and slides will be taken and retained permanently as part of the medical record.
Give parents the opportunity to donate tissues and organs
Inform them that the involvement of the police does not imply that they are being blamed for their child's death

Parents offered to see and hold their baby → Parents should be offered the opportunity to see and hold their child. Encourage as helps them accept the reality of their child's death. They may wish to see the child again within the next few days. The family may wish a minister of religion to be called.

Initial strategy discussion → SUDI paediatrician and supervising police officer
Social services review to identify if previously involved or any child protection issues

Home visit within 24 hours → Police visit the home to talk with the parents and examine the place where the baby died
SUDI paediatrician may also attend
Detailed history obtained
Report compiled for the coroner

Postmortem → Performed by paediatric pathologist
Preliminary postmortem result

Case discussion → Multi-agency meeting, including SUDI paediatrician, police, GP/health visitor and, where appropriate, the social worker
All relevant information reviewed
Possibility of abuse or neglect considered
Report is sent to the coroner
Paediatrician writes a detailed letter to the parents providing information about the cause of the infant's death and arranges to meet them

Follow-up and bereavement counselling → Follow-up to provide family an opportunity to discuss the final results of the postmortem and consider its implications for future pregnancies. Genetic counselling may be indicated.
Bereavement counselling – available from health professionals and other agencies

Figure 6.17 A recommended approach to the management of the sudden unexpected death of an infant. There are local variations in its implementation. (Adapted from RCPCH. 2004. *Sudden Unexpected Death in Infancy*. The report of a working group convened by the Royal College of Pathologists and The Royal College of Paediatrics and Child Health. RCPCH, London. Available at: www.rcpath.org and www.rcpch.ac.uk (Accessed January 2011).

Paediatric emergencies

95

- Parents should not smoke near their infants
- Parents should seek medical advice promptly if their infant becomes unwell.
- Parents should have the baby in their bedroom for the first 6 months of life

- Parents should avoid bringing the baby into their bed when they are tired or have taken alcohol, sedative medicines or drugs
- Parents should avoid sleeping with their infant on a sofa, settee or armchair.

Summary

Sudden infant death syndrome (SIDS)

- SIDS is the commonest cause of death in children aged 1 month to 1 year.
- The peak age is 2–4 months.
- SIDS has been dramatically reduced by lying babies on their back to sleep.

Following the sudden death of a child

The sudden death of a child is one of the most distressing events that can happen to a family. If close family members are absent, arrangements should be made for them to come, if this is possible. The family should be spoken to sympathetically and in private (see Ch. 5). An outline of the recommended management after an infant has died suddenly and unexpectedly is shown in Figure 6.17.

Summary

Following an unexpected death

- The parents should be offered the opportunity to see and hold their child.
- The coroner must be informed and a postmortem performed.
- The parents should be informed about the postmortem, that investigations will be performed and that the police will be involved and they should be reassured that this is standard practice.
- Follow-up and bereavement counselling should be offered.

Further reading

Advanced Life Support Group: *Advanced Paediatric Life Support. The Practical Approach*, ed 4, Blackwell BMJ Books, 2005, London.

Goldman A, Hain R, Lieben S: *The Oxford Textbook of Palliative Care in Children*, ed 2, Oxford, 2011, Oxford University Press.

Medical, psychological and practical issues of caring for terminally ill children and their families.

RCPCH: *Sudden Unexpected Death in Infancy.* The report of a working group convened by the Royal College of Pathologists and The Royal College of Paediatrics and Child Health, London, 2004, RCPCH. Available at: www.rcpath.org and www.rcpch.ac.uk (Accessed May 2011).

Resuscitation Council (UK): Updated guidelines on paediatric life support, London, 2008, 2010. Resuscitation Council (UK).

7

Accidents, poisoning and child protection

Accidents	97
Poisoning	102
Child protection	106

Children need a safe, healthy and nurturing environment to achieve their full potential. Environmental hazards include accidents and poisons. Protecting children and young people from harm is a primary responsibility of parents, families and carers, but all members of society, including doctors, teachers and other professionals, play an important role in advocating for safe environments for children.

The risk of accidents, poisons and abuse is increased by:

- Poverty
- Poor-quality, overcrowded homes
- Lack of a safe environment for play
- Poor parenting skills, which may be due to parental psychiatric illness, drug and alcohol abuse, violent temperament, poor education or lack of social support.

Accidents

Accidents (now often called 'unintentional injuries') are extremely common. In the UK, one in four children attend an A&E department each year; about half because of an accident. They are more common in boys. Most accidents cause only minor injury but can also be fatal. Injuries, mostly accidents, and poisoning are the major cause of death in children 1–14 years of age in the UK (Figs 7.1, 7.2). Accidents also cause significant disability and suffering, including post-traumatic stress disorder. Head injury with brain damage is the major cause of disability from accidents. Cosmetic damage following burns, scalds and other accidents may cause the child profound psychological harm.

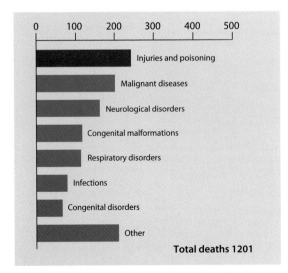

Figure 7.1 Causes of death in children aged 1–14 years in England and Wales (2008).

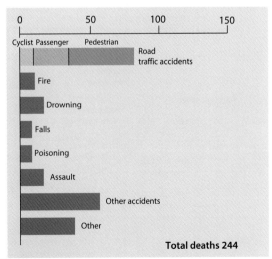

Figure 7.2 Causes of fatal injuries and poisoning in children in England and Wales (2008). The most common cause of injuries is road traffic accidents.

Injuries are the most common cause of death in children over 1 year of age.

Types of accident affecting children

Most accidents affecting children depend on the child's age and development.

In babies and toddlers they can usually be anticipated by an observant adult and may be prevented by vigilant supervision.

Accident prevention

The prevention of childhood accidents is clearly important. Doctors and nurses who treat children and see the effects of accidents are particularly well placed to provide the community with advice on appropriate preventive measures (Fig. 7.3). In order to prevent accidents:

- The relationship between an individual type of accident and the child's developmental level must be considered
- Specific solutions should be based on detailed epidemiology, e.g. child-resistant containers are the best method to limit children's access to medicines
- Changes backed by legislation are the most successful.

Organisations such as the Royal Society for the Prevention of Accidents and the Children Accident Prevention Trust are important resources in helping reduce accidents by providing education and lobbying for legislative changes, e.g. bicycle helmet wearing.

 The number of children killed in accidents has declined markedly over the past 20 years.

Road traffic accidents

Road traffic accidents (RTAs) are the most common cause of accidental death or serious injury in childhood and in 2008 accounted for 23 000 children killed or injured on the UK's roads. RTAs can be divided into several types.

Pedestrian road traffic accidents

Children's involvement in road traffic accidents is mostly as pedestrians. Boys between the ages of 5 and 9 years are at maximum risk, particularly after school. Children are unable to estimate the speed or dangers of traffic and to foresee dangerous situations. Social and economic factors play a part, with children in social class 5 being 5 times more likely to be killed as a pedestrian than children in social class 1.

Child passengers in cars

Unrestrained children become missiles inside cars during crashes, even at low speeds. There is good evidence that child restraint systems prevent injury and

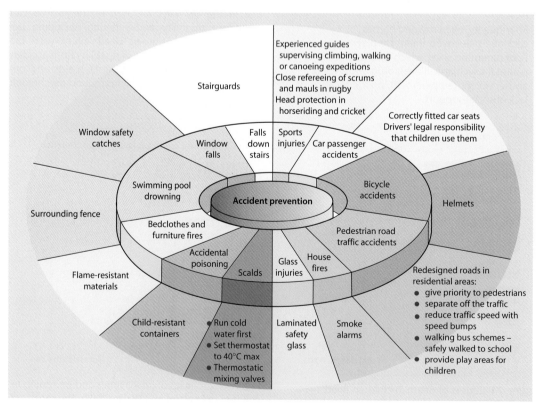

Figure 7.3 Examples of accident prevention.

death and they are required by law in the UK for all children <135 cm tall.

Bicycle accidents

Bicycle accidents are common during childhood. A boy has a 1 in 80 chance of having a cycling-related head injury severe enough to warrant admission to hospital during childhood. Although 70% of cycle deaths involve a head injury, only 1 in 5 children >10 years wear a helmet.

Head injuries

Minor head injuries in childhood are common, and the vast majority of children recover without suffering any ill effects. However, about 1 in 800 of these children develop serious problems. The aim of the management of head injuries is to identify those children requiring treatment and to avoid secondary damage to the brain from hypoxia or poor cerebral perfusion (Fig. 7.4).

Head injury may result in concussion, a reversible impairment of consciousness, a subdural or extradural haematoma or intracerebral contusion (see Ch. 27).

In infants, as their skull sutures have not fused, cranial volume may increase from an extradural or sub-dural bleed before neurological signs or symptoms develop. The haemoglobin concentration may fall and they may become shocked.

> ### Summary
>
> **Accidental head injury management**
> - Mild – discharge home with written advice
> - Potentially severe – monitor to avoid secondary damage
> - Severe – resuscitate, CT scan and neurosurgical referral.

Internal injuries

Children may suffer internal injuries associated with severe trauma. These include:

- Abdominal injuries, including a ruptured spleen, ruptured liver, kidney and bowel. There should be a high index of suspicion for these internal injuries if there has been abdominal trauma or if the clinical setting suggests significant inflicted, i.e. abusive, injury. The child needs close observation. Abdominal ultrasound (focused abdominal sonography in trauma – FAST scan) and X-rays, including CT scan, may be helpful. If there is any doubt, a laparotomy/laparoscopy is undertaken. Intra-abdominal injuries such as a contained splenic bleed are increasingly managed conservatively with close monitoring, but paediatric surgical support must be available immediately in case surgery is required.
- Chest injuries, including pneumothorax and haemopericardium, may require emergency treatment. These children should be managed in a paediatric intensive care unit.

Burns and scalds

Burns and scalds are a significant accidental (and non-accidental) cause of death, although most of the deaths occurring in house fires are caused by gas and smoke inhalation rather than thermal injury. Scalds in toddlers are common; children are scalded at lower temperatures than adults, as their skin is thinner. It is important to exclude inflicted burns.

Management

The severity of the injury is assessed:

- Is the *airway, breathing and circulation* satisfactory?
- *Was there any smoke inhalation*? If this has occurred, there is a danger of subsequent respiratory complications and carbon monoxide poisoning. All affected children should be observed and managed in hospital, with a low threshold to protect the airway before secondary problems develop.
- *Depth of the burn*. In superficial burns, the skin will be epithelialised from surviving cells. In partial thickness burns, there is some damage to the dermis with blistering, and the skin is pink or mottled; regeneration for superficial and partial thickness burns is from the margins of the wound and from the residual epithelial layer surrounding the hair follicles deep within the dermis. In deep (full thickness) burns, the skin is destroyed down to and including the dermis and looks white or charred, is painless and involves hair follicles, hence skin grafting is often required. Deep burns need assessment and treatment in hospital.
- *Surface area of the burn*. This should be calculated from a surface area chart (Fig. 7.5). The palm and adducted fingers cover about 1% of the body surface. Burns covering more than 5% full thickness and 10% partial thickness need assessment by burns specialists. Involvement of more than 70% of the body surface carries a poor chance of survival.
- *Involvement of special sites*. Burns to the face may be disfiguring, those to the mouth may compromise the airway from oedema, and those to the hand/joints may cause functional loss from scarring. Burns to the perineum and other special sites should all be referred to a burns unit.

Treatment

This should be directed at:

- relieving pain, assessed with a pain score; may require the use of strong analgesics such as intravenous morphine
- treating shock with intravenous fluids, preferably plasma expanders, and close monitoring of haematocrit and urinary output. Children with more than 10% burns will require intravenous fluids
- providing wound care. Burns should be covered with cling film (plastic wrapping), which reduces pain from contact with cold air and reduces the risk of infection. Blisters should be left alone. Irrigation

Accidents, poisoning and child protection

Head injuries in children

Damage caused by head injuries

Primary damage

Cerebral contusions
or lacerations
Dural tears
Diffuse axonal damage

Secondary damage

Hypoxia from:
• airway obstruction or
  inadequate ventilation
Hypoglycaemia and
hyperglycaemia

Reduced cerebral
perfusion:
• hypotension from bleeding
• raised intracranial pressure

Haematoma: extradural,
subdural, intracranial
Infection: from open
wound or CSF leak

Outline of initial management

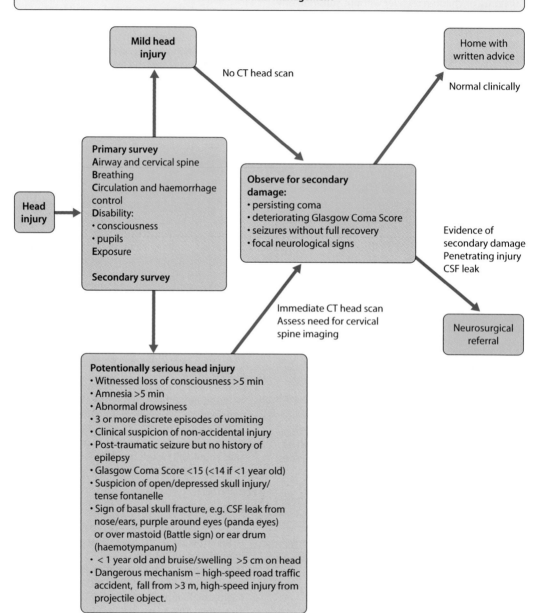

Mild head injury

No CT head scan

Home with written advice

Normal clinically

Head injury

Primary survey
Airway and cervical spine
Breathing
Circulation and haemorrhage
control
Disability:
• consciousness
• pupils
Exposure

Secondary survey

Observe for secondary damage:
• persisting coma
• deteriorating Glasgow Coma Score
• seizures without full recovery
• focal neurological signs

Evidence of
secondary damage
Penetrating injury
CSF leak

Immediate CT head scan
Assess need for cervical
spine imaging

Neurosurgical referral

Potentionally serious head injury
• Witnessed loss of consciousness >5 min
• Amnesia >5 min
• Abnormal drowsiness
• 3 or more discrete episodes of vomiting
• Clinical suspicion of non-accidental injury
• Post-traumatic seizure but no history of
  epilepsy
• Glasgow Coma Score <15 (<14 if <1 year old)
• Suspicion of open/depressed skull injury/
  tense fontanelle
• Sign of basal skull fracture, e.g. CSF leak from
  nose/ears, purple around eyes (panda eyes)
  or over mastoid (Battle sign) or ear drum
  (haemotympanum)
• < 1 year old and bruise/swelling >5 cm on head
• Dangerous mechanism – high-speed road traffic
  accident, fall from >3 m, high-speed injury from
  projectile object.

Figure 7.4 Head injuries in children. (Adapted from NICE Guideline, 2007.)

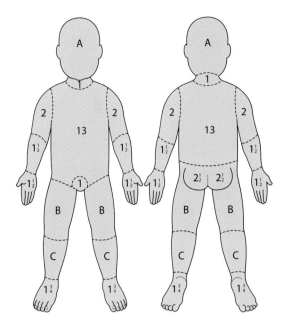

Area indicated	Surface area at			
	1 year	**5 years**	**10 years**	**15 years**
A	8.5	6.5	5.5	4.5
B	3.25	4.0	4.5	4.5
C	2.5	2.75	3.0	3.25

Figure 7.5 Method of calculating the surface area of a burn (Lund and Browder chart).

with cold water should only be used briefly to superficial or partial thickness burns covering less than 10% of the body as it may rapidly cause excessive cooling. Tetanus immunisation status must be ascertained and a booster given if required. Ongoing care involves removal of dead tissue and placement of sterile dressings.

Severe burns or significant burns to special sites are best dealt with in specialist units. Plastic surgeons will often need to embark on a programme of skin grafts and treatment of contractures. The psychological sequelae of severe burns are often marked and long-lasting, and appropriate psychological support is required.

Summary

Burns and scalds

- Assess: need for resuscitation, if any smoke inhalation, depth and surface area of burns and if special sites involved
- Management: pain control, treat shock, provide wound care (cling film), refer to specialist centre if more than 5% full thickness, 10% partial thickness or significant burns to special sites.

Drowning and near-drowning

Drowning is a significant cause of accidental death in children in the UK. Most victims are young children. Drowning is three times more common in boys than in girls. Warmer, affluent countries tend to have a higher incidence of drowning than in the UK, particularly because of drowning in domestic swimming pools. Babies may drown in the bath, toddlers may wander into domestic ponds or swimming pools, and older children may get into difficulty in swimming pools, rivers, canals, lakes and in the sea. Children should always be supervised when swimming.

Near-drowning

Up to 30% of fatalities can be prevented by skilled on-site resuscitation. Even children who are unconscious with fixed dilated pupils can survive near-drowning episodes, particularly if the water is cold, due to the protective effect of hypothermia against hypoxic brain injury. Children who are unconscious with fixed dilated pupils should therefore be fully resuscitated until their temperature is nearly normal. Immediate management at the waterside is with mouth-to-mouth resuscitation and chest compressions. Heat loss should be prevented by covering and warming. Children who may have inhaled water should be admitted to hospital to be observed for signs of respiratory distress from pulmonary oedema after 1–72 h from secondary surfactant. Some aspirate water and develop pneumonia with secondary infection. It is now thought that there is no difference in outlook for fresh- and salt-water drowning.

Choking, suffocation and strangulation

Children may choke on vomit, toys or food. Some children may strangle themselves accidentally on curtain cords, bedding and necklaces. Most are accidents but some such injuries are inflicted deliberately as a form of child abuse. Some adolescents deliberately hang themselves.

In airway obstruction from an aspirated foreign body, the actions outlined in Figures 7.6 and 7.7 should be followed.

Dog bites

Most dog bites are minor, but severe lacerations, particularly to the face, do occur, especially in the toddler age group.

Wound management is as important as antimicrobials in preventing infection:

- Copious wound irrigation, toilet and debridement
- Removal of foreign bodies
- Delayed wound closure, especially on limbs, due to increased incidence of infection
- Raise and immobilise limb
- Regular wound review
- Tetanus booster
- Prophylactic antibiotics if wounds or child is at increased infection risk, i.e. puncture wounds, bites to hands/wrists, crush wounds with devitalised

Inhaled foreign body

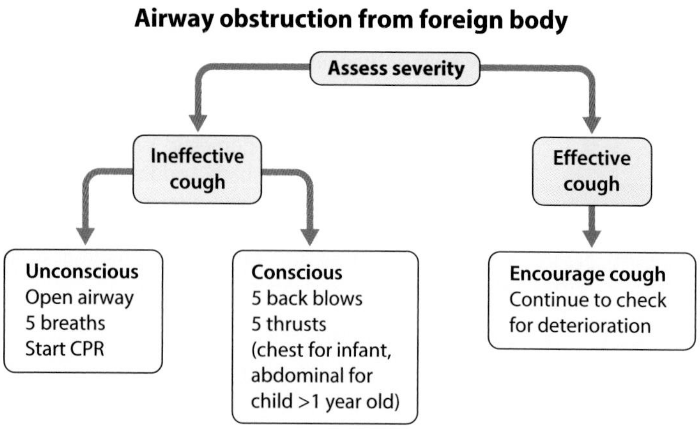

Airway obstruction from foreign body

Figure 7.6 Management of a foreign body.

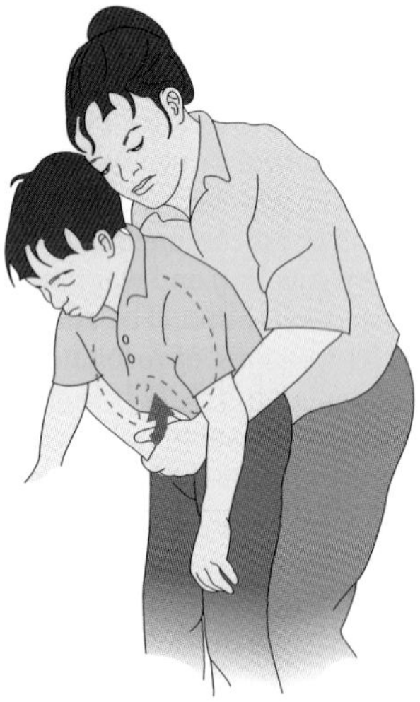

```
                    Assess severity
              ┌───────────┴───────────┐
         Ineffective                Effective
           cough                      cough
      ┌──────┴──────┐                   │
 Unconscious     Conscious        Encourage cough
 Open airway     5 back blows     Continue to check
 5 breaths       5 thrusts        for deterioration
 Start CPR       (chest for infant,
                 abdominal for
                 child >1 year old)
```

Figure 7.7a Abdominal thrusts using the Heimlich manoeuvre in older children to expel an inhaled foreign body. One hand is formed into a fist and placed against the child's abdomen above the umbilicus and below the xiphisternum. The other hand is placed over the fist. Both hands are thrust into the abdomen. This is repeated several times. The child can be standing, kneeling, sitting or supine.

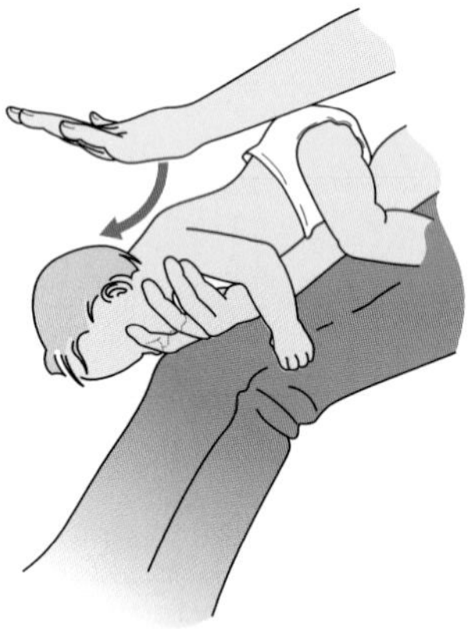

Figure 7.7b In infants, back blows and chest thrusts are recommended to expel an inhaled foreign body. Abdominal thrusts are best avoided in infants as they may cause intra-abdominal injury.

tissue, bites to genitals, child has diabetes mellitus, immunosuppression and in all bites after primary closure.

The antibiotic of choice is co-amoxiclav, as this also covers *Pasteurella* infection.

Although there has been much publicity about fierce dog breeds, such as Rottweilers, attacking children in parks or public places, most attacks are by dogs known to the child.

Poisoning

Poisoning in children may be:

- accidental – the vast majority
- deliberate self-poisoning in older children

- non-accidental as a form of child abuse
- iatrogenic.

Accidental poisoning

Although many thousands of young children are rushed to doctors' surgeries or hospital for urgent medical attention following accidental ingestion, most do not develop serious symptoms, as they ingest only a small quantity of poison or take relatively non-toxic substances (Table 7.1). However, a small percentage of children become seriously ill and a very few children die from poisoning each year.

Most accidental poisoning is in young children, with a peak age of 30 months. Inquisitive toddlers are unaware of the potential danger of taking medicines,

Table 7.1 Potential toxicity in accidental poisoning in infants and young children, with some examples

Toxicity	Medicines	Household products	Plants
Low	Oral contraceptives, most antibiotics	Chalk and crayons, washing powder	Cyclamen, sweet pea
Intermediate	Paracetamol elixir, salbutamol	Bleach, disinfectants, window cleaners	Fuchsia, holly
High	Alcoholic drinks, digoxin, iron, salicylate, tricyclic antidepressants	Acids, alkalis, petroleum distillates, organophosphorus insecticides	Deadly nightshade, laburnum, yew

household products and eating plants. Most ingestions occur in the child's own home, when supervision is inadequate. Supervision of toddlers entails not only reacting to a dangerous situation but also prevention through anticipation.

The aim of management of poisoning should be to prevent unnecessary admissions to hospital while maintaining safety. There has been a marked reduction in the hospital admission rate for poisoning. Reasons for this include:

- The introduction of child-resistant containers – in the UK they must be used for paracetamol and salicylate preparations, and certain household products, such as white spirit; an alternative container for tablets is opaque blister packs
- The reduction in the number of tablets per pack
- A reduction in prescriptions of potentially harmful medicines, e.g. aspirin and iron.

Management

Clinical features that may alert one to poisoning are shown in Table 7.2; however, in young children parents usually know the identity of tablets or other poisons taken (Table 7.3). Management is outlined in Figure 7.8.

Summary

Accidental poisoning in children
- Common in toddlers and young children
- Most do not cause serious illness
- When an ingestion has occurred, identify the agent and assess its toxicity to plan management
- Potentially harmful poisons in children are alcohol, acids and alkalis, bleach, digoxin, batteries, iron, paracetamol, petroleum distillates, salicylates and tricyclic antidepressants
- Assess the social circumstances behind why it happened.

Deliberate poisoning in older children

Older children are more likely to take significant amounts of poison than younger children. Substances that can be regarded as having intermediate toxicity

Table 7.2 Clinical features of poisons

Tachypnoea	Aspirin, carbon monoxide
Slow respiratory rate	Opiates, alcohol
Hypertension	Amphetamines, cocaine
Hypotension	Tricyclics, opiates, β-blockers, iron (secondary to shock)
Convulsions	Tricyclics, organophosphates
Tachycardia	Cocaine, antidepressants, amphetamines
Bradycardia	β-blockers
Large pupils	Tricyclics, cocaine, cannabis, amphetamines
Small pupils	Opiates, organophosphates

when taken accidentally should be regarded as potentially toxic when taken deliberately. Poisoning in older children should be recognised as a serious symptom and an indication of child and family disturbance, so all children who take poisons deliberately should ideally be assessed by a child and adolescent psychiatrist and a social worker.

Chronic poisoning

Children can be poisoned by chronic exposure to chemicals and pollutants. An example from the past is mercury poisoning from teething powders, which used to cause 'pink disease', so-called because it resulted in red painful extremities. It also caused anorexia, weight loss and hypotonia. Now the commonest causes are lead ingestion and smoking.

Lead poisoning

Environmental lead levels are now much reduced. In the past, certain paints contained lead. Children are liable to be poisoned from chewing such paintwork or from inhalation when the paint is removed. This is still a problem in parts of the USA. Lead fumes from burning

103

Table 7.3 Potentially harmful poisons

Poison	Adverse effects	Management
Alcohol (accidental or experimenting by older children)	Hypoglycaemia Coma Respiratory failure	Monitor blood glucose. Intravenous glucose if necessary. Blood alcohol levels for severity
Acids and alkalis	Inflammation and ulceration of upper gastrointestinal tract leading to stenosis	No emesis/gastric lavage No chemical antidotes as they produce heat Early endoscopy
Digoxin	Arrhythmias, hyperkalaemia	Activated charcoal if <1 h after ingestion ECG monitoring, serum digoxin concentration
Disc or button batteries	Mild gastrointestinal symptoms Oesophageal stricture with large batteries (>20 mm) Corrosion of gut wall and perforation Break open with release of mercury – rare	Monitor progress with chest and abdominal X-rays – almost all passed within 2 days, no symptoms Remove batteries if in oesophagus or signs of disintegration. Some authorities recommend removal if not passed within 48 h to avoid danger of disintegration
Iron	*Initial*: vomiting, diarrhoea, haematemesis, melaena, acute gastric ulceration *Latent period of improvement* *Hours later*: drowsiness, coma, shock, liver failure with hypoglycaemia and convulsions *Long term*: gastric strictures	Serious toxicity if >60 mg/kg elemental iron Abdominal X-ray to count the number of tablets Serum iron levels Gastric lavage considered in severe cases if <1 h after ingestion Intravenous desferrioxamine for chelation
Paracetamol – large ingestion uncommon in young children as tablets are difficult to swallow and elixir is too sweet	Gastric irritation Liver failure after 3–5 days	Check plasma concentration after 4 h after ingestion. If >150 mg/kg paracetamol is thought to have been taken, or the plasma concentration is high, start intravenous acetylcysteine Monitor prothrombin time, liver function tests and plasma creatinine
Petroleum distillates (paraffin/kerosene, white spirit)	Aspiration causing pneumonitis	Emesis and gastric lavage contraindicated Usually no treatment required
Salicylates	Tinnitus, deafness, nausea, vomiting, dehydration Hyperventilation causing respiratory alkalosis. Later, metabolic acidosis. Hypoglycaemia. Disorientation	Measure plasma salicylate concentration Gastric lavage if <1 h. Give activated charcoal Monitor fluid and electrolyte balance Correct dehydration, electrolyte imbalance and acidosis. Dialysis
Tricyclic antidepressants	Sinus tachycardia Conduction disorders Dry mouth, blurred vision Agitation, confusion, convulsions, coma Hypotension Respiratory depression	Activated charcoal if within 1 h Cardiac monitoring. Treat arrhythmias conservatively with sodium bicarbonate Correct metabolic acidosis Treat convulsions with diazepam

Management of poisoning

Identification of the agent → Parents usually know the identity or can provide container or tablets

Assessment of the agent's toxicity (Table 7.1): check via TOXBASE → Toxicity – low, intermediate or high?
Contact the Regional Poisons Information Centre if in doubt about a substance's identity or toxicity

Activated charcoal (by mouth or nasogastric tube)
Most effective of the methods available
Absorbs some drugs
Ineffective for iron, hydrocarbons and insecticides
Black, unpalatable and gritty, but can be disguised in flat cola
Aspiration causes pneumonitis

Is removal of poison indicated?
Little evidence effective if > 1 hour after ingestion →

Gastric lavage
Rarely used in children. Only considered if large quantity of toxic drug ingested in the previous hour
A cuffed tracheal tube must be used if the patient is drowsy

Induced vomiting with ipecac
Now rarely used as ineffective. May be considered in young children if toxic substance and charcoal cannot be used

Are investigations indicated? →
Blood glucose for alcohol ingestion
Blood levels helpful only for alcohol, paracetamol, salicylate, iron, digoxin
Toxicology screen – when ingestion suspected but cause uncertain or non-accidental poisoning is suspected

Plan clinical management →
Mainly determined by toxicity of poison:
- Low – allow home
- Intermediate – observe for the recommended time, then discharge home unless symptoms develop
- High – admit to hospital
Also consider maximum dose that could have been ingested

Specific therapy or antidotes available for only a limited number of poisons (Table 7.2)
Observation and supportive care is the mainstay of management

Assess social circumstances →
Required in order to prevent further poisoning or accidents
The general practitioner and other health professionals should be informed; a home visit by the health visitor may be helpful

Figure 7.8 Outline of the management of poisoning. TOXBASE is an online database of the National Poisons Information Service for registered users.

batteries, lead shot for fishing and lead from old water pipes are other potential sources. Children from the Indian subcontinent may be poisoned by *surma*, the lead-containing eye make-up sometimes used even on young babies. Lead from vehicle exhaust fumes results in higher blood levels in children living in urban compared with rural areas. The change to unleaded petrol was in response to concern about its potential as an environmental hazard.

Children present with pica (compulsive eating of substances other than food), anorexia, colicky abdominal pain, irritability and failure to thrive and pallor from anaemia. Severe lead poisoning may present with neurological symptoms, including drowsiness, convulsions and coma from lead encephalopathy. Raised intracranial pressure with papilloedema may be present. There is increasing evidence that chronic exposure to relatively low lead levels may be harmful to cognitive development.

The diagnosis is confirmed by elevated blood lead levels. There may be a hypochromic anaemia and basophilic stippling of neutrophils. Radiographs of the

Accidents, poisoning and child protection

105

knee or wrist may show 'lead lines', which are dense metaphyseal bands. The source of lead should be identified and removed. Chelating agents are used to form non-toxic lead compounds. In mild cases, D-penicillamine is given orally, and in severe cases sodium calcium edetate (EDTA) is indicated.

Smoking

The harmful effects of smoking are well documented, with a greatly increased risk of developing chronic bronchitis, lung cancer and cardiovascular disease. Unfortunately, many children become regular smokers while still at school. Children should be given appropriate health education, although its effectiveness is limited by the poor example set by the widespread smoking of adults and the difficulties of health education in secondary school age children. When parents or carers smoke, children have been shown to have a higher incidence of bronchitis, asthma, pneumonia and serous otitis media (glue ear). This particularly applies to babies and young children. Maternal smoking places the infant at increased risk of sudden infant death syndrome (SIDS).

 Parents' smoking adversely affects their children's health.

Child protection

Children and young people require parents or carers who love, look after, provide shelter and protect them from harm. Unfortunately, this is not the case for all children. Emotional, physical, sexual abuse and neglect of children by parents, carers and others has occurred throughout history. Abuse and neglect seriously decrease the likelihood that a child will reach his or her full potential, although this is not inevitable; some resilient individuals manage despite very difficult circumstances.

Society, including the medical profession, was largely reluctant to accept that child abuse and neglect occurred until the second half of the twentieth century, when attention was drawn by two American paediatricians to the 'battered child'. In many countries, it is now accepted that child abuse and neglect exist and legislation is in place making them a criminal offence.

Following the Second World War, in parallel with the recognition of child abuse, came increasing recognition of human rights. The UN Convention on the Rights of the Child (see Ch. 1) specifically refers to the child's right to be protected from mistreatment, both physical and mental. It gives governments the responsibility to ensure that children are properly cared for and protected from violence, exploitation, abuse and neglect.

In the UK, a series of high profile cases of child abuse, most recently Victoria Climbie and Baby P (Box 7.1), have highlighted the difficulties faced by all professionals involved with the welfare of children, whether social workers, teachers, police, healthcare professionals or others, in recognising and responding appropriately to the alerting signs of child abuse.

Box 7.1 Two high profile cases of child abuse in the UK

Victoria Climbie

- An 8-year-old girl, abused and murdered by her guardians in London in 2000
- Postmortem – 128 separate injuries
- Public outrage led to public inquiry, which resulted in the 'Every Child Matters' initiative, where all organisations involved with providing services to children were instructed to share information and work together to protect children and young people from harm.

Peter Connelly (Baby P)

- The 17-month-old baby died in 2007 following physical abuse throughout his life
- At death – 50 injuries
- He had 35 contacts with healthcare professionals

A report (Laming report) highlighted the need for better information sharing in both cases.

 High profile cases of child abuse:
- **can make some doctors frightened to deal with child protection or become oversuspicious from fear of missing cases. However, specialist advice and assistance should always be available.**
- **have led to improved guidelines and procedures**
- **have resulted in better child protection training for all health professionals.**

However, fear of missing child abuse has to be weighed against the damage of falsely accusing parents of abusing their children. This requires sensible judgement, excellent communication with the parents and a professional culture in which any concern that a child is being maltreated can be readily discussed with senior members of the team.

Summary

- Child abuse has existed for centuries but societies have been slow to acknowledge it as a problem.
- Children are vulnerable and cannot protect themselves – the basis of children's rights.
- Protecting children from harm is a key role of parents or carers and all involved with children.
- All healthcare professionals, social workers, teachers, police and others have a duty to ensure that they know what to do if they have concerns that a child may be being abused.

Types of child abuse and neglect

Abuse and neglect are both forms of maltreatment of a child. Somebody may abuse or neglect a child by inflicting harm, or by failing to act to prevent harm. Children may be abused in a family at home or in an institution or community, usually by someone known to them or, rarely, by a stranger. They may be abused by one or more adults or another child or children. Conventionally, child abuse is categorised into:

- Physical abuse
- Emotional abuse
- Sexual abuse
- Neglect
- Fabricated or induced illness (FII).

Physical abuse

Physical abuse may involve hitting, shaking, throwing, poisoning, burning or scalding, drowning, suffocating, or otherwise causing physical harm to a child.

Emotional abuse

Emotional abuse is the persistent emotional maltreatment of a child resulting in severe and persistent adverse effects on the child's emotional development. It may involve conveying to children that they are worthless or unloved, inadequate, or valued only insofar as they meet the needs of another person. It may feature developmentally inappropriate expectations being imposed on children. These may include interactions that are beyond the child's developmental capability, as well as overprotection and abnormal social interaction. It may involve seeing or hearing the ill treatment of another. It may also involve serious bullying that causes children to feel frightened or in danger, or the exploitation or corruption of children. Some level of emotional abuse is involved in all types of maltreatment of a child, although it may occur alone.

Sexual abuse

Sexual abuse involves forcing or enticing a child or young person to take part in sexual activities, including prostitution, whether or not the child is aware of what is happening. The activities may involve physical contact, including penetrative acts such as rape, buggery or oral sex, and/or non-contact activities, such as involving children in looking at or producing pornographic material or watching sexual activities or encouraging children to behave in sexually inappropriate ways.

Neglect

Neglect is the persistent failure to meet a child's basic physical and/or psychological needs, likely to result in the serious impairment of the child's health or development. It may involve a parent or carer failing to provide:

- adequate food and clothing
- shelter, including exclusion from home or abandonment
- protection from physical and emotional harm or danger
- adequate supervision, including the use of inadequate caregivers
- access to appropriate medical care or treatment. It may also include neglect or unresponsiveness to a child's basic emotional needs.

Fabricated or induced illness (FII)

This is a broad term to describe a group of behaviours by parents (or carers), but usually the mother (>80%), which cause harm to children. It fulfils the parents (or carers) own needs. It may consist of:

Verbal fabrication – parents fabricate (i.e. invent) symptoms and signs in the child, telling a false story to healthcare professionals, leading them to believe the child is ill and requires investigation and treatment. Medical and nursing staff are used as the instrument to harm the child through unnecessary interventions, including medication, hospital stays, intrusive tests and surgery. In community settings, the false stories may lead to medication, special diets and a restricted lifestyle or special schools.

Induction of illness may involve:

- suffocation of the child, which may present as an acute life-threatening event (ALTE)
- administration of noxious substances or poisons
- excessive or unnecessary administration of ordinary substances (e.g. excess salt)
- excess or unnecessary use of medication (prescribed for the child or others)
- the use of medically provided portals of entry (such as gastrostomy buttons, central lines).

Organic illness, may coexist with fabricated or induced illness in a child, making the fabrication more difficult to identify. It may manifest as overprotection, imposing unwarranted restrictions or giving treatment that is inappropriate or excessive.

A clue may be that the condition only occurs when the offending parent/carer is present or following a hospital visit. The condition can be extremely difficult to diagnose, but may be suspected if the child has frequent unexplained illnesses and multiple hospital admissions with symptoms that only occur in the carer's presence and are not substantiated by clinical findings. This disorder can be very damaging to the child, as unnecessary investigations and potentially harmful treatment are likely to be given. The child also learns to live with a pattern of illness rather than health. In induced poisoning, the diagnosis is often difficult but can usually be made by identifying the drug in the blood or urine.

Risk factors

Child maltreatment occurs across socioeconomic, religious, cultural, racial and ethnic groups. While no specific causes have been definitively identified that lead a parent or other caregiver to abuse or neglect a child, research has recognised a number of risk factors commonly associated with maltreatment (Box 7.2). Children within families and environments in which these factors exist have a higher probability of experiencing maltreatment. It must be emphasised, however, that while certain factors are often present among

Box 7.2 Risk factors for child abuse

In the child

- Failure to meet parental expectations and aspirations, e.g. disabled, wrong gender
- Resulted from forced, coercive or commercial sex

Parent/carer

- Mental health problems
- Parental indifference, intolerance or over-anxiousness
- Alcohol, drug abuse

In the family

- Step-parents
- Domestic violence
- Multiple/closely spaced births
- Social isolation or a perceived lack of social support
- Young parental age

Environment

- Poverty, poor housing
- Unsavoury neighbourhood.

families where maltreatment occurs, this does not mean that the presence of these factors will *always* result in child abuse and neglect. For example, there is a relationship between poverty and maltreatment, yet most people living in poverty do not harm their children.

Presentation

Child abuse and neglect

Child abuse may present with one or more of:

- Physical symptoms and signs
- Psychological symptoms and signs
- A concerning interaction observed between the child and the parent or carer
- The child may tell someone about the abuse
- The abuse may be observed.

Identification of child abuse in children with disabilities may be more difficult; disability is also a risk factor for child abuse.

In order to diagnose child abuse or neglect, a detailed history and thorough examination are crucial. In most instances where child abuse is considered, seeking advice from colleagues, e.g. more experienced members of the team, paediatric radiologists, paediatric surgeons, is essential.

Factors to consider in the presentation of a physical injury are:

- The child's age and stage of development
- The history given by the child (if they can communicate)
- The plausibility and/or reasonableness of the explanation for the injury

- Any background, e.g. previous child protection concerns, multiple attendances to A&E or general practitioner
- Delay in reporting the injury
- Inconsistent histories from caregivers
- Inappropriate reaction of parents or caregivers who are vague, evasive, unconcerned or excessively distressed or aggressive.

It is often not clear whether an injury is inflicted or non-inflicted. Table 7.4 gives examples of injuries and a guide as to the likelihood that it is due to an inflicted injury. The context and observations of the family are very important in evaluating injuries which may be inflicted.

Key features of bruising

- **The age of a bruise cannot be accurately estimated.**
- **Bruising is hard to detect on children with dark skin.**
- **Mongolian spots can be mistaken for bruises, as they may still be present at several years of age (see Fig. 9.13d).**

Neglect

Consider the possibility of neglect when the child:

- consistently misses important medical appointments
- lacks needed medical or dental care, immunisations or glasses
- seems ravenously hungry
- is dirty
- is wearing inadequate clothing in cold weather
- is abusing alcohol or other drugs
- says there is no one at home to provide care.

Consider the possibility of neglect when the parent or other adult caregiver:

- appears to be indifferent to the child
- seems apathetic or depressed
- behaves irrationally or in a bizarre manner
- is abusing alcohol or other drugs.

Emotional abuse

This damaging form of abuse is the hardest form of abuse to identify in a healthcare setting. Some clues may be found by noting how the parent or caregiver perceives the child. Is the child:

- the 'wrong' gender
- born at a time of parental separation or violence
- seen as unduly 'difficult'?

There may be clues from the behaviour of the child. This depends on the child's age:

- Babies:
  - Apathetic, delayed development, non-demanding
  - Described by the mother as 'spoiled, attention seeking, in control, not loving her'.
- Toddlers and preschool children:
  - Violent, apathetic, fearful.

Table 7.4 Examples of injuries and a guide as to how likely it is due to an inflicted injury

Injury	More likely to be inflicted	May be inflicted or accidental	Less likely or unlikely to be inflicted
Fractures	Any fracture in a non-mobile child (excluding those with a medical condition predisposing to fragile bones) Rib fractures Multiple fractures (unless due to significant accidental trauma, e.g. a road traffic accident) Multiple fractures of different ages	Skull fracture in young child Long bone fractures in a young but mobile child	Fracture in school-age child with witnessed trauma, e.g. fall from swing
Bruises	Bruising in the shape of a hand (Fig. 7.9a) or object Bruises on the neck that look like attempted strangulation Bruises around the wrists or ankles that look like ligature marks Bruise to the buttocks in a child less than 2 years or any age without a good explanation	Bruising to the trunk with a vague history	Bruises on the shins of a mobile child
Burns	Any burn in a child who is not mobile A burn in the shape of an implement – cigarette, iron A 'glove or stocking' burn consistent with forced immersion (Fig. 7.9b)		A burn to the chest of a mobile toddler with splash marks, a history of pulling a cup of hot tea onto himself
Bites	Bruising in the shape of a bite thought unlikely to have been caused by a young child (Fig. 7.9c)		A witnessed biting of one toddler by another

Physical injuries that can be caused by child abuse

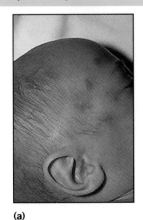

(a)

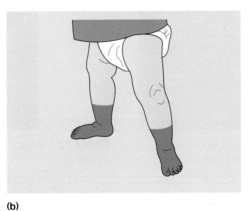

(b)

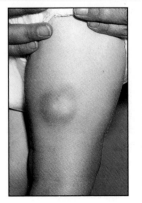

(c)

Figure 7.9 (a) Bruising from finger trauma to a baby's head. **(b)** Scald with stocking distribution including the soles from forced immersion in hot water. **(c)** A bite mark on an infant's leg. Adult bite marks may be seen in abuse, but bites from other children are not uncommon.

Accidents, poisoning and child protection

Case History

7.1 Severe child abuse

A 2-month-old boy was brought into A&E by ambulance, with unexplained loss of consciousness. His mother accompanying him appeared to have learning difficulties and could not explain what had happened. His father arrived soon after and said that he had been changing the child's nappy on the floor when suddenly he 'went all floppy and asleep'.

The child was unresponsive and had shallow breathing. His pupils were dilated. He appeared well nourished and was dressed only in a nappy. There were no obvious injuries seen.

Medical management was rapidly instituted. CT head scan showed subdural haemorrhages (Fig. 7.10). A chest X-ray obtained following intubation showed old posterior rib fractures (Fig. 7.11). Subsequent ophthalmological examination showed bilateral retinal haemorrhages (Fig. 7.12).

The child was transferred to an intensive care unit where, sadly, he died. A postmortem skeletal survey showed metaphyseal fractures (Fig. 7.13).

The parents maintained their story, despite the compelling evidence of inflicted head injury and shaking. The case went to the criminal court and both were sentenced on a number of charges.

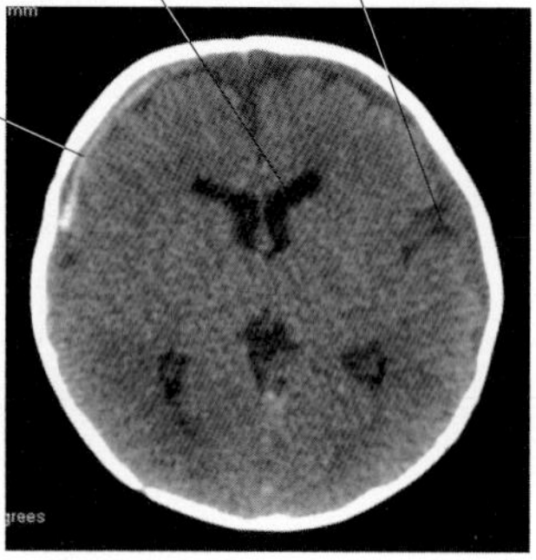

Mixed density blood, either older subdural bleed or active bleeding

Normal CSF density

Acute blood in subdural space

Figure 7.10 Subdural haemorrhage.

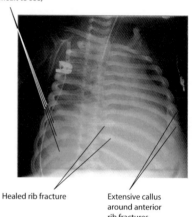

Fracture lines with no healing (difficult to see)

Healed rib fracture

Extensive callus around anterior rib fractures

Figure 7.11 Multiple rib fractures of different ages.

> ❋ **Severe physical child abuse resulting in death gains considerable attention from the media but is rare. Many more children suffer permanent injury. Most have been seen previously by health professionals. Early recognition and response to child protection concerns could prevent severe injury.**

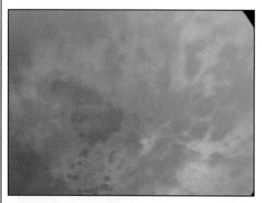

Figure 7.12 Retinal haemorrhages from trauma to the head. (Courtesy of Ms Clare Roberts.)

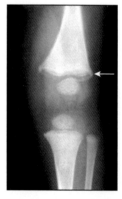

Figure 7.13 Metaphyseal fracture of distal humerus.

- School children:
  - Wetting , soiling, relationship difficulties, non-attendance, anti-social behaviour.
- Adolescents:
  - Self-harm, depression, oppositional, aggressive and delinquent behaviour

  - Being bullied is increasingly recognised as an important form of emotional abuse. Every school should have a written bullying policy which needs to be implemented when necessary.

The assessment of sexual abuse

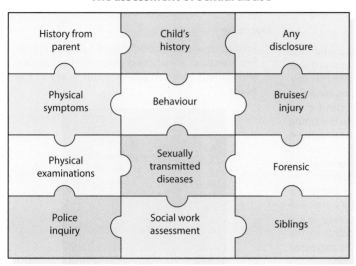

Figure 7.14 The assessment of sexual abuse is like a jigsaw puzzle. Many different pieces of information need to be pieced together to make an informed opinion. (From: *Child Protection Companion,* Royal College of Paediatrics and Child Health, 2005. After Hobbs CJ, Wynne JM, The sexually abused battered child. *Archives of Disease in Childhood* 1990; 65: 423-427. Reproduced with permission from the BMJ Publishing Group.)

Sexual abuse

In suspected sexual abuse, information from different sources needs to be pieced together (Fig. 7.14).

Recognition

The child or young person may:

- tell someone about the abuse
- be identified in pornographic material
- be pregnant (by legal definition this is due to sexual abuse for a girl under the age of 13 years)
- have a sexually transmitted infection with no clear explanation (but some sexually transmitted infections can be passed from the mother to the baby during pregnancy or birth).

Physical symptoms

- Vaginal bleeding, itching, discharge
- Rectal bleeding.

Behavioural symptoms

- Soiling, secondary enuresis
- Self-harm, aggressive or sexualised behaviours, regression, poor school performance.

Signs

There are few clearly diagnostic signs of sexual abuse on examination. This is because sexual abuse of children often comprises touching or kissing or other activities that do not involve significant physical force. Furthermore, the genital area heals very quickly in young children, so signs may be absent even a few days after significant trauma. Forensic material also decays rapidly.

Examination of children suspected of having been sexually abused requires a doctor with specific expertise and training, facilities for photographic documentation, sexually transmitted infection screening and management and, where indicated, forensic testing (Fig. 7.14). Forensic testing of swabs from the child or his/her clothing/bedding may reveal DNA from the sperm of the perpetrator.

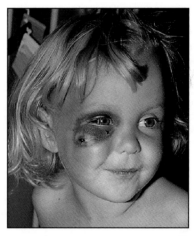

Figure 7.15 A thorough medical assessment is required in all children when non-accidental injury is suspected. This girl's large bruise followed what was said to be a minor bump. Non-accidental injury was suspected, but examination showed multiple bruises and petechiae. She had immune thrombocytopenic purpura (ITP).

Investigation

In physical abuse, fractures in young children may not be detectable clinically and X-rays are required to identify them. Bruising overlying a fracture is rarely seen on presentation. A full radiographic skeletal survey with oblique views of the ribs should be performed in all children with suspected physical abuse under 30 months of age. Some lesions may be inconspicuous initially but, if indicated, become evident on a repeat X-ray 1–2 weeks later. Other medical conditions which need to be considered and excluded in suspected child abuse are:

- Bruising – coagulation disorders (Fig. 7.15), Mongolian blue spots on the back or thighs

111

Case History

7.2 Possible child abuse

Parents brought their 8-month-old daughter into paediatric A&E department. They were worried that she had not been moving her right arm for that day. The family remembered that at the evening meal two evenings before, father was bringing dishes for the family meal to a low corner coffee table in the sitting room. Mother was sitting with baby on her knee, next to the table, trying to control the older siblings, when father had accidentally dropped a heavy serving bowl of food. Mother automatically reached out to try to catch it, dropping the baby in doing so and in the confusion, the serving bowl hit the baby's arm. The baby cried very loudly for about 10 minutes or so but then seemed to settle. The next day she didn't use the right arm but the family thought this was explained by the injury causing a 'strain' as they couldn't see any bruising on the arm. An X-ray showed a fracture of the right radius and ulna (Fig. 7.16).

Child protection concerns

- Baby under 1 year with fracture
- Delayed presentation.

Positive features

- Plausible, consistent story
- Good parent–child interaction observed by medical and nursing staff
- Well-nourished, well-cared-for appearance of baby
- No other injuries on full examination
- Skeletal survey showed no other fractures
- Personal child health record showed regularly weighed, thriving baby up to date with immunisations
- No GP or HV concerns about the family
- Not previously known to local Children's Social Services.

Outcome

- Strategy meeting – no additional concerns identified. Decision – increased Health Visitor contact and parents received advice about safety in the home.

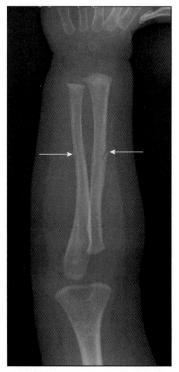

Figure 7.16 X-ray of right arm showing fracture of radius and ulna.

 In child protection, conclusive evidence is often not available.

- Fractures – osteogenesis imperfecta, commonly referred to as brittle bone disease. The type commonly involved with unexplained fractures is type I, which is an autosomal dominant disorder, so there may be a family history. Blue sclerae are a key clinical finding and there may be generalised osteoporosis and wormian bones in the skull (extra bones within skull sutures) on skeletal survey.
- Scalds and cigarette burns – may be misinterpreted in children with bullous impetigo or scalded skin syndrome.

Where brain injury is suspected all children require:

- An immediate CT head scan followed later by a MRI head scan
- A skeletal survey to exclude fractures
- An expert ophthalmological examination to identify retinal haemorrhages
- A coagulation screen.

Management

Abused children may present to doctors in the hospital or to medical or nursing staff in the community. They may also be brought for a medical opinion by social services or the police. In all cases, the procedures of the local safeguarding children board should be followed. The medical consultation should be the same as for any medical condition, with a detailed history and full examination. It is usually most productive when this is conducted in a sensitive and concerned way without being accusatory or condemning. Any injuries or medical findings should be carefully noted, measured, recorded and drawn on a body map and photographed (with consent). The height, weight and head circumference (where appropriate) should be recorded and plotted on a centile chart. The interaction between the child and parents should be noted. All notes must be meticulous, dated, timed and signed on each page. Treatment of specific injuries should be instigated and blood tests and X-rays undertaken.

If abuse is suspected or confirmed, a decision needs to be made as to whether the child needs immediate protection from further harm. If this is the case, this may be achieved by admission to hospital, which also allows investigations and multidisciplinary assessment. If sympathetically handled, most parents are willing to accept medical advice for hospital admission for observation and investigation. Occasionally, this is not possible and legal enforcement is required. If medical treatment is not necessary but it is felt to be unsafe for the child to return home, a placement may be found in a foster home.

When dealing with any child suspected of having been abused, the safety of any other siblings or children at home must be considered; the police and/or social services should be alerted to any concerns.

In addition to a detailed medical assessment, evaluation by social workers and other health professionals will be required. A strategy meeting and later a child protection conference may be convened in accordance with local procedures. Members may include social workers, health visitors, police, general practitioner, paediatricians, teachers and lawyers. Parents attend all or part of the case conference. Details of the incident leading to the conference and the family background will be discussed. Good communication and a trusting working relationship between the professionals are vital, as it can be extremely difficult to evaluate the likelihood that injuries were inflicted deliberately and the possible outcome of legal proceedings. The conference will decide:

- whether the child should be provided with a Child Protection Plan and under what category (see Case History 7.1)
- whether there should be an application to the Court to protect the child
- what follow-up is needed.

 Why is child protection so difficult?
Child protection:

- **goes against the assumption that parents usually have their children's best interests at heart**
- **can involve confronting parents who may be manipulative or aggressive**
- **requires detailed evaluation of the history and examination to identify inconsistencies and interpret subtle findings**
- **depends on genuinely good multi-professional teamwork and respect of colleagues.**

Summary

Child abuse

- Child abuse is the responsibility of all doctors, and must not be avoided or ignored because it raises difficult issues and possible appearance in Court.
- It takes various forms – physical abuse, emotional abuse, sexual abuse, neglect, fabricated or induced illness.

- The interests of the child should be kept uppermost to ensure protection from harm.
- In many instances it is uncertain whether or not the problem is one of child abuse. Good communication with the parents and child is vital.

Further reading

HM Government: *Working Together to Safeguard Children: Every Child Matters*, London, 2006, HM Government.

HM Government: *Children Act*, London, 1989, HM Government.

Laming Report 2003, 2009.

Local Safeguarding Children Board. Policies and Procedures.

NICE: *NICE Guideline – Child Maltreatment*, London, 2009, NICE.

Royal College of Paediatrics and Child Health: *Child Protection Companion and Reader.* UK.

Lancet Series: Child Maltreatment, 2008.

Accidents, poisoning and child protection

8

Genetics

Genetic disorders are:

- common, with 2% of live-born babies having a significant congenital malformation and about 5% a genetic disorder
- burdensome to the affected individual, family and society, as many are associated with severe and permanent disability.

There has recently been an unprecedented growth in knowledge about the genetic basis of diseases :

- The Human Genome Project resulted in the first publication of the human genome sequence in 2001.
- It is now estimated that the human genome contains 20 000–25 000 genes, although the function of many of them remains unknown. Greater diversity and complexity at the protein level is achieved by alternative mRNA splicing and post-translational modification of gene products.
- Microarray techniques and high throughput sequencing are increasing the volume and speed of genetic investigations and reducing their costs, leading to a greater understanding of the impact of genetics on health and disease.
- Access to genome browser databases containing DNA sequence and protein structure has greatly enhanced progress in scientific research and the interpretation of clinical test results (Fig. 8.1).
- Genetic databases are available on thousands of multiple congenital anomaly syndromes, on chromosomal variations and disease phenotypes and on all Mendelian disorders.
- Clinical application of these advances is available to families through specialist genetic centres that offer investigation, diagnosis, counselling and antenatal diagnosis for an ever-widening range of disorders.
- Gene-based knowledge is entering mainstream medical and paediatric practice, especially in diagnosis and in therapeutic guidance, such as for the treatment of malignancies.

Genetically determined diseases include those resulting from:

- chromosomal abnormalities
- the action of a single gene (Mendelian disorders)
- unusual genetic mechanisms
- interaction of genetic and environmental factors (polygenic, multifactorial, or complex disorders).

Chromosomal abnormalities

Genes are composed of DNA that is wound around a core of histone proteins and packaged into a succession of supercoils to form the chromosomes. The human chromosome complement was confirmed as 46 in 1956. The chromosomal abnormalities in Down, Klinefelter and Turner syndromes were recognised in 1959 and thousands of chromosome defects have now been documented.

Chromosomal abnormalities are either numerical or structural. They occur in approximately 10% of spermatozoa and 25% of mature oöcytes and are a common cause of early spontaneous miscarriage. The estimated incidence of chromosomal abnormalities in live-born infants is about 1 in 150; they usually cause multiple congenital anomalies and cognitive difficulties. Acquired chromosomal changes play a significant role in carcinogenesis and tumour progression.

Down syndrome (trisomy 21)

This is the most common autosomal trisomy and the most common genetic cause of severe learning difficulties. The incidence (without antenatal screening) in live-born infants is about 1 in 650.

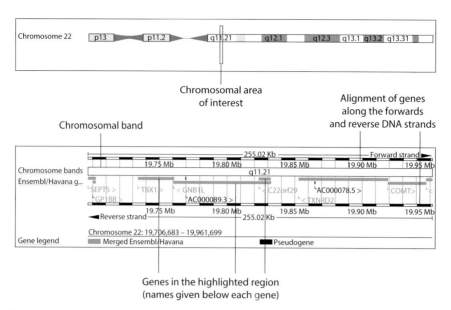

Figure 8.1 Ensembl Genome Browser. The image shows part of chromosome region 22q11, involved in 22q11 deletion syndrome (Di George syndrome). Although only part of the commonly deleted region is shown, the image shows several genes that are deleted in 22q11 deletion syndrome. The online Ensembl browser can be used to 'zoom in' on specific areas, showing the genes present in different chromosome regions, and can also be used to show the gene sequence itself.

Clinical features

Down syndrome is usually suspected at birth because of the baby's facial appearance. Most affected infants are hypotonic and other useful clinical signs include a flat occiput, single palmar creases, incurved fifth finger and wide 'sandal' gap between the big and second toe (Fig. 8.2a–c, Box 8.1). The diagnosis can be difficult to make when relying on clinical signs alone and a suspected diagnosis should be confirmed by a senior paediatrician. Before blood is sent for analysis, parents should be informed that a test for Down syndrome is being performed. The results may take 1–2 days, using rapid FISH (fluorescent in situ hybridisation) techniques. Parents need information about the short- and long-term implications of the diagnosis. They are also likely, at some stage in the future, to appreciate the opportunity to discuss how and why the condition has arisen, the risk of recurrence and the possibility of antenatal diagnosis in future pregnancies.

It is difficult to give a precise long-term prognosis in the neonatal period, as there is individual variation in the degree of learning difficulty and the development of complications. Over 85% of infants with trisomy 21 survive to 1 year of age. Congenital heart disease is present in 30% and, particularly atrioventricular canal defect, is a major cause of early mortality. At least 50% of affected individuals live longer than 50 years. Parents also need to know what assistance is available from both professionals and family support groups. Counselling may be helpful to assist the family to deal with feelings of grief, anger or guilt.

The Child Development Service will provide or coordinate care for the parents. This will include regular review of the child's development and health. Children with Down syndrome are at increased risk of hypothyroidism, impairment of vision and hearing and of atlanto-axial instability.

Cytogenetics

The extra chromosome 21 may result from meiotic non-disjunction, translocation or mosaicism.

Meiotic non-disjunction (94%)

In non-disjunction trisomy 21:

- most cases result from an error at meiosis
- the pair of chromosome 21s fails to separate, so that one gamete has two chromosome 21s and one has none (Fig. 8.3)
- fertilisation of the gamete with two chromosome 21s gives rise to a zygote with trisomy 21
- parental chromosomes do not need to be examined.

The incidence of trisomy 21 due to non-disjunction is related to maternal age (Table 8.1). However, as the proportion of pregnancies in older mothers is small, most affected babies are born to younger mothers. Furthermore, meiotic non-disjunction can occur in spermatogenesis so that the extra 21 can be of paternal origin. All pregnant women are now offered screening tests measuring biochemical markers in blood samples and often also nuchal thickening on ultrasound (thickening of the soft tissues at the back of the neck) to identify an increased risk of Down syndrome in the fetus. When an increased risk is identified, amniocentesis is offered to check the fetal karyotype. After having one child with trisomy 21 due to non-disjunction, the risk of recurrence of Down syndrome is given as 1 in 200 for mothers under the age of 35 years, but remains similar to their age-related population risk for those over the age of 35 years.

Down syndrome

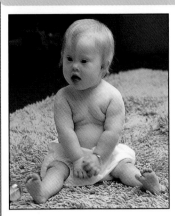

Figure 8.2a Characteristic facies seen in Down syndrome. Her posture is due to hypotonia.

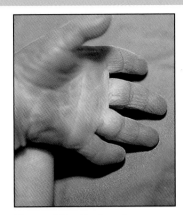

Figure 8.2b Single palmar crease.

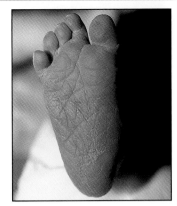

Figure 8.2c Pronounced 'sandal' gap between the big and second toe.

Box 8.1 Characteristic clinical manifestations of Down syndrome

Typical craniofacial appearance

- Round face and flat nasal bridge
- Upslanted palpebral fissures
- Epicanthic folds (a fold of skin running across the inner edge of the palpebral fissure)
- Brushfield spots in iris (pigmented spots)
- Small mouth and protruding tongue
- Small ears
- Flat occiput and third fontanelle

Other anomalies

- Short neck
- Single palmar creases, incurved fifth finger and wide 'sandal' gap between toes
- Hypotonia
- Congenital heart defects (40%)
- Duodenal atresia
- Hirschsprung disease

Later medical problems

- Delayed motor milestones
- Moderate to severe learning difficulties
- Small stature
- Increased susceptibility to infections
- Hearing impairment from secretory otitis media
- Visual impairment from cataracts, squints, myopia
- Increased risk of leukaemia and solid tumours
- Risk of atlanto-axial instability
- Increased risk of hypothyroidism and coeliac disease
- Epilepsy
- Alzheimer's disease.

Translocation (5%)

When the extra chromosome 21 is joined onto another chromosome (usually chromosome 14, but occasionally chromosome 15, 22 or 21), this is known as a Robertsonian translocation. This may be present in a phenotypically normal carrier with 45 chromosomes (two being 'joined together') or in someone with Down syndrome and a set of 46 chromosomes but with three copies of chromosome 21 material. In this situation, parental chromosomal analysis is recommended, since one of the parents may well carry the translocation in balanced form (in 25% of cases) (Fig. 8.4).

In translocation Down syndrome:

- The risk of recurrence is 10–15% if the mother is the translocation carrier and about 2.5% if the father is the carrier.
- If a parent carries the rare 21:21 translocation, all the offspring will have Down syndrome.
- If neither parent carries a translocation (75% of cases), the risk of recurrence is <1%.

Mosaicism (1%)

In mosaicism, some of the cells are normal and some have trisomy 21. This usually arises after the formation of the chromosomally normal zygote by non-disjunction at mitosis but can arise by later mitotic non-disjunction in a trisomy 21 conception. The phenotype is sometimes milder in Down syndrome mosaicism.

Inheritance of Down syndrome

Non-disjunction

Parents

Chromosome 21s

Non-disjunction
at meiosis

Gametes

Not viable

Fertilisation

Offspring

Trisomy 21 Down syndrome

Figure 8.3 Non-disjunction Down syndrome.

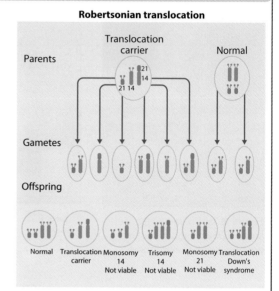

Robertsonian translocation

Translocation
carrier

Normal

Parents

21
14

21 14

Gametes

Offspring

Normal | Translocation carrier | Monosomy 14 Not viable | Trisomy 14 Not viable | Monosomy 21 Not viable | Translocation Down's syndrome

Figure 8.4 Translocation Down syndrome. There is a Robertsonian translocation involving chromosomes 21 and 14, which has been inherited from a parent.

Table 8.1 Risk of Down syndrome (live births) with maternal age at delivery, prior to screening in pregnancy

Maternal age (years)	Risk of Down syndrome
All ages	1 in 650
20	1 in 1530
30	1 in 900
35	1 in 385
37	1 in 240
40	1 in 110
44	1 in 37

Summary

Down syndrome (trisomy 21)

- Natural incidence ~1.5 per 1000 infants
- Cytogenetics – non-disjunction (most common, related to maternal age), translocation (one parent may carry a balanced translocation) or mosaicism (rare)
- Presentation – antenatal screening, prenatal diagnosis or clinical presentation; confirmed on chromosome analysis
- Immediate medical complications – increased risk of duodenal atresia, congenital heart disease
- Clinical manifestations (see Box 8.1).

Edwards syndrome (trisomy 18) and Patau syndrome (trisomy 13)

Although rarer than Down syndrome (1 in 8000 and 1 in 14000 live births, respectively), particular constellations of severe multiple abnormalities suggest these diagnoses at birth; most affected babies die in infancy (Fig. 8.5, Boxes 8.2 and 8.3). The diagnosis is confirmed by chromosome analysis. Many affected fetuses are detected by ultrasound scan during the second trimester of pregnancy and diagnosis can be confirmed antenatally by amniocentesis and chromosome analysis. Recurrence risk is low, except when the trisomy is due to a balanced chromosome rearrangement in one of the parents.

Turner syndrome (45, X)

Usually (>95%), Turner syndrome results in early miscarriage and is increasingly detected by ultrasound antenatally when fetal oedema of the neck, hands or feet or a cystic hygroma may be identified. In live-born females, the incidence is about 1 in 2500. Figure 8.6 and Box 8.4 show the clinical features of Turner syndrome, although short stature may be the only clinical abnormality in children.

Edwards syndome and Patau syndrome

Box 8.2 Clinical features of Edwards syndrome (trisomy 18)

- Low birthweight
- Prominent occiput
- Small mouth and chin
- Short sternum
- Flexed, overlapping fingers (Fig. 8.5)
- 'Rocker-bottom' feet
- Cardiac and renal malformations.

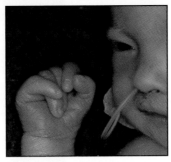

Figure 8.5 Overlapping of the fingers in Edwards syndrome.

Box 8.3 Clinical features of Patau syndrome (trisomy 13)

- Structural defect of brain
- Scalp defects
- Small eyes (microphthalmia) and other eye defects
- Cleft lip and palate
- Polydactyly
- Cardiac and renal malformations.

Turner syndrome

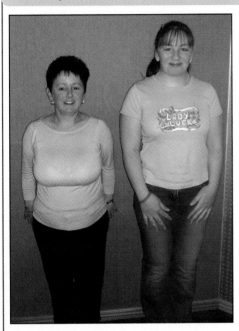

Figure 8.6 Turner syndrome. The woman on the left has marked short stature but no other clinical features; the adolescent female on the right has neck webbing and has received growth hormone and is 150 cm in height.

Box 8.4 Clinical features of Turner syndrome

- Lymphoedema of hands and feet in neonate, which may persist
- Spoon-shaped nails
- Short stature – a cardinal feature
- Neck webbing or thick neck
- Wide carrying angle (cubitus valgus)
- Widely spaced nipples
- Congenital heart defects (particularly coarctation of the aorta)
- Delayed puberty
- Ovarian dysgenesis resulting in infertility, although pregnancy may be possible with in vitro fertilisation (IVF) using donated ova
- Hypothyroidism
- Renal anomalies
- Pigmented moles
- Recurrent otitis media
- Normal intellectual function in most.

Treatment is with:

- Growth hormone therapy
- Oestrogen replacement for development of secondary sexual characteristics at the time of puberty (but infertility persists).

In about 50% of girls with Turner syndrome, there are 45 chromosomes, with only one X chromosome. The other cases have a deletion of the short arm of one X chromosome, an isochromosome that has two long arms but no short arm, or a variety of other structural defects of one of the X chromosomes. The presence of a Y chromosome sequence may increase the risk of gonadoblastoma.

The incidence does not increase with maternal age and risk of recurrence is very low.

Klinefelter syndrome (47, XXY)

This disorder occurs in about 1–2 per 1000 live-born males. For clinical features, see Box 8.5. Recurrence risk is very low.

Reciprocal translocations

An exchange of material between two different chromosomes is called a reciprocal translocation. When this exchange involves no loss or gain of chromosomal

Box 8.5 Clinical features of Klinefelter syndrome

- Infertility – most common presentation
- Hypogonadism with small testes
- Pubertal development may appear normal (some males benefit from testosterone therapy)
- Gynaecomastia in adolescence
- Tall stature
- Intelligence usually in the normal range, but some have educational and psychological problems.

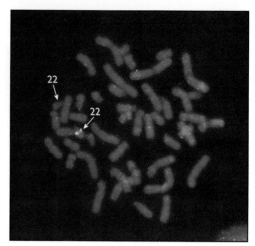

Figure 8.7 Fluorescent in situ hybridisation (FISH) demonstrating a microdeletion on chromosome 22 associated with DiGeorge syndrome. Hybridisation signals are seen on one chromosome 22 but not on the other because of the presence of a deletion. (Courtesy of L. Gaunt, St Mary's Hospital, Manchester.)

material, the translocation is 'balanced' and usually has no phenotypic effect. Balanced reciprocal translocations are relatively common, occurring in 1 in 500 of the general population. A translocation that appears balanced on conventional chromosome analysis may still involve the loss of a few genes or the disruption of a single gene at one of the chromosomal breakpoints and result in an abnormal phenotype, often including cognitive difficulties. Studying the breakpoints in such individuals has been one way of identifying the location of specific genes.

Unbalanced reciprocal translocations contain an 'incorrect' amount of chromosomal material and often impair both physical and cognitive development, leading to dysmorphic features, congenital malformations, developmental delay and learning difficulties. In a newborn baby, the prognosis is difficult to predict but the effect is usually severe. The parents' chromosomes should be checked to determine whether the abnormality has arisen *de novo*, or as a consequence of a parental rearrangement. Finding a balanced translocation in one parent indicates a recurrence risk for future pregnancies, so that antenatal diagnosis by chorionic villus sampling or amniocentesis should be offered as well as testing relatives who might be carriers.

Deletions

Deletions are another type of structural abnormality. Loss of part of a chromosome usually results in physical abnormalities and cognitive impairment. The deletion may involve loss of the terminal or an interstitial part of a chromosome arm.

An example of a deletion syndrome involves loss of the tip of the short arm of chromosome 5, hence the name 5p- or monosomy 5p. Because affected babies have a high-pitched mewing cry in early infancy, it is also known as *cri du chat* syndrome. Parental chromosomes should be checked to see if one parent carries a balanced chromosomal rearrangement. The clinical severity varies greatly, depending upon the extent of the deletion. It is now possible to specify the genes involved in chromosomal deletions as molecular methods are replacing standard cytogenetic investigations.

An increasing number of syndromes are now known to be due to chromosome deletions too small to be seen by conventional cytogenetic analysis. Submicroscopic deletions can be detected by FISH studies using DNA probes specific to particular chromosome regions. FISH studies are useful when a specific chromosome deletion is suspected.

DiGeorge syndrome is associated with a deletion of band q11 on chromosome 22 (i.e. 22q11) (Fig. 8.7). Williams syndrome is another example of a microdeletion syndrome due to loss of chromosomal material at band q11 on the long arm of chromosome 7 (i.e. 7q11) (Fig. 8.18, see also Box 8.12).

Mendelian inheritance

Mendelian inheritance, described by Mendel in garden peas in 1866, is the transmission of inherited traits or diseases caused by variation in a single gene in a characteristic pattern. These Mendelian traits or disorders are individually rare but collectively numerous and important: over 6000 have been described. For many disorders, the Mendelian pattern of inheritance is known. If the diagnosis of a condition is uncertain, its pattern of inheritance may be evident on drawing a family tree (pedigree), which is an essential part of genetic evaluation (Fig. 8.8).

Autosomal dominant inheritance

This is the most common mode of Mendelian inheritance (Box 8.6). Autosomal dominant conditions are caused by alterations in only one copy of a gene pair, i.e. the condition occurs in the heterozygous state despite the presence of an intact copy of the relevant gene. Autosomal dominant genes are located on the autosomes (chromosomes 1–22) so males and females are equally affected. Each child from an affected parent has a 1 in 2 (50%) chance of inheriting the abnormal gene (Fig. 8.9a,b). This appears to be straightforward, but complicating factors include the following factors.

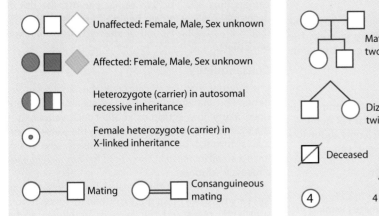

Figure 8.8 Examples of pedigree symbols.

Autosomal dominant inheritance

Box 8.6 Examples of autosomal dominant disorders

- Achondroplasia
- Ehlers–Danlos syndrome
- Familial hypercholesterolaemia
- Huntington disease
- Marfan syndrome
- Myotonic dystrophy
- Neurofibromatosis
- Noonan syndrome
- Osteogenesis imperfecta
- Otosclerosis
- Polyposis coli
- Tuberous sclerosis.

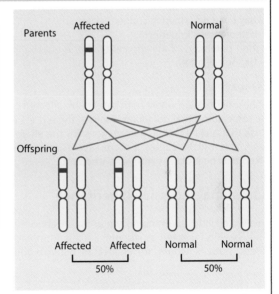

Figure 8.9a Autosomal dominant inheritance.

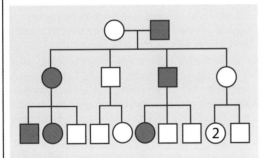

Figure 8.9b Typical pedigree of an autosomal dominant disorder.

Summary

Autosomal dominant inheritance

- Most common mode of Mendelian inheritance
- Affected individual carries the abnormal gene on one of a pair of autosomes
- 1 in 2 chance of inheriting the abnormal gene from affected parent, but there may be variation in expression, non-penetrance, no family history (new mutation, parental mosaicism, non-paternity) or homozygosity (rare).

Genetics

121

Variation in expression

Within a family, some affected individuals may manifest the disorder mildly and others more severely. This may be the result of variation at other genes, environmental effects, or sheer chance.

Non-penetrance

Refers to the lack of clinical signs and symptoms in an individual who has inherited the abnormal gene. An example of this is otosclerosis, in which only about 40% of gene carriers develop deafness (Fig. 8.10).

No family history of the disorder

It therefore may be due to:

- A new mutation in one of the gametes leading to the conception of the affected person. This is the most common reason for absence of a family history in dominant disorders, e.g. >80% of individuals with achondroplasia have unaffected parents.
- Parental mosaicism – very occasionally a healthy parent harbours the mutation only in some of their cells, e.g. in their gonads. This can account for recurrences of autosomal dominant disorders in siblings born to apparently unaffected parents. It has been described in congenital lethal osteogenesis imperfecta.
- Non-paternity – if the apparent father is not the biological father.

Homozygosity

In the rare situation where both parents are affected by the same autosomal dominant disorder, there is a 1 in 4 risk that a child will be homozygous for the altered gene. This usually causes a more severe phenotype which may be lethal, as with achondroplasia.

Autosomal recessive inheritance

An affected individual is homozygous for the abnormal gene, having inherited an abnormal allele from each parent, both of whom are unaffected heterozygous carriers (Box 8.7). For two carrier parents, the risk of each child, male or female, being affected is 1 in 4 (25%) (Fig. 8.11a,b). All offspring of affected individuals will be carriers.

Consanguinity

It is thought that we all carry 6–8 abnormal recessive genes. Fortunately, our partners usually carry different ones. Marrying a cousin or another relative increases the chance of both partners carrying the same abnormal autosomal recessive gene. Cousins who marry have a small increase in the risk of having a child with a recessive disorder.

The frequencies of disease alleles at recessive gene loci vary between racial groups. When the gene occurs sufficiently often and the gene or its effect can be detected, population-based carrier screening can be performed and antenatal diagnosis offered for high-risk pregnancies where both parents are carriers. Disorders that can be screened for in this way include sickle cell disease in black Africans and Afro-Americans, the thalassaemias in those from Mediterranean or Asian populations and Tay–Sachs disease in Ashkenazi Jews.

X-linked inheritance

X-linked conditions are caused by alterations in genes found on the X chromosome. These may be inherited as X-linked recessive or X-linked dominant traits but the distinction between these is much less clear than in autosomal traits because of the variable pattern of X chromosome inactivation in females.

In X-linked recessive inheritance (Box 8.8, Fig. 8.12a,b):

- Males are affected
- Female carriers are usually healthy
- Occasionally a female carrier shows mild signs of the disease (manifesting carrier)
- Each son of a female carrier has a 1 in 2 (50%) risk of being affected
- Each daughter of a female carrier has a 1 in 2 (50%) risk of being a carrier
- Daughters of affected males will all be carriers
- Sons of affected males will not be affected, since a man passes a Y chromosome to his son.

The family history may be negative, since new mutations and (gonadal) mosaicism are fairly common. Identification of carrier females in a family requires interpretation of the pedigree, the search for mild clinical manifestations and performing specific biochemical

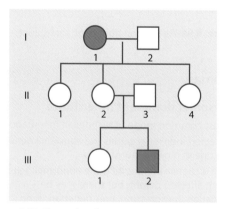

Figure 8.10 Example of non-penetrance. I1 and III2 have otosclerosis. II2 has normal hearing but must have the gene (a new mutation event is most unlikely to arise independently for a second time in the family). The gene is non-penetrant in II2.

Summary

X-linked recessive inheritance

- Males are affected; females can be carriers but are usually healthy or have mild disease
- Family history may be negative – new mutations and gonadal mosaicism
- Identifying female carriers is important to be able to provide genetic counselling.

Autosomal recessive inheritance

Box 8.7 Examples of autosomal recessive disorders

- Congenital adrenal hyperplasia
- Cystic fibrosis
- Friedreich ataxia
- Galactosaemia
- Glycogen storage diseases
- Hurler syndrome
- Oculocutaneous albinism
- Phenylketonuria
- Sickle cell disease
- Tay–Sachs disease
- Thalassaemia
- Werdnig–Hoffmann disease (SMA I).

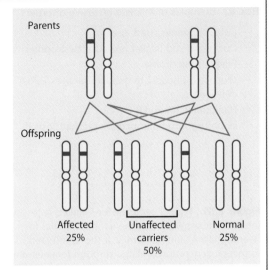

Figure 8.11a Autosomal recessive inheritance.

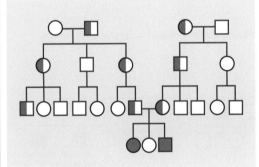

Figure 8.11b Pedigree to show autosomal recessive inheritance.

Summary

Autosomal recessive inheritance

- Affected individuals are homozygous for the abnormal gene; each unaffected parent will be a heterozygous carrier
- Two carrier parents have a 1 in 4 risk of having an affected child
- Risk of these disorders is increased by consanguinity and within specific populations
- Autosomal recessive disorders often affect metabolic pathways, whereas autosomal dominant disorders often affect structural proteins.

or molecular tests. Identifying carriers is important because a female carrier has a 50% risk of having an affected son regardless of who her partner is, and X-linked recessive disorders are often very severe.

X-linked dominant inheritance

X-linked disorders where the mutation has a dominant effect are rare. Both males and females are affected, e.g. hypophosphataemic (vitamin D-resistant) rickets. In some disorders, male lethality is expected and the only affected individuals seen will be female, e.g. incontinentia pigmenti. In others, the condition may affect females because it arises predominantly through mutations at spermatogenesis.

Y-linked inheritance

Y-linked traits are extremely rare. Y-linked inheritance would result in only males being affected, with transmission from an affected father to all his sons.

Y-linked genes determine sexual differentiation and spermatogenesis, and mutations are associated with infertility and so are rarely transmitted.

Unusual genetic mechanisms

Trinucleotide repeat expansion mutations

This is a class of unstable mutations caused by unstable expansions of trinucleotide repeat sequences inherited in Mendelian fashion. Fragile X syndrome and myotonic dystrophy were among the first disorders found to be due to such mutations. Other disorders include Huntington disease, spinocerebellar ataxia and Friedreich's ataxia. These disorders follow different patterns of inheritance but share certain unusual properties due to the nature of the underlying mutation. Clinical anticipation is often seen, with the disorders presenting at an earlier age and becoming more severe in successive

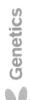

Genetics

Box 8.8 Examples of X-linked recessive disorders

- Colour blindness (red–green)
- Duchenne and Becker muscular dystrophies
- Fragile X syndrome
- Glucose-6-phosphate dehydrogenase (G6PD) deficiency
- Haemophilia A and B
- Hunter syndrome (mucopolysaccharidosis II).

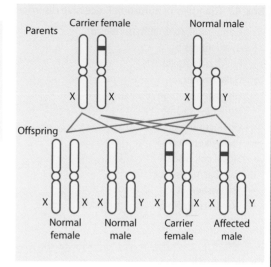

Figure 8.12a X-linked recessive inheritance.

Figure 8.12b Typical pedigree for X-linked recessive inheritance, showing Queen Victoria, a carrier for haemophilia A, and her family. It shows affected males in several generations, related through females, and that affected males do not have affected sons (contrast with autosomal dominant inheritance).

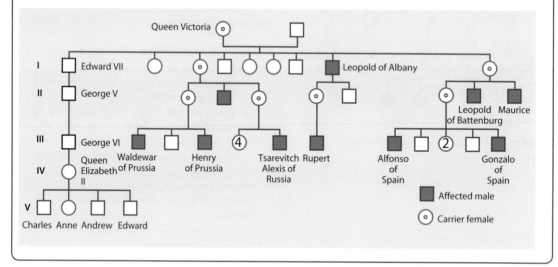

generations of a family as the triplet expands, and with entirely new mutations being exceptionally rare. There are two major categories of triplet repeat disorder, depending upon whether or not the triplet repeat is in the coding sequence of the gene.

Fragile X syndrome

The prevalence of significant learning difficulties in males due to fragile X syndrome is about 1 in 4000 (Fig. 8.13 and Box 8.9). This condition was initially diagnosed on the basis of the appearance of an apparent gap or break (a fragile site) in the distal part of the long arm of the X chromosome. Diagnosis is now achieved by molecular analysis of the CGG trinucleotide repeat expansion in the relevant gene (*FMR1*).

Although it is inherited as an X-linked recessive disorder, a substantial proportion of obligate female carriers have learning difficulties (usually mild to moderate) and around one-fifth of males who inherit the mutation are phenotypically normal but may pass the disorder on to their grandsons through their daughters.

These unusual findings are explained by the nature of the mutation, which occurs in 'pre-mutation' and 'full mutation' forms. The normal copy of the gene contains fewer than 50 copies of the CGG trinucleotide repeat sequence and is stable when transmitted to offspring. Genes with the pre-mutation contain 55–199 copies of the repeat sequence. This expansion causes no intellectual disability in male or female carriers, but is unstable and may become larger during transmission through females. Genes with the full mutation contain more than 200 copies of the repeat sequence. This affects gene function, causing the clinical features of fragile X syndrome in virtually all males and around half of female carriers. These full mutations always arise from expansion of pre-mutations, and never arise directly from normal genes. Hence all mothers of affected males are carriers.

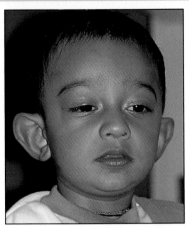

Box 8.9 Clinical findings in males in fragile X syndrome

- Moderate–severe learning difficulty (IQ 20–80, mean 50)
- Macrocephaly
- Macro-orchidism – postpubertal
- Characteristic facies – long face, large everted ears, prominent mandible and broad forehead, most evident in affected adults
- Other features – mitral valve prolapse, joint laxity, scoliosis, autism, hyperactivity.

Figure 8.13 A child with fragile X syndrome. At this age, the main physical feature is often the prominent ears.

 Fragile X syndrome is the commonest familial form of learning difficulties and the second most common genetic cause of severe learning difficulties after Down syndrome.

Mitochondrial or cytoplasmic inheritance

Mitochondria are cytoplasmic organelles that function as major energy producers for the cell and contain their own DNA (mtDNA). Each cell contains thousands of copies of the mitochondrial genome. Inherited disorders of the mitochondria may result from mutations in the nuclear genome (the chromosomal genome of the cell nucleus) or in the mitochondria's own genome. In disorders of the mtDNA, the mutation may be present in all or only some of the mitochondria, so that the tissues affected and the severity of the condition can be highly variable. Large deletions of the mtDNA can only be present in a proportion of the mitochondria as they would otherwise be lethal to the cell. Mutations in mtDNA cause overlapping clusters of disease phenotypes (e.g. Leber hereditary optic neuropathy and various mitochondrial myopathies and encephalopathies, MERFF, MELAS, NARP). Mitochondrial DNA mutations show only maternal transmission, since only the egg contributes mitochondria to the zygote.

Imprinting and uniparental disomy

In the past, it was assumed that the activity of a gene is the same regardless of whether it is inherited from the mother or father. It has been shown that the expression of some genes is influenced by the sex of the parent who had transmitted it. This phenomenon is called 'imprinting'. An example involves Prader–Willi syndrome (PWS) (hypotonia, developmental delay, hyperphagia and obesity). The PWS chromosomal region is found at 15q11–13 (i.e. at bands 11–13 on the long arm of chromosome 15). The paternal copy of this chromosomal region has to function for normal development; in its absence, a child will develop PWS. Failure to inherit a functioning maternal copy of this chromosomal region results in an entirely different condition, Angelman syndrome (AS) (causing severe cognitive impairment, a characteristic facial appearance, ataxia and epilepsy), because only the maternal copy of one particular gene in this region is able to function (the paternal copy is inactive because of imprinting). There are two main ways that a child can develop one or other condition:

- De novo *deletion* (Fig. 8.14). Parental chromosomes are normal, and a deletion occurs as a new mutation in the child. If the deletion occurs on the paternal chromosome 15, the child has Prader–Willi syndrome. If the deletion affects the maternal chromosome 15, the child has Angelman syndrome.
- *Uniparental disomy* (Fig. 8.15). This is when a child inherits two copies of a chromosome from one parent and none from the other parent. In Prader–Willi syndrome the affected child has no paternal (but two maternal) copies of chromosome 15q11–13. In Angelman syndrome, the affected child has no maternal (but two paternal) copies of chromosome 15q11–13. This can be detected with DNA analysis.
- There exist other mechanisms that can lead to these conditions.

 Imprinting is the unusual property of some genes that express only the copy derived from the parent of a given sex.

Genetics

Imprinting

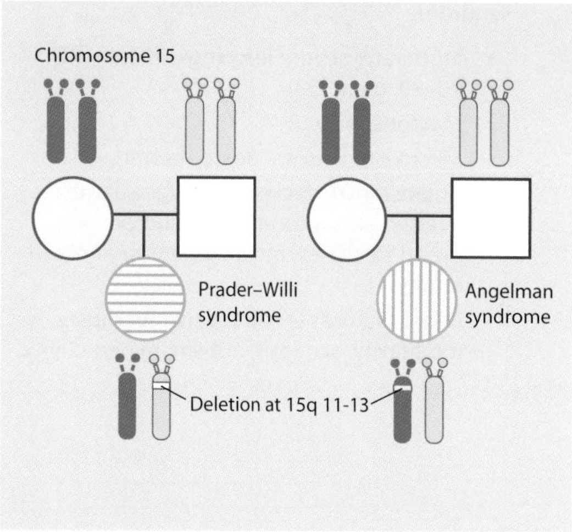

Figure 8.14 Genetic disorder resulting from deletion of an imprinted gene. If the deletion occurs on chromosome 15 inherited from the father, the child has Prader–Willi syndrome. If the deletion occurs on chromosome 15 from the mother, the child has Angelman syndrome.

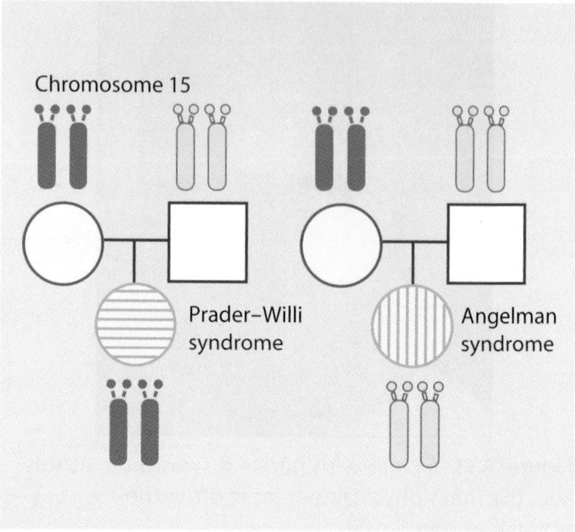

Figure 8.15 Genetic disorder resulting from uniparental disomy affecting imprinted chromosome region. A child who inherits two maternal chromosome 15s will have Prader–Willi syndrome. A child who inherits two paternal chromosome 15s will have Angelman syndrome.

Polygenic, multifactorial or complex inheritance

There is a spectrum in the aetiology of disease, from environmental factors (e.g. trauma) at one end to purely genetic causes (e.g. Mendelian disorder) at the other. Between these two extremes are many disorders which result from the interacting effects of several genes (hence the term polygenic) with or without the influence of environmental or other unknown factors, including chance (multifactorial or complex). The terms are used interchangeably (Box 8.10).

Normal quantitative traits such as height and intelligence are inherited in this fashion, with many relevant influences including genetic constitution, environmental exposures and early life (including intrauterine) experiences. These parameters show a Gaussian (or 'normal') distribution in the population. Similarly, the liability of an individual to develop a disease of multifactorial or polygenic aetiology has a Gaussian distribution. The condition occurs when a certain threshold level of liability is exceeded. Relatives of an affected person show an increased liability due to inheritance of genes conferring susceptibility, and so a greater proportion of them than in the general population will fall beyond the threshold and will manifest the disorder (Fig. 8.16). The risk of recurrence of a polygenic disorder in a family is usually low and is most significant for first-degree relatives. Empirical recurrence risk data are used for genetic counselling. They are derived from family studies that have reported the frequency at which various family members are affected. Factors that increase the risk to relatives are:

- having a more severe form of the disorder, e.g. the risk of recurrence to siblings is greater in bilateral cleft lip and palate than in unilateral cleft lip alone
- close relationship to the affected person, e.g. overall risk to siblings or children is greater than to more distant relatives
- multiple affected family members, e.g. the more siblings already affected, the greater the risk of recurrence
- sex difference in prevalence, with the recurrence risk greater in the more commonly affected sex and if the affected individual is of the less commonly affected sex.

The phenotype (clinical picture) of a disorder may have a heterogeneous (mixed) basis in different families; e.g. hyperlipidaemia leading to atherosclerosis and coronary heart disease can be due to a single gene disorder such as autosomal dominant familial hypercholesterolaemia, but some forms of hyperlipidaemia are polygenic and result from an interaction of the effect of several genes and dietary factors on various lipoproteins.

In some complex disorders, such as Hirschprung disease, the molecular genetic basis and the important contribution of new mutations is becoming clear.

In many multifactorial disorders, the 'environmental factors' remain obscure. Clear exceptions include dietary fat intake and smoking in atherosclerosis, and viral infection in insulin-dependent diabetes mellitus.

Multifactorial, polygenic or complex inheritance

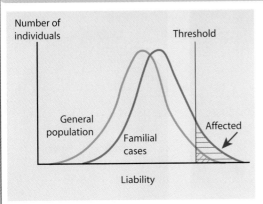

Figure 8.16 Diagram showing the increased liability to a multifactorial disorder in relatives of an affected person.

Box 8.10 Conditions often associated with multifactorial (polygenic, complex) inheritance

Congenital malformations
- Neural tube defects (anencephaly and spina bifida)
- Congenital heart disease
- Cleft lip and palate
- Pyloric stenosis
- Congenital dislocation of the hip
- Talipes equinovarus
- Hypospadias

Childhood
- Atopy (especially asthma and eczema)
- Epilepsy
- Diabetes mellitus type 1 (insulin-dependent diabetes)

Adult life
- Atherosclerosis and coronary artery disease
- Diabetes mellitus type 2
- Alzheimer's disease
- Malignancy (especially the common cancers, e.g. breast and colorectal cancer)
- Hypertension
- Cerebrovascular disease (especially stroke).

For neural tube defects, the risk of recurrence to siblings is lowered from about 4% to 1% or less in future pregnancies if the mother takes folic acid before conception and in the early weeks of pregnancy.

Dysmorphology

The term 'dysmorphology' literally means 'the study of abnormal form' and refers to the assessment of birth defects and unusual physical features that have their origin during embryogenesis.

Pathogenic mechanisms

Malformation

A primary structural defect occurring during the development of a tissue or organ, e.g. spina bifida, cleft lip and palate.

Deformation

Implies an abnormal intrauterine mechanical force that distorts a normally formed structure, e.g. joint contractures or pulmonary hypoplasia due to fetal compression caused by severe oligohydramnios.

Disruption

Involves destruction of a fetal part which initially formed normally, e.g. amniotic membrane rupture may lead to amniotic bands which may cause limb reduction defects.

Dysplasia

Refers to abnormal cellular organisation or function of specific tissue types, e.g. skeletal dysplasias, dysplastic kidney disease.

Clinical classification of birth defects

Single-system defects

These include single congenital malformations, such as spina bifida, which are often multifactorial in nature with fairly low recurrence risks.

Sequence

Refers to a pattern of multiple abnormalities occurring after one initiating defect. Potter syndrome (fetal compression and pulmonary hypoplasia) is an example of a sequence in which all abnormalities may be traced to one original malformation, renal agenesis.

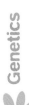

Genetics

127

Syndromes recognised by 'Gestalt' (clinical recognition)

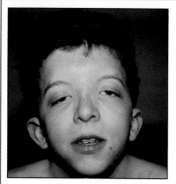

Figure 8.17 Noonan syndrome affects males and females. There are some similarities to the phenotype in Turner syndrome, but it is caused by mutation in an autosomal dominant gene and the karyotype is normal.

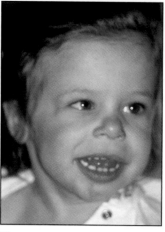

Figure 8.18 Williams syndrome is usually sporadic.

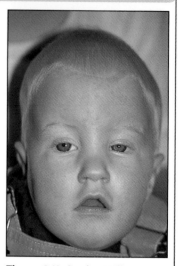

Figure 8.19 Prader–Willi syndrome.

Box 8.11 Clinical features of Noonan syndrome

- Characteristic facies
- Occasional mild learning difficulties
- Short webbed neck with trident hair line
- Pectus excavatum
- Short stature
- Congenital heart disease (especially pulmonary stenosis, atrial septal defect).

Box 8.12 Clinical features of Williams syndrome

- Short stature
- Characteristic facies
- Transient neonatal hypercalcaemia (occasionally)
- Congenital heart disease (supravalvular aortic stenosis)
- Mild to moderate learning difficulties.

Box 8.13 Clinical features of Prader–Willi syndrome

- Characteristic facies
- Hypotonia
- Neonatal feeding difficulties
- Failure to thrive in infancy
- Obesity in later childhood
- Hypogonadism
- Developmental delay
- Learning difficulties.

Association

A group of malformations that occur together more often than expected by chance, but in different combinations from case to case, e.g. VACTERL association (Vertebral anomalies, Anal atresia, Cardiac defects, Tracheo-oEsophageal fistula, Renal anomalies, Limb defects).

Syndrome

When a particular set of multiple anomalies occurs repeatedly in a consistent pattern and there is known or thought to be a common underlying causal mechanism, this is called a 'syndrome'. Multiple malformation syndromes are often associated with moderate or severe cognitive impairment and may be due to:

- chromosomal defects
- a single gene defect (dominant, recessive or sex-linked)
- exposure to teratogens such as alcohol, drugs (especially anticonvulsants such as valproate, carbamazepine and phenytoin) or viral infections during pregnancy
- unknown cause.

Syndrome diagnosis

Although most syndromes are individually rare, recognition of a dysmorphic syndrome is worthwhile as it may give information regarding:

- risk of recurrence
- prognosis
- likely complications which can be sought and perhaps treated successfully if detected early
- the avoidance of unnecessary investigations
- experience and information which parents can share with other affected families through family support groups.

Examples of syndromes recognisable by facial appearance are shown in Figures 8.17–8.19 (see also Boxes 8.11–8.13). The importance and impact of syndrome diagnosis is demonstrated in Case History 8.1. Databases are available to assist with the recognition of thousands of multiple congenital anomaly syndromes (e.g. London Dysmorphology Database (LDDB) & POSSUM).

Summary

Dysmorphology

- comprises birth defects and abnormal clinical features originating during embryogenesis
- may be a malformation, deformation, disruption or dysplasia
- may be classified as a single-system defect, sequence, association or syndrome
- syndromes are recognised by 'Gestalt' (clinical recognition).

Gene-based therapies

The treatment of most genetic disorders is based on conventional therapeutic approaches.

Gene therapy involves the repair, suppression or artificial introduction of genes into genetically abnormal cells with the aim of curing the disease and is at an experimental stage for most genetic conditions being studied. There are still many technical and safety issues to be resolved. Gene therapy has been initiated in adenosine deaminase deficiency (a rare recessive immune disorder), malignant melanoma and cystic fibrosis, and

Case History

8.1 Syndrome diagnosis and genetic counselling

Sean, the second child of healthy parents, was born at term by emergency caesarean section for fetal distress. The pregnancy had been uneventful and no abnormalities were detected on antenatal ultrasound scan. He developed respiratory distress and investigation for a cardiac murmur revealed an interrupted aortic arch and ventricular septal defect that required surgical correction in the neonatal period.

The parents asked about recurrence risk for congenital heart disease and were referred to the genetic clinic. At that time, Sean was thriving and early developmental progress appeared normal. On examination, there were minor dysmorphic features, including a short philtrum, thin upper lip and prominent ears (Fig. 8.20). There was no family history of congenital heart disease or other significant problems and no abnormalities were detected on examination of the parents.

Because of an association between outflow tract abnormalities of the heart and deletions of chromosome 22, cytogenetic analysis was performed using fluorescent in situ hybridisation (FISH). A submicroscopic deletion of the long arm of one chromosome 22 (band 22q11) was detected. Other features of DiGeorge syndrome (hypocalcaemia and T-cell deficiency), which occurs with the same chromosome deletion, were excluded by appropriate tests but could have been important in Sean's medical management.

Parental chromosome analysis showed no deletion at chromosome 22q11 in either parent, indicating a low recurrence risk for future pregnancies since gonadal mosaicism for this deletion is very rare. The older sibling was also normal on testing. Because the parents had normal karyotypes, their own brothers and sisters did not need to be offered tests.

Identification of a 22q11 deletion indicated that other associated problems were likely. Subsequently, Sean required assessment by a multidisciplinary child development team (for developmental delay), that

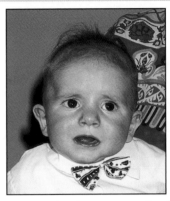

Figure 8.20 Sean's facial appearance showing the short philtrum (vertical groove in the upper lip), thin upper lip and prominent ears.

led to educational statementing and recommendation for appropriate placement in a school for children with special educational needs (learning difficulty), input from a clinical psychologist when behavioural problems appeared (ritualistic behaviour and obsessional tendencies), input from speech therapist and plastic surgeon (indistinct speech due to velopharyngeal incompetence) and audiology review (conductive hearing loss due to recurrent otitis media).

The impact of the diagnosis and its implications was considerable for the family and the parents needed support from a variety of professionals while coming to terms with the various problems as they became apparent. Written information and details of the 22q11 support group were given to the parents. Medical care was coordinated by the paediatrician.

There was the additional worry for the family about a subsequent pregnancy. Fetal echocardiography showed no evidence of congenital heart disease, but invasive tests for cytogenetic analysis were declined because of the low recurrence risk. The baby was born unaffected, with chromosome studies performed on a cord blood sample revealing no abnormality.

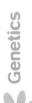

Genetics

some clinical benefit has been reported in a few patients. At present, it is generally accepted that gene therapy should be limited to somatic (not germline) cells, so that the risk of adversely affecting future generations is minimised.

However, other treatments based upon a genetic understanding of disease are being introduced into practice. Two examples are:

- Suppressors of nonsense (stop codon, chain-terminating) mutations, which are under trial in patients with cystic fibrosis and Duchenne muscular dystrophy caused by the appropriate mutations.
- Antisense oligo-DNA molecules that cause the skipping of specific exons in the Duchenne muscular dystrophy gene, i.e. complementary DNA molecules that bind and block exons around the faulty part of the gene (often deletions or duplications in Duchenne muscular dystrophy). This approach can restore the reading frame of the message downstream of the causal deletion; it is hoped that this will result in a milder form of the disease.

Genetic services

In the UK, all health regions have a clinical genetics centre where specialist genetic services are provided by consultants and other medical staff, genetic counsellors and laboratory scientists. Specialist genetic investigations and counselling are provided at the centre and at secondary and primary care. Increased recognition of disorders antenatally has necessitated expansion of perinatal genetic services in addition to paediatric and adult services.

Genetic investigations

For many years genetic investigation relied on determining the karyotype by visualisation under the microscope. This has been transformed by the tremendous advances in molecular testing.

DNA analysis using polymerase chain reaction (PCR) allows rapid analysis on small samples. Its main impact for genetic counselling is:

- Confirmation of a clinical diagnosis of an increasing number of single gene disorders
- Detection of female carriers in X-linked disorders, e.g. Duchenne and Becker muscular dystrophies, haemophilia A and B
- Carrier detection in autosomal recessive disorders, e.g. cystic fibrosis
- Presymptomatic diagnosis in autosomal dominant disorders, e.g. Huntington disease, myotonic dystrophy, familial cancer syndromes
- Antenatal diagnosis of an increasing number of Mendelian conditions.

These are accomplished by the following.

Mutation analysis

For an increasing number of Mendelian disorders, it is possible to directly detect the actual mutation causing the disease. This provides very accurate results for confirmation of diagnosis, and presymptomatic or predictive testing. Identifying the mutation in an affected individual may be very time-consuming, but once this has been done, testing other relatives is usually fairly simple. Examples are:

- *Deletions*: large deletion mutations are common in a variety of disorders including Duchenne and Becker muscular dystrophies, alpha-thalassaemia and 21-hydroxylase deficiency (congenital adrenal hyperplasia).
- *Point mutations and small deletions*: these can be readily identified if the same mutation causes all cases of the disorder, as in sickle cell disease. For most disorders, however, there is a spectrum of mutations. About 78% of cystic fibrosis carriers in the UK possess the ΔF508 mutation, but over 900 other mutations have been identified. Most laboratories test for a certain number of the most common mutations in the population they serve.
- *Trinucleotide repeat expansion mutations*: these are readily tested for because the mutation in a given disease is virtually always at the same site and can be amplified from the same oligo-DNA primers used in the amplification by PCR: the only difference is the size of the repeat sequence, which can be determined from the size of the DNA fragment containing the repeat.

Genetic linkage

If mutation analysis is not available, it may be possible to use DNA sequence variations (markers) located near to, or within, the disease gene to track the inheritance of this gene through a family. This type of analysis requires a suitable family structure and several key members need to be tested to identify appropriate markers before linkage testing can be used in diagnostic, predictive or prenatal testing.

Some of the genetic investigations now available are summarised in Table 8.2.

Genetic counselling

The main aims of genetic counselling are supportive and educational. Genetic counselling aims to support and provide information for individuals, couples and families:

- To understand their situation
- To make their own decisions about managing the disease or risk of disease, including decisions about genetic testing and reproduction
- To adjust to their situation of being affected by or at risk of the genetic condition.

A primary goal of genetic counselling is to provide information to allow for greater autonomy and choice in reproductive decisions and other areas of personal life. Avoiding additional cases of genetic disease in a family may be a consequence of genetic counselling but is not the primary aim. The elements of genetic counselling include:

- Listening to the questions and concerns of the patient, client or family.

Table 8.2 Genetic investigations

Investigation	Application
Cytogenetic analysis – karyotype	Chromosomes stained and visualised under a microscope
	Detects alterations in chromosome number and structural rearrangements; this method is being replaced by molecular methods such as CGH.
Molecular cytogenetic analysis – FISH (fluorescent in situ hybridisation)	Fluorescent-labelled DNA probes to detect the presence, number and chromosomal location of specific chromosomal sequences
	Useful for microdeletion syndromes
Microarray comparative genomic hybridisation (aCGH)	Detects chromosomal imbalances using thousands of DNA probes to investigate a whole genome with much greater sensitivity than cytogenetic methods
DNA analysis	Polymerase chain reaction (PCR) to amplify the DNA and determine the sequence of the relevant gene
High throughput DNA sequencing	Rapid sequencing of whole genomes or many loci within the genome
Linkage disequilibrium and genome-wide association studies (GWAS)	Comparing the frequency of combinations of alleles at nearby loci in a given population to identify genetic variants associated with complex diseases

- Establishing the correct diagnosis. This involves detailed history, examination and appropriate investigations that may include chromosome or DNA or other molecular genetic analysis, biochemical tests, X-rays and clinical photographs. Despite extensive investigation, including searching databases, the diagnosis may remain unknown, e.g. in children with learning disability and mild or non-specific dysmorphic features.
- Risk estimation. This requires both diagnostic and pedigree information. Drawing a pedigree of three generations is an essential part of a clinical genetic assessment. The mode of inheritance may be apparent from the pedigree even when the precise diagnosis is not known. In some cases it may not be possible to define a precise recurrence risk and uncertainty may remain, e.g. conditions that only affect one member of a family and are known to follow autosomal dominant inheritance in some families and autosomal recessive inheritance in others (genetic heterogeneity).
- Communication. Information must be presented in an understandable and unbiased way. Families often find written information helpful to refer back to and diagrams are often used to explain patterns of inheritance. The impact of saying 'the recurrence risk is 5% or 1 in 20' may be different from saying 'the chance of an unaffected child is 95% or 19 out of 20', and so both should be presented.
- Discussing options for management and prevention. If there appears to be a risk to offspring, all reproductive options should be discussed. These include not having (any more)

Box 8.14 Influences on decisions regarding options for genetic counselling

- Magnitude of risk
- Perceived severity of disorder
- Availability of treatment
- Person's experience of the disorder
- Family size
- Availability of a safe and reliable prenatal diagnostic test
- Parental cultural, religious or ethical values.

children, reducing intended family size, taking the risk and proceeding with pregnancy or having antenatal diagnosis and selective termination of an affected fetus. For some couples donor insemination or ovum donation may be appropriate and for others achieving a pregnancy through IVF (in vitro fertilisation) and preimplantation diagnosis may be possible.

Counselling should be non-directive, but should also assist in the decision-making process (Box 8.14). Information from lay support groups may also be helpful.

 Genetic counselling aims to allow parents greater autonomy and choice in reproductive decisions.

Pre-symptomatic (predictive) testing

Children may be referred because they are at increased risk of developing a genetic disorder in childhood or adult life.

If the condition is likely to manifest in childhood (e.g. Duchenne muscular dystrophy) or if there are useful medical interventions available in childhood (e.g. screening by colonoscopy for colorectal tumours in children at risk of familial adenomatosis poly-posis coli), then genetic testing is appropriate in childhood.

If the child is at risk of a late-onset and untreatable disorder (e.g. Huntington disease) or if the genetic test result is only relevant to reproductive questions in the future (the child's genetic carrier status), then there is a case for deferring genetic testing until the child can be actively involved in making the decision. These difficult issues are often best handled through a process of genetic counselling supporting open and sustained communication within the family and especially between parents and children.

 Pre-symptomatic testing of disorders which manifest in adult life should not be performed until the individual can give informed consent.

Further reading

Firth HV, Hurst JA, Hall JG: *Oxford Desk Reference – Clinical Genetics*, Oxford, 2005, Oxford University Press.

Harper PS: *Practical Genetic Counselling*, ed 7, London, 2010, Arnold.

Book on the clinical approach to genetics and genetic counselling

Jones KL: *Smith's Recognisable Patterns of Human Malformation*, ed 5, Philadelphia, 2005, WB Saunders.

Diagnosing syndromes

Kingston HM: *ABC of Clinical Genetics*, ed 3, London, 2002, BMJ Books.

Read A, Donnai D: *The New Clinical Genetics* ed 2, Bloxham, 2010, Scion.

Strachan T, Read AP: *Human Molecular Genetics*, ed 4, London, 2010, Garland.

Turnpenny P, Ellard S: *Emery's Elements of Medical Genetics*, ed 13, Edinburgh, 2007, Churchill Livingstone.

General introduction to medical genetics

Young ID: *Medical Genetics*, Oxford (Oxford Core Texts), 2005, Oxford University Press.

Websites (Accessed January 2011)

Contact-a-family: Available at: www.cafamily.org.uk.

UK family support group alliance.

Decipher: Available at: http://decipher.sanger.ac.uk.

Database of Chromosome Imbalance and Phenotype in Humans using Ensembl Resources.

E!Ensembl: Available at: http://www.ensembl.org.

Genome browser

GeneTests: http://www.genetests.org.

Review articles on selected genetic disorders.

NCBI MapViewer: Available at: http://www.ncbi.nlm.nih.gov/projects/mapview.

Genome browser

OMIM (Online Mendelian Inheritance in Man): Available at: http://www.ncbi.nlm.nih.gov/omim.

The British, European and American Societies of Human Genetics: Available at: http://www.bshg.org.uk, http://www.eshg.org and http://www.ashg.org.

Websites include professional and policy pages.

Your Genes, Your Health: Available at: http://www.ygyh.org.

Cold Spring Harbor website giving information on some common genetic disorders and links to DNA tutorials.

Perinatal medicine

The term 'perinatal medicine' refers to medical care of the infant before, during and after birth, acknowledging the continuity of fetal and neonatal life. Using modern technology, such as high-resolution ultrasound and DNA analysis, detailed information about the fetus can now be obtained for a large and increasing number of conditions. Close cooperation is important between the professionals involved in the care of the pregnant mother and fetus and those caring for the newborn infant.

Some definitions used in perinatal medicine are:

- Stillbirth – fetus born with no signs of life ≥24 weeks of pregnancy
- Perinatal mortality rate – stillbirths + deaths within the first week per 1000 live births and stillbirths
- Neonatal mortality rate – deaths of liveborn infants within the first 4 weeks after birth per 1000 live births
- Neonate – infant ≤28 days old
- Preterm – gestation <37 weeks of pregnancy
- Term – 37–41 weeks of pregnancy
- Post-term – gestation ≥42 weeks of pregnancy
- Low birthweight (LBW) – <2500 g
- Very low birthweight (VLBW) – <1500 g
- Extremely low birthweight (ELBW) – <1000 g
- Small for gestational age – birthweight <10th centile for gestational age
- Large for gestational age – birthweight >90th centile for gestational age.

Pre-pregnancy care

The better a mother's state of health and nutrition, and the higher her socioeconomic living standard and the quality of healthcare she receives, the greater is the chance of a successful outcome to her pregnancy.

Couples planning to have a baby often ask what they should do to optimise their chances of having a healthy child. They can be informed that for the mother:

- *Smoking* reduces birthweight, which may be of critical importance if born preterm. On average, the babies of smokers weigh 170 g less than those of non-smokers, but the reduction in birthweight is related to the number of cigarettes smoked per day. Smoking is also associated with an increased risk of miscarriage and stillbirth. The infant has a greater risk of sudden infant death syndrome (SIDS).
- *Pre-pregnancy folic acid* supplements reduce the risk of neural tube defects in the fetus. Low-dose folic acid supplementation is recommended for all women planning a pregnancy. A higher dose is recommended for women with, or have a close relative with, a previously affected fetus.
- Any long-term conditions, such as diabetes and epilepsy, must be reviewed and management changed if necessary.
- *Certain medications* such as retinoids, warfarin and sodium valproate must be avoided because of teratogenic effects.
- *Alcohol* ingestion and *drug abuse* (opiates, cocaine) may damage the fetus.
- *Congenital rubella* is preventable by maternal immunisation before pregnancy.
- *Exposure to toxoplasmosis* should be minimised by avoiding eating undercooked meat and by wearing gloves when handling cat litter.
- *Listeria infection* can be acquired from eating unpasteurised dairy products, soft ripened

cheeses, e.g. brie, camembert and blue veined varieties, patés and ready-to-eat poultry, unless thoroughly re-heated.

- *Eating liver* during pregnancy is best avoided as it contains a high concentration of vitamin A.

Any pre-existing maternal medical condition (e.g. hypertension, HIV) or obstetric risk factors for complications of pregnancy or delivery (e.g. recurrent miscarriage or previous preterm delivery) should be identified and treated or monitored. Obesity increases the risk of developing gestational diabetes and pregnancy-induced hypertension.

Couples at increased risk of inherited disorders should receive genetic counselling before pregnancy. They can then be fully informed, decide whether or not to proceed, and consider antenatal diagnosis if available. Pregnancies at increased risk of fetal abnormality include those in which:

- the mother is older (if she is >35 years old, the risk of Down syndrome is >1 in 380), although screening is now available for all mothers
- there is previous congenital abnormality
- there is a family history of an inherited disorder
- the parents are identified as carriers of an autosomal recessive disorder, e.g. thalassaemia
- a parent carries a chromosomal rearrangement
- parents are close blood relatives.

 Pre-pregnancy folic acid supplements reduce the risk of neural tube defects in the fetus.

Antenatal diagnosis

Antenatal diagnosis has become available for an increasing number of disorders. Screening tests performed on maternal blood and ultrasound of the fetus are listed in Box 9.1. The main diagnostic techniques for antenatal diagnosis are maternal serum screening, detailed ultrasound scanning, chorionic villus sampling (at >10 weeks of pregnancy) and amniocentesis (>15 weeks) (Fig. 9.1). In some rare conditions, preimplantation genetic diagnosis (PGD) allows genetic analysis of cells from a developing embryo before transfer to the uterus. The structural malformations and other lesions which can be identified on ultrasound are listed in Box 9.2, with an example in Figure 9.2.

Antenatal screening for disorders affecting the mother or fetus allows:

- reassurance where disorders are not detected
- optimal obstetric management of the mother and fetus
- interventions for a limited number of conditions, such as relieving bladder obstruction or draining pleural effusions, to improve perinatal outcome
- counselling and neonatal management to be planned in advance
- the option of termination of pregnancy to be offered for severe disorders affecting the fetus (see Case History 9.1) or compromising maternal health.

Parents require accurate medical advice and counselling to help them with these difficult decisions. Many

Box 9.1 Screening tests for antenatal diagnosis

Maternal blood	Blood group and antibodies – for rhesus and other red cell incompatibilities
	Hepatitis B
	Syphilis
	Rubella
	HIV infection
	Neural tube defects – raised maternal serum alphafetoprotein (MSAFP) with spina bifida or anencephaly, but ultrasound alone increasingly used
	Down syndrome – risk estimate calculated from age, biochemical markers combined with ultrasound screening for nuchal translucency (back of neck). Aim is to detect >75% with <3% false-positive rate. If high risk, fetal chromosome analysis is offered
Ultrasound screening	Gestational age – can be estimated reliably if early in pregnancy
	Multiple pregnancies – can be identified
	Structural malformation – 50–70% of major congenital malformations can be detected. If a significant abnormality is suspected, a more detailed scan by a specialist is indicated
	Fetal growth – can be monitored by serial measurement of abdominal circumference, head circumference and femur length
	Amniotic fluid volume – oligohydramnios may result from reduced fetal urine production (because of dysplastic or absent kidneys or obstructive uropathy), from prolonged rupture of the membranes or associated with severe intrauterine growth restriction. It may cause pulmonary hypoplasia and limb and facial deformities from pressure on the fetus (Potter syndrome)
	Polyhydramnios – is associated with maternal diabetes and structural gastrointestinal abnormalities, e.g. atresia in the fetus

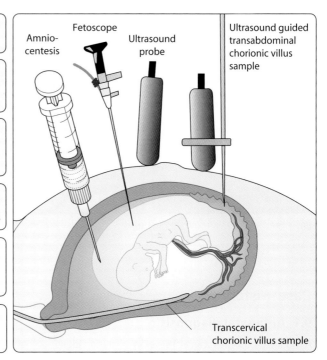

| **Amniocentesis** |
| Chromosome/micro-array and DNA analysis |
| Fetal infection – PCR |

| **Fetal blood sampling** |
| Fetal haemoglobin for anaemia |
| Fetal infection serology |
| Fetal blood transfusion |

| **Chorionic villus sampling** |
| Chromosome/micro-array and DNA analysis |
| Fetal infection – PCR |
| Enzyme analysis of inborn error of metabolism |

| **Preimplantation genetic diagnosis (PGD)** |
| In vitro fertilisation allows genetic analysis of cells from developing embryo before transfer to the uterus |

| **Fetoscopy** |
| Minimally invasive surgery, e.g. laser photo-coagulation of communicating vessels in twin–twin transfusion syndrome. |

| **Non-invasive genetic diagnosis – free fetal DNA from maternal blood** |
| Identification of fetal gender and rhesus status |

Figure 9.1 Some of the techniques used for antenatal diagnosis.

Box 9.2 Main structural malformations and other lesions detectable by ultrasound

CNS	Anencephaly – always detected
	Spina bifida
	Hydrocephalus, microcephaly, encephalocele
Cardiac	About 50% of severe malformations detected on 'routine' screening, over 90% at specialist centres
Intrathoracica	Diaphragmatic hernia, congenital cystadenomatoid lung malformation (CCAM)
	Oesophageal atresia
Facial	Cleft lip
Gastrointestinal	Bowel obstruction, e.g. duodenal atresia
	Exomphalos and gastroschisis
Genitourinary	Dysplastic or cystic kidneys
	Obstructive disorders of kidneys or urinary tract (hydronephrosis, distended bladder)
Skeletal	Skeletal dysplasias, e.g. achondroplasia and limb reduction deformities
Hydrops	Oedema of the skin, pleural effusions and ascites
Chromosomal	Down syndrome – suspected from thickened back of neck (nuchal translucency), duodenal atresia or an atrioventricular canal defect of the heart. Other chromosomal disorders – from identifying multiple abnormalities

transient or minor structural disorders of the fetus are also detected, which may cause considerable anxiety.

 Antenatal diagnosis allows many congenital malformations which used to be diagnosed at birth or during infancy to be identified before birth.

Fetal medicine

The fetus can sometimes be treated by giving medication to the mother. Examples include:

- *Glucocorticoid therapy* before preterm delivery accelerates lung maturity and surfactant production. This has been tested in over 15 randomised trials and markedly reduces

Example of antenatal diagnosis-gastroschisis

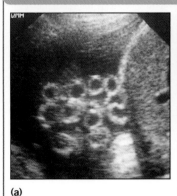
(a)

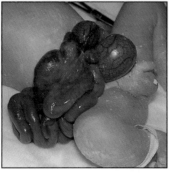
(b)

Figure 9.2 Gastroschisis on antenatal ultrasound showing free loops of small bowel in the amniotic fluid **(a)** and following delivery **(b)**. Antenatal diagnosis allowed the baby to be delivered at a paediatric surgical unit and the parents to be forewarned about the need for surgery. Satisfactory surgical repair was achieved. (Courtesy of Mr Karl Murphy.)

Case History

9.1 Antenatal diagnosis

A routine ultrasound scan at 18 weeks' gestation identified an abnormal 'lemon-shaped' skull (Fig. 9.3). This, together with an abnormal appearance of the cerebellum, is the Arnold–Chiari malformation, which is associated with spina bifida. An extensive spinal defect was confirmed on ultrasound. Dilatation of the cerebral ventricles and talipes already present in this fetus suggested a severe spinal lesion. After counselling, the parents decided to terminate the pregnancy.

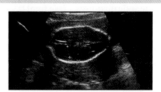

Figure 9.3 Transverse section showing a 'lemon-shaped' skull on ultrasound instead of the normal oval shape. This is associated with spina bifida. (Courtesy of Mr Guy Thorpe-Beeston.)

the incidence of respiratory distress syndrome (RDS) (relative risk 0.66), of intraventricular haemorrhage (relative risk 0.54) and neonatal mortality (relative risk 0.69) in preterm infants. For optimal effect, a completed course needs to be given at least 24 h before delivery.

- *Digoxin or flecainide* can be given to the mother to treat fetal supraventricular tachycardia.

There are a few conditions where therapy can be given to the fetus directly:

- *Rhesus isoimmunisation.* Severely affected fetuses become anaemic and may develop *hydrops fetalis*, with oedema and ascites. Infants at risk are identified by maternal antibody screening. Regular ultrasound of the fetus is performed to detect fetal anaemia non-invasively using Doppler velocimetry of the fetal middle cerebral artery. Fetal blood transfusion via the umbilical vein may be required regularly from about 20 weeks' gestation. The incidence of rhesus haemolytic disease has fallen markedly since anti-D immunisation of mothers was introduced but hydrops fetalis is still seen due to other red blood cell antibodies such as Kell.
- *Perinatal isoimmune thrombocytopenia.* This condition is analogous to rhesus isoimmunisation but involves maternal antiplatelet antibodies crossing the placenta. It is rare, affecting about 1

in 5000 births. Intracranial haemorrhage secondary to fetal thrombocytopenia occurs in up to 25%. The problem may be anticipated if there was a previously affected infant, when prenatal intravenous immunoglobulin can be given or repeated intrauterine platelet transfusions performed.

> *Maternal glucocorticoid therapy before preterm delivery markedly reduces morbidity and mortality in the neonate.*

Fetal surgery

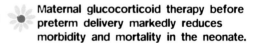

Fetal surgery is a relatively new development with varying results. Procedures which have been performed include:

- Catheter shunts inserted under ultrasound guidance. This is to drain fetal pleural effusions (pleuro-amniotic shunts), often from a chylothorax (lymphatic fluid) or congenital cystic adenomatous malformation of the lung. One end of a looped catheter lies in the chest, the other end in the amniotic cavity.
- Laser therapy to ablate placental anastomoses which lead to the twin–twin transfusion syndrome (TTTS)

- Intrauterine shunting for obstruction to urinary outflow as with posterior urethral valves
- Dilatation of stenotic heart valves via a transabdominal catheter inserted under ultrasound guidance into the fetal heart. Results appear promising
- Endotracheal balloon occlusion for congenital diaphragmatic hernia, as tracheal obstruction in utero may promote lung growth
- Surgical correction by hysterotomy. This is when the uterus is opened at 22–24 weeks' gestation. It has been performed in a few specialist centres for spina bifida but may precipitate preterm delivery and its efficacy remains highly uncertain. Results of fetal surgery to close spina bifida suggest that hydrocephalus may be reduced but does not improve the prognosis of the spinal lesion.

Outcome has mostly been very poor because of the severity of the conditions treated. Careful case selection and follow-up are required to ensure that these novel forms of treatment are of long-term benefit.

Obstetric conditions affecting the fetus

Pre-eclampsia

Mothers with pre-eclampsia may require preterm delivery because of the maternal risks of eclampsia and of cerebrovascular accident or the fetal risks associated with placental insufficiency and growth restriction. Determining the optimal time for preterm delivery requires an evaluation of the risk to the mother and fetus of allowing the pregnancy to continue compared with the neonatal complications associated with preterm birth.

Placental insufficiency and intrauterine growth restriction (IUGR)

Fetal growth may be progressively restricted because of placental insufficiency. Transfer of oxygen and nutrients is reduced. The growth-restricted fetus will need to be monitored closely to prevent intrauterine death. This is done by measuring growth parameters, the biophysical profile (amniotic fluid volume, fetal movement, fetal tone, fetal breathing movements, fetal heart activity) and Doppler blood flow velocity (umbilical and middle cerebral artery). Absence or reversal of flow velocity during diastole carries an increased risk of morbidity from hypoxic damage to the gut or brain, or of intrauterine death. These measurements assist in deciding the optimal time for delivery of a growth-restricted fetus.

Multiple births

Twins occur naturally in the UK in 1 in 90 deliveries, triplets in 1 in 90^2, i.e. approximately 1 in 8000, and quadruplets in 1 in 90^3, i.e. approximately 1 in every 700 000 deliveries. Over the last decade, the number of triplets and higher-order births has more than doubled, mainly from assisted reproduction programmes and advancing maternal age. One in 70 births is now a multiple birth, although the number of triplets and higher-order births has recently declined in the UK.

The main problems for the infant associated with multiple births are:

- *Preterm labour.* The median gestation for twins is 37 weeks, for triplets 34 weeks and for quads 32 weeks. Preterm delivery is the most important cause of the greater perinatal mortality of multiple births, especially for triplets and higher-order pregnancies. When a higher-order pregnancy is identified, embryo reduction may be offered.
- *Intrauterine growth restriction (IUGR).* Fetal growth in one or more fetuses may deteriorate and needs to be monitored regularly.
- *Congenital abnormalities.* These occur twice as frequently as in a singleton, but the risk is increased four-fold in monochorionic twins.
- *Twin–twin transfusion syndrome (TTTS) in monochorionic twins (shared placenta).* May cause extreme preterm delivery, fetal death and discrepancy in growth.
- *Complicated deliveries*, e.g. due to malpresentation of the second twin at vaginal delivery.

Finding sufficient intensive care cots for preterm multiple births can be problematic.

Although multiple births may look endearing, the families may need additional assistance and support:

- Practical – with their care and housework (requires about 200 h/week for triplets in infancy!)
- Emotional and physical exhaustion
- Loss of privacy as a couple
- Additional financial costs
- Increased behavioural problems in the infants and their siblings. While being a multiple birth may provide companionship, affection and stimulation between each other, it may also engender domination, dependency and jealousy.

There are local and national support groups for parents of multiple births.

Summary

Multiple births

- have markedly increased over the last 20 years
- are associated with an increased risk of prematurity, intrauterine growth restriction (IUGR), congenital malformations and twin–twin transfusion syndrome (in monochorionic twins)
- are responsible for 30% of very low birthweight infants (<1.5 kg birthweight)
- provide many additional problems for their parents to care for them.

Maternal conditions affecting the fetus

Diabetes mellitus

Women with insulin-dependent diabetes find it more difficult to maintain good diabetic control during pregnancy and have an increased insulin requirement. Poorly-controlled maternal diabetes is associated with polyhydramnios and pre-eclampsia, increased rate of early fetal loss, congenital malformations and late unexplained intrauterine death. Ketoacidosis carries a high fetal mortality. With meticulous attention to diabetic control, the perinatal mortality rate is now only slightly greater than in non-diabetics. The National Institute for Health and Clinical Excellence (NICE) has produced guidance on the management of diabetes and its complications from preconception to the postnatal period. The emphasis is on aiming for good control of blood glucose.

Fetal problems associated with maternal diabetes are:

- *Congenital malformations.* Overall, there is a 6% risk of congenital malformations, a three-fold increase compared with the non-diabetic population. The range of anomalies is similar to that for the general population, apart from an increased incidence of cardiac malformations, sacral agenesis (caudal regression syndrome) and hypoplastic left colon, although the latter two conditions are rare. Studies show that good diabetic control periconceptionally reduces the risk of congenital malformations.
- *Intrauterine growth restriction (IUGR).* There is a three-fold increase in growth restriction in mothers with long-standing microvascular disease.
- *Macrosomia* (Fig. 9.4). Maternal hyperglycaemia causes fetal hyperglycaemia as glucose crosses the placenta. As insulin does not cross the placenta, the fetus responds with increased secretion of insulin, which promotes growth by increasing both cell number and size. About 25% of such infants have a birthweight greater than 4 kg compared with 8% of non-diabetics. The macrosomia

predisposes to cephalopelvic disproportion, birth asphyxia, shoulder dystocia and brachial plexus injury.

Neonatal problems include:

- *Hypoglycaemia.* Transient hypoglycaemia is common during the first day of life from fetal hyperinsulinism, but can often be prevented by early feeding. The infant's blood glucose should be closely monitored during the first 24 h and hypoglycaemia treated
- *Respiratory distress syndrome (RDS).* More common as lung maturation is delayed
- *Hypertrophic cardiomyopathy.* Hypertrophy of the cardiac septum occurs in some infants. It regresses over several weeks but may cause heart failure from reduced left ventricular function
- *Polycythaemia* (venous haematocrit >0.65). Makes the infant look plethoric. Treatment with partial exchange transfusion to reduce the haematocrit and normalise viscosity may be required.

Gestational diabetes is when carbohydrate intolerance occurs only during pregnancy. Its definition and method of identification remain controversial. It is more common in women who are obese and in those of Afro-Caribbean and Asian ethnicity. The incidence of macrosomia and its complications is similar to that of the insulin-dependent diabetic mother, but the incidence of congenital malformations is not increased. However, there are an increasing number of mothers with type 2 non-insulin dependent diabetes, associated with the increase in obesity in the population. Their fetuses are also at increased risk of congenital malformations.

Summary

Maternal diabetes

- Meticulous control pre-conceptually and during pregnancy markedly reduces fetal and neonatal morbidity and mortality.
- The fetus may be macrosomic because of fetal hyperglycaemia resulting in hyperinsulinism, or growth-restricted secondary to maternal microvascular disease, and is at increased risk of congenital malformations.
- The macrosomic infant is at increased risk of asphyxia and birth trauma from obstructed labour or delivery.
- The newborn infant is prone to hypoglycaemia and polycythaemia.

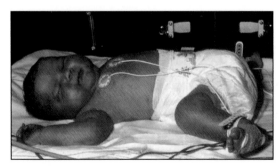

Figure 9.4 Infant of a diabetic mother showing macrosomia and plethora. Born vaginally at 36 weeks' gestation, she weighed 5.5 kg and suffered a right-sided brachial plexus injury.

Hyperthyroidism

If mothers have had Graves' disease, 1–2% of their newborn infants are hyperthyroid, due to circulating thyroid-stimulating antibody, which crosses the placenta and stimulates the fetal thyroid. Hyperthyroidism in the fetus is suggested by fetal tachycardia on the CTG trace, and fetal goitre may be evident on ultrasound; in the neonate it is suggested by irritability, weight loss, tachycardia, heart failure, diarrhoea and exophthalmos. Treatment with anti-thyroid drugs may be necessary for several months until the condition resolves.

Systemic lupus erythematosus

Systemic lupus erythematosus (SLE) with antiphospholipid syndrome is associated with recurrent miscarriage, intrauterine growth restriction, pre-eclampsia, placental abruption and preterm delivery. Some of the infants born to mothers with antibodies to the Ro (SS-A) or La (SS-B) antigens develop neonatal lupus syndrome, in which there is a self-limiting rash and, rarely, heart block.

Autoimmune thrombocytopenic purpura

In maternal autoimmune thrombocytopenic purpura (AITP), the fetus may become thrombocytopenic because maternal IgG antibodies cross the placenta and damage fetal platelets. Severe fetal thrombocytopenia places the fetus at risk of intracranial haemorrhage following birth trauma. Infants with severe thrombocytopenia or petechiae at birth should be given intravenous immunoglobulin. Platelet transfusions may be required if there is acute bleeding.

Maternal drugs affecting the fetus

Relatively few drugs are known definitely to damage the fetus (Table 9.1), but it is clearly advisable for pregnant women to avoid taking medicines unless it is essential. While the teratogenicity of a drug may be recognised if it causes malformations which are severe and distinctive, as with limb shortening following thalidomide ingestion, milder and less distinctive abnormalities may go unrecognised.

The problem of establishing a link may be compounded by a delay of months or years before any problems present. An example of this is diethylstilboestrol (DES), given in the past for threatened miscarriage, and its subsequent association with vaginal adenosis and carcinoma of the vagina and cervix in female offspring during adolescence or early adult life.

Alcohol and smoking

Excessive alcohol ingestion during pregnancy is sometimes associated with the 'fetal alcohol syndrome'. Its clinical features are growth restriction, characteristic face (Fig. 9.5), developmental delay and cardiac defects (up to 70%). The effects of less severe ingestion and binge-drinking remain uncertain but may affect growth and development, and mothers are advised to avoid alcohol (Department of Health, London, UK). Maternal

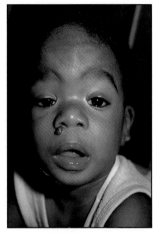

Figure 9.5 Characteristic facies of fetal alcohol syndrome with: a saddle-shaped nose; maxillary hypoplasia; absent philtrum between the nose and upper lip; and short, thin upper lip. This child also has a strawberry naevus below the right nostril.

Table 9.1 Maternal medication which may adversely affect the fetus

Medication	Adverse effect on fetus
Anticonvulsant therapy with carbamazepine, valproic acid (sodium valproate) or hydantoins (phenytoin)	Fetal carbamazepine/valproate/hydantoin syndrome – midfacial hypoplasia, CNS, limb and cardiac malformations, developmental delay
Cytotoxic agents	Congenital malformations
Diethylstilboestrol (DES)	Clear-cell adenocarcinoma of vagina and cervix
Iodides/propylthiouracil	Goitre, hypothyroidism
Lithium	Congenital heart disease
Tetracycline	Enamel hypoplasia of the teeth
Thalidomide	Limb shortening (phocomelia)
Vitamin A and retinoids	Increased spontaneous abortions, abnormal face
Warfarin	Interferes with cartilage formation (nasal hypoplasia and epiphyseal stippling); cerebral haemorrhages and microcephaly

cigarette smoking is associated in the fetus with an increased risk of miscarriage and stillbirth, a reduction in birthweight and IUGR (see pre-pregnancy care, earlier in this chapter).

Drug abuse

Maternal drug abuse with opiates is associated with an increased risk of prematurity and growth restriction. Many narcotic abusers take multiple drugs. Infants of mothers abusing heroin, methadone and other opiates during pregnancy often show evidence of drug withdrawal, with jitteriness, sneezing, yawning, poor feeding, vomiting, diarrhoea, weight loss and seizures during the first 2 weeks of life. Cocaine abuse is associated with placental abruption and preterm delivery, but rarely with withdrawal in the infant, although it may result in cerebral infarction. Amphetamine abuse is also associated with gastrointestinal and cerebral infarction. Mothers who abuse drugs, and their infants, are also at increased risk of hepatitis B and C and HIV infection. Hepatitis B vaccine is given to babies when indicated. Social and child protection aspects must be considered and Social Services involved.

Infants who develop significant features of drug withdrawal require admission to the Neonatal Unit and treatment. Oral morphine, methadone and diazepam are used at different centres. One of the major problems in managing these infants is that the parents' lifestyle and temperament are often not conducive to the needs of babies and young children. Close supervision or alternative caregivers are often required.

 If there are unexplained clinical signs in an infant, consider drug withdrawal.

Drugs given during labour

Potential adverse effects to the fetus of drugs given during labour are:

- *Opioid analgesics/anaesthetic agents*. May suppress respiration at birth
- *Epidural anaesthesia*. May cause maternal pyrexia during labour. It is often difficult to differentiate this from fever caused by an infection. There is an increase in the rate of forceps deliveries
- *Sedatives, e.g. diazepam*. May cause sedation, hypothermia and hypotension in the newborn
- *Oxytocin and prostaglandin F2*. May cause hyperstimulation of the uterus leading to fetal hypoxia. It is also associated with a small increase in bilirubin levels in the neonate
- *Intravenous fluids*. May cause neonatal hyponatraemia unless they contain an adequate concentration of sodium.

Congenital infections

Intrauterine infection is usually from maternal primary infection during pregnancy. Those that can damage the fetus are:

Congenital infections

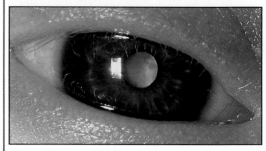

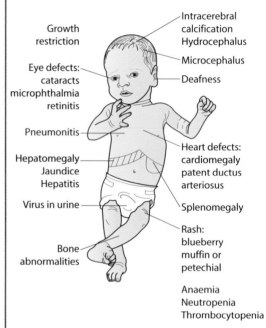

Figure 9.6a Cataract from congenital rubella. Congenital heart disease and deafness are the other common defects.

Growth restriction

Eye defects: cataracts microphthalmia retinitis

Pneumonitis

Hepatomegaly Jaundice Hepatitis

Virus in urine

Bone abnormalities

Intracerebral calcification Hydrocephalus

Microcephalus

Deafness

Heart defects: cardiomegaly patent ductus arteriosus

Splenomegaly

Rash: blueberry muffin or petechial

Anaemia Neutropenia Thrombocytopenia

Figure 9.6b Clinical features of congenital rubella, cytomegalovirus (CMV), toxoplasmosis and syphilis.

- Rubella
- Cytomegalovirus (CMV)
- *Toxoplasma gondii*
- Parvovirus
- Varicella zoster
- Syphilis.

Rubella

The diagnosis of maternal infection must be confirmed serologically as clinical diagnosis is unreliable. The risk and extent of fetal damage are mainly determined by the gestational age at the onset of maternal infection. Infection before 8 weeks' gestation causes deafness, congenital heart disease and cataracts in over 80% (Fig. 9.6a). About 30% of fetuses of mothers infected at 13–16 weeks' gestation have impaired hearing; beyond 18 weeks' gestation, the risk to the fetus is minimal.

Box 9.3 Diagnosis of congenital rubella, cytomegalovirus (CMV) and *Toxoplasma* infection

Mother	Seroconversion on screening serology
Fetus	Amniocentesis or chorionic villus sample, PCR
Placenta	Microscopy for syphilis, PCR
Urine from infant	Rubella, CMV – culture, PCR
Blood, CSF, other samples from infant	Culture, PCR
Blood serology	Rubella-specific IgM, CMV-specific IgM, *Toxoplasma*-specific IgM and persistently raised *Toxoplasma* IgG

Viraemia after birth continues to damage the infant. Tests used to confirm the diagnosis are shown in Box 9.3. The range of clinical features characteristic of congenital infections is shown in Figure 9.6b.

Congenital rubella is preventable. In the UK, it has become extremely rare since the measles/mumps/rubella (MMR) vaccine was introduced into the childhood immunisation programme, but this is dependent on the maintenance of a high vaccine uptake rate.

Cytomegalovirus

CMV is the most common congenital infection, affecting 3–4/1000 live births in the UK, with higher rates reported in parts of the USA. In Europe, 50% of pregnant women are susceptible to CMV. About 1% of susceptible women will have a primary infection during pregnancy, and in about 40% of them the infant becomes infected. The infant may also become infected following an episode of recurrent infection in the mother, but this is much less likely to damage the fetus. When an infant is infected:

- 90% are normal at birth and develop normally
- 5% have clinical features at birth, such as hepatosplenomegaly and petechiae (Fig. 9.6b), most of whom will have neurodevelopmental disabilities such as sensorineural hearing loss, cerebral palsy, epilepsy and cognitive impairment
- 5% develop problems later in life, mainly sensorineural hearing loss.

Infection in the pregnant woman is usually asymptomatic or causes a mild non-specific illness. There is no CMV vaccine and pregnant women are not screened for CMV. Antiviral therapy for infected infants with ganciclovir is under investigation in randomised controlled trials.

Toxoplasmosis

Acute infection with *Toxoplasma gondii*, a protozoan parasite, may result from the consumption of raw or undercooked meat and from contact with the faeces of recently infected cats. In the UK, fewer than 20% of pregnant women have had past infection, in contrast to 80% in France and Austria. Transplacental infection may occur during the parasitaemia of a primary infection, and about 40% of fetuses become infected. In the UK, the incidence of congenital infection is only about 0.1 per 1000 live births. Most infected infants are asymptomatic. About 10% have clinical manifestations (Fig. 9.6b), of which the most common are:

- Retinopathy, an acute fundal chorioretinitis which sometimes interferes with vision
- Cerebral calcification
- Hydrocephalus.

These infants usually have long-term neurological disabilities. Infected newborn infants are usually treated (pyrimethamine and sulfadiazine) for 1 year. Asymptomatic infants remain at risk of developing chorioretinitis into adulthood.

Varicella zoster

A total of 15% of pregnant women are susceptible to varicella (chickenpox). Usually, the fetus is unaffected but will be at risk if the mother develops chickenpox:

- in the first half of pregnancy (<20 weeks), when there is a <2% risk of the fetus developing severe scarring of the skin and possibly ocular and neurological damage and digital dysplasia
- within 5 days before or 2 days after delivery, when the fetus is unprotected by maternal antibodies and the viral dose is high. About 25% develop a vesicular rash. The illness has a mortality as high as 30%.

Exposed susceptible mothers can be protected with varicella zoster immune globulin (VZIG) and treated with aciclovir. Infants born in the high-risk period should also receive zoster immune globulin and are often also given aciclovir prophylactically.

 If a mother develops chickenpox shortly before or after delivery, the infant needs protection from infection.

Syphilis

Congenital syphilis is rare in the UK. The clinical features are shown in Figure 9.6b. Those specific to congenital syphilis include a characteristic rash on the soles of the feet and hands and bone lesions. If mothers with syphilis identified on antenatal screening are fully treated 1 month or more before delivery, the infant does not require treatment and has an excellent prognosis. If there is any doubt about the adequacy of maternal treatment, the infant should be treated with penicillin.

Adaptation to extrauterine life

In the fetus, the lungs are filled with fluid, and oxygen is supplied by the placenta. The blood vessels that supply and drain the lungs are constricted (high

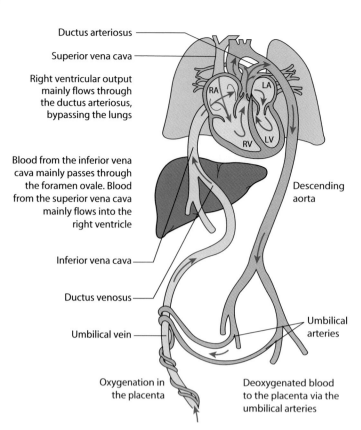

Ductus arteriosus

Superior vena cava

Right ventricular output mainly flows through the ductus arteriosus, bypassing the lungs

Blood from the inferior vena cava mainly passes through the foramen ovale. Blood from the superior vena cava mainly flows into the right ventricle

RA   LA

RV   LV

Descending aorta

Inferior vena cava

Ductus venosus

Umbilical vein

Umbilical arteries

Oxygenation in the placenta

Deoxygenated blood to the placenta via the umbilical arteries

Figure 9.7 The fetal circulation.

pulmonary vascular resistance), so most blood from the right side of the heart bypasses the lungs and flows through the ductus arteriosus into the aorta, and some flows across the foramen ovale (Fig. 9.7). Shortly before and during labour, lung liquid production is reduced. During descent through the birth canal, the infant's chest is squeezed and some lung liquid drained. Multiple stimuli, including thermal, tactile and hormonal (with a particularly dramatic increase in catecholamine levels), initiate breathing. On average, the first breath occurs 6 s after delivery. Lung expansion is generated by intrathoracic negative pressure and a functional residual capacity is established. The mean time to establish regular breathing is 30 s. Once the infant gasps, the majority of the remaining lung fluid is absorbed into the lymphatic and pulmonary circulation.

Pulmonary expansion at birth is associated with a rise in oxygen tension, and with falling pulmonary vascular resistance the pulmonary blood flow increases. Increased left atrial filling results in a rise in the left atrial pressure with closure of the foramen ovale. The flow of oxygenated blood through the ductus arteriosus causes physiological, and eventual anatomical, ductal closure. After an elective caesarean section, when the mother has not been in labour and the infant's chest has not been squeezed through the birth canal, it may take several hours for the lung fluid to be completely absorbed, causing rapid, laboured breathing (transient tachypnoea of the newborn).

Some infants do not breathe at birth. This may be due to asphyxia, when the fetus experiences a lack of oxygen during labour and/or delivery. It does not necessarily mean that the brain has been injured but asphyxia can lead to brain injury or death. A fetus

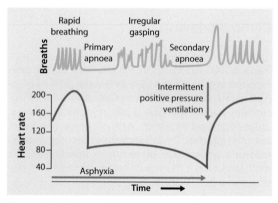

Rapid breathing   Irregular gasping

Primary apnoea   Secondary apnoea

Breaths

Intermittent positive pressure ventilation

Heart rate

200
160
120
80
40

Asphyxia

Time

Figure 9.8 Changes in respiration and heart rate with continuous asphyxia. Once the infant has stopped gasping in secondary apnoea, resuscitation with lung expansion is required to establish regular respiration and restore the circulation.

deprived of oxygen in utero will attempt to breathe, but if this is unsuccessful (as it will be in utero), it will then become apnoeic (primary apnoea), during which time the heart rate is maintained. If oxygen deprivation continues, primary apnoea is followed by irregular gasping and then a second period of apnoea (secondary or terminal apnoea), when the heart rate and blood pressure fall. If delivered at this stage, the infant will only recover if help with lung expansion is provided, e.g. by positive pressure ventilation by mask or tracheal tube (Fig. 9.8).

The human fetus rarely experiences a continuous asphyxial insult, except after placental abruption or

Table 9.2 The Apgar score

	Score		
	0	**1**	**2**
Heart rate	Absent	<100 beats/min	≥100 beats/min
Respiratory effort	Absent	Gasping or irregular	Regular, strong cry
Muscle tone	Flaccid	Some flexion of limbs	Well flexed, active
Reflex irritability	None	Grimace	Cry, cough
Colour	Pale/blue	Body pink, extremities blue	Pink

complete occlusion of umbilical blood flow in a cord prolapse. More commonly, asphyxia, which occurs during labour and delivery is intermittent, e.g. from prolonged and frequent uterine contractions. Although birth asphyxia is an important cause of failure to establish breathing requiring resuscitation at birth, there are other causes, including birth trauma, maternal analgesic or anaesthetic agents, retained lung fluid, preterm infant or a congenital malformation which interferes with breathing.

The Apgar score is used to describe a baby's condition at 1 and 5 min after delivery (Table 9.2). It is also measured at 5-min intervals thereafter, if the infant's condition remains poor. The most important components are the heart rate and respiration.

Neonatal resuscitation

Most infants do not require any resuscitation. Shortly after birth, the baby will take a breath or cry, establish regular breathing and become pink. The baby can be handed directly to his or her mother, and covered with a warm towel to avoid becoming cold. However, a newborn infant who does not establish normal respiration directly will need to be transferred to a resuscitation table for further assessment (Fig. 9.9a). There should be an overhead radiant heater and the infant should be dried and partially covered and kept warm. Suction of the mouth and nose is normally unnecessary and vigorous suction of the back of the throat may provoke bradycardia from vagal stimulation. If the infant's breathing in the first minute of life is irregular or shallow, but the heart rate is satisfactory (>100 beats/min), breathing is encouraged with airway opening manoeuvres.

If the infant does not start to breathe, or if the heart rate drops below 100 beats/min, airway positioning and lung inflation by breathing by mask ventilation are started (Fig. 9.9b–f). If the baby's condition does not improve promptly, or if the infant is clearly in very poor condition at birth, additional assistance should be summoned immediately while continuing to maintain ventilation. If an attendant has the appropriate skills, tracheal intubation can be performed (Fig. 9.9g).

After tracheal intubation, if the heart rate does not increase and adequate chest movement is not achieved, consider 'DOPE':

- **D**isplaced tube: often in the oesophagus or right main bronchus
- **O**bstructed tube: especially meconium
- **P**atient:
  - tracheal obstruction
  - lung disorders: lung immaturity or respiratory distress syndrome, pneumothorax, diaphragmatic hernia, lung hypoplasia, pleural effusion
  - shock from blood loss
  - birth asphyxia or trauma
  - upper airways obstruction: choanal atresia.
- **E**quipment failure: gas supply exhausted or disconnected.

If there is any uncertainty about the adequacy of ventilation in an intubated baby, consider removing the tracheal tube, give mask ventilation and then re-intubate.

If at any time the heart rate drops below 60 beats/min, provided adequate breathing has been achieved, chest compressions should be given (Fig. 9.9h–j). If the response to ventilation and chest compression remains inadequate, drugs should be given (Fig. 9.9k). Evidence for their efficacy is very poor.

 Providing lung inflation, evidenced by good chest wall movement, is the key to successful neonatal resuscitation.

Meconium aspiration

The passage of meconium becomes increasingly common the greater the infant's gestational age, particularly when post-term. Infants who also become acidotic may inhale thick meconium and develop meconium aspiration syndrome. Attempting to aspirate meconium from the nose and mouth while the infant's head is on the perineum is not recommended, as it is ineffective. If the infant cries at birth and establishes regular respiration, no resuscitation is required. If respiration is not established, the larynx should be inspected under direct vision and any thick meconium aspirated by suctioning with a large-bore suction catheter, but if the infant becomes bradycardic, positive pressure ventilation will be needed despite the presence of meconium.

Preparation

- All health professionals dealing with newborn infants should be proficient in basic resuscitation; i.e. **A**irway, **B**reathing with mask ventilation, **C**irculation with cardiac compressions
- Additional skilled assistance is needed if the baby does not respond rapidly and should be called without delay
- A person proficient in advanced resuscitation (**A**irway, **B**reathing via tracheal ventilation, **C**irculation, **D**rugs) should be on site and available at short notice in a maternity unit at all times
- The need for resuscitation can usually be anticipated and a person proficient in advanced resuscitation should be in attendance at all high-risk deliveries
- A clock should be started at birth for accurate timing of changes in the infant's condition
- Keep the infant warm. Dry, remove wet towel and replace with dry one. This will also provide stimulation. Can place directly on mother's chest and covered if crying, good tone and colour and desired by the mother
- Resuscitation should be performed under a radiant warmer
- If preterm and <30 weeks' gestation, to avoid heat loss, place the infant in a plastic bag without drying but under a radiant warmer and on a warming mattress. Leave the head exposed and cover with a woollen hat.
- Assess the infant's condition. Is the baby breathing or crying, good heart rate (120–160 beats/min, best assessed by listening with a stethoscope), good colour and muscle tone?
- If not, commence neonatal resuscitation

Overview

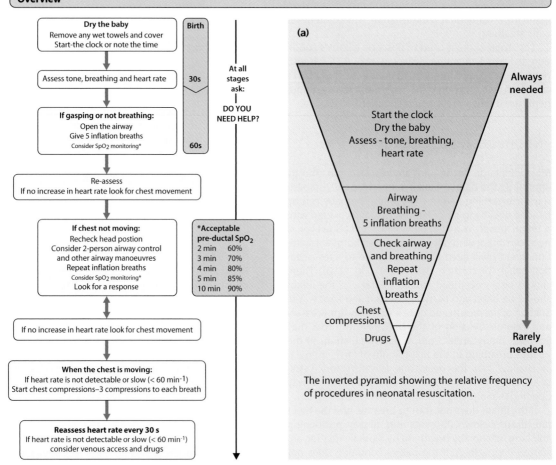

Figure 9.9 Neonatal resuscitation. (*Newborn Life Support,* 3rd ed. 2011, Resuscitation Council (UK). Reproduced with the kind permission of the Resuscitation Council (UK).)

Airway and Breathing

Airway
- Opened by placing the infants's head in a neutral position **(b)**
- Provide chin lift or jaw thrust if necessary **(c)**
- Suction any blood or secretions
- Consider placing a Guedel airway

Breathing – mask ventilation
- If not breathing adequately, start mask ventilation
- Mask is placed over mouth and nose **(d)** and connected to flow-controlled pressure-limited circuit (e.g. mechanical ventilator or Neopuff) or self-inflating bag **(e)**
- Head in neutral position
- Give 5 inflation breaths, inflation time 2–3 seconds at inspiratory pressure of 30 cm H_2O in term infants to expand lungs
- If heart rate increases, but breathing does not start, continue with peak inspiratory pressure to achieve chest wall movement (15–25 cm H_2O, 0.5 second inflation time) and rate of 30–40 breaths/min
- Begin ventilatory resuscitation in air to avoid excessive tissue oxygenation. If giving additional oxygen, use air/oxygen blender to titrate oxygen concentration with oxygen saturation on pulse oximeter. (Acceptable pre-ductal saturations – 2 min 60%; 3 min 70%; 4 min 80%; 5 min 85%; 10 min 90%.)
- Reassess every 30 seconds. If heart rate not responding, check mask position, neck position, is jaw thrust needed, is circuit all right, ensure adequate chest movement. Consider using two-person airway control **(f)**. Call for help

Intubation
- Intubation and mechanical ventilation **(g)** are indicated if: mask ventilation is ineffective, tracheal suction needed to clear an obstructed airway, congenital upper airway abnormality, extreme prematurity-for giving surfactant.
- Limit intubation attempts to 20–30 seconds.

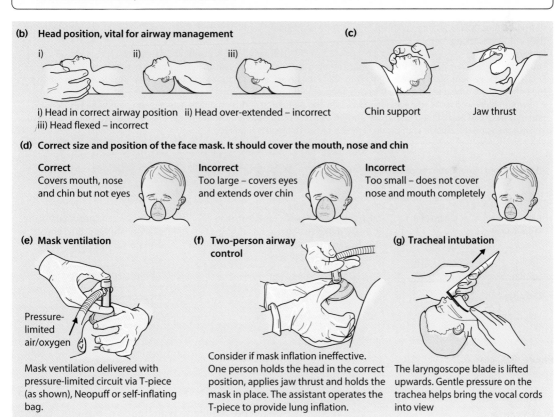

(b) Head position, vital for airway management

i) Head in correct airway position ii) Head over-extended – incorrect
iii) Head flexed – incorrect

(c) Chin support   Jaw thrust

(d) Correct size and position of the face mask. It should cover the mouth, nose and chin

Correct Covers mouth, nose and chin but not eyes

Incorrect Too large – covers eyes and extends over chin

Incorrect Too small – does not cover nose and mouth completely

(e) Mask ventilation

Pressure-limited air/oxygen

Mask ventilation delivered with pressure-limited circuit via T-piece (as shown), Neopuff or self-inflating bag.

(f) Two-person airway control

Consider if mask inflation ineffective. One person holds the head in the correct position, applies jaw thrust and holds the mask in place. The assistant operates the T-piece to provide lung inflation.

(g) Tracheal intubation

The laryngoscope blade is lifted upwards. Gentle pressure on the trachea helps bring the vocal cords into view

Figure 9.9, cont'd.

Perinatal medicine

145

Circulation

Chest compression (h, i and j)
- Start if heart rate < 60 beats/min in spite of effective lung inflation
- Ratio of compression: lung inflation of 3:1, rate of 90 compressions: 30 breaths/min (120 events/min)
- Recheck heart rate every 30 seconds; stop when heart rate >60 beats/min

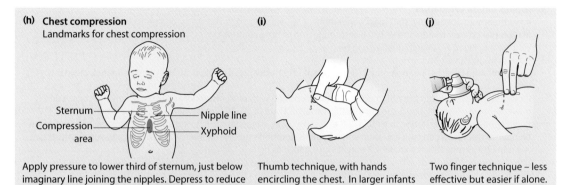

(h) Chest compression
Landmarks for chest compression

Sternum
Compression area
Nipple line
Xyphoid

Apply pressure to lower third of sternum, just below imaginary line joining the nipples. Depress to reduce antero-posterior diameter by one-third (1–1.5 cm).

(i)

Thumb technique, with hands encircling the chest. In larger infants thumbs can be placed side by side.

(j)

Two finger technique – less effective but easier if alone.

Volume and drugs

Consider drugs **(k)** if heart rate <60 beats/min in spite of adequate ventilation and chest compression, though evidence for their efficacy is lacking
Rarely needed.
Drugs should be given via an umbilical venous catheter, or, if not possible, via an intra-osseous needle.
Drugs given via a peripheral vein are unlikely to reach the heart. Giving standard doses of epinephrine (adrenaline) down the endotracheal tube does not appear to be effective, so drug dosage is increased for this route.
A newborn baby who looks white and has poor skin and peripheral perfusion due to acidosis and peripheral vasoconstriction may have had acute blood loss. There may be a history of antepartum haemorrhage or acute twin-to-twin transfusion. Immediate blood transfusion with Group O rhesus negative blood is required.

(k) Drugs used in neonatal resuscitation

Drug	Concentration	Route/dosage	Indications
Epinephrine (adrenaline)	1:10 000	IV: 0.1 ml/kg (10 micrograms/kg), then 0.1– 0.3 ml/kg (10–30 micrograms/kg) ET: 1ml/kg (100 micrograms/kg) i.e. 10 times the IV dose, whilst IV access is obtained	Heart rate <60 beats/min in spite of adequate ventilation and external cardiac compression
Sodium bicarbonate	4.2%	2–4 ml/kg (1–2 mmol/kg)	Severe lactic acidosis
Dextrose	10%	2.5 ml/kg (250 mg/kg)	Hypoglycaemia
Volume expander	Normal saline Blood	10 ml/kg, repeat if necessary	Blood loss

Figure 9.9, cont'd.

Naloxone

Infants born to mothers who have received opiate analgesia within a few hours of delivery may occasionally develop respiratory depression, which can be reversed by naloxone. It is only given if respiration continues to be depressed following initial resuscitation. As the half-life of naloxone is shorter than that of the maternal opiate, the infant's breathing must be monitored for several hours, as further doses of naloxone may be required. With modern obstetric practice, naloxone is rarely needed. Naloxone should not be given to babies of opiate abusing mothers as acute withdrawal symptoms may be precipitated.

Resuscitation of the preterm infant

Preterm infants are particularly liable to hypothermia, and every effort must be made to keep them warm during resuscitation. Infants of <30 weeks' gestation

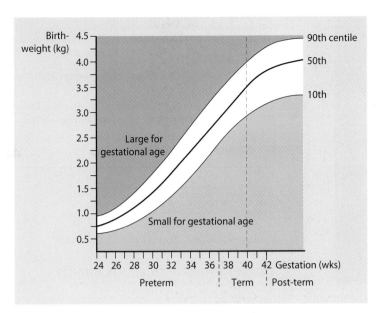

Figure 9.10 The birthweight of small-for-gestational-age infants is below the 10th centile for their gestation. Small-for-gestational-age infants may be preterm, term or post-term.

should, with the exception of the face, be placed into a plastic bag or wrapped in plastic sheeting. Excessive tissue oxygenation may cause tissue damage to the brain, lungs and eyes from oxygen free radicals. Ideally, an air/oxygen mixer should be used and any additional oxygen given titrated against oxygen saturation. Avoid exceeding a pre-ductal saturation of 95%. Very premature infants often develop respiratory distress syndrome, and early endotracheal administration of artificial surfactant may be indicated. Resuscitation of infants at the threshold of viability, at 22–24 weeks' gestation, raises particularly difficult ethical and management issues. An experienced paediatrician should be responsible for counselling the parents before delivery, if possible, and lead the management of the baby after birth.

Failure to respond to resuscitation

The decision to stop resuscitation is always difficult and should be made by a senior paediatrician. The longer it takes a baby to respond to resuscitation, the less likely is survival. If there is no breathing or cardiac output after 10 min of effective resuscitation, further efforts are likely to be fruitless and resuscitation should be stopped. If prolonged resuscitation has been required, the infant should be transferred to the neonatal unit for assessment and monitoring.

Size at birth

An infant's gestation and birthweight influence the nature of the medical problems likely to be encountered in the neonatal period. In the UK, 7% of babies are of low birthweight (<2.5 kg). However, they account for about 70% of neonatal deaths.

Definitions

Babies with a birthweight below the 10th centile for their gestational age are called small for gestational age or small-for-dates (Fig. 9.10). The majority of these infants are normal, but small. The incidence of congenital abnormalities and neonatal problems is higher in those whose birthweight falls below the second centile (approximately two standard deviations (SD) below the mean), and some authorities restrict the term to this group of babies. An infant's birthweight may also be low because of preterm birth, or because the infant is both preterm and small for gestational age.

Small-for-gestational-age infants may have grown normally but are small, or they may have experienced intrauterine growth restriction (IUGR), i.e. they have failed to reach their full genetically determined growth potential and appear thin and malnourished. Babies with a birthweight above the 10th centile may also be malnourished, e.g. a fetus growing along the 80th centile who develops growth failure and whose weight falls to the 20th centile.

Patterns of growth restriction

Growth restriction in both the fetus and infant has traditionally been classified as symmetrical or asymmetrical. In the more common asymmetrical growth restriction, the weight or abdominal circumference lies on a lower centile than that of the head. This occurs when the placenta fails to provide adequate nutrition late in pregnancy but brain growth is relatively spared at the expense of liver glycogen and skin fat (Fig. 9.11). This form of growth restriction is associated with uteroplacental dysfunction secondary to maternal pre-eclampsia, multiple pregnancy, maternal smoking or it may be idiopathic. These infants rapidly put on weight after birth.

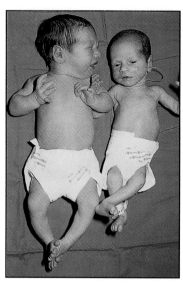

Figure 9.11 Severe intrauterine growth restriction in a twin.

In symmetrical growth restriction, the head circumference is equally reduced. It suggests a prolonged period of poor intrauterine growth starting in early pregnancy (or that the gestational age is incorrect). It is usually due to a small but normal fetus, but may be due to a fetal chromosomal disorder or syndrome, a congenital infection, maternal drug and alcohol abuse or a chronic medical condition or malnutrition. These infants are more likely to remain small permanently.

In practice, distinction between asymmetrical and symmetrical growth restriction often cannot be made.

Monitoring the growth-restricted fetus

The fetus with IUGR is at risk from:

- intrauterine hypoxia and 'unexplained' intrauterine death
- asphyxia during labour and delivery.

The growth-restricted fetus will need to be monitored closely to determine the optimal time for delivery. Progressive uteroplacental failure results in:

- reduced growth in femur length and abdominal circumference
- abnormal umbilical artery Doppler waveforms – absent or reversed end diastolic flow velocity
- redistribution of blood flow in the fetus – increased to the brain, reduced to gastrointestinal tract, liver, skin and kidneys
- reduced amniotic fluid volume
- reduced fetal movements and abnormal CTG (cardiotocography).

The growth-restricted infant

After birth, these infants are liable to:

- hypothermia because of their relatively large surface area
- hypoglycaemia from poor fat and glycogen stores

Summary

Size at birth

- Small for gestational age – birthweight <10th centile
- Intrauterine growth restriction (IUGR) – fails to reach genetically determined growth potential
- Growth restriction – symmetrical or asymmetrical, but often mixed.

- hypocalcaemia
- polycythaemia (venous haematocrit >0.65).

Large-for-gestational-age infants

Large-for-gestational-age infants are those above the 90th weight centile for their gestation. Macrosomia is a feature of infants of mothers with either permanent or gestational diabetes, or a baby with a congenital syndrome (e.g. Beckwith–Wiedemann syndrome). The problems associated with being large for gestational age are:

- Birth asphyxia from a difficult delivery
- Breathing difficulty from an enlarged tongue in Beckwith–Wiedemann syndrome
- Birth trauma, especially from shoulder dystocia at delivery (difficulty delivering the shoulders from impaction behind maternal symphysis pubis)
- Hypoglycaemia due to hyperinsulinism
- Polycythaemia.

Routine examination of the newborn infant

Immediately after a baby is born, parents are naturally anxious to know if their baby is alright and appears normal. To answer this, the midwife (or the paediatrician or obstetrician, if present) will briefly but carefully check that the baby is pink, breathing normally and has no major abnormalities. If a significant problem is identified, an experienced paediatrician must explain the situation to the parents. If the baby is markedly preterm, small or ill, admission to a neonatal unit will be required. Should there be any uncertainty about the child's sex, it is important not to guess but to explain to the parents that further tests are necessary. Babies are given vitamin K at birth to prevent haemorrhagic disease of the newborn unless parents will not give consent.

Within 24 h of birth every baby should have a full and thorough examination, the 'routine examination of the newborn infant'. Its purpose is to:

- detect congenital abnormalities not already identified at birth, e.g. congenital heart disease, developmental dysplasia of the hip (DDH)
- check for potential problems arising from maternal disease or familial disorders

Birthweight, gestational age and birthweight centile are noted.

General observation of the baby's appearance, posture and movements provides valuable information about many abnormalities. The baby must be fully undressed during the examination.

The head circumference is measured with a paper tape measure and its centile noted. This is a surrogate measure of brain size.

The fontanelle and sutures are palpated. The fontanelle size is very variable. The sagittal suture is often separated and the coronal sutures may be overriding. A tense fontanelle when the baby is not crying may be due to raised intracranial pressure and cranial ultrasound should be performed to check for hydrocephalus. A tense fontanelle is also a late sign of meningitis.

The face is observed. If abnormal, this may represent a syndrome, particularly if other anomalies are present. Down syndrome is the most common, but there are hundreds of syndromes. When the diagnosis is uncertain, a book or a computer database may be consulted and advice should be sought from a senior paediatrician or geneticist.

If plethoric or pale, the haematocrit should be checked to identify polycythaemia or anaemia. Central cyanosis, which always needs urgent assessment, is best seen on the tongue.

Jaundice within 24 h of birth requires further evaluation.

The eyes are checked for red reflex with an ophthalmoscope. If absent, may be from cataracts, retinoblastoma and corneal opacity. This reflex is

not present in infants with pigmented skin, but the retinal vessels can be visualised.

The palate needs to be inspected, including posteriorly to exclude a posterior cleft palate, and palpated to detect an indentation of the posterior palate from a submucous cleft.

Breathing and chest wall movement are observed for signs of respiratory distress.

On auscultating the heart, the normal rate is 110–160 beats/min in term babies, but may drop to 85 beats/min during sleep.

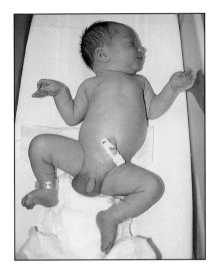

Figure 9.12 Term newborn. Median measurements:
- birthweight 3.5 kg;
- head circumference 35 cm;
- length 50 cm.

On palpating the abdomen, the liver normally extends 1–2 cm below the costal margin, the spleen tip may be palpable, as may the kidney on the left side. Any intra-abdominal masses, which are usually renal in origin, need further investigation.

The femoral pulses are palpated. Their pulse pressure is:
- reduced in coarctation of the aorta. This can be confirmed by measuring the blood pressure in the arms and legs
- increased if there is a patent ductus arteriosus.

The genitalia and anus are inspected on removing the nappy. Patency of the anus is confirmed. In boys, the presence of testes in the scrotum is checked by palpation.

Muscle tone is assessed by observing limb movements. Most babies will support their head briefly when the trunk is held vertically.

The whole of the back and spine is observed, looking for any midline defects of the skin.

The hips are checked for developmental dysplasia of the hips (DDH). This is left until last as the procedure is uncomfortable.

Box 9.4 Routine examination of the newborn.

- provide an opportunity for the parents to discuss any questions about their baby.

Before approaching the mother and baby, the obstetric and neonatal notes must be checked to identify relevant information. The examination (Fig. 9.12a and b) should be performed with the mother or ideally both parents present. Many findings in the newborn resolve spontaneously (Box 9.5, Fig. 9.13). Common significant abnormalities detectable at birth are listed in Box 9.6. A serious congenital anomaly is present at birth in

about 10–15/1000 live births (Table 9.3). In addition, many congenital anomalies, especially of the heart, present clinically at a later age.

Testing for developmental dysplasia of the hip (DDH)

To test for developmental dysplasia of the hip (DDH), also called congenital dislocation of the hip (CDH), the infant needs to be relaxed, as kicking or crying results

Box 9.5 Lesions in newborn infants that resolve spontaneously

Peripheral cyanosis of the hands and feet – common in the first day

Traumatic cyanosis from a cord round the baby's neck or from a face or brow presentation – causes blue discoloration of the skin, petechiae over the head and neck or affected part but not the tongue

Swollen eyelids and distortion of shape of the head from the delivery

Subconjunctival haemorrhages – occur during delivery

Small white pearls along the midline of the palate (Epstein pearls)

Cysts of the gums (epulis) or floor of the mouth (ranula)

Breast enlargement – may occur in newborn babies of either sex (Fig. 9.13a). A small amount of milk may be discharged

White vaginal discharge or small withdrawal bleed in girls. There may be a prolapse of a ring of vaginal mucosa

Capillary haemangioma or 'stork bites' – pink macules on the upper eyelids, mid-forehead and nape of the neck are common and arise from distension of the dermal capillaries. Those on the eyelids gradually fade over the first year; those on the neck become covered with hair

Neonatal urticaria (erythema toxicum) – a common rash appearing at 2–3 days of age, consisting of white pinpoint papules at the centre of an erythematous base (Fig. 9.13b). The fluid contains eosinophils. The lesions are concentrated on the trunk; they come and go at different sites

Milia – white pimples on the nose and cheeks, from retention of keratin and sebaceous material in the pilaceous follicles (Fig. 9.13c)

Mongolian blue spots – blue/black macular discoloration at the base of the spine and on the buttocks (Fig. 9.13d); occasionally occur on the legs and other parts of the body. Usually but not invariably in Afro-Caribbean or Asian infants. They fade slowly over the first few years. They are of no significance unless misdiagnosed as bruises

Umbilical hernia – common, particularly in Afro-Caribbean infants. No treatment is indicated as it usually resolves within the first 2–3 years

Positional talipes – the feet often remain in their in-utero position. Unlike true talipes equinovarus, the foot can be fully dorsiflexed to touch the front of the lower leg (Fig. 9.13e,f)

Caput succedaneum (see Fig. 10.6).

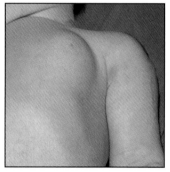

Figure 9.13a Breast enlargement in a newborn infant.

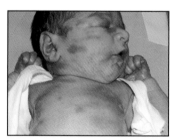

Figure 9.13b Erythema toxicum (neonatal urticaria), often has a raised pale centre. (Courtesy of Dr Nim Subhedar.)

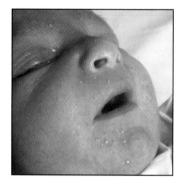

Figure 9.13c Milia. (Courtesy of Dr Rodney Rivers.)

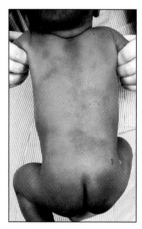

Figure 9.13d Mongolian blue spot.

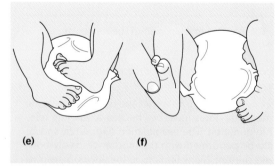

(e)   (f)

Figure 9.13e Positional talipes. Appearance at birth.
Figure 9.13f The foot can be fully dorsiflexed to touch the front of the lower leg. In true talipes equinovarus this is not possible.

Some significant abnormalities detected on routine examination

Box 9.6 Some significant abnormalities detected on routine examination

Port-wine stain (naevus flammeus). Present from birth and usually grows with the infant (Fig. 9.14a). It is due to a vascular malformation of the capillaries in the dermis. Rarely, if along the distribution of the trigeminal nerve, it may be associated with intracranial vascular anomalies (Sturge–Weber syndrome), or severe lesions on the limbs with bone hypertrophy (Klippel–Trenaunay syndrome). Disfiguring lesions can now be improved with laser therapy.

Strawberry naevus (cavernous haemangioma). Often not present at birth, but appear in the first month of life and may be multiple (Fig. 9.14b). It is more common in preterm infants. It increases in size until 3–15 months old, then gradually regresses. No treatment is indicated unless the lesion interferes with vision or the airway. Ulceration or haemorrhage may occur. Thrombocytopenia may occur with large lesions, when therapy with systemic steroids or interferon-α may be required.

Natal teeth consisting of the front lower incisors – may be present at birth. If loose, they should be removed to avoid the risk of aspiration.

Extra digits – are sometimes connected by a thin skin tag but may be completely attached

containing bone (Fig. 9.14c) and should ideally be removed by a plastic surgeon or else tied off at its base. Skin tags anterior to the ear and accessory auricles should be removed by a plastic surgeon.

Heart murmur – poses a difficult problem, as most murmurs audible in the first few days of life resolve shortly afterwards. However, some are caused by congenital heart disease. If there are any features of a significant murmur (see Ch. 17), upper and lower limb blood pressures, and pre- and post-ductal pulse oximetry should be checked followed by an echocardiogram. Otherwise, a follow-up examination is arranged and the parents warned to seek medical assistance if their baby feeds poorly, develops laboured breathing or becomes cyanosed.

Midline abnormality over the spine or skull, such as a tuft of hair, swelling or naevus – requires further evaluation as it may indicate an underlying abnormality of the vertebrae, spinal cord or brain.

Palpable and large bladder – if there is urinary outflow obstruction, particularly in boys with posterior urethral valves. Requires prompt evaluation with ultrasound.

Talipes equinovarus – which cannot be corrected as in positional talipes.

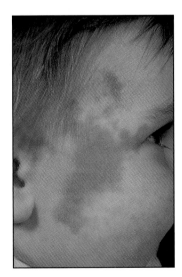

Figure 9.14a Port-wine stain in an infant.

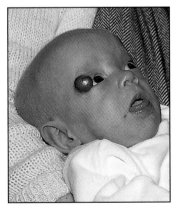

Figure 9.14b Strawberry naevus.

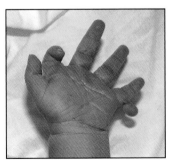

Figure 9.14c Extra digits.

Table 9.3 Prevalence of serious congenital anomalies per 1000 live births (England and Wales)

Anomaly	Prevalence
Congenital heart disease	6–8 (0.8 on the first day of life)
Developmental dysplasia of the hip	1.5 (but about 6/1000 have an abnormal initial clinical examination)
Talipes	1.0
Down syndrome	1.0
Cleft lip and palate	0.8
Urogenital (hypospadias, undescended testes)	1.2
Spina bifida/anencephaly	0.1

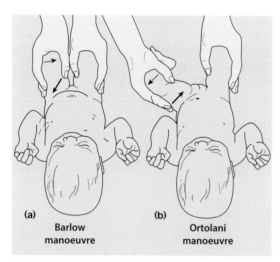

(a) Barlow manoeuvre

(b) Ortolani manoeuvre

Figure 9.15 (a) The hip is dislocated posteriorly out of the acetabulum (Barlow manoeuvre). **(b)** The dislocated hip is relocated back into the acetabulum (Ortolani manoeuvre).

in tightening of the muscles around the hip and prevents satisfactory examination. The pelvis is stabilised with one hand. With the other hand, the examiner's middle finger is placed over the greater trochanter and the thumb around the distal medial femur. The hip is held flexed and adducted. The femoral head is gently pushed downwards. If the hip is dislocatable, the femoral head will be pushed posteriorly out of the acetabulum (Fig. 9.15a).

The next part of the examination is to see if the hip can be returned from its dislocated position back into the acetabulum. With the hip abducted, upward leverage is applied (Fig. 9.15b). A dislocated hip will return with a 'clunk' into the acetabulum. Ligamentous clicks without any movement of the head of femur are of no

significance. It should also be possible to abduct the hips fully, but this may be restricted if the hip is dislocated. Clinical examination does not identify some infants who have hip dysplasia from lack of development of the acetabular shelf. DDH is more common in girls (six-fold increase), if there is a positive family history (20% of affected infants), if the birth is a breech presentation (30% of affected infants) or if the infant has a neuromuscular disorder.

Early recognition of DDH is important as early splinting in abduction reduces long-term morbidity. A specialist orthopaedic opinion should be sought in the management of this condition. Ultrasound examination of the hip joint is performed increasingly in many hospitals, either following an abnormal examination or to screen babies at increased risk (breech presentation or positive family history). Ultrasound examination can be performed to screen all babies, but is not currently recommended in the UK as it is expensive, requires considerable expertise and there are many false positives. It will, however, identify some babies missed on clinical examination.

Vitamin K therapy

Vitamin K deficiency may result in haemorrhagic disease of the newborn. This disorder can occur early, during the first week of life, or late, from 1 to 8 weeks of age. In most affected infants, the haemorrhage is mild, such as bruising, haematemesis and melaena, or prolonged bleeding of the umbilical stump or after a circumcision. However, some suffer from intracranial haemorrhage, half of whom are permanently disabled or die.

Breast milk is a poor source of vitamin K, whereas infant formula milk has a much higher vitamin K content. Haemorrhagic disease of the newborn may occur in infants who are wholly breast-fed but not if fed with an infant formula. Infants of mothers taking anticonvulsants, which impair the synthesis of vitamin K-dependent clotting factors, are at increased risk of haemorrhagic disease, both during delivery and soon after birth. Infants with liver disease are also at increased risk.

The disease can be prevented if vitamin K is given by intramuscular injection, and in the UK, it was widely given to all newborn infants immediately after birth. In the early 1990s, one study suggested a possible association between vitamin K given intramuscularly and the development of cancer in childhood, but this has not been found in other, much larger studies. It is still recommended that all newborn infants are given intramuscular vitamin K. However, parents may request oral vitamin K as an alternative. As absorption via the oral route is variable, three doses are needed over the first 4 weeks of life to achieve adequate liver storage. Mothers on anticonvulsant therapy should receive oral prophylaxis from 36 weeks' gestation and the baby should be given intramuscular vitamin K.

 Vitamin K should be given to all newborn infants to prevent haemorrhagic disease of the newborn.

Biochemical screening (Guthrie test)

Biochemical screening is performed on every baby. A blood sample, usually a heel prick, is taken when feeding has been established on day 5–9 of life. In the UK, all infants are screened for:

- phenylketonuria
- hypothyroidism
- haemoglobinopathies (sickle cell and thalassaemia)
- cystic fibrosis
- MCAD (medium-chain acyl-CoA dehydrogenase) deficiency – a rare inborn error of mitochondrial fatty acid metabolism causing acute illness and hypoglycaemia following fasting, which may also present as an ALTE (acute life-threatening episode).

Screening for cystic fibrosis is performed by measuring the serum immunoreactive trypsin, which is raised if there is pancreatic duct obstruction. If raised, DNA analysis is also performed to reduce the false-positive rate (see Ch. 16).

 In the UK, biochemical screening is performed on all babies to identify phenylketonuria, congenital hypothyroidism, haemoglobinopathies, cystic fibrosis and MCAD deficiency.

Newborn hearing screening

Universal screening has been introduced in the UK to detect severe hearing impairment in newborn infants. Early detection and intervention improves speech and language. Evoked otoacoustic emission (EOAE) testing, when an earphone is placed over the ear and a sound is emitted which evokes an echo or emission from the ear if cochlear function is normal, is used as the initial screening test. If a normal test is not achieved, testing with automated auditory brainstem response (AABR) audiometry, using computer analysis of EEG waveforms evoked in response to a series of clicks, is performed, with referral to a paediatric audiologist if abnormal (see Ch. 3 for further details).

 Newborn hearing screening is performed on all infants to detect severe hearing impairment.

Further reading

Lissauer T, Fanaroff A: *Neonatology at a Glance*, ed 2, Oxford, 2011, Blackwell.

Rennie JM: *Roberton's Textbook of Neonatology*, Edinburgh, 2011, Churchill Livingstone.

Resuscitation Council, UK: *Newborn Life Support*, 3rd ed, 2011, Resuscitation Council (UK).

Website (Accessed May 2011)

Newborn Life Support: Resuscitation Council, UK. Available at: www.resus.org.uk.

Perinatal medicine

10

Neonatal medicine

The dramatic reduction in neonatal mortality throughout the developed world has resulted from advances in the management of newborn infants together with improvements in maternal health and obstetric care. Neonatal intensive care became increasingly available in the UK from 1975, and it is since that time that the mortality of very low birthweight (VLBW) infants has fallen (Fig. 10.1).

About 8–10% of babies born in the UK are admitted to a neonatal unit for special medical and nursing care, although whenever possible babies are cared for on postnatal wards to avoid separating mothers from their babies. About 1–3% of babies require intensive care.

In the UK, neonatal units are organised as networks, with units providing either:

- special care (level 1)
- short-term intensive care (level 2)
- long-term intensive care (level 3), usually linked to specialist fetal and obstetric care to form a specialist tertiary perinatal centre.

Modern technology allows even tiny preterm infants to benefit from the full range of intensive care, anaesthesia and surgery. If it is anticipated during pregnancy that the infant is likely to require long-term intensive care or surgery, it is preferable for the transfer to the

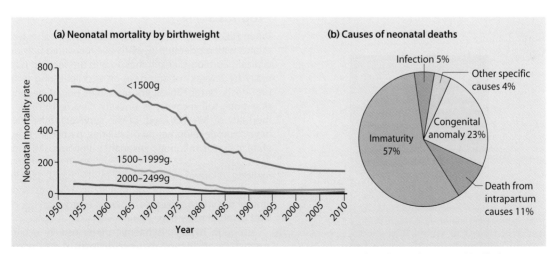

Figure 10.1 (a) The dramatic fall in neonatal mortality rate in England and Wales in the second half of the twentieth century, according to birthweight. In very low birthweight infants (<1500 g), the marked fall in the mortality occurred after the introduction of intensive care. (b) Causes of neonatal deaths in England and Wales, 2008. (Adapted from the Audit Commission and ONS 2010).

tertiary centre to be made in utero. When a baby requires transfer postnatally, transport should be by an experienced team of doctors and nurses. Arrangements should also be made for parents to be close to their infant during this stressful time.

Hypoxic-ischaemic encephalopathy

In perinatal asphyxia, gas exchange, either placental or pulmonary, is compromised or ceases altogether, resulting in cardiorespiratory depression. Hypoxia, hypercarbia and metabolic acidosis follow. Compromised cardiac output diminishes tissue perfusion, causing hypoxic-ischaemic injury to the brain and other organs. The neonatal condition is called hypoxic-ischaemic encephalopathy (HIE). It remains an important cause of brain damage, resulting in disability (Fig. 10.2) or death, and its prevention is one of the key aims of modern obstetric care. In developed countries, approximately 0.5–1/1000 liveborn term infants develop HIE and 0.3/1000 have significant neurologic disability. The incidence is higher in developing countries.

Most cases of hypoxic-ischaemic encephalopathy (HIE) follow a significant hypoxic event immediately before or during labour or delivery. These include:

- Failure of gas exchange across the placenta – excessive or prolonged uterine contractions, placental abruption, ruptured uterus
- Interruption of umbilical blood flow – cord compression including shoulder dystocia, cord prolapse
- Inadequate maternal placental perfusion, maternal hypotension or hypertension – often with intrauterine growth restriction
- Compromised fetus – anemia, intrauterine growth restriction
- Failure of cardiorespiratory adaptation at birth – failure to breathe.

The clinical manifestations start immediately or up to 48 h after asphyxia, and can be graded:

- Mild – the infant is irritable, responds excessively to stimulation, may have staring of the eyes and hyperventilation and has impaired feeding
- Moderate – the infant shows marked abnormalities of tone and movement, cannot feed and may have seizures
- Severe – there are no normal spontaneous movements or response to pain; tone in the limbs may fluctuate between hypotonia and hypertonia; seizures are prolonged and often refractory to treatment; multi-organ failure is present.

The neuronal damage may be immediate from primary neuronal death or may be delayed from reperfusion injury causing secondary neuronal death. This delay offers the opportunity for neuroprotection with mild hypothermia.

Management

Skilled resuscitation and stabilisation of sick infants will minimise neuronal damage. Infants with HIE may need:

- respiratory support
- recording of amplitude-integrated electroencephalogram (aEEG, cerebral function monitor) to detect abnormal background activity to confirm early encephalopathy or identify seizures
- treatment of clinical seizures with anticonvulsants
- fluid restriction because of transient renal impairment
- treatment of hypotension by volume and inotrope support
- monitoring and treatment of hypoglycaemia and electrolyte imbalance, especially hypocalcaemia.

Recent randomised clinical trials have shown that mild hypothermia (cooling to a rectal temperature of 33–34°C for 72 h by wrapping the infant in a cooling blanket) reduces brain damage if started within 6 h of birth.

Prognosis

When HIE is mild, complete recovery can be expected. Infants with moderate HIE who have recovered fully on clinical neurological examination and are feeding normally by 2 weeks of age have an excellent long-term prognosis, but if clinical abnormalities persist beyond that time, full recovery is unlikely. Severe HIE has a mortality of 30–40%, and, of the survivors, over 80% have neurodevelopmental disabilities, particularly cerebral palsy. If magnetic resonance imaging (MRI) at 4–14 days in a term infant shows significant abnormalities (bilateral abnormalities in the basal ganglia and thalamus and lack of myelin in the posterior limb of the internal capsule), there is a very high risk of later cerebral palsy (Fig. 10.3).

Although hypoxic-ischaemic injury usually occurs antenatally or during labour or delivery, it may occur postnatally or be caused by a neonatal condition (e.g. inborn error of metabolism or kernicterus). The diagnosis 'birth asphyxia' has potentially serious medicolegal implications; it has been recommended that infants

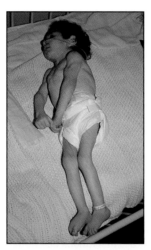

Figure 10.2 Brain damage from severe birth asphyxia.

Summary

Hypoxic-ischaemic encephalopathy (HIE)

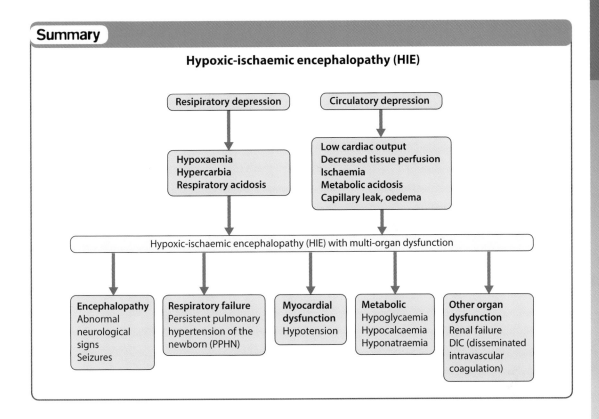

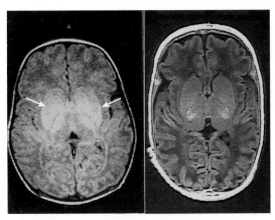

Figure 10.3 Magnetic resonance image of the brain at term. Left: hypoxic-ischaemic encephalopathy (HIE) showing abnormal (white) signal in the basal ganglia and thalami (arrows) and absence of signal in the internal capsule bilaterally. Right: normal scan showing grey basal ganglia and a white signal from myelin in the posterior limb of the internal capsule.

who have the clinical features of HIE should only be considered to have birth asphyxia if there is:

- evidence of severe hypoxia antenatally or during labour or at delivery
- resuscitation needed at birth
- features of encephalopathy
- evidence of hypoxic damage to other organs such as liver, kidney, or heart
- no other prenatal or postnatal cause identified
- characteristic findings on MRI neuroimaging.

Mild hypothermia for moderate and severe HIE reduces death and severe disability and increases the likelihood of survival with normal neurological function.

Birth injuries

Infants may be injured at birth, particularly if they are malpositioned or too large for the pelvic outlet. Injuries may also occur during manual manoeuvres, from forceps blades or at Ventouse deliveries. Fortunately, now that Caesarean section is available in every maternity unit, heroic attempts to achieve a vaginal delivery with resultant severe injuries to the infant have become extremely rare.

Soft tissue injuries

These include:

- Caput succedaneum (Fig. 10.4) – bruising and oedema of the presenting part extending beyond the margins of the skull bones; resolves in a few days
- Cephalhaematoma (Figs 10.4, 10.5) – haematoma from bleeding below the periosteum, confined within the margins of the skull sutures. It usually involves the parietal bone. The centre of the haematoma feels soft. It resolves over several weeks
- Chignon (Fig. 10.6) – oedema and bruising from Ventouse delivery
- Bruising to the face after a face presentation and to the genitalia and buttocks after breech delivery.

Neonatal medicine

157

Soft tissue injuries

- Caput succedaneum, cephalhaematoma, chignon, bruises and abrasions
- Subaponeurotic haemorrhage

Nerve palsies

- Brachial plexus – Erb palsy
- Facial nerve palsy

Fractures

- Clavicle, humerus, femur

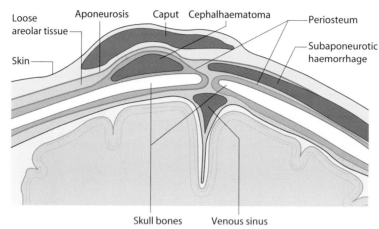

Figure 10.4 Location of extracranial haemorrhages.

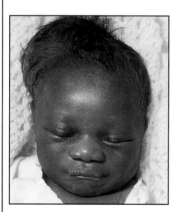

Figure 10.5 A large cephalhaematoma.

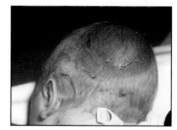

Figure 10.6 Chignon.

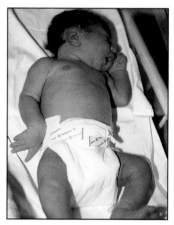

Figure 10.7 Erb palsy. The affected arm lies straight, limp and with the hand pronated and the fingers flexed (waiter's tip position).

Preterm infants bruise readily from even mild trauma
- Abrasions to the skin from scalp electrodes applied during labour or from accidental scalpel incision at Caesarean section
- Forceps marks to face from pressure of blades – transient
- Subaponeurotic haemorrhage (Fig. 10.4) (very uncommon) – diffuse, boggy swelling of scalp on examination, blood loss may be severe and lead to hypovolaemic shock and coagulopathy.

Nerve palsies

Brachial nerve palsy results from traction to the brachial plexus nerve roots. They may occur at breech deliveries or with shoulder dystocia. Upper nerve root (C5 and C6) injury results in an Erb palsy (Fig. 10.7). It may be accompanied by phrenic nerve palsy causing an elevated diaphragm. Most palsies resolve completely, but should be referred to an orthopaedic or plastic surgeon if not resolved by 2–3 months. Most recover by 2 years. A facial nerve palsy may result from compression of the facial nerve against the mother's ischial spine. It is unilateral, and there is facial weakness on crying but the eye remains open. It is usually transient, but methylcellulose drops may be needed for the eye. Rarely, nerve palsies may be from damage to the cervical spine, when there is lack of movement below the level of the lesion.

Fractures

Clavicle

Usually from shoulder dystocia. A snap may be heard at delivery or the infant may have reduced arm movement on the affected side, or a lump from callus formation may be noticed over the clavicle at several days of age. The prognosis is excellent and no specific treatment is required.

Humerus/femur

Usually mid-shaft, occurring at breech deliveries, or fracture of the humerus at shoulder dystocia. There is deformity, reduced movement of the limb and pain on movement. They heal rapidly with immobilisation.

Stabilising the preterm or sick infant

Preterm infants of <34 weeks' gestation and newborn infants who become seriously ill require their condition to be stabilised and monitored (Fig. 10.8). Many of them will need respiratory and circulatory support.

The preterm infant

The appearance, the likely clinical course, chances of survival and long-term prognosis depend on the gestational age at birth. The appearance and maturational changes of very preterm infants are described in Table 10.1 and the importance of parental involvement shown in Figures 10.10a and b. The external appearance and neurological findings can be scored to provide an estimate of an infant's gestational age (see Appendix).

The rate and severity of problems associated with prematurity decline markedly with increasing gestation. Infants born at 23–26 weeks' gestation encounter many problems (Box 10.1), require many weeks of intensive and special care in hospital and have a high overall mortality. With modern intensive care, the prognosis is excellent after 32 weeks' gestational age. The severity of an infant's respiratory disease and of any episodes of infection largely determine the neonatal course and outcome.

Box 10.1 Medical problems of preterm infants

- Need for resuscitation at birth
- Respiratory
  - Respiratory distress syndrome (RDS)
  - Pneumothorax
  - Apnoea and bradycardia
- Hypotension
- Patent ductus arteriosus
- Temperature control
- Metabolic
  - Hypoglycaemia
  - Hypocalcaemia
  - Electrolyte imbalance
  - Osteopenia of prematurity
- Nutrition
- Infection
- Jaundice
- Intraventricular haemorrhage/periventricular leukomalacia
- Necrotising enterocolitis
- Retinopathy of prematurity
- Anaemia of prematurity
- Iatrogenic
- Bronchopulmonary dysplasia (chronic lung disease)
- Inguinal hernias.

Respiratory distress syndrome

In respiratory distress syndrome (RDS), (also called hyaline membrane disease), there is a deficiency of surfactant, which lowers surface tension. Surfactant is a mixture of phospholipids and proteins excreted by the type II pneumocytes of the alveolar epithelium. Surfactant deficiency leads to widespread alveolar collapse and inadequate gas exchange. The more preterm the infant, the higher the incidence of RDS; it is common in infants born before 28 weeks' gestation and tends to be more severe in boys than girls. Surfactant deficiency is rare at term but may occur in infants of diabetic mothers. The term hyaline membrane disease derives from a proteinaceous exudate seen in the airways on histology. Glucocorticoids, given antenatally to the mother, stimulate fetal surfactant production and are given if preterm delivery is anticipated (see Ch. 9.)

The development of surfactant therapy has been a major advance. The preparations are natural, derived from extracts of calf or pig lung. They are instilled directly into the lung via a tracheal tube. Multinational placebo-controlled trials show that surfactant treatment reduces mortality from RDS by about 40%, without increasing the morbidity rate (Fig. 10.11).

At delivery or within 4 h of birth, babies with RDS develop clinical signs of:

- tachypnoea >60 breaths/min
- laboured breathing with chest wall recession (particularly sternal and subcostal indrawing) and nasal flaring

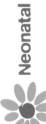

Stabilising preterm or sick infants

Airway, breathing

- Respiratory distress: tachypnoea, laboured breathing with chest wall recession, nasal flaring, expiratory grunting, cyanosis
- Apnoea

Management, as required:

- Clear the airway
- Oxygen
- High-flow humidified oxygen therapy
- CPAP (continuous positive airway pressure)
- Mechanical ventilation

Monitoring

- Oxygen saturation (maintain at 88–95% if preterm)
- Heart rate
- Respiratory rate
- Temperature
- Blood pressure
- Blood glucose
- Blood gases
- Weight

Temperature control

- Place in plastic bag at birth to keep warm if extremely preterm
- Perform stabilisation under a radiant warmer or in a humidified incubator to avoid hypothermia.

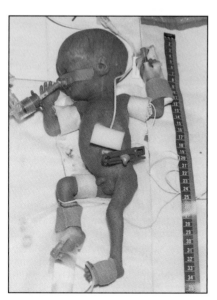

Figure 10.8 Stabilising preterm or sick infants is important to prevent complications. This preterm infant has leads on his limbs for monitoring heart rate and respiratory rate, temperature and oxygen saturation. There are arterial and intravenous cannulae and a nasotracheal tube for artificial ventilation.

Venous and arterial lines

Peripheral intravenous line

Required for intravenous fluids, antibiotics and other drugs.

Umbilical venous catheter

May be used for intravenous access at resuscitation, in extremely preterm infants for the first few days or to administer high osmolality fluids (e.g. high-concentration dextrose) or medications needing central delivery (e.g. inotropes).

Arterial line

- Inserted if frequent blood gas analysis, blood tests and continuous blood pressure monitoring are required. Usually umbilical artery catheter (UAC), sometimes peripheral cannula if for short period or no umbilical artery catheter possible.
- The arterial oxygen tension is maintained at 8–12 kPa (60–90 mmHg) and the CO_2 tension at 4.5–6.5 kPa (35–50 mmHg). Continuous non-invasive transcutaneous arterial blood gas monitoring may also be used.

Central venous line for parenteral nutrition, if indicated

Inserted peripherally when infant is stable.

Chest X-ray with or without abdominal X-ray

Assists in the diagnosis of respiratory disorders and to confirm the position of the tracheal tube and central lines.

Investigations

- Haemoglobin, neutrophil count, platelet count
- Blood urea, creatinine, electrolytes and lactate
- Culture – blood ± CSF ± urine
- Blood glucose
- CRP/acute phase reactant
- Coagulation screen if indicated

Antibiotics

Broad-spectrum antibiotics are given.

Minimal handling

All procedures, especially painful ones, adversely affect oxygenation and the circulation. Handling the infant is kept to a minimum and done as gently, rapidly and efficiently as possible. Analgesia should be provided to prevent pain as necessary.

Parents

Although medical and nursing staff are usually fully occupied stabilising the baby, time must be found for parents and immediate relatives to allow them to see and touch their baby and to be kept fully informed.

The preterm infant: maturational changes in appearance and development

Figure 10.9
(a) Preterm infant.
(b) Term infant.

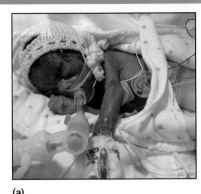

(a)

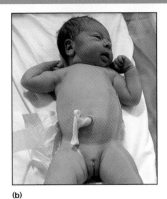

(b)

Table 10.1 The preterm infant compared with the term infant

Gestation	23–27 weeks	Term (37–42 weeks)
Birthweight (50th centile)	At 24 weeks – male 700 g, female 620 g	At 40 weeks – male 3.55 kg, female 3.4 kg
Skin	Very thin (Fig. 10.9a)	Thick skin (Fig. 10.9b)
	Dark red colour all over body	Pale pink colour
Ears	Pinna soft, no recoil	Pinna firm, cartilage to edge, immediate recoil
Breast tissue	No breast tissue palpable	One or both nodules >1 cm
Genitalia	Male – scrotum smooth, no testes in scrotum	Male – scrotum has rugae, testes in scrotum
	Female – prominent clitoris, labia majora widely separated, labia minora protruding	Female – labia minora and clitoris covered
Breathing	Needs respiratory support. Apnoea common	Rarely needs respiratory support. Apnoea rare
Sucking and swallowing	No coordinated sucking	Coordinated (from 34–35 weeks)
Feeding	Usually needs TPN (total parenteral nutrition), then tube feeding	Cries when hungry. Feeds on demand
Cry	Faint	Loud
Vision, interaction	Eyelids may be fused. Infrequent eye movements. Not available for interaction	Makes eye contact, alert wakefulness
Hearing	Startles to loud noise	Responds to sound
Posture	Limbs extended, jerky movements	Flexed posture, smooth movements

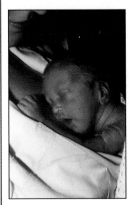

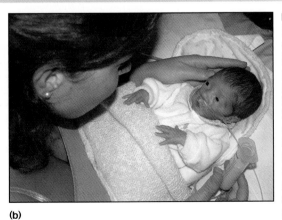

(a)

(b)

Figure 10.10a Parental involvement in neonatal care. Skin-to-skin contact between infant and parent (Kangaroo care) promotes bonding.
Figure 10.10b Parental involvement in neonatal care. Mother giving her baby expressed breast milk (in syringe) via nasogastric tube, allowing close eye and skin contact between mother and baby.

Respiratory distress syndrome

- Common in very preterm infants
- Caused by surfactant deficiency
- Antenatal corticosteroids and surfactant therapy markedly reduce morbidity and mortality.

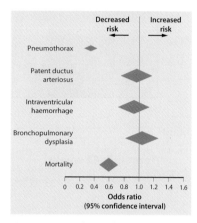

Figure 10.11 Meta-analysis of treatment of preterm infants with natural surfactant, showing a dramatic reduction in pneumothoraces and mortality.

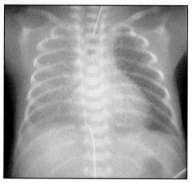

Figure 10.12 Chest X-ray in respiratory distress syndrome showing a diffuse granular or 'ground glass' appearance of the lungs and an air bronchogram, where the larger airways are outlined. The heart border becomes indistinct or obscured completely with severe disease. A tracheal tube and an umbilical artery catheter are present.

- expiratory grunting in order to try to create positive airway pressure during expiration and maintain functional residual capacity
- cyanosis if severe.

The characteristic chest X-ray appearance is shown in Figure 10.12. Treatment with raised ambient oxygen is required, which may need to be supplemented with continuous positive airway pressure (delivered via nasal cannulae) or artificial ventilation via a tracheal tube. The ventilatory requirements need to be adjusted according to the infant's oxygenation (which is measured continuously), chest wall movements and blood gas analyses. Mechanical ventilation (with intermittent positive pressure ventilation or high-frequency oscillation) may be required. High-flow humidified oxygen therapy, via nasal cannulae, may be used to wean babies from added oxygen therapy.

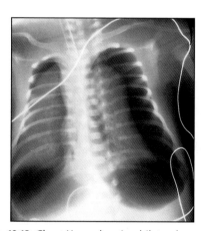

Figure 10.13 Chest X-ray showing bilateral pneumothoraces in a preterm infant with respiratory distress syndrome.

 Surfactant therapy reduces morbidity and mortality of preterm infants with respiratory distress syndrome.

Pneumothorax

In respiratory distress syndrome, air from the overdistended alveoli may track into the interstitium, resulting in pulmonary interstitial emphysema (PIE). In up to 10% of infants ventilated for RDS, air leaks into the pleural cavity and causes a pneumothorax (Fig. 10.13). When this occurs, the infant's oxygen requirement usually increases, and the breath sounds and chest movement on the affected side are reduced, although this can be difficult to detect clinically. A pneumothorax may be demonstrated by transillumination with a bright fibre-optic light source applied to the chest wall. A tension pneumothorax is treated by inserting a chest drain. In order to try and prevent pneumothoraces, infants are ventilated with the lowest pressures that provide adequate chest movement and satisfactory blood gases.

Apnoea and bradycardia and desaturation

Episodes of apnoea and bradycardia and desaturation are common in very low birthweight infants until they reach about 32 weeks' gestational age. Bradycardia may occur either when an infant stops breathing for over 20–30 s or when breathing continues but against a closed glottis. An underlying cause (hypoxia, infection, anaemia, electrolyte disturbance, hypoglycaemia, seizures, heart failure or aspiration due to gastro-oesophageal reflux) needs to be excluded, but in many instances, the cause is immaturity of central respiratory control. Breathing will usually start again after gentle physical stimulation. Treatment with the respiratory stimulant caffeine often helps. Continuous positive airways pressure (CPAP) may be necessary if apnoeic episodes are frequent.

Temperature control

Hypothermia causes increased energy consumption and may result in hypoxia and hypoglycaemia, failure to gain weight and increased mortality. Preterm infants are particularly vulnerable to hypothermia, as:

- they have a large surface area relative to their mass, so there is greater heat loss (related to surface area) than heat generation (related to mass)
- their skin is thin and heat permeable, so transepidermal water loss is important in the first week of life
- they have little subcutaneous fat for insulation
- they are often nursed naked and cannot conserve heat by curling up or generate heat by shivering.

There is a neutral temperature range in which an infant's energy consumption is at a minimum level. In the very immature baby, this neutral temperature is highest during the first few days of life and subsequently declines. The temperature of these small babies is maintained using incubators (Fig. 10.14) or initially with overhead radiant heaters. Incubators also allow ambient humidity to be provided, which reduces transepidermal heat loss.

Patent ductus arteriosus

The ductus arteriosus remains patent in many preterm infants. Shunting of blood across the ductus, from the left to the right side of the circulation, is most common in infants with RDS. It may produce no symptoms or it may cause apnoea and bradycardia, increased oxygen requirement and difficulty in weaning the infant from artificial ventilation. The pulses are 'bounding' from an increased pulse pressure, the precordial impulse becomes prominent and a systolic murmur may be audible. With increasing circulatory overload, signs of heart failure may develop. More accurate assessment of the infant's circulation can be obtained on echocardiography. If the infant is symptomatic, pharmacological closure with a prostaglandin synthetase inhibitor, indometacin or ibuprofen, is used. If these measures fail to close a symptomatic duct, surgical ligation will be required.

Fluid balance

A preterm infant's fluid requirements will vary with gestational and chronological age. On the first day of life, about 60–90 ml/kg is usually required. This is adjusted according to the infant's clinical condition, plasma electrolytes, urine output and weight change. Subsequent

---

Temperature control

Prevention of heat loss in newborn infants

1. **Convection**
   - Raise temperature of ambient air in incubator
   - Clothe, including covering head
   - Avoid draughts
2. **Radiation**
   - Cover baby
   - Double walls for incubators
3. **Evaporation**
   - Dry and wrap at birth; if extremely preterm place baby's body directly into plastic bag at birth
   - Humidify incubator
4. **Conduction**
   - Nurse on heated mattress.

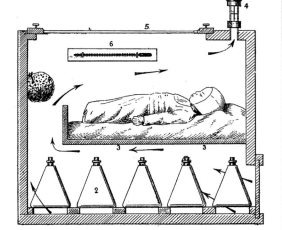

Figure 10.14 The importance of avoiding hypothermia in newborn infants has long been recognised. This incubator was used in the late nineteenth century to keep newborn infants warm. The sponge is to increase ambient humidity.

fluid volume is increased by 20–30 ml/kg per day to 150–180 ml/kg per day.

Nutrition

Preterm infants have a high nutritional requirement because of their rapid growth. Preterm infants at 28 weeks' gestation double their birthweight in 6 weeks and treble it in 12 weeks, whereas term babies double their weight in only 4.5 months and treble it in a year.

Infants of 35–36 weeks' gestational age are mature enough to suck and swallow milk. Less mature infants will need to be fed via an oro- or nasogastric tube. Even in very preterm infants, enteral feeds, preferably breast milk, are introduced as soon as possible. In these infants, breast milk needs to be supplemented with phosphate and may need supplementation with protein and calories (in breast milk fortifier) and calcium. In some neonatal units, extremely preterm infants are initially fed on donor breast milk if maternal breast milk is not available. If formula feeding is required, special infant formulas are available which are designed to meet the increased nutritional requirements of preterm infants but, in contrast to breast milk, do not provide protection against infection or other benefits of breast milk. In the very immature or sick infant, parenteral nutrition is often required. This is usually given through a central venous catheter, inserted peripherally (PICC lines, peripherally inserted central catheters), paying strict attention to aseptic technique both during insertion and when fluids are changed. However, PICC lines carry a significant risk of septicaemia; other risks include thrombosis of a major vein. For this reason, parenteral nutrition may sometimes be given via a peripheral vein, but extravasation may cause skin damage with scarring. Because of the significant risk of septicaemia from parenteral nutrition and the increased risk of necrotising enterocolitis with cow's milk based formula, mothers should be encouraged and supported to provide breast milk.

Poor bone mineralisation (osteopenia of prematurity) was previously common but is prevented by provision of adequate phosphate, calcium and vitamin D. Because iron is mostly transferred to the fetus during the last trimester, preterm babies have low iron stores and are at a risk of iron deficiency. This is in addition to loss of blood from sampling and an inadequate erythropoietin response. Iron supplements are started at several weeks of age and continued after discharge home.

Infection

Preterm infants are at increased risk of infection, as IgG is mostly transferred across the placenta in the last trimester and no IgA or IgM is transferred. In addition, infection in or around the cervix is often a reason for preterm labour and may cause infection shortly after birth. Most infections in preterm infants occur after several days of age and are nosocomial (hospital-derived); they are often associated with indwelling catheters or artificial ventilation. Infection is considered in more detail later in this chapter.

 Infection in preterm infants is a major cause of death and contributes to bronchopulmonary dysplasia (chronic lung disease), white matter injury in the brain and later disability.

Preterm brain injury

Haemorrhages in the brain occur in 25% of very low birthweight infants and are easily recognised on cranial ultrasound scans (Fig. 10.15a). Typically, they occur in the germinal matrix above the caudate nucleus, which contains a fragile network of blood vessels. Most haemorrhages occur within the first 72 h of life. They are more common following perinatal asphyxia and in infants with severe respiratory distress syndrome. Pneumothorax is a significant risk factor. Small haemorrhages confined to the germinal matrix do not increase the risk of cerebral palsy. Haemorrhage may occur in the ventricles. The most severe haemorrhage is unilateral haemorrhagic infarction involving the parenchyma of the brain; this usually results in hemiplegia (Fig. 10.15b).

A large intraventricular haemorrhage may impair the drainage and reabsorption of cerebrospinal fluid (CSF), thus allowing CSF to build up under pressure. This dilatation (Fig. 10.15c) may resolve spontaneously or progress to hydrocephalus, which may cause the cranial sutures to separate, the head circumference to increase rapidly and the anterior fontanelle to become tense. A ventriculoperitoneal shunt may be required, but initially symptomatic relief may be provided by removal of CSF by lumbar puncture or ventricular tap. About half of infants with progressive post-haemorrhagic ventricular dilatation have cerebral palsy, a higher proportion if parenchymal infarction is also present.

Periventricular white matter brain injury may occur following ischaemia or inflammation and may occur in the absence of haemorrhage. It is more difficult to detect by cranial ultrasound. Initially there may be an echodense area or 'flare' within the brain parenchyma. This may resolve within a week (in which case the risk of cerebral palsy is not increased), but if cystic lesions become visible on ultrasound 2–4 weeks later, there is definite loss of white matter. Bilateral multiple cysts, called periventricular leukomalacia (PVL), have an 80–90% risk of spastic diplegia, often with cognitive impairment, if posteriorly sited (Fig. 10.15d).

Both intraventricular haemorrhage and periventricular leukomalacia may occur in the absence of abnormal clinical signs.

Necrotising enterocolitis

Necrotising enterocolitis is a serious illness mainly affecting preterm infants in the first few weeks of life. It is associated with bacterial invasion of ischaemic bowel wall. Preterm infants fed cow's milk formula are more likely to develop this condition than if they are fed only breast milk. The infant stops tolerating feeds, milk is aspirated from the stomach and there may be vomiting, which may be bile-stained. The abdomen becomes distended (Fig. 10.16a) and the stool

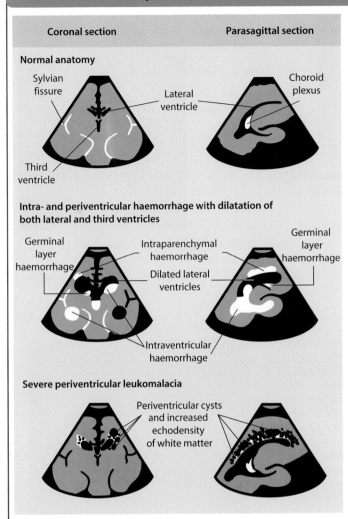

Coronal section   **Parasagittal section**

Normal anatomy

Sylvian fissure
Lateral ventricle
Choroid plexus
Third ventricle

Intra- and periventricular haemorrhage with dilatation of both lateral and third ventricles

Germinal layer haemorrhage
Intraparenchymal haemorrhage
Germinal layer haemorrhage
Dilated lateral ventricles
Intraventricular haemorrhage

Severe periventricular leukomalacia

Periventricular cysts and increased echodensity of white matter

Figure 10.15a Cranial ultrasound in preterm infants.

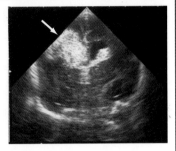

Figure 10.15b Large intraventricular haemorrhage with parenchymal haemorrhagic infarction on the right.

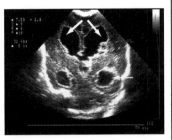

Figure 10.15c Dilatation of lateral ventricles following intraventricular haemorrhage.

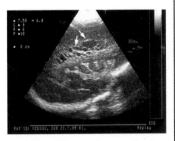

Figure 10.15d Widespread cysts in periventricular leukomalacia.

sometimes contains fresh blood. The infant may rapidly become shocked and require artificial ventilation because of abdominal distension and pain. The characteristic X-ray features are distended loops of bowel and thickening of the bowel wall with intramural gas, and there may be gas in the portal tract (Fig. 10.16b). The disease may progress to bowel perforation, which can be detected by X-ray or by transillumination of the abdomen.

Treatment is to stop oral feeding and give broad-spectrum antibiotics to cover both aerobic and anaerobic organisms. Parenteral nutrition is always needed

and artificial ventilation and circulatory support are often needed. Surgery is performed for bowel perforation. The disease has significant morbidity and a mortality of about 20%. Long-term sequelae include the development of strictures and malabsorption if extensive bowel resection has been necessary.

Retinopathy of prematurity

Retinopathy of prematurity (ROP) affects developing blood vessels at the junction of the vascular and non-vascularised retina. There is vascular proliferation

Neonatal medicine

165

Necrotising enterocolitis

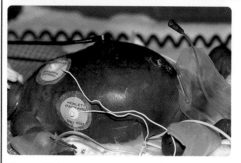

Figure 10.16a Necrotising enterocolitis showing gross abdominal distension and tense and shiny skin over the abdomen.

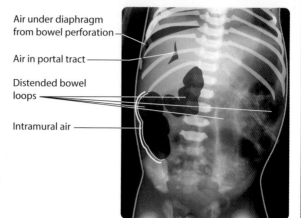

Air under diaphragm from bowel perforation

Air in portal tract

Distended bowel loops

Intramural air

Figure 10.16b Diagram of characteristic features of necrotising enterocolitis on abdominal X-ray.

which may progress to retinal detachment, fibrosis and blindness. It was initially recognised that the risk is increased by uncontrolled use of high concentrations of oxygen. Now, even with careful monitoring of the infant's oxygenation, retinopathy of prematurity is still found in about 35% of all very low birthweight infants. As laser therapy reduces visual impairment, the eyes of susceptible preterm infants (<1500 g birthweight or <32 weeks' gestation) are screened every week by an ophthalmologist. Severe bilateral visual impairment occurs in about 1% of very low birthweight infants, mostly in infants of <28 weeks' gestation.

Bronchopulmonary dysplasia

Infants who still have an oxygen requirement at a postmenstrual age of 36 weeks are described as having bronchopulmonary dysplasia (BPD) or chronic lung disease. The lung damage comes from pressure and volume trauma from artificial ventilation, oxygen toxicity and infection. The chest X-ray characteristically shows widespread areas of opacification, sometimes with cystic changes (Fig. 10.17). Some infants need prolonged artificial ventilation, but most are weaned onto continuous positive airways pressure (CPAP) followed by additional ambient oxygen, sometimes over several months. Corticosteroid therapy may facilitate earlier weaning from the ventilator and often reduces the infant's oxygen requirements in the short term, but concern about increased risk of abnormal neurodevelopment including cerebral palsy limits use to those at highest risk and only short courses are given. Some babies go home while still receiving additional oxygen. A few infants with severe disease may die of intercurrent infection or pulmonary hypertension. Subsequent pertussis and RSV (respiratory syncytial virus) infection may cause respiratory failure necessitating intensive care.

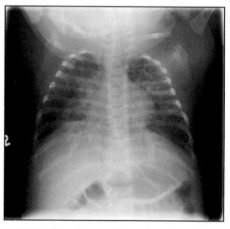

Figure 10.17 Chest X-ray of bronchopulmonary dysplasia (BPD) showing fibrosis and lung collapse, cystic changes and overdistension of the lungs.

Problems following discharge

To prevent anaemia of prematurity, additional iron as supplementation or in preterm formula is given until 6 months corrected age, when iron becomes available from solid foods. Multivitamins are also recommended. The standard immunisations should be given.

Medical problems include increased risk of:

- poor growth – at discharge, over 90% of VLBW infants are below the 10th centile for weight, length and head circumference. Many show some catch-up growth in the first 2–3 years
- pneumonia/wheezing/asthma
- bronchiolitis from RSV (respiratory syncytial virus) infection (hospitalisation reduced

by giving RSV monoclonal antibody, palivizumab)
- bronchopulmonary dysplasia – may require additional oxygen therapy for many months, when it may be provided at home
- gastro-oesophageal reflux – especially with bronchopulmonary dysplasia
- complex nutritional and gastrointestinal disorders – following necrotising enterocolitis or gastrointestinal surgery
- inguinal hernias – require surgical repair.

Readmission to hospital during the first year of life is increased approximately four-fold – mainly for respiratory disorders and surgical repair of inguinal hernias.

Summary

Summary of problems of very low birthweight infants (<1.5 kg)

Respiratory

Respiratory distress syndrome (surfactant deficiency)(74%)
- respiratory distress within 4 hours of birth
- antenatal corticosteroids and surfactant therapy reduce morbidity and mortality
- oxygen therapy, but excess may damage the retina
- nasal CPAP (continuous positive airway pressure) (67%) and mechanical ventilation (64%) - often required to expand lungs and prevent lung collapse

Pneumothorax (4%)
Apnoea and bradycardia and desaturations
Bronchopulmonary dysplasia (chronic lung disease) – O_2 requirement at 36 weeks post-menstrual age (27%)

Circulation

Hypotension – may require volume support, intropes or corticosteroids
Patent ductus arteriosus – needing medical treatment (34%) or surgical ligation (8%)

Nutrition

Nasogastric tube feeding – until 35–36 weeks post-menstrual age
Feeding intolerance - TPN (total parenteral nutrition) often required

Gastrointestinal

Necrotising enterocolitis (6%) – serious, management is medical or surgery for bowel necrosis or perforation

Metabolic

Hypoglycaemia – common
Electrolyte disturbances
Osteopenia of prematurity from phosphate deficiency

Hearing

Checked before discharge

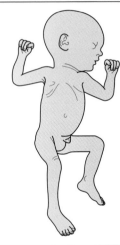

Jaundice – common, low treatment threshold

Anaemia
Often need blood transfusions

Eyes
Retinopathy of prematurity – may need laser therapy (4%)

Temperature control

Avoid hypothermia
Nurse in neutral thermal environment
Nurse in incubator or under radiant warmer
Clothe if possible
Humidity reduces evaporative heat loss

Infection

Common and potentially serious (25%)
Increased risk of early-onset infection – group B streptococcus
Main problem is nosocomial infection – mainly coagulase-negative staphylococcus, also fungal and other infections

Brain injury

Haemorrhage (25%) - germinal layer, intraventricular, parenchymal
Ventricular dilatation – may need ventriculo-peritoneal shunt
Periventricular leukomalacia (3%) – ischaemic white matter injury

Following discharge
Specialist community nursing support helpful, if available
Increased risk of respiratory infection and wheezing – especially from bronchiolitis (caused by respiratory syncitial virus, RSV) and pertussis; may need intensive care
Consider prophylaxis against RSV infection
Increased rehospitalisation – respiratory disorders, inguinal hernias
Monitor growth, development (for learning disorders, co-ordination, cerebral palsy), behaviour, attention, vision, hearing – increased risk of impairment

About 5–10% of very low birthweight infants develop cerebral palsy, but the most common impairments are learning difficulties. The prevalence of cognitive impairment and of other associated difficulties increases with decreasing gestational age at birth, and is greatest if born at very early gestational age (<26 weeks' gestation) (Fig. 10.18a,b). It becomes increasingly evident when the individual child is compared to their peers at nursery or school. In addition, children may have difficulties with:

- fine motor skills, e.g. threading beads
- concentration, with short attention span
- behavior problems, especially attention deficit disorders
- abstract reasoning, e.g. mathematics
- processing several tasks simultaneously.

A small proportion also have hearing impairment, with 1–2% requiring amplification, or visual impairment, with 1% blind in both eyes. A greater proportion have refraction errors and squints and therefore require glasses.

Jaundice

Over 50% of all newborn infants become visibly jaundiced. This is because:

- there is marked physiological release of haemoglobin from the breakdown of red cells because of the high Hb concentration at birth (Fig. 10.19)
- the red cell life span of newborn infants (70 days) is markedly shorter than that of adults (120 days)
- hepatic bilirubin metabolism is less efficient in the first few days of life.

Neonatal jaundice is important as:

- it may be a sign of another disorder, e.g. haemolytic anaemia, infection, metabolic disease, liver disease.
- unconjugated bilirubin can be deposited in the brain, particularly in the basal ganglia, causing kernicterus.

Kernicterus

This is the encephalopathy resulting from the deposition of unconjugated bilirubin in the basal ganglia and brainstem nuclei (Fig. 10.20). It may occur when the level of unconjugated bilirubin exceeds the albumin-binding capacity of bilirubin of the blood. As this free bilirubin is fat-soluble, it can cross the blood–brain barrier. The neurotoxic effects vary in severity from transient disturbance to severe damage and death. Acute manifestations are lethargy and poor feeding. In severe cases, there is irritability, increased muscle tone causing the baby to lie with an arched back (opisthotonos), seizures and coma. Infants who survive may develop choreoathetoid cerebral palsy (due to damage to the basal ganglia), learning difficulties and sensorineural deafness. Kernicterus used to be an important cause of brain damage in infants with severe rhesus haemolytic disease, but has become rare since the introduction of prophylactic anti-D

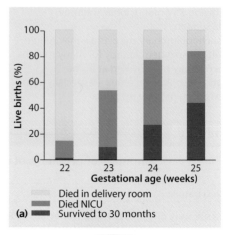

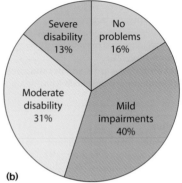

(b)

Figure 10.18 The EPICure study, a population-based study of mortality and disability in the UK and Ireland in 1995 of all infants born alive at 22–25 weeks' gestation. **(a)** Survival. (Adapted from Wood NS, et al. 2000. Neurologic and developmental disability after extremely preterm birth. EPICure Study Group. *New England Journal of Medicine* 343:378–384). **(b)** Proportion of survivors with disability at 11 years of age. (Adapted from Johnson S et al. 2009. Neurodevelopmental disability through 11 years of age in children born before 26 weeks of gestation. *Pediatrics* 124:e249–e257). Preterm babies born in 2006 show a 30% increase in numbers born at <26 weeks and increased survival. Long-term follow-up is in progress.

immunoglobulin for rhesus-negative mothers. However, a few cases continue to occur, especially in slightly preterm infants (35–37 weeks), which has led NICE to issue guidelines on the management of neonatal jaundice.

Clinical evaluation

Babies become clinically jaundiced when the bilirubin level reaches about 80 µmol/L. Management varies according to the infant's gestational age, age at onset, bilirubin level and rate of rise, and the overall clinical condition.

Age at onset

The age of onset is a useful guide to the likely cause of the jaundice (Table 10.2).

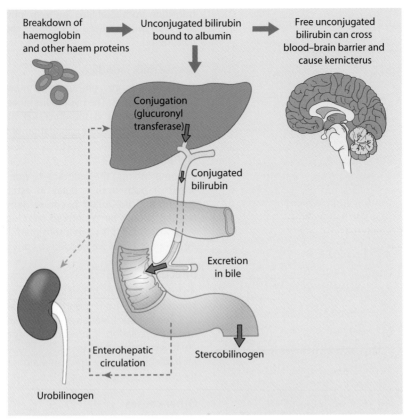

Figure 10.19 The breakdown product of haemoglobin is unconjugated bilirubin (indirect bilirubin), which is insoluble in water but soluble in lipids. It is carried in the blood bound to albumin. When the albumin binding is saturated, free unconjugated bilirubin can cross the blood–brain barrier, as it is lipid soluble. Unconjugated bilirubin bound to albumin is taken up by the liver and conjugated by the enzyme glucuronyl transferase to conjugated bilirubin (direct bilirubin), which is water-soluble and excreted in bile into the gut and is detectable in urine when blood levels rise. Reabsorption of bilirubin from the gut (enterohepatic circulation) is increased when milk intake is low.

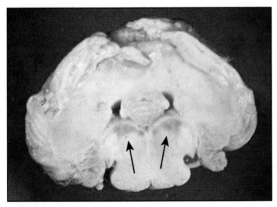

Figure 10.20 Postmortem brainstem and cerebellum showing kernicterus with yellow bilirubin staining of brainstem nuclei (arrows).

Jaundice <24 h of age

Jaundice starting within 24 h of birth usually results from haemolysis. This is particularly important to identify as the bilirubin is unconjugated and can rise very rapidly and reach extremely high levels.

Haemolytic disorders

Rhesus haemolytic disease – Affected infants are usually identified antenatally and monitored and treated if necessary (see Ch. 9). The birth of a severely affected infant, with anaemia, hydrops and hepatosplenomegaly with rapidly developing severe jaundice, has become rare. Antibodies may develop to rhesus antigens other than D and to the Kell and Duffy blood groups, but haemolysis is usually less severe.

ABO incompatibility – This is now more common than rhesus haemolytic disease. Most ABO antibodies are IgM and do not cross the placenta, but some group O women have an IgG anti-A-haemolysin in the blood which can cross the placenta and haemolyse the red cells of a group A infant. Occasionally, group B infants are affected by anti-B haemolysins. Haemolysis can cause severe jaundice but it is usually less severe than in rhesus disease. The infant's haemoglobin level is usually normal or only slightly reduced and, in contrast to rhesus disease, hepatosplenomegaly is absent. The direct antibody test (Coombs' test), which demonstrates antibody on the surface of red cells, is positive. The jaundice usually peaks in the first 12–72 h.

G6PD deficiency (see Ch. 22) – Mainly in people originating in the Mediterranean, Middle-East and Far East

Table 10.2 Causes of neonatal jaundice

Jaundice starting at <24 h of age	*Haemolytic disorders*: 　Rhesus incompatibility 　ABO incompatibility 　G6PD deficiency 　Spherocytosis, pyruvate kinase deficiency 　Congenital infection *(conjugated)*
Jaundice at 24 h to 2 weeks of age	Physiological jaundice Breast milk jaundice Infection, e.g. urinary tract infection Haemolysis, e.g. G6PD deficiency, ABO incompatibility Bruising Polycythaemia Crigler–Najjar syndrome *(Glucoronyl transferase def)*
Jaundice at >2 weeks of age	*Unconjugated*: 　Physiological or breast milk jaundice 　Infection (particularly urinary tract) 　Hypothyroidism 　Haemolytic anaemia, e.g. G6PD deficiency 　High gastrointestinal obstruction, e.g. pyloric stenosis *Conjugated (>25 µmol/L)*: 　Bile duct obstruction 　Neonatal hepatitis

Investigations:
- Bilirubin (Total, direct & indirect)
- CBC & reticulocytes
- Maternal & fetal Blood groups
- Coomb's test.

or in African-Americans. Mainly affects male infants , but some females develop significant jaundice. Parents of affected infants should be given a list of drugs to be avoided, as they may precipitate haemolysis.

Spherocytosis – This is considerably less common than G6PD deficiency (see Ch. 22). There is often, but not always, a family history. The disorder can be identified by recognising spherocytes on the blood film.

Congenital infection

Jaundice at birth can also be from congenital infection. In this case, the bilirubin is conjugated and the infants have other abnormal clinical signs, such as growth restriction, hepatosplenomegaly and thrombocytopenic purpura.

Jaundice at 2 days to 2 weeks of age

Physiological jaundice

Most babies who become mildly or moderately jaundiced during this period have no underlying cause and the bilirubin has risen as the infant is adapting to the transition from fetal life. The term 'physiological jaundice' can only be used after other causes have been considered.

Breast milk jaundice

Jaundice is more common and more prolonged in breast-fed infants. The hyperbilirubinaemia is unconjugated. The cause is multifactorial but may involve increased enterohepatic circulation of bilirubin.

Dehydration

In some infants, the jaundice is exacerbated if milk intake is poor from a delay in establishing breast-feeding and the infant becomes dehydrated. Breast-feeding should be continued, although the bilirubin level would fall if it were interrupted. In some infants, intravenous fluids are needed to correct dehydration.

Infection

An infected baby may develop an unconjugated hyperbilirubinaemia from poor fluid intake, haemolysis, reduced hepatic function and an increase in the enterohepatic circulation. If infection is suspected, appropriate investigations and treatment should be instigated. In particular, urinary tract infection may present in this way.

Other causes

Although jaundice from haemolysis usually presents in the first day of life, it may occur during the first week. Bruising and polycythaemia (venous haematocrit is >0.65) will exacerbate the infant's jaundice. The very rare Crigler–Najjar syndrome, in which the enzyme glucuronyl transferase is deficient or absent, may result in extremely high levels of unconjugated bilirubin.

The causes and management of jaundice at >2 weeks of age (persistent neonatal jaundice), (3 weeks if preterm), are different and are considered separately below.

Severity of jaundice

Jaundice can be observed most easily by blanching the skin with one's finger. The jaundice tends to start on the head and face and then spreads down the trunk and limbs. If the baby is clinically jaundiced, the bilirubin should be checked with a transcutaneous bilirubin meter or blood sample. It is easy to underestimate in Afro-Caribbean, Asian and preterm babies, and a low threshold should be adopted for measuring the bilirubin of these infants. A high transcutaneous bilirubin level must be checked with a blood laboratory measurement. It is now recommended in the UK that all babies should be checked clinically for jaundice in the first 72 h of life, whether at hospital or home, and if clinically jaundiced, a transcutaneous measurement made.

Rate of change

The rate of rise tends to be linear until a plateau is reached, so serial measurements can be plotted on a chart and used to anticipate the need for treatment before it rises to a dangerous level.

Gestation

Preterm infants are more susceptible to damage from raised bilirubin, so the intervention threshold is lower.

Clinical condition

Infants who experience severe hypoxia, hypothermia or any serious illness may be more susceptible to damage from severe jaundice. Drugs which may displace bilirubin from albumin, e.g. sulphonamides and diazepam, are therefore avoided in newborn infants.

Management

Poor milk intake and dehydration will exacerbate jaundice and should be corrected, but studies have failed to show that routinely supplementing breast-fed infants with water or dextrose solution reduces jaundice. Phototherapy is the most widely used therapy, with exchange transfusion for severe cases.

Phototherapy

Light (wavelength 450 nm) from the blue–green band of the visible spectrum converts unconjugated bilirubin into a harmless water-soluble pigment excreted predominantly in the urine. It is delivered with an overhead light source placed the optimal distance above the infant to achieve high irradiance. Although no long-term sequelae of phototherapy from overhead light have been reported, it is disruptive to normal nursing of the infant and should not be used indiscriminately. The infant's eyes are covered, as bright light is uncomfortable. Phototherapy can result in temperature instability as the infant is undressed, a macular rash and bronze discoloration of the skin if the jaundice is conjugated.

[handwritten annotations: ① ② ③ 4. Eye Injury 5. Diarrhea.]

Continuous multiple ('intensive') phototherapy is given if the bilirubin is rising rapidly or has reached a high level.

Exchange transfusion

Exchange transfusion is required if the bilirubin rises to levels which are considered potentially dangerous. Blood is removed from the baby in small aliquots, (usually from an arterial line or the umbilical vein) and replaced with donor blood (via peripheral or umbilical vein). Twice the infant's blood volume (2×80 ml/kg) is exchanged. Donor blood should be as fresh as possible and screened to exclude CMV, hepatitis B and C and HIV infection. The procedure does carry some risk of morbidity and mortality.

Phototherapy has been very successful in reducing the need for exchange transfusion. In infants with rhesus haemolytic disease or ABO incompatibility unresponsive to intensive phototherapy, intravenous immunoglobulin reduces the need for exchange transfusion.

There is no bilirubin level known to be safe or which will definitely cause kernicterus. In rhesus haemolytic disease, it was found that kernicterus could be prevented if the bilirubin was kept below 340 μmol/L (20 mg/dl). As there is no consensus among paediatricians in the UK on the bilirubin levels for phototherapy and exchange transfusion, guidelines have been published by NICE to ensure uniform practice.

Jaundice at >2 weeks of age

Jaundice in babies more than 2 weeks old (3 weeks if preterm), is called persistent or prolonged neonatal jaundice. The key feature is that it may be caused by biliary atresia, and it is important to diagnose

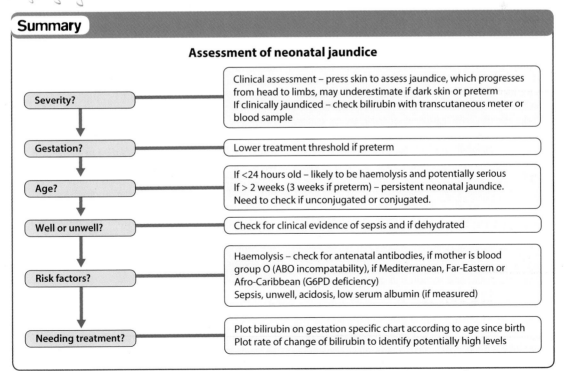

Summary

Assessment of neonatal jaundice

Severity?	Clinical assessment – press skin to assess jaundice, which progresses from head to limbs, may underestimate if dark skin or preterm. If clinically jaundiced – check bilirubin with transcutaneous meter or blood sample
Gestation?	Lower treatment threshold if preterm
Age?	If <24 hours old – likely to be haemolysis and potentially serious. If > 2 weeks (3 weeks if preterm) – persistent neonatal jaundice. Need to check if unconjugated or conjugated.
Well or unwell?	Check for clinical evidence of sepsis and if dehydrated
Risk factors?	Haemolysis – check for antenatal antibodies, if mother is blood group O (ABO incompatability), if Mediterranean, Far-Eastern or Afro-Caribbean (G6PD deficiency). Sepsis, unwell, acidosis, low serum albumin (if measured)
Needing treatment?	Plot bilirubin on gestation specific chart according to age since birth. Plot rate of change of bilirubin to identify potentially high levels

Neonatal medicine

biliary atresia promptly, as delay in surgical treatment adversely affects outcome (see Ch. 20 for further details).

However, in most infants with persistent neonatal jaundice, the hyperbilirubinaemia is unconjugated, but this needs to be confirmed on laboratory testing.

In prolonged unconjugated hyperbilirubinaemia:

- 'Breast milk jaundice' is the most common cause, affecting up to 15% of healthy breast-fed infants; the jaundice gradually fades and disappears by 4–5 weeks of age.
- Infection, particularly of the urinary tract, needs to be considered.
- Congenital hypothyroidism may cause prolonged jaundice before the clinical features of coarse facies, dry skin, hypotonia and constipation become evident. Affected infants should be identified on routine neonatal biochemical screening (Guthrie test).

Conjugated hyperbilirubinaemia (>25 µmol/L) is suggested by the baby passing dark urine and unpigmented pale stools. Hepatomegaly and poor weight gain are other clinical signs that may be present. Its causes include neonatal hepatitis syndrome and biliary atresia, with improved prognosis of biliary atresia with early diagnosis (see Ch. 20 for further details).

Respiratory distress in term infants

Newborn infants with respiratory problems develop the following signs of respiratory distress:

- tachypnoea (>60 breaths/min)
- laboured breathing, with chest wall recession (particularly sternal and subcostal indrawing) and nasal flaring
- expiratory grunting
- cyanosis if severe.

The causes in term infants are listed in Table 10.3.

Affected infants should be admitted to the neonatal unit for monitoring of heart and respiratory rates, oxygenation and circulation. A chest X-ray will be required to help identify the cause, especially those causes which may need immediate treatment, e.g. pneumothorax or diaphragmatic hernia. Additional ambient oxygen, mechanical ventilation and circulatory support are given as required.

Transient tachypnoea of the newborn

This is by far the commonest cause of respiratory distress in term infants. It is caused by delay in the resorption of lung liquid and is more common after birth by Caesarean section. The chest X-ray may show fluid in the horizontal fissure. Additional ambient oxygen may be required. The condition usually settles within the first day of life but can take several days to resolve completely. This is a diagnosis made after consideration and exclusion of other causes.

Table 10.3 Causes of respiratory distress in term infants

Pulmonary	
Common	Transient tachypnoea of the newborn
Less common	Meconium aspiration
	Pneumonia
	Respiratory distress syndrome
	Pneumothorax
	Persistent pulmonary hypertension of the newborn
	Milk aspiration
Rare	Diaphragmatic hernia
	Tracheo-oesophageal fistula (TOF)
	Pulmonary hypoplasia
	Airways obstruction, e.g. choanal atresia
	Pulmonary haemorrhage
Non-pulmonary	
	Congenital heart disease
	Intracranial birth trauma/ encephalopathy
	Severe anaemia
	Metabolic acidosis

Meconium aspiration

Meconium is passed before birth by 8–20% of babies. It is rarely passed by preterm infants, and occurs increasingly the greater the gestational age, affecting 20–25% of deliveries by 42 weeks. It may be passed in response to fetal hypoxia. At birth these infants may inhale thick meconium. Asphyxiated infants may start gasping and aspirate meconium before delivery. Meconium is a lung irritant and results in both mechanical obstruction and a chemical pneumonitis, as well as predisposing to infection. In meconium aspiration the lungs are over-inflated, accompanied by patches of collapse and consolidation. There is a high incidence of air leak, leading to pneumothorax and pneumomediastinum. Artificial ventilation is often required. Infants with meconium aspiration may develop persistent pulmonary hypertension of the newborn which may make it difficult to achieve adequate oxygenation despite high pressure ventilation (see below for management). Severe meconium aspiration is associated with significant morbidity and mortality.

Pneumonia

Prolonged rupture of the membranes, chorioamnionitis and low birthweight predispose to pneumonia. Infants with respiratory distress will usually require investigation to identify any infection. Broad-spectrum antibiotics are started early until the results of the infection screen are available.

Pneumothorax

A pneumothorax may occur spontaneously in up to 2% of deliveries. It is usually asymptomatic but may cause respiratory distress. Pneumothoraces also occur secondary to meconium aspiration, respiratory distress syndrome or as a complication of ventilation. (Management is described earlier in this chapter.)

Milk aspiration

This occurs more frequently in preterm infants and those with respiratory distress or neurological damage. Babies with bronchopulmonary dysplasia often have gastro-oesophageal reflux, which predisposes to aspiration. Infants with a cleft palate are prone to aspirate respiratory secretions or milk.

Persistent pulmonary hypertension of the newborn

This life-threatening condition is usually associated with birth asphyxia, meconium aspiration, septicaemia or respiratory distress syndrome. It sometimes occurs as a primary disorder. As a result of the high pulmonary vascular resistance, there is right-to-left shunting within the lungs and at atrial and ductal levels. Cyanosis occurs soon after birth. Heart murmurs and signs of heart failure are often absent. A chest X-ray shows that the heart is of normal size and there may be pulmonary oligaemia. An urgent echocardiogram is required to establish that the child does not have congenital heart disease.

Most infants require mechanical ventilation and circulatory support in order to achieve adequate oxygenation. Inhaled nitric oxide, a potent vasodilator, is often beneficial. Another vasodilator, sildenafil (Viagra), has been introduced more recently. High-frequency or oscillatory ventilation is sometimes helpful. Extracorporeal membrane oxygenation (ECMO), where the infant is placed on heart and lung bypass for several days, is indicated for severe but reversible cases, but is only performed in a few specialist centres.

Diaphragmatic hernia

This occurs in about 1 in 4000 births. Many are now diagnosed on antenatal ultrasound screening. In the newborn period, it usually presents with failure to respond to resuscitation or as respiratory distress. In most cases, there is a left-sided herniation of abdominal contents through the posterolateral foramen of the diaphragm. The apex beat and heart sounds will then be displaced to the right side of the chest, with poor air entry in the left chest. Vigorous resuscitation may cause a pneumothorax in the normal lung, thereby aggravating the situation. The diagnosis is confirmed by X-ray of the chest and abdomen (Fig. 10.21). Once the

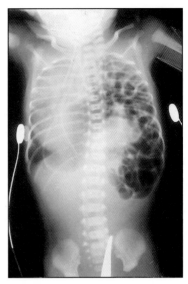

Figure 10.21 Chest X-ray of diaphragmatic hernia showing loops of bowel in the left chest and displacement of the mediastinum.

diagnosis is suspected, a large nasogastric tube is passed and suction is applied to prevent distension of the intrathoracic bowel. After stabilisation, the diaphragmatic hernia is repaired surgically, but in most infants with this condition the main problem is pulmonary hypoplasia – where compression by the herniated viscera throughout pregnancy has prevented development of the lung in the fetus. If the lungs are hypoplastic, mortality is high.

Other causes

Other causes of respiratory distress are listed in Table 10.3. When due to heart failure, abnormal heart sounds and/or heart murmurs may be present on auscultation. An enlarged liver from venous congestion is a helpful sign. The femoral arteries must be palpated in all infants with respiratory distress, as coarctation of the aorta and interrupted aortic arch are important causes of heart failure in newborn infants.

Infection

The time of highest risk in childhood for acquiring a serious invasive bacterial infection is the neonatal period. Infections fall into two broad categories, early- and late-onset sepsis.

Early-onset infection

In early-onset sepsis (<48 h after birth), bacteria have ascended from the birth canal and invaded the amniotic fluid. The fetus is secondarily infected because the fetal lungs are in direct contact with infected amniotic fluid. These infants have pneumonia and secondary bacteraemia/septicaemia. In contrast, congenital viral infections and early-onset infection with *Listeria*

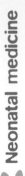

modes of infection:
- Birth canal → amniotic fluid
- Placenta

173

Box 10.2 Clinical features of neonatal sepsis

- Fever or temperature instability or hypothermia
- Poor feeding
- Vomiting
- Apnoea and bradycardia
- Respiratory distress
- Abdominal distension
- Jaundice
- Neutropenia
- Hypo-/hyperglycaemia
- Shock
- Irritability
- Seizures
- Lethargy, drowsiness
- *In meningitis:*
- Tense or bulging fontanelle
- Head retraction (opisthotonos)

monocytogenes, fetal infection is acquired via the placenta following maternal infection.

The risk of early-onset infection is increased if there has been prolonged or premature rupture of the amniotic membranes, and when chorioamnionitis is clinically evident such as when the mother has fever during labour. Presentation is with respiratory distress, apnoea and temperature instability (Box 10.2). A chest X-ray is performed, together with a septic screen. A full blood count is performed to detect neutropenia, as well as blood cultures. An acute-phase reactant (C-reactive protein) is helpful but takes 12–24 h to rise, so one normal result does not exclude infection, but two consecutive normal values are strong evidence against infection. Antibiotics are started immediately without waiting for culture results. Intravenous antibiotics are given to cover group B streptococci, *Listeria monocytogenes* and other Gram-positive organisms (usually benzylpenicillin or amoxicillin), combined with cover for Gram-negative organisms (usually an aminoglycoside such as gentamicin). If cultures and CRP are negative and the infant has recovered clinically, antibiotics can be stopped after 48 h. If the blood culture is positive or if there are any neurological signs, CSF must be examined and cultured.

Late-onset infection (infant environment)

In late-onset infection (>48 h after birth), the source of infection is often the infant's environment. The presentation is usually non-specific (Box 10.2). Nosocomially acquired infections are an inherent risk in a neonatal unit, and all staff must adhere strictly to effective hand hygiene measures to prevent cross-infection. In neonatal intensive care, the main sources of infection are indwelling central venous catheters for parenteral nutrition, invasive procedures which break the protective barrier of the skin, and tracheal tubes. Coagulase-negative staphylococcus (*Staphylococcus epidermidis*) is the most common pathogen, but the range of organisms is broad, and includes Gram-positive bacteria (*Staphylococcus aureus* and *Enterococcus faecalis*) and Gram-negative bacteria (*Escherichia coli* and *Pseudomonas*, *Klebsiella* and *Serratia* species). Initial therapy (e.g. with flucloxacillin and gentamicin) is aimed to cover most staphylococci and Gram-negative bacilli. If the organism is resistant to these antibiotics or the infant's condition does not improve, specific antibiotics (e.g. vancomycin for coagulase-negative staphylococci or enterococci) or broad-spectrum antibiotics (e.g. meropenem) may be indicated. Use of prolonged or broad-spectrum antibiotics predisposes to invasive fungal infections (e.g. *Candida albicans*) in premature babies. Serial measurements of an acute-phase reactant (CRP) are useful to monitor response to therapy.

Neonatal meningitis, although uncommon, has a mortality of 20–50%, with one-third of survivors having serious sequelae. Presentation is non-specific (Box 10.2); a bulging fontanelle and hyperextension of neck and back (opisthotonos) are late signs and rarely seen in newborn infants. If meningitis is thought likely, ampicillin or penicillin and a third-generation cephalosporin (e.g. cefotaxime, which has CSF penetration) are given. Complications include cerebral abscess, ventriculitis, hydrocephalus, hearing loss and neurodevelopmental impairment.

Some specific infections

Group B streptococcal infection

Around 10–30% of pregnant women have faecal or vaginal carriage of group B streptococci. The organism causes early- and late-onset sepsis. In early-onset sepsis, the newborn baby has respiratory distress and pneumonia. In the UK, approximately 0.5–1 in 1000 babies have early-onset infection; most have pneumonia only, but it may cause septicaemia and meningitis. The severity of the neonatal presentation depends on the duration of the infection in utero. Mortality in babies with positive blood or CSF cultures is up to 10%.

Up to half of infants born to mothers who carry group B streptococcus are colonised on their mucous membranes or skin. Some of these babies develop late-onset disease, up to 3 months of age. It usually presents with meningitis, or occasionally with focal infection (e.g. osteomyelitis or septic arthritis).

In colonised mothers, risk factors for infection are preterm, prolonged rupture of membranes, maternal fever during labour (>38°C), maternal chorioamnionitis or previously infected infant. Prophylactic intrapartum antibiotics given intravenously to the mother can prevent group B streptococcus infection in the newborn baby. There are two approaches to the use of intrapartum antibiotics – universal screening at 35–38 weeks to identify mothers who carry the organism (as practiced in the USA and Australia) and a risk-based approach, in which mothers with risk factors for infection are offered antibiotics (as in the UK).

Listeria monocytogenes *infection*

Fetal or newborn *Listeria* infection is uncommon but serious. The organism is transmitted to the mother in food, such as unpasteurised milk, soft cheeses and undercooked poultry. It causes a bacteraemia, often with mild, influenza-like illness in the mother, and passage to the fetus via the placenta. Maternal infection may cause spontaneous abortion, preterm delivery or fetal/neonatal sepsis. Characteristic features are meconium staining of the liquor, unusual in preterm infants, a widespread rash, septicaemia, pneumonia and meningitis. The mortality is 30%.

Late-onset disease also occurs, most often with meningitis, and has a better prognosis.

Gram-negative infections

Early-onset infection is acquired in the same way as group B streptococcal infection. Late-onset infection is usually from infected central venous lines, but occasionally from seeding to the circulation from the intestines.

Conjunctivitis

Sticky eyes are common in the neonatal period, starting on the 3rd or 4th day of life. Cleaning with saline or water is all that is required and the condition resolves spontaneously. A more troublesome discharge with redness of the eye may be due to staphylococcal or streptococcal infection and can be treated with a topical antibiotic eye ointment, e.g. neomycin.

Purulent discharge with conjunctival injection and swelling of the eyelids within the first 48 h of life may be due to gonococcal infection. The discharge should be Gram-stained urgently, as well as cultured, and treatment started immediately, as permanent loss of vision can occur. In countries such as the UK and the USA where penicillin resistance is a problem, a third-generation cephalosporin is given intravenously. The eye needs to be cleansed frequently.

Chlamydia trachomatis eye infection usually presents with a purulent discharge, together with swelling of the eyelids (Fig. 10.22), at 1–2 weeks of age, but may also present shortly after birth. The organism can be identified with immunofluorescent staining. Treatment is with oral erythromycin for 2 weeks. The

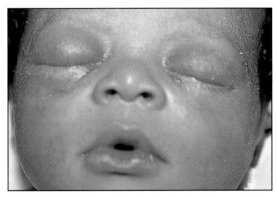

Figure 10.22 Purulent discharge, together with swollen eyelids, in an 8-day-old infant. This is the characteristic presentation of conjunctivitis from *Chlamydia trachomatis*. *Neisseria gonorrhoeae* was absent.

mother and partner also need to be checked and treated.

Umbilical infection

The umbilicus dries and separates during the first few days of life. If the skin surrounding the umbilicus becomes inflamed, systemic antibiotics are indicated. Sometimes the umbilicus continues to be sticky, as it is prevented from involuting by an umbilical granuloma. This can be removed by applying silver nitrate while protecting the surrounding skin to avoid chemical burns, or by applying a ligature around the base of the exposed stump.

Herpes simplex virus (HSV) infections

Neonatal HSV infection is uncommon, occurring in 1 in 3000 to 1 in 20 000 live births. HSV infection is usually transmitted during passage through an infected birth canal or occasionally by ascending infection. The risk to an infant born to a mother with a primary genital infection is high, about 40%, while the risk from recurrent maternal infection is less than 3%. In most infants who develop HSV infection, the condition is unexpected as the mother does not know that she is infected (asymptomatic or non-specific illness).

Infection is more common in preterm infants. Presentation is at any time up to 4 weeks of age, with localised herpetic lesions on the skin or eye, or with encephalitis or disseminated disease. Mortality due to localised disease is low, but, even with aciclovir treatment, disseminated disease has a high mortality with considerable morbidity after encephalitis. If the mother is recognised as having primary disease or develops genital herpetic lesions at the time of delivery, elective Caesarean section is indicated. Women with a history of recurrent genital infection can be delivered vaginally as the risk of neonatal infection is low and maternal treatment before delivery minimises the presence of virus at delivery. Aciclovir can be given prophylactically to the baby during the at-risk period, but its efficacy is unproven.

Hepatitis B

Infants of mothers who are hepatitis B surface antigen (HBsAg)-positive should receive hepatitis B vaccination shortly after birth to prevent vertical transmission. The vaccination course needs to be completed during infancy and antibody response checked. Babies are at highest risk of becoming chronic carriers when their mothers are 'e' antigen-positive but have no 'e' antibodies. Infants of 'e' antigen-positive mothers should also be given passive immunisation with hepatitis B immunoglobulin within 24 h of birth.

 Infants of HBsAg-positive mothers should be vaccinated against hepatitis B.

Hypoglycaemia

Hypoglycaemia is particularly likely in the first 24 h of life in babies with intrauterine growth restriction, who are preterm, born to mothers with diabetes mellitus, are large-for-dates, hypothermic, polycythaemic or ill for any reason. Growth-restricted and preterm infants have poor glycogen stores, whereas the infants of a diabetic mother have sufficient glycogen stores, but hyperplasia of the islet cells in the pancreas causes high insulin levels. Symptoms are jitteriness, irritability, apnoea, lethargy, drowsiness and seizures.

There is no agreed definition of hypoglycaemia in the newborn. Many babies tolerate low blood glucose levels in the first few days of life, as they are able to utilise lactate and ketones as energy stores. Recent evidence suggests that blood glucose levels above 2.6 mmol/L are desirable for optimal neurodevelopmental outcome, although during the first 24 h after birth many asymptomatic infants transiently have blood glucose levels below this level. There is good evidence that prolonged, symptomatic hypoglycaemia can cause permanent neurological disability.

Hypoglycaemia can usually be prevented by early and frequent milk feeding. In infants at increased risk of hypoglycaemia, blood glucose is regularly monitored at the bedside. If an asymptomatic infant has two low glucose values (i.e. below 2.6 mmol/L) in spite of adequate feeding or one very low value (<1.6 mmol/L) or becomes symptomatic, glucose is given by intravenous infusion aiming to maintain the glucose >2.6 mmol/L. The concentration of the intravenous dextrose may need to be increased from 10% to 15% or even 20%. Abnormal blood glucose results should be confirmed in the laboratory. High-concentration intravenous infusions of glucose should be given via a central venous catheter to avoid extravasation into the tissues, which may cause skin necrosis and reactive hypoglycaemia. If there is difficulty or delay in starting the infusion, or a satisfactory response is not achieved, glucagon or hydrocortisone can be given.

Neonatal seizures

Many babies startle or have tremors when stimulated or make strange jerks during active sleep. Seizures, on the other hand, are unstimulated. Typically, there are repetitive, rhythmic (clonic) movements of the limbs which persist despite restraint and are often accompanied by eye movements and changes in respiration. Many neonatal units now use continuous single channel EEG (amplified integrated EEG, also called a cerebral function monitor) to be able to confirm changes in electrical discharges in the brain. The causes of seizures are listed in Box 10.3.

Whenever seizures are observed, hypoglycaemia and meningitis need to be excluded or treated urgently. A cerebral ultrasound is performed to identify haemorrhage or cerebral malformation. Identification of some cerebral ischaemic lesions or cerebral malformations will require MRI scans of the brain. Treatment is directed at the cause, whenever possible. Ongoing or repeated seizures are treated with an anticonvulsant, although their efficacy in suppressing seizures is much poorer than in older children. The prognosis depends on the underlying cause.

Box 10.3 Causes of neonatal seizures

- Hypoxic-ischaemic encephalopathy
- Cerebral infarction
- Septicaemia/meningitis
- Metabolic
  - Hypoglycaemia
  - Hypo-/hypernatraemia
  - Hypocalcaemia
  - Hypomagnesaemia
  - Inborn errors of metabolism
  - Pyridoxine dependency
- Intracranial haemorrhage
- Cerebral malformations
- Drug withdrawal, e.g. maternal opiates
- Congenital infection
- Kernicterus

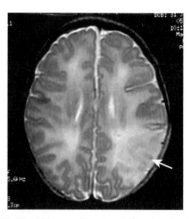

Figure 10.23 MRI scan showing infarction in the territory of a branch of the left middle cerebral artery.

Cerebral infarction (neonatal stroke)

Infarction in the territory of the middle cerebral artery may present with seizures at 12–48 h in a term infant. The seizures may be focal or generalised. In contrast to infants with hypoxic-ischaemic encephalopathy, there are no other abnormal clinical features. The diagnosis is confirmed by MRI (Fig. 10.23). The mechanism is thought to be thrombotic, either thromboembolism from placental vessels or sometimes secondary to inherited thrombophilia. In spite of pronounced abnormalities on the MRI scans, the prognosis is relatively good, with only 20% having hemiparesis or epilepsy presenting later in infancy or early childhood.

Craniofacial disorders

Cleft lip and palate

A cleft lip (Fig. 10.24a) may be unilateral or bilateral. It results from failure of fusion of the frontonasal and maxillary processes. In bilateral cases the premaxilla is

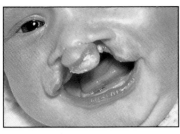

(a)

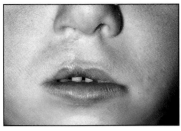

(b)

Figure 10.24 Before **(a)** and after **(b)** operation for cleft lip. Photographs showing the impressive results of surgery help many patients cope with the initial distress at having an affected infant. (Courtesy of Mr N. Waterhouse.)

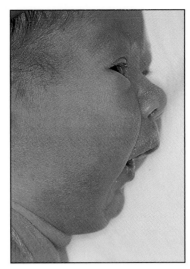

Figure 10.25 Micrognathia in Pierre Robin sequence.

anteverted. Cleft palate results from failure of fusion of the palatine processes and the nasal septum. Cleft lip and palate affect about 0.8 per 1000 babies. Most are inherited polygenically, but they may be part of a syndrome of multiple abnormalities, e.g. chromosomal disorders. Some are associated with maternal anticonvulsant therapy. They may be detected on antenatal ultrasound scanning.

Surgical repair of the lip (Fig. 10.24b) may be performed within the first week of life for cosmetic reasons, although some surgeons feel that better results are obtained if surgery is delayed. The palate is usually repaired at several months of age. A cleft palate may make feeding more difficult, but some affected infants can still be breast-fed successfully. In bottle-fed babies, if milk is observed to enter the nose and cause coughing and choking, special teats and feeding devices may be helpful. Orthodontic advice and a dental prosthesis may help with feeding. Secretory otitis media is relatively common and should be sought on follow-up. Infants are also prone to acute otitis media. Adenoidectomy is best avoided, as the resultant gap between the abnormal palate and nasopharynx will exacerbate feeding problems and the nasal quality of speech. A multidisciplinary team approach is required, involving plastic and ENT surgeons, paediatrician, orthodontist, audiologist and speech therapist. Parent support groups can provide valuable support and advice for families (Cleft Lip and Palate Association, CLAPA).

Pierre Robin sequence

The Pierre Robin sequence is an association of micrognathia (Fig. 10.25), posterior displacement of the tongue (glossoptosis) and midline cleft of the soft palate. There may be difficulty feeding and, as the tongue falls back, there is obstruction to the upper airways which may result in cyanotic episodes. The infant is at risk of failure to thrive during the first few months. If there is upper airways obstruction, the infant may need to lie prone, allowing the tongue and small mandible to fall forward. Persistent obstruction can be treated using a nasopharyngeal airway. Eventually the mandible grows and these problems resolve. The cleft palate can then be repaired.

Gastrointestinal disorders

Oesophageal atresia

Oesophageal atresia is usually associated with a tracheo-oesophageal fistula (Fig. 10.26). It occurs in 1 in 3500 live births and is associated with polyhydramnios during pregnancy. If suspected, a wide-calibre feeding tube is passed and checked by X-ray to see if it reaches the stomach. If not diagnosed at birth, clinical presentation is with persistent salivation and drooling from the mouth after birth. If the diagnosis is not made at this stage, the infant will cough and choke when fed, and have cyanotic episodes. There may be aspiration into the lungs of saliva (or milk) from the upper airways and acid secretions from the stomach. Almost half of the babies have other congenital malformations, e.g. as part of the VACTERL association (**V**ertebral, **A**norectal, **C**ardiac, **T**racheo-o**E**sophageal, **R**enal and Radial **L**imb anomalies). Continuous suction is applied to a tube passed into the oesophageal pouch to reduce aspiration of saliva and secretions pending transfer to a neonatal surgical unit.

Small bowel obstruction

This may be recognised antenatally on ultrasound scanning. Otherwise, small bowel obstruction presents with persistent vomiting, which is bile-stained unless the obstruction is above the ampulla of Vater.

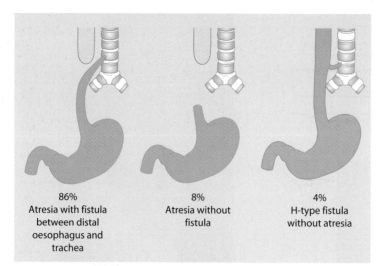

Figure 10.26 Oesophageal atresia and tracheo-oesophageal fistula.

86%
Atresia with fistula between distal oesophagus and trachea

8%
Atresia without fistula

4%
H-type fistula without atresia

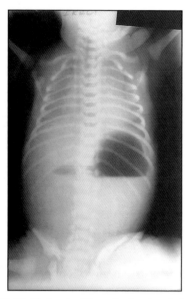

Figure 10.27 Abdominal X-ray in duodenal atresia showing a 'double bubble' from distension of the stomach and duodenal cap. There is absence of air distally.

Meconium may initially be passed, but subsequently its passage is usually delayed or absent. Abdominal distension becomes increasingly prominent the more distal the bowel obstruction. High lesions will present soon after birth, but lower obstruction may not present for some days.

Small bowel obstruction may be caused by:

* Atresia or stenosis of the duodenum (Fig. 10.27) – one-third have Down syndrome and it is also associated with other congenital malformations
* Atresia or stenosis of the jejunum or ileum – there may be multiple atretic segments of bowel
* Malrotation with volvulus – a dangerous condition as it may lead to infarction of the entire midgut
* Meconium ileus – thick inspissated meconium, of putty-like consistency, becomes impacted in the

lower ileum; almost all affected neonates have cystic fibrosis
* Meconium plug – a plug of inspissated meconium causes lower intestinal obstruction.

The diagnosis is made on clinical features and abdominal X-ray showing intestinal obstruction. Atresia or stenosis of the bowel and malrotation are treated surgically, after correction of fluid and electrolyte depletion. A meconium plug will usually pass spontaneously. Meconium ileus may be dislodged using Gastrografin contrast medium.

Large bowel obstruction

This may be caused by:

* *Hirschsprung disease.* Absence of the myenteric nerve plexus in the rectum which may extend along the colon. The baby often does not pass meconium within 48 h of birth and subsequently the abdomen distends. About 15% present as an acute enterocolitis (see Ch. 13).
* *Rectal atresia.* Absence of the anus at the normal site. Lesions are high or low, depending whether the bowel ends above or below the levator ani muscle. In high lesions, there is a fistula to the bladder or urethra in boys, or adjacent to the vagina or to the bladder in girls. Treatment is surgical.

 Bile-stained vomiting is from intestinal obstruction until proved otherwise.

Exomphalos/gastroschisis

These lesions are often diagnosed antenatally (see Ch. 9). In exomphalos (also called omphalocele), the abdominal contents protrude through the umbilical ring, covered with a transparent sac formed by the amniotic membrane and peritoneum (Fig. 10.28). It is often associated with other major congenital abnormalities. In gastroschisis, the bowel protrudes through a defect in the anterior abdominal wall, adjacent to

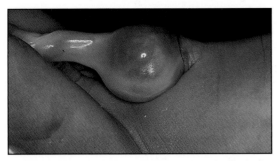

Figure 10.28 Small exomphalos with loops of bowel confined to the umbilicus. Care needs to be taken not to put a cord clamp across these lesions.

the umbilicus, and there is no covering sac (see Fig. 9.2). It is not associated with other congenital abnormalities.

Gastroschisis carries a much greater risk of dehydration and protein loss, so the abdomen of affected infants should be wrapped in several layers of clingfilm to minimise fluid and heat loss. A nasogastric tube is passed and aspirated frequently and an intravenous infusion of dextrose established. Colloid support is often required to replace protein loss. Many lesions can be repaired by primary closure of the abdomen. With large lesions, the intestine is enclosed in a silastic sac sutured to the edges of the abdominal wall and the contents gradually returned into the peritoneal cavity.

Further reading

Lissauer T, Fanaroff AA: *Neonatology at a Glance*, ed 2, Oxford, 2011, Blackwell Science.
Short, illustrated textbook.

Rennie JM: *Roberton's Textbook of Neonatology*, ed 4, Edinburgh, 2011, Elsevier/Churchill Livingstone.
Comprehensive textbook.

Websites (Accessed May 2011)

BLISS. For parents of infants born too early, too small or too sick: Available at: http://www.bliss.org.uk/.

Sands. Stillbith and neonatal death charity: Available at: http://www.uk-sands.org/.

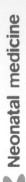

Growth and puberty

In contrast to adults, growth of all body parameters and, later, the development of puberty are key features of childhood and adolescence. Deviation from the norm needs to be recognised and the underlying cause identified and treated. This requires knowledge concerning normal growth and puberty.

There are four phases of normal human growth (Fig. 11.1).

Fetal

This is the fastest period of growth, accounting for about 30% of eventual height. Size at birth is determined by the size of the mother and by placental nutrient supply, which in turn modulates fetal growth factors (IGF-2, human placental lactogen and insulin). Optimal placental nutrient supply is dependent on an adequate maternal diet. Size at birth is largely independent of the father's height and of growth hormone. Severe intrauterine growth restriction and extreme prematurity when accompanied by poor postnatal growth can result in permanent short stature. Paradoxically, low birthweight increases the later metabolic risk of childhood obesity.

The infantile phase

Growth during infancy to around 18 months of age is also largely dependent on adequate nutrition. Good health and normal thyroid function are also necessary. This phase is characterised by a rapid but decelerating growth rate, and accounts for about 15% of eventual height. By the end of this phase, children have changed from their fetal length, largely determined by the uterine environment, to their genetically determined height. An inadequate rate of weight gain during this period is called 'failure to thrive' (see Ch. 12).

Childhood phase

This is a slow, steady but prolonged period of growth that contributes 40% of final height. Pituitary growth hormone (GH) secretion acting to produce insulin-like growth factor 1 (IGF-1) at the epiphyses is the main determinant of a child's rate of growth, provided there is adequate nutrition and good health. Thyroid hormone, vitamin D and steroids also affect cartilage cell division and bone formation. Profound chronic unhappiness can decrease GH secretion and accounts for psychosocial short stature.

Pubertal growth spurt

Sex hormones, mainly testosterone and oestradiol, cause the back to lengthen and boost GH secretion. This adds 15% to final height. The same sex steroids cause fusion of the epiphyseal growth plates and a cessation of growth. If puberty is early, which is not uncommon in girls, the final height is reduced because of early fusion of the epiphyses (see below).

Measurement

Growth must be measured accurately, with attention to correct technique and accurate plotting of the data:

- Weight – readily and accurately determined with electronic scales but must be performed on a naked infant or a child dressed only in underclothing as an entire month's or year's weight gain can be represented by a wet nappy or heavy jeans, respectively.
- Height – the equipment must be regularly calibrated and maintained. In children over 2 years

Determinants of childhood growth

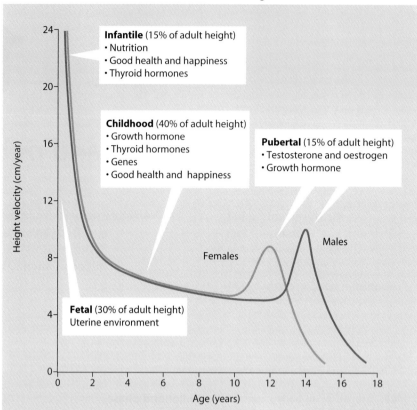

Infantile (15% of adult height)
- Nutrition
- Good health and happiness
- Thyroid hormones

Childhood (40% of adult height)
- Growth hormone
- Thyroid hormones
- Genes
- Good health and happiness

Pubertal (15% of adult height)
- Testosterone and oestrogen
- Growth hormone

Females

Males

Fetal (30% of adult height)
Uterine environment

Height velocity (cm/year)

Age (years)

Figure 11.1 Male and female height velocity charts (50th percentile) showing the determinants of childhood growth. The fetal and infantile phases are mainly dependent on adequate nutrition, whereas the childhood and pubertal phases are dependent on growth hormone and other hormones. Adult males are taller than females as they have a longer childhood growth phase, their peak height velocity is higher and their growth ceases later.

of age, the standing height is measured as illustrated in Figure 11.2. In children under 2 years, length is measured lying horizontally (Fig. 11.3), using the mother to assist. Accurate length measurement in infants can be difficult to obtain, as the legs need to be held straight and infants often dislike being held still. For this reason, routine measurement of length in infancy is often omitted from child surveillance, but it should always be performed whenever there is doubt about an infant's growth.

- Head circumference – the occipitofrontal circumference is a measure of head and hence brain growth. The maximum of three measurements is used. It is of particular importance in developmental delay or suspected hydrocephalus

These measurements should be plotted as a simple dot on an appropriate growth centile chart. Standards for a population should be constructed and updated every generation to allow for the trend towards earlier puberty and taller adult stature from improved childhood nutrition. In 2009, the UK adopted the World Health Organization (WHO) new global Child Growth Standards for infants and children 0–4 years old (See Appendix Fig. A1). The new charts are based on the optimal growth of healthy children totally

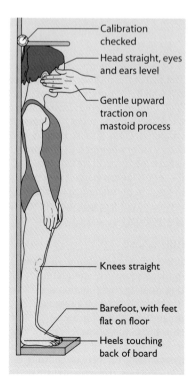

Calibration checked

Head straight, eyes and ears level

Gentle upward traction on mastoid process

Knees straight

Barefoot, with feet flat on floor

Heels touching back of board

Figure 11.2 Measuring height accurately in children.

breast-fed up to the age of 6 months. These charts allow for the lower weight of totally breast-fed infants and are therefore less likely to identify some breast-fed babies as underweight and may also allow early identification of bottle-fed babies gaining weight too rapidly.

Height in a population is normally distributed and the deviation from the mean can be measured as a centile or standard deviation (Fig. 11.4). The bands on the growth reference charts have been chosen to be two-thirds of a standard deviation apart and correspond approximately to the 25th, 9th, 2nd and 0.4th centiles below the mean, and the 75th, 91st, 98th and 99.6th centiles above the mean. The further these centiles lie from the mean, the more likely it is that a child has a pathological cause for his short or tall stature. For instance, values below the 0.4th or above the 99.6th centile will occur by chance in only 4 per 1000 children and can be used as a criterion for referral from primary to specialist care. A single growth parameter should not be assessed in isolation from the other growth parameters: e.g. a child's low weight may be in proportion to the height if short, but abnormal if tall. Serial measurements are used to show the pattern and determine the rate of growth. This is helpful in diagnosing or monitoring many paediatric conditions. The WHO charts include an adult height predictor and a BMI centile ready-reckoner.

Summary

Measurement of children

- Measurement must be accurate for meaningful monitoring of growth
- Growth parameters should be plotted on charts
- Significant abnormalities of height are:
  - measurements outside the 0.4th or 99.6th centiles if the mid-parental height is not short or tall
  - if markedly discrepant from weight
  - serial measurements which cross growth centile lines after the first year of life.

Puberty

Puberty follows a well-defined sequence of changes that may be assigned stages, as shown in Figures 11.5 and 11.6. Over the last 20 years, the mean age at which puberty starts in girls has lowered. However, the age at which menarche occurs has remained stable. Therefore, females now remain in puberty for longer.

In *females* the features of puberty are:

- Breast development – the first sign, usually starting between 8.5 and 12.5 years
- Pubic hair growth and a rapid height spurt – occur almost immediately after breast development
- Menarche – occurs on average 2.5 years after the start of puberty and signals that growth is coming to an end, with only around 5 cm height gain remaining.

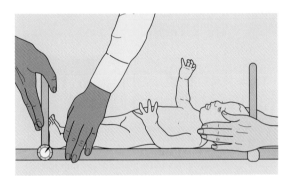

Figure 11.3 Measuring length in infants and young children. An assistant is required to hold the legs straight.

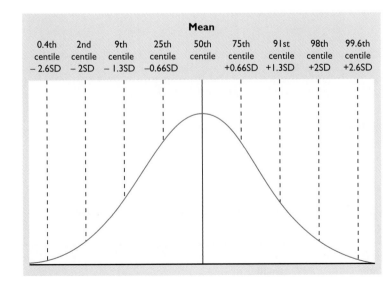

Figure 11.4 Interpretation of the UK growth reference charts. The lines show the mean and bands which are two-thirds of a standard deviation (SD) apart. The centiles are shown in the diagram.

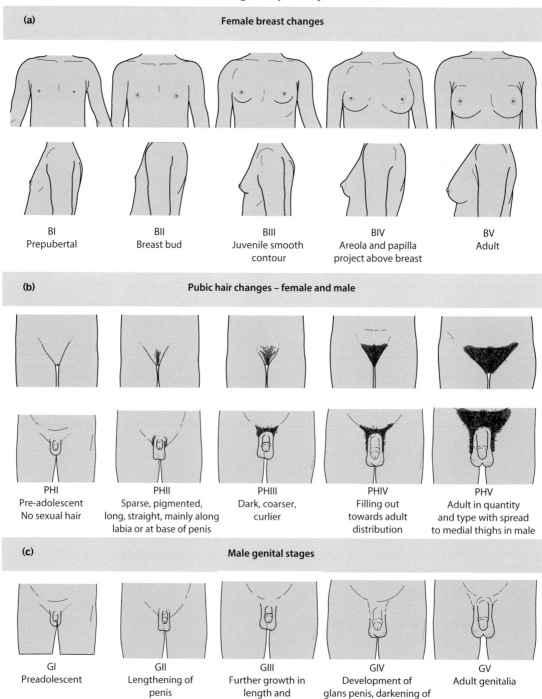

Figure 11.5 Schematic drawings of male and female stages of puberty. Pubertal changes are shown according to the Tanner stages of puberty.

In *males*:

- Testicular enlargement to >4 ml volume measured using an orchidometer (Fig. 11.7) – the first sign of puberty
- Pubic hair growth – follows testicular enlargement, usually between 10 and 14 years of age

- Height spurt – when the testicular volume is 12–15 ml, after a delay of around 18 months.

The height spurt in males occurs later and is of greater magnitude than in females, accounting for the greater final average height of males than females.

Timing of puberty

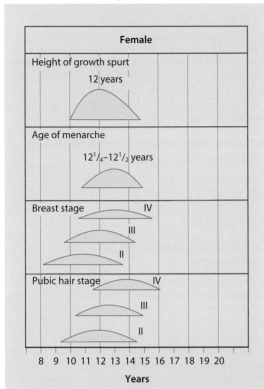

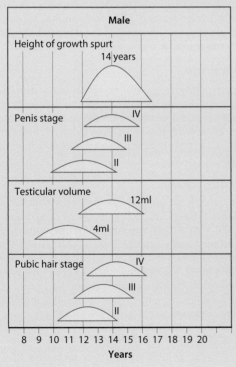

Figure 11.6 Timing of puberty. Pubertal changes are shown according to the Tanner stages of puberty. (Diagrams based on Zitelli BJ, Davis HW. 1992. *Atlas of Pediatric Physical Diagnosis,* 2nd edn. Lippincott, Philadelphia; Johnson TR, Moore WM, Jeffries JE. 1978. *Children are Different,* 2nd edn. Ross Laboratories, Division of Abbot Laboratories, Columbus, OH.)

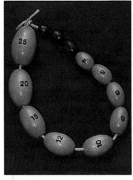

Figure 11.7 Orchidometer to assess testicular volume (in ml). (From Wales JKH, Rogol AD, Wit JM. 2003. *Pediatric Endocrinology and Growth.* Mosby-Wolfe, London, with permission.)

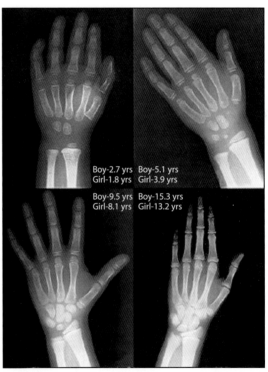

Boy-2.7 yrs Boy-5.1 yrs
Girl-1.8 yrs Girl-3.9 yrs

Boy-9.5 yrs Boy-15.3 yrs
Girl-8.1 yrs Girl-13.2 yrs

Figure 11.8 X-rays of the left wrist and hand to determine bone ages. This technique allows assessment of skeletal maturation from the time of appearance or maturity of the epiphyseal centres, using a standardised rating system. The child's height can be compared with skeletal maturation and an adult height prediction made. The ages show bone age of each X-ray.

In *both sexes*, there will be development of acne, axillary hair, body odour and mood changes.

If puberty is abnormally early or late, it can be further assessed:

- Bone age measurement from a hand and wrist X-ray to determine skeletal maturation (Fig. 11.8)
- In females, pelvic ultrasound can be used to assess uterine size and endometrial thickness.

Menstruation has a wide range of normal variation. The normal cycle length varies between 21 and 45 days. The length of blood loss varies between 3 and 7 days and the average blood loss per cycle is <80 ml – passage of blood clots or the use of more than six pads per day implies heavy bleeding, which needs evaluation. Rarely, it can indicate clotting disorders such as von Willebrand disease.

Summary

Puberty

- The first sign in females is breast development; in males it is testicular enlargement.
- In females the height spurt occurs shortly after breast development; in males it starts almost 18 months after the first signs of puberty.

Short stature

Short stature is usually defined as a height below the second centile (i.e. two standard deviations (SD) below the mean) or 0.4th centile (−2.6 SD). Only 1 in 50 children will be shorter than the 2nd centile and 1 in 250 (4 in 1000) shorter than the 0.4th centile. Most of these children will be normal, though short, with short parents, but the further the child is below these centiles, the more likely it is that there will be a pathological cause. However, the rate of growth (measured as height velocity; Fig. 11.1) may be abnormal long before a child's height falls below these values. This growth failure can be identified from the child's height falling across centile lines plotted on a height velocity chart (Fig. 11.1). This allows growth failure to be identified earlier, even though the child's height is still above the 2nd centile.

Measuring height velocity is a sensitive indicator of growth failure. Two *accurate* measurements at least 6 months but preferably a year apart allow calculation of height velocity in cm/year (Fig. 11.1). This is plotted at the midpoint in time on a height/velocity chart. A height velocity persistently below the 25th centile is abnormal and that child will eventually become short. A disadvantage of using height velocity calculations is that they are highly dependent on the accuracy of the height measurements and so tend not to be used outside specialist growth units.

The height centile of a child must be compared with the weight centile and an estimate of their genetic target centile and range calculated from the height of their parents. This is calculated as the mean of the father's and mother's height with 7 cm added for the mid-parental target height of a boy, and 7 cm subtracted for a girl. The 9th–91st centile range of this estimate is given by ±10 cm in a boy and ±8.5 cm in a girl (see examples in Fig. 11.9).

Most short children are psychologically well adjusted to their size. However, there may be problems from being teased or bullied at school, poor self-esteem and they are at a considerable disadvantage in most competitive sport. They are also assumed by adults to be younger than their true age and may be treated inappropriately.

Familial

Most short children have short parents and fall within the centile target range allowing for mid-parental height. Care needs to be taken, though, that both the child and a parent do not have a dominantly inherited growth disorder.

Intrauterine growth restriction (IUGR) and extreme prematurity

About one-third of children born with severe intra-uterine growth restriction or who were extremely premature remain short. Growth hormone treatment may be indicated.

Constitutional delay of growth and puberty

These children have delayed puberty, which is often familial, usually having occurred in the parent of the same sex. It is commoner in males. It is a variation of the normal timing of puberty rather than an abnormal condition. It may also be induced by dieting or excessive physical training. An affected child will have delayed sexual changes compared with his peers, and bone age would show moderate delay. The legs will be long in comparison to the back. Eventually the target height will be reached. The condition may cause psychological upset. The onset of puberty can be induced with androgens or oestrogens.

Endocrine

Hypothyroidism, growth hormone (GH) deficiency, IGF-1 (insulin-like growth factor 1) deficiency and steroid excess are uncommon causes of short stature. They are associated with children being relatively over-weight, i.e. their weight on a higher centile than their height.

Hypothyroidism

This is usually caused by autoimmune thyroiditis during childhood (see Ch. 25). This produces growth failure, usually with excess weight gain. It may go undiagnosed for many years and lead to short stature. When treated, catch-up growth rapidly occurs but often with a rapid entry into puberty that can limit final height. Congenital hypothyroidism is diagnosed soon after birth by screening and so does not result in any abnormality of growth.

Growth hormone deficiency

This may be an isolated defect or secondary to pan-hypopituitarism. Pituitary function may be abnormal in congenital mid-facial defects or as a result of a cranio-pharyngioma (a tumour affecting the pituitary region), a hypothalamic tumour or trauma such as head injury, meningitis and cranial irradiation. Craniopharyngioma usually presents in late childhood and may result in abnormal visual fields (characteristically a bitemporal hemianopia as it impinges on the optic chiasm), optic atrophy or papilloedema on fundoscopy. In growth hormone deficiency, the bone age is markedly delayed. Laron syndrome is a condition due to defective growth hormone receptors resulting in growth hormone insensitivity. Patients with this condition have high growth hormone levels but low levels of the downstream active product of growth hormone known as insulin-like growth factor 1 (IGF-1) produced at the growth plate and in the liver. Rare abnormalities in the gene producing IGF-1 have also recently been discovered in children.

Corticosteroid excess, Cushing syndrome

This is usually iatrogenic, as corticosteroid therapy is a potent growth suppressor. This effect is greatly reduced by alternate day therapy, but some growth suppression may be seen even with relatively low doses of inhaled or topical steroids in susceptible individuals. Non-iatrogenic Cushing syndrome is very unusual in childhood and may be caused by pituitary or adrenal pathology. Growth failure may be very severe, usually with excess weight gain, although normalisation of body shape and height occurs on withdrawal of treatment or treatment of the underlying steroid excess. Cushing syndrome during puberty can result in permanent loss of height (see Ch. 25).

Nutritional/chronic illness

This is a relatively common cause of abnormal growth. These children are usually short and underweight: i.e. their weight is on the same or a lower centile than their height. Inadequate nutrition may be due to insufficient food, restricted diets or poor appetite associated with a chronic illness, or from the increased nutritional requirement from a raised metabolic rate. Chronic illnesses which may present with short stature include:

- Coeliac disease, which usually presents in the first 2 years of life, but can present late with growth failure. Coeliac disease may result in short stature without gastrointestinal symptoms
- Crohn disease
- Chronic renal failure – may be present in the absence of a history of renal disease.

Psychosocial deprivation

Children subjected to physical and emotional deprivation may be short and underweight and show delayed puberty. This condition may be extremely difficult to identify, but affected children show catch-up growth if placed in a nurturing environment.

Chromosomal disorder/syndromes

Many chromosomal disorders and syndromes are associated with short stature. Down syndrome is usually diagnosed at birth, but Turner (Fig. 8.6 and see Ch. 8), Noonan (Fig. 8.17) and Russell–Silver syndromes may present with short stature. Turner syndrome may be particularly difficult to diagnose clinically and *should be considered in all short females.*

Extreme short stature

There are a few rare conditions that cause extreme short stature in children. These include absolute resistance to growth hormone (Laron syndrome), and primordial dwarfism. Idiopathic short stature (ISS) refers to short stature that does not have Growth hormone resistance Primordial dwarfism Idiopathic short stature (ISS) a diagnostic explanation. In addition, abnormalities in a gene called *SHOX* (short stature homeobox) located on the X chromosome lead to severe short stature with skeletal abnormalities when present on both copies of the gene. Absence of one *SHOX* gene in Turner syndrome is thought to be the cause of short stature in this condition (and additional copies in Klinefelter syndrome produce taller than normal stature). Polymorphisms in this gene probably account for a proportion of idiopathic short stature.

Disproportionate short stature

This is confirmed by measuring:

- Sitting height – base of spine to top of head
- Subischial leg length – subtraction of sitting height from total height
- Limited radiographic skeletal survey to identify the skeletal abnormality.

Charts exist to assess the normality of body proportions. Conditions with abnormal body proportions are rare and may be caused by disorders of the formation of bone (skeletal dysplasias). They include achondroplasia and other short-limbed dysplasias. If the legs are extremely short, treatment by surgical leg lengthening may be appropriate. The back may be short from severe scoliosis or some storage disorders, such as the mucopolysaccharidoses.

Examination and investigation

Plotting present and previous heights and weights on appropriate growth charts, together with the clinical features, usually allows the cause to be identified without any investigations (Fig. 11.9a-i). Previous height and weight measurements should be available from the parent-held personal child health record. The bone age may be helpful, as it is markedly delayed in some endocrine disorders, e.g. hypothyroidism and growth hormone deficiency, and is used to estimate adult height potential. Investigations that may be indicated are shown in Table 11.1.

Growth hormone treatment of short stature

Growth hormone deficiency is treated with biosynthetic growth hormone, which is given by subcutaneous injection, usually daily. It is expensive and the management of growth hormone deficiency is undertaken at specialist centres. The best response is seen in children with the most severe hormone deficiency. Other indications include Turner syndrome, Prader–Willi syndrome (Fig. 8.19), chronic renal failure, *SHOX* (short stature homeobox) deficiency and intrauterine growth restriction (IUGR). In Prader–Willi syndrome (an imprinting disorder resulting in early hypotonia and feeding difficulties followed by short stature, obesity and learning difficulties), growth hormone improves muscular

Causes & evaluation of short stature

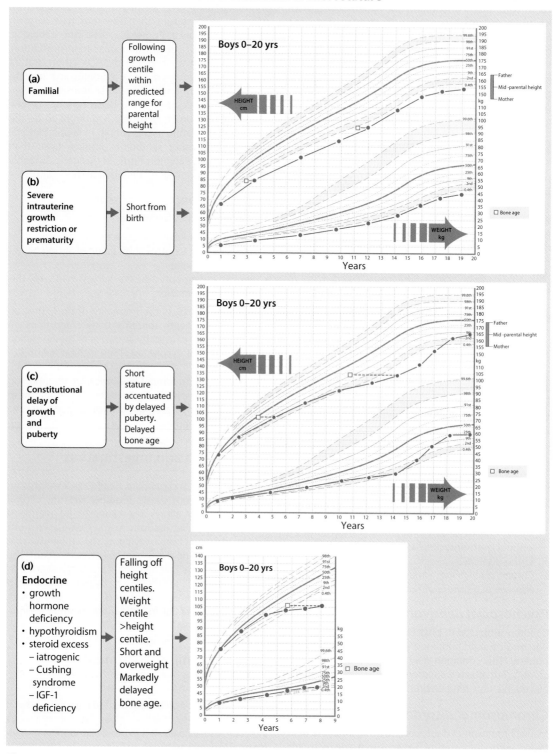

Figure 11.9 Causes of short stature.
Charts © Child Growth Foundation, reproduced with permission. Further supplies and information from www.healthforallchildren.co.uk.

Causes & evaluation of short stature

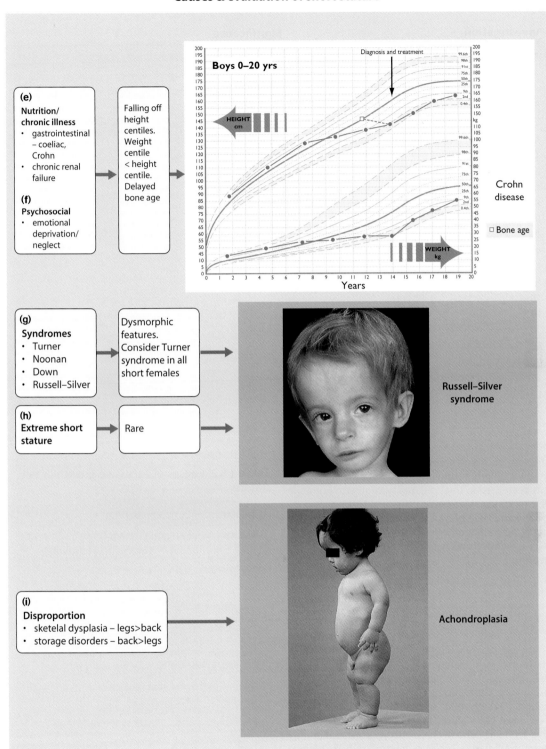

(e)

Nutrition/ chronic illness
- gastrointestinal – coeliac, Crohn
- chronic renal failure

(f)

Psychosocial
- emotional deprivation/ neglect

Falling off height centiles. Weight centile < height centile. Delayed bone age

Boys 0–20 yrs

Diagnosis and treatment

HEIGHT cm

WEIGHT kg

Years

Crohn disease

□ Bone age

(g)

Syndromes
- Turner
- Noonan
- Down
- Russell–Silver

Dysmorphic features. Consider Turner syndrome in all short females

Russell–Silver syndrome

(h)

Extreme short stature

Rare

(i)

Disproportion
- sketelal dysplasia – legs>back
- storage disorders – back>legs

Achondroplasia

Figure 11.9, cont'd.

Table 11.1 Investigations considered for short stature

Investigation	Significance
X-ray of wrist and hand for bone age	Some delay in constitutional delay of growth and puberty
	Marked delay for hypothyroidism or growth hormone deficiency or other endocrine causes
Full blood count	Anaemia in coeliac or Crohn disease
Creatinine and electrolytes	Creatinine raised in chronic renal failure
Calcium, phosphate, alkaline phosphatise	Renal and bone disorders
Thyroid-stimulating hormone (TSH)	Raised in primary hypothyroidism
Karyotype	Turner syndrome shows 45XO, other chromosomal disorders
Endomysial and anti-tissue transglutaminase IgA antibodies	Usually present in coeliac disease
CRP (acute-phase reactant) and erythrocyte sedimentation rate (ESR)	Raised in Crohn disease
Growth hormone provocation tests (using insulin, glucagon, clonidine or arginine in specialist centres)	Growth hormone deficiency
IGF-1	Disorders of the growth hormone axis, including IGF-1 deficiency
0900 cortisol and dexamethasone suppression test	Cushing syndrome
MRI scan if neurological symptoms/signs	Craniopharyngioma or intracranial tumour
Limited skeletal survey	Skeletal dysplasia, scoliosis

strength and body composition as well as modestly improving final height. Recently, recombinant IGF-1 has been used to treat children with growth hormone resistance (e.g. Laron syndrome) and IGF-1 deficiency who would have previously not responded to growth hormone treatment. Recombinant IGF-1 therapy is still very expensive and is confined to a few specialised centres.

Tall stature

This is a less common presenting complaint than short stature, as many parents are proud that their child is tall. However, some adolescents (mainly females) become concerned about excessive height during their pubertal growth spurt. The causes are shown in Table 11.2. Most tall stature is inherited from tall parents. Obesity in childhood 'fuels' early growth and may result in tall stature; however, because puberty is often somewhat earlier than average, it does not increase final height.

Secondary endocrine causes are rare. Both congenital adrenal hyperplasia and precocious puberty lead to early epiphyseal fusion so that eventual height is reduced after an early excessive growth rate.

Marfan (a disorder of loose connective tissue) and Klinefelter (XXY – an excess of *SHOX* dose) syndromes

Table 11.2 Causes of excessive growth or tall stature

Familial	Most common cause
Obesity	Puberty is advanced, so final height centile is less than in childhood
Secondary	Hyperthyroidism
	Excess sex steroids – precocious puberty from whatever cause
	Excess adrenal androgen steroids – congenital adrenal hyperplasia
	True gigantism (excess GH secretion)
Syndromes	Long-legged tall stature:
	Marfan syndrome
	Homocystinuria
	Klinefelter syndrome (47 XXY and XXY karyotype)
	Proportionate tall stature at birth:
	Maternal diabetes
	Primary hyperinsulinism
	Beckwith syndrome
	Sotos syndrome – associated with large head, characteristic facial features and learning difficulties

Summary

Assessment of a child with short stature

Examination of the growth chart:
- Following growth centile lines for length/height, weight and head circumference?
  Consider familial, low birthweight, constitutional delay of growth and puberty, syndromes and skeletal dysplasias
- Growth failure with crossing of centile lines?
  Consider endocrine (including therapeutic corticosteroids), nutrition/chronic illness, psychosocial deprivation

Determine the mid-parental height
- For genetic target range

History
- Birth length, weight, head circumference and gestational age
- Pregnancy history: infection, intrauterine growth restriction, drug use, alcohol/smoking
- Feeding history
- Developmental milestones
- Family history of constitutional delay of growth and puberty or other diseases?
- Consanguinity pertaining to inherited conditions
- Features of chronic illness, endocrine causes, e.g. hypothyroidism, pituitary tumour, Cushing syndrome or psychosocial deprivation?
- Medications, e.g. corticosteroids?

Examination
- Dysmorphic features – chromosome/syndrome present? (But in Turner syndrome other stigmata may be absent)
- Chronic illness, e.g. Crohn, cystic fibrosis, coeliac disease?
- Evidence of endocrine causes?
- Disproportionate short stature from skeletal dysplasia?
- Pubertal stage?

Diagnosis
Cause can usually be determined from the above and no tests are required

both cause long-legged tall stature, and in XXY there is also infertility and learning difficulties.

Tall children may be disadvantaged by being treated as older than their chronological age. Excessive height in prepubertal or early pubertal adolescent females and males can be treated with oestrogen therapy and testosterone therapy, respectively, to induce premature fusion of the epiphyses, but as it produces variable results and has potentially serious side-effects, it is seldom undertaken. Surgical destruction of the epiphyses in the legs may also be considered in extreme cases.

Abnormal head growth

Most head growth occurs in the first 2 years of life and 80% of adult head size is achieved before the age of 5 years. This largely reflects brain growth, but small or large heads may be familial and the mid-parental head percentile may need to be calculated. At birth, the sutures and fontanelle are open. During the first few months of life, the head circumference may increase across centiles, especially if small for gestational age. The posterior fontanelle has closed by 8 weeks, and the anterior fontanelle by 12–18 months. If there is a rapid increase in head circumference, raised intracranial pressure should be excluded.

Microcephaly

Microcephaly, a head circumference below the 2nd centile, may be:

- Familial – when it is present from birth and development is often normal
- An autosomal recessive condition – when it is associated with developmental delay

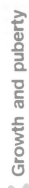

Growth and puberty

191

Case History

11.1 Microcephaly

Figure 11.10 shows the head circumference chart of Tim, who was healthy and was developing normally. At 9 months of age, he was rushed to hospital as he was unrousable from profound hypoglycaemia secondary to the deliberate administration of insulin by his mother, who had diabetes. Although Tim was taken into care and had no further hypoglycaemic episodes, his head circumference shows cessation of growth. He has developed moderate learning difficulties and mild cerebral palsy.

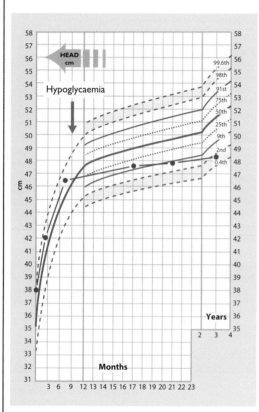

Figure 11.10 Tim's head circumference chart. Chart © Child Growth Foundation, reproduced with permission. Further supplies and information from www.healthforallchildren.co.uk.

- Caused by a congenital infection
- Acquired after an insult to the developing brain, e.g. perinatal hypoxia, hypoglycaemia or meningitis, when it is often accompanied by cerebral palsy and seizures (see Case History 11.1).

Macrocephaly

Macrocephaly is a head circumference above the 98th centile. The causes of a large head are listed in Box 11.1. Most are normal children and often the parents have

Box 11.1 Causes of a large head

- Tall stature
- Familial macrocephaly
- Raised intracranial pressure
- Hydrocephalus – progressive or arrested
- Chronic subdural haematoma
- Cerebral tumour
- Neurofibromatosis
- Cerebral gigantism (Sotos syndrome)
- CNS storage disorders, e.g. mucopolysaccharidosis (Hurler syndrome).

large heads. A rapidly increasing head circumference, even if the head circumference is still below the 98th centile, suggests raised intracranial pressure and may be due to hydrocephalus, subdural haematoma or brain tumour. It must be investigated promptly by intracranial ultrasound if the anterior fontanelle is still open, otherwise by CT or MRI scan.

 If an infant's head circumference is enlarging and crossing centile lines – check for raised intracranial pressure.

Asymmetric heads

Skull asymmetry may result from an imbalance of the growth rate at the coronal, sagittal or lambdoid sutures, although the head circumference increases normally. Occipital plagiocephaly, a parallelogram-shaped head with flattening of the back of the skull, is seen with increased frequency since the advice to parents that babies should sleep lying on their back to reduce the risk of sudden infant death syndrome. It improves with time as the infant becomes more mobile. Plagiocephaly is also seen in infants with hypotonia. Preterm infants may develop long, flat heads from lying on their sides for long periods on the hard surface of incubators unless provided with a soft surface to lie on and their head position is changed frequently (see Fig. 11.11). Under these circumstances, it is not associated with abnormal development.

Craniosynostosis

The sutures of the skull bones start to fuse during infancy but do not finally fuse until late childhood. Premature fusion of one or more sutures (craniosynostosis) may lead to distortion of the head shape. Craniosynostosis is usually localised (Box 11.2). It most often affects the sagittal suture, when it results in a long narrow skull (Fig. 11.12). Rarely it affects the lambdoid suture to result in skull asymmetry, which needs to be differentiated from plagiocephaly, where there is asymmetric flattening of one side of the skull from positional moulding.

Abnormal head shape

Box 11.2 Forms of craniosynostosis

Localised
- Sagittal suture – long narrow skull
- Coronal suture – asymmetrical skull
- Lambdoid suture – flattening of skull

Generalised
- Multiple sutures resulting in microcephaly and developmental delay
- Genetic syndromes, e.g. with syndactyly in Apert syndrome, with exophthalmos in Crouzon syndrome.

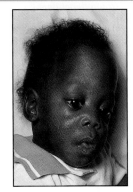

Figure 11.11 Long flat head of a preterm infant. This can be avoided by lying preterm infants on a soft surface and regularly changing their head position.

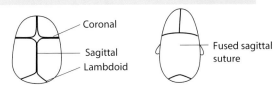

Normal skull sutures — Coronal, Sagittal, Lambdoid

Sagittal craniosynostosis — Fused sagittal suture

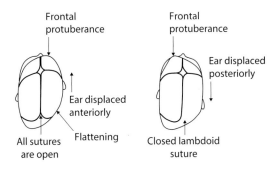

Plagiocephaly (positional moulding) — Frontal protuberance, Ear displaced anteriorly, Flattening, All sutures are open

Lambdoidal synostosis — Frontal protuberance, Ear displaced posteriorly, Closed lambdoid suture

Figure 11.12 Differentiating craniosynostosis from plagiocephaly.

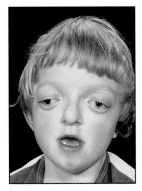

Figure 11.13 Crouzon syndrome showing the typical shallow orbits and exophthalmos. Craniofacial reconstructive surgery is required to prevent visual loss and cerebral damage from raised intracranial pressure and for cosmetic appearance.

Craniosynostosis may be generalised (Box 11.2), when it may be a feature of a syndrome (Fig. 11.13). The fused suture may be felt or seen as a palpable ridge and confirmed on skull X-ray or cranial CT scan. If necessary, the condition can be treated surgically because of raised intracranial pressure or for cosmetic reasons. Such operations are performed in specialist centres for craniofacial reconstructive surgery.

Premature sexual development

The development of secondary sexual characteristics before 8 years old in females and 9 years old in males is defined as outside the normal range in the UK. It may be due to:

- Precocious puberty when it is accompanied by a growth spurt
- Premature breast development (thelarche)
- Premature pubic hair development (pubarche).

Precocious puberty

Precocious puberty (PP) may be categorised according to the levels of the pituitary-derived gonadotropins, follicle-stimulating hormone (FSH) and luteinising hormone (LH), (Fig. 11.14) as:

- Gonadotropin-dependent (central, 'true' PP) from premature activation of the hypothalamic–pituitary–gonadal axis
- Gonadotropin-independent (pseudo, 'false' PP) from excess sex steroids.

Females

This is usually idiopathic or familial and follows the normal sequence of puberty. Organic causes are rare and are associated with:

- dissonance, when the sequence of pubertal changes is abnormal, e.g. isolated pubic hair with virilisation of the genitalia, suggesting excess

Causes of precocious puberty

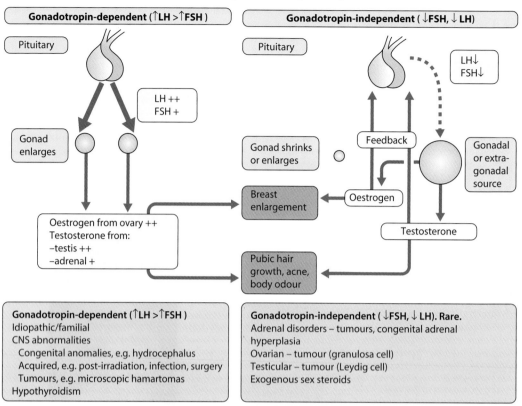

Figure 11.14 Causes of precocious puberty. (Courtesy of Dr Emma Rhodes.)

androgens from either congenital adrenal hyperplasia or an androgen-secreting tumour

- rapid onset
- neurological symptoms and signs, e.g. neurofibromatosis.

Ultrasound examination of the ovaries and uterus is helpful in establishing the cause of precocious puberty. In the premature onset of normal puberty, multicystic ovaries and an enlarging uterus will be identified.

Precocious puberty in females is commonly due to the premature onset of normal puberty.

Males (see Case History 11.2)

This is uncommon and usually has an organic cause, particularly intracranial tumours. Examination of the testes may be helpful:

- Bilateral enlargement suggests gonadotropin release, usually from an intracranial lesion
- Small testes suggest an adrenal cause (e.g. a tumour or adrenal hyperplasia)
- A unilateral enlarged testis suggests a gonadal tumour.

Tumours in the hypothalamic region are best investigated by cranial MRI scan.

Central precocious puberty in males more often has an organic cause.

Management

The management of precocious puberty is directed towards:

- detection and treatment of any underlying pathology, e.g. intracranial tumour in males, and reducing the rate of skeletal maturation if necessary. Skeletal maturation is assessed by bone age. An early growth spurt may result in early cessation of growth and a reduction in adult height.
- addressing psychological/behavioural difficulties associated with early progression through puberty.

Deciding whether to treat a girl who is simply going through puberty early needs further consideration. If treatment is required for gonadotropin-dependent disease, gonadotropin-releasing hormone (GnRH) analogues are the treatment of choice. In gonadotropin-independent cases, the source of excess sex steroids needs to be identified. Inhibitors of androgen or oestrogen production or action (e.g. medroxyprogesterone acetate, cyproterone acetate, testolactone, ketoconazole) may be used.

Premature breast development (thelarche)

This usually affects females between 6 months and 2 years of age. The breast enlargement may be asymmetrical and rarely progresses beyond stage 3. It is

11.2 Precocious puberty in a boy

This 6-year-old boy presented with precocious puberty (Fig. 11.15a,b). He was noted to have multiple café-au-lait spots consistent with a diagnosis of neurofibromatosis type 1. An MRI scan showed a mass in the hypothalamus which proved to be an optic glioma. He was treated with radiotherapy, although full remission was not possible to achieve. The site of injection of gonadotropin super-agonist treatment to suppress his sexual development is covered by the plaster.

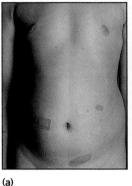 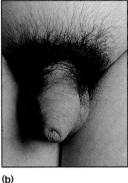

(a) (b)

Figure 11.15 (a) Multiple café-au-lait spots. Neurofibromatosis type 1 was diagnosed. **(b)** Genitalia showing stage 3 genitalia and pubic hair with 12 ml testicles bilaterally. He also had adult body odour. (From Wales JKH, Rogol AD, Wit JM. 2003. *Pediatric Endocrinology and Growth*. Saunders, London, with permission.)

differentiated from precocious puberty by the absence of axillary and pubic hair and of a growth spurt. It is non-progressive and self-limiting. Investigations are not usually required (see Case History 11.3).

Premature pubarche (adrenarche)

This occurs when pubic hair develops before 8 years of age in females and before 9 years in males but with no other signs of sexual development. It is most commonly caused by an accentuation of the normal maturation of androgen production by the adrenal gland (adrenarche). It is more common in Asian and Afro-Caribbean children. There may be a slight increase in growth rate. It is usually self-limiting. An ultrasound scan of the ovaries and uterus and a bone age should be obtained to exclude central precocious puberty. A more aggressive course of virilisation would suggest late-onset non-salt-losing congenital adrenal hyperplasia (CAH) or an adrenal tumour. Obtaining a urinary steroid profile helps differentiate premature pubarche from late onset CAH or an adrenal tumour. Children who develop premature pubarche are at an increased risk of developing polycystic ovarian syndrome (PCOS) in later life.

Delayed puberty

Delayed puberty is often defined as the absence of pubertal development by 14 years of age in females and 15 years in males. The causes of delayed puberty are listed in Box 11.3.

In contrast to precocious puberty, the problem is more common in males, in whom it is mostly due to constitutional delay in growth and puberty (CDGP). This is often familial, usually having occurred in the parent of the same sex. It may also be induced by

11.3 Premature thelarche

This 18-month-old female developed enlargement of both breasts (Fig. 11.16). There was no pubic hair growth, sweatiness or body odour and her height was in the mid-parental range. Her bone age was only mildly advanced (21 months) and a pelvic ultrasound showed a prepubertal uterus, small volume ovaries with two cysts in the left ovary. Her subsequent growth rate was normal. A diagnosis of premature thelarche was made.

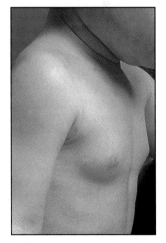

Figure 11.16 Premature breast development in an 18-month-old girl. The absence of a growth spurt and axillary and pubic hair differentiates it from precocious puberty. It is self-limiting and often resolves. (From Wales JKH, Rogol AD, Wit JM. 2003. *Pediatric Endocrinology and Growth*. Saunders, London, with permission.)

Growth and puberty

195

Box 11.3 Causes of delayed puberty

Constitutional delay of growth and puberty/familial

By far the commonest

Low gonadotropin secretion (hypogonadotropic hypogonadism)

- Systemic disease
  - Cystic fibrosis, severe asthma, Crohn disease, organ failure, anorexia nervosa, starvation, excess physical training
- Hypothalamo-pituitary disorders
  - Panhypopituitarism
  - Isolated gonadotropin or growth hormone deficiency
  - Intracranial tumours (including craniopharyngioma)
  - Kallmann syndrome (LHRH deficiency and inability to smell)
- Acquired hypothyroidism

High gonadotropin secretion (hypergonadotropic hypogonadism)

- Chromosomal abnormalities
  - Klinefelter syndrome (47 XXY)
  - Turner syndrome (45 XO)
- Steroid hormone enzyme deficiencies
- Acquired gonadal damage
  - Post-surgery, chemotherapy, radiotherapy, trauma, torsion of the testis, autoimmune disorder.

dieting or excessive physical training. Children affected with constitutional delay in growth and puberty are short during childhood, with a delay in sexual maturation and have delayed skeletal maturity on bone age. The legs will be long in comparison to the back (eunuchoid body habitus). Eventually the target height will be reached as growth in affected children will continue for longer than in their peers. The condition may cause considerable psychological upset from teasing, poor self-esteem and disadvantage in competitive sport.

In boys, assessment includes:

- Pubertal staging, especially testicular volume
- Identification of chronic systemic disorders.

In girls, karyotype should be performed to identify Turner syndrome, and thyroid and sex steroid hormones should be measured. The aims of management are to:

- identify and treat any underlying pathology
- ensure normal psychological adaptation to puberty and adulthood
- accelerate growth and promote entry into puberty if necessary.

Following reassurance that puberty will occur, treatment is usually not required. Should treatment be wanted, oral oxandrolone can be used in young males.

This weakly androgenic anabolic steroid will induce some catch-up growth but not secondary sexual characteristics. In older boys, low-dose intramuscular testosterone will accelerate growth as well as inducing secondary sexual characteristics. Females may be treated with oestradiol.

Disorders of sexual differentiation (DSD)

The fetal gonad is initially bipotential (Fig. 11.17). In the male, a testis-determining gene on the Y chromosome (*SRY*) is responsible for the differentiation of the gonad into a testis. The production of testosterone and its metabolite, dihydrotestosterone, results in the development of male genitalia. In the absence of *SRY*, the gonads become ovaries and the genitalia female.

Rarely, newborn infants may be born with a disorder of sexual differentiation and there may be uncertainty about the infant's sex. A disorder of sexual differentiation may be secondary to:

- Excessive androgens producing virilisation in a female – the commonest cause of this is congenital adrenal hyperplasia
- Inadequate androgen action, producing under-virilisation in a male – this can result from inability to respond to androgens (a receptor problem – androgen insensitivity syndrome, which may be complete or partial) or to convert testosterone to dihydrotestosterone (5α-reductase deficiency) or abnormalities of the synthesis of androgens from cholesterol
- Gonadotrophin insufficiency, also seen in several syndromes such as Prader–Willi syndrome and congenital hypopituitarism, which results in a small penis and cryptorchidism
- Ovotesticular disorder of sex development (DSD) (previously known as true hermaphroditism), caused by both XX- and Y-containing cells being present in the fetus leading to both testicular and ovarian tissue being present and a complex external phenotype; this is rare.

All parents and their relatives are desperate to know the sex of their newborn baby. However, if the genitalia are abnormal, the infant's sex must not be assigned until detailed assessment by medical, surgical and psychological specialists has been performed followed by full discussion with the parents. Birth registration must be delayed until this has been completed.

Sexuality is complex and depends on more than the phenotype, chromosomes and hormone levels. Before the most appropriate sex of rearing is decided upon, the karyotype needs to be determined, adrenal and sex hormone levels measured, and ultrasound of the internal structures and gonads performed. Sometimes laparoscopic imaging and biopsy of internal structures are necessary. In many disorders of sexual differentiation, it has been usual to raise the child as a female, as it is easier to fashion female external genitalia, whereas it is not possible surgically to create an adequately functioning penis. However, it may be impossible to predict the sexual identity of the child in eventual adult

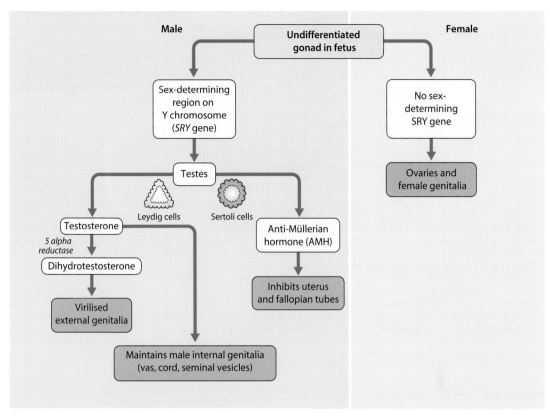

Figure 11.17 Sexual differentiation in the fetus.

life and further support or gender reassignment may be required. For this reason, there is a move toward delaying definitive surgery to allow the affected individual to give informed consent to any reconstructive procedures. This is a controversial area and is best managed by experienced multidisciplinary teams.

 If there is abnormal sexual differentiation at birth:

- **Do not guess the infant's gender**
- **The most common cause of a disorder of sexual development is female virilisation from congenital adrenal hyperplasia.**

Congenital adrenal hyperplasia (CAH)

A number of autosomal recessive disorders of adrenal steroid biosynthesis result in congenital adrenal hyperplasia. Its incidence is about 1 in 5000 births, and it is commoner in the offspring of consanguineous marriages. Over 90% have a deficiency of the enzyme 21-hydroxylase, which is needed for cortisol biosynthesis. About 80% are also unable to produce aldosterone, leading to salt loss (low sodium and high potassium) (Fig. 11.18). In the fetus, the resulting cortisol deficiency stimulates the pituitary to produce adrenocorticotrophic hormone (ACTH), which drives overproduction of adrenal androgens.

Presentation:

- Virilisation of the external genitalia in female infants, with clitoral hypertrophy and variable fusion of the labia (see Case History 11.4)
- In the infant male, the penis may be enlarged and the scrotum pigmented, but these changes are seldom identified
- A salt-losing adrenal crisis in the 80% of males who are salt losers; this occurs at 1–3 weeks of age, presenting with vomiting and weight loss, floppiness and circulatory collapse
- Tall stature in the 20% of male non-salt losers; both male and female non-salt losers also develop a muscular build, adult body odour, pubic hair and acne from excess androgen production, leading to precocious pubarche.

There may be a family history of neonatal death if a salt-losing crisis had not been recognised and treated.

Diagnosis

This is made by finding markedly raised levels of the metabolic precursor 17α-hydroxyprogesterone in the blood. In salt losers, the biochemical abnormalities are:

- Low plasma sodium
- High plasma potassium
- Metabolic acidosis
- Hypoglycaemia.

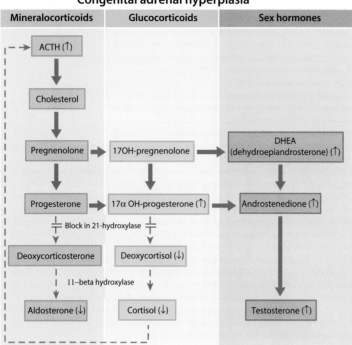

Congenital adrenal hyperplasia

Mineralocorticoids	Glucocorticoids	Sex hormones

ACTH (↑)

Cholesterol

Pregnenolone → 17OH-pregnenolone → DHEA (dehydroepiandrosterone) (↑)

Progesterone → 17α OH-progesterone (↑) → Androstenedione (↑)

Block in 21-hydroxylase

Deoxycorticosterone   Deoxycortisol (↓)

11–beta hydroxylase

Aldosterone (↓)   Cortisol (↓)   Testosterone (↑)

Figure 11.18 Abnormal adrenal steroid biosynthesis from 21-hydroxylase deficiency is the commonest form of congenital adrenal hyperplasia. ACTH, adrenocorticotrophic hormone.

Case History

11.4 Abnormal genitalia at birth

The appearance of this newborn infant's genitalia is shown in Figure 11.19.

Investigation revealed:

- A normal female karyotype, 46XX
- The presence of a uterus on ultrasound examination
- A markedly raised plasma 17α-hydroxy-progesterone concentration, confirming congenital adrenal hyperplasia.
- A low sodium and a high potassium level
- A low bicarbonate (metabolic acidosis) and high urea (dehydration).

Plasma electrolytes identified a low sodium and a high potassium, indicating that the baby had the salt-losing form of CAH. After detailed explanation with her parents, she was started on oral hydrocortisone and fludrocortisone replacement therapy and oral salt replacement (NaCl). Surgery was performed at 9 months of age to reduce clitoral size and separate the labia. Her growth, biochemistry and bone age were monitored frequently at follow-up and she attained normal adult height. Psychological counselling and support were offered around puberty and further genital surgery was needed before she became sexually active.

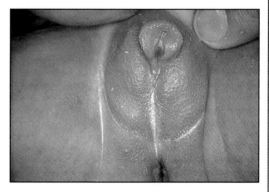

Figure 11.19 Abnormal genitalia at birth. Investigation established that this was a female infant with congenital adrenal hyperplasia causing clitoral hypertrophy with fusion of the labia.

 Severe hypospadias and bilateral undescended testes – a male or virilised female? The karyotype and a pelvic ultrasound are required.

Management

Affected females will sometimes require corrective surgery to their external genitalia within the first year but as they have a uterus and ovaries they should usually be reared as girls and are able to have children. Definitive surgical reconstruction is usually delayed until late puberty. Males in a salt-losing crisis require saline, dextrose and hydrocortisone intravenously.

The long-term management of both sexes is with:

- Lifelong glucocorticoids to suppress ACTH levels (and hence testosterone) to allow normal growth and maturation
- Mineralocorticoids (fludrocortisone) if there is salt loss; before weaning, infants may need added sodium chloride
- Monitoring of growth, skeletal maturity and plasma androgens and 17α-hydroxyprogesterone – insufficient hormone replacement results in increased ACTH secretion and androgen excess, which will cause rapid initial growth and skeletal maturation at the expense of final height; excessive hormonal replacement will result in skeletal delay and slow growth
- Additional hormone replacement to cover illness or surgery, as they are unable to mount a cortisol response.

Death can occur from adrenal crisis at the time of illness or injury. Females require surgery to reduce clitoromegaly and a vaginoplasty before sexual intercourse is attempted. Females often experience psychosexual problems, which may relate to the high androgen levels experienced in utero prior to diagnosis.

Prenatal diagnosis and treatment are possible when a couple have had a previously affected child. Dexamethasone may be given to the mother around the time of conception, and continued if the fetus is found to be female, in order to reduce fetal ACTH drive and hence the virilisation.

Summary

Congenital adrenal hyperplasia

- Autosomal recessive disorder of adrenal steroid biosynthesis
- Females present with virilisation of the external genitalia
- Males present with salt loss (80%) or tall stature and precocious puberty (20%)
- Long-term medical management with lifelong glucocorticoids, mineralocorticoids/sodium chloride if salt loss
- Additional corticosteroids to cover illness or surgery
- Salt-losing adrenal crisis needs urgent treatment with hydrocortisone, saline and glucose given intravenously
- Monitor growth, skeletal maturity, plasma androgens and 17α-hydroxyprogesterone
- Surgery for females.

Further reading

Brook C, Clayton P, Brown R: *Brook's Clinical Paediatric Endocrinology*, ed 6, Oxford, 2009, Blackwell.

Lifshitz F, editor: *Pediatric Endocrinology*, ed 5, New York, 2007, Marcel Dekker.

Wales JKH, Rogol AD, Wit JM: *Pediatric Endocrinology and Growth*. London, 2003, Saunders.

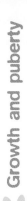

Growth and puberty

Nutrition

Notable features of nutrition in children are:

- The optimal nutrition for newborn infants is from breast-feeding.
- Inadequate nutrition in infants and young children rapidly leads to weight loss followed by growth failure, commonly called failure to thrive, which if severe and prolonged leads to malnutrition
- Whereas malnutrition is a major cause of morbidity and death in developing countries, obesity is the major nutritional problem in developed countries.

The nutritional vulnerability of infants and children

Infants and children are more vulnerable to poor nutrition than are adults. There are a number of reasons for this.

Low nutritional stores

Newborn infants, particularly those born before term, have poor stores of fat and protein (Fig. 12.1). The smaller the child, the less the calorie reserve and the shorter the period the child will be able to withstand starvation.

High nutritional demands for growth

The nourishment children require, per unit body size, is greatest in infancy (Table 12.1), because of their rapid growth during this period. At 4 months of age, 30% of an infant's energy intake is used for growth, but by 1 year of age, this falls to 5%, and by 3 years to 2%. The risk of growth failure from restricted energy intake is therefore greater in the first 6 months of life than in later childhood. Even small but recurrent deficits in early childhood will lead to a cumulative deficit in weight and height.

Rapid neuronal development

The brain grows rapidly during the last trimester of pregnancy and throughout the first 2 years of life. The complexity of interneuronal connections also increases substantially during this time. This process appears to be sensitive to undernutrition. Even modest energy deprivation during periods of rapid brain growth and differentiation is thought to lead to an increased risk of adverse neurodevelopmental outcome. This is not surprising when one considers that at birth the brain accounts for approximately two-thirds of basal

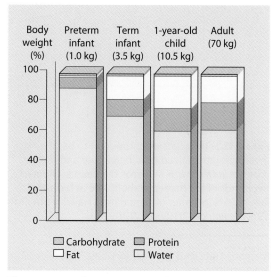

Figure 12.1 Body composition of preterm and term infants, children and adults. Newborn infants, particularly the preterm, have poor stores of fat and protein.

Table 12.1 Reference values for energy and protein requirements

Age	Energy (kcal/kg per 24 h)	Protein (g/kg per 24 h)
0–6 months	115	2.2
6–12 months	95	2.0
1–3 years	95	1.8
4–6 years	90	1.5
7–10 years	75	1.2
Adolescence	(male/female)	
11–14 years	65/55	1.0
15–18 years	60/40	0.8

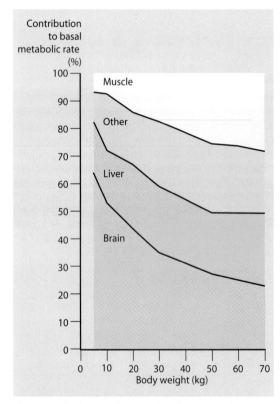

Figure 12.2 The relative contribution to basal metabolic rate derived from brain, liver and muscle changes with growth. Whereas the brain accounts for two-thirds of the basal metabolic rate at birth, this falls to 25% in adults. (Adapted from Halliday MA. 1971. *Pediatrics* 47(1 Suppl 2):169.)

metabolic rate, and at 1 year for about 50% (Fig. 12.2). Many studies have drawn attention to the delayed development seen in children suffering from protein-energy malnutrition due to inadequate food intake, although inadequate psychosocial stimulation may also contribute.

Acute illness or surgery

A child's nutrition may be compromised following an acute illness or surgery. Infants are prone to recurrent infections, which reduce food intake and increase nutritional demands. Following surgery, after a brief anabolic phase, catecholamine secretion is increased, causing the metabolic rate and energy requirement to increase. Urinary nitrogen losses may become so great that it is impossible to achieve a positive nitrogen balance and weight is lost. After uncomplicated surgery, this phase may last for a week, but it can last several weeks after extensive burns, complicated surgery or severe sepsis. Thereafter, previously lost tissue is replaced and a positive energy and nitrogen balance can be achieved. However, infants may not show catch-up growth unless their energy intake is as high as 150–200 kcal/kg per day compared with the normal of 95–115 kcal/kg per day.

Long-term outcome of early nutritional deficiency

Linear growth of populations

Growth and nutrition are closely related, such that the mean height of a population reflects its nutritional status. Thus, in the developed world, people have become taller. Height is adversely affected by lower socioeconomic status and increasing number of children in families. Children's size increases amongst populations emigrating from poor to more affluent countries.

Disease in adult life

Evidence suggests that undernutrition in utero resulting in growth restriction is associated with an increased incidence of coronary heart disease, stroke, non-insulin-dependent diabetes and hypertension in later life (Fig. 12.3). There is also a similar but weaker association with low weight at 1 year of age. The mechanism is unclear, but it is recognised that fetal undernutrition leads to redistribution of blood flow and changes in fetal hormones, such as insulin-like growth factors and cortisol. Alternatively, it may be the rapid, postnatal growth (catch-up) seen in babies suffering from intrauterine growth restriction that is the causal factor.

Summary

Nutritional vulnerability

Infants are more vulnerable to poor nutrition because of:
- Poor stores of fat and protein
- Extra nutritional demands for growth – the weight of a term infant doubles by 4 months and trebles by 1 year.
- More frequent intercurrent illnesses that reduce food intake and increase nutritional demands.

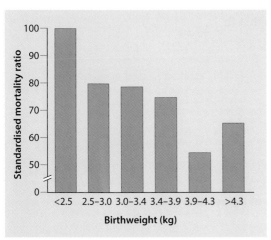

Figure 12.3 Death rates from coronary heart disease according to birthweight showing increased rate in low birthweight babies. (After Barker DJ. 1999. Fetal origins of adult disease. *Growing up in Britain: Ensuring the Healthy Future for our Children.* A Study of 4–5 year olds. BMJ Books, London.)

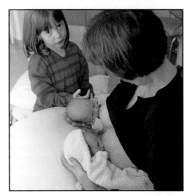

Figure 12.4 Successful breast-feeding of preterm twins.

Infant feeding

Breast-feeding

There can be no doubt that breastmilk is the best diet for babies, although the popularity of breast-feeding has frequently reflected fashion. The prevalence of breast-feeding in the UK has increased, and 78% of mothers breast-feed their infants at birth. The Department of Health guidelines in the UK, endorsing the World Health Organization recommendation, is that mothers should breast-feed exclusively for the first 6 months of life, though most are weaned to solid food before this age.

Advantages (see Box 12.1)

In developing countries, where the environment is often highly contaminated, breast-feeding dramatically improves survival during infancy as a result of reduced gastrointestinal infection. Consequently, breast-feeding is one of the four most important World Health Organization strategies for improving infant and child survival. The superiority of breast milk over modern adapted cow's milk formulae is less easy to prove in developed countries. This is partly because it is impossible to conduct randomised studies and partly because of confounders such as social class, education and smoking.

However, there is convincing evidence that gastrointestinal infection is less common in breast-fed infants even in developed countries. There is also evidence that human milk feeds reduce the incidence of necrotising enterocolitis in preterm infants.

Many mothers who breast-feed find that it helps them establish an intimate, loving relationship with their baby. However, establishing breast-feeding is not always straightforward, and many mothers need help and encouragement.

Breast-feeding is associated with a reduced incidence of obesity, diabetes mellitus and hypertension in later life. There is also a reduction in breast cancer in mothers who breast-feed.

 Exclusive breast-feeding in early infancy is life-saving in developing countries.

Potential complications (Box 12.2)

As one cannot readily tell how much milk a baby is taking from the breast, the baby's weight should be checked regularly, every few days in the first couple of weeks, then weekly until feeding is well established. Successful breast-feeding of twins can be achieved, but is more difficult (Fig. 12.4). It is rarely possible to totally breast-feed triplets and higher-order births. Preterm infants can be breast-fed, but the milk will need to be expressed from the breast until the infant can suck. Maintaining the supply of milk can be a problem for mothers of preterm babies.

While two-thirds of mothers in the UK initially breast-feed, this proportion rapidly declines during the first few months (Fig. 12.5). Nearly 90% of social class I mothers start breast-feeding, but only 60% of mothers from social class V. Breast-feeding is restrictive for the mother, as others cannot take charge of her baby for any length of time. This is particularly important if she goes to work and may delay her return, which may cause financial hardship for the family. Facilities for breast-feeding in public places remain limited. Failure to establish breast-feeding will sometimes cause significant emotional upset in the mother.

Establishing breast-feeding

Colostrum, rather than milk, is produced for the first few days. Colostrum differs from mature milk in that the content of protein and immunoglobulin is much higher. Volumes are low, but water or formula supplements are not required while the supply of breast milk is becoming established.

The first breast-feed should take place as soon as possible after birth. Subsequently, frequent suckling is beneficial as it enhances the secretion of the hormones initiating and promoting lactation (Fig. 12.6).

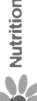

203

Box 12.1 Why breast is best – the advantages of breast milk

Advantages of breast-feeding for the infant are that it:

- provides the ideal nutrition for infants during the first 4–6 months of life
- is life-saving in developing countries
- reduces the risk of gastrointestinal infection, and, in preterm infants, of necrotising enterocolitis
- enhances mother–child relationship
- reduces risk of insulin-dependent diabetes, hypertension and obesity in later life.

Advantages for the mother are that it:

- promotes close attachment between mother and baby
- increases the time interval between children, which is important in reducing birth rate in developing countries
- helps with a possible reduction in premenopausal breast cancer.

Scientific explanation of some of the properties of breast milk

Anti-infective properties

Humoral

Secretory IgA	Comprises 90% of immunoglobulin in human milk. Provides mucosal protection, but of uncertain benefit
Bifidus factor	Promotes growth of *Lactobacillus bifidus*, which metabolises lactose to lactic and acetic acids. The resulting low pH may inhibit growth of gastrointestinal pathogens
Lysozyme	Bacteriolytic enzyme
Lactoferrin	Iron-binding protein. Inhibits growth of *Escherichia coli*
Interferon	Antiviral agent

Cellular

Macrophages	Phagocytic. Synthesise lysozyme, lactoferrin, C3, C4
Lymphocytes	T cells may transfer delayed hypersensitivity responses to infant. B cells synthesise IgA

Nutritional properties

Protein quality	More easily digested curd (60:40 whey:casein ratio)
Lipid quality	Rich in oleic acid (with palmitate in C-2 position). Improved digestibility and fat absorption. Enhanced lipolysis lipase.
Calcium: phosphorus ratio of 2:1	Prevents hypocalcaemic tetany and improves calcium absorption
Renal solute load	Low
Iron content	Bioavailable (40–50% absorption)
Long-chain polyunsaturated fatty acids	Structural lipids; important in retinal development

Box 12.2 Potential complications of breast-feeding

Unknown intake	Volume of milk intake not known
Transmission of infection	Maternal CMV, hepatitis B and HIV – increases risk of transmission to the baby
Breast-milk jaundice	Mild, self-limiting, unconjugated hyperbilirubinaemia; continue breast-feeding
Transmission of drugs	Antimetabolites and some other drugs contra-indicated. Check formulary
Nutrient inadequacies	Breast-feeding beyond 6 months without timely introduction of appropriate solids may lead to poor weight gain and rickets
Vitamin K deficiency	Insufficient vitamin K in breast milk to prevent haemorrhagic disease of the newborn. Supplementation is required
Potential transmission of environmental contaminants	Nicotine, alcohol, caffeine, etc.
Less flexible	Other family members cannot help or take part. More difficult in public places
Emotional upset	If difficulties or lack of success can be upsetting

Primates probably do not breast-feed instinctively. Monkeys bred in captivity in zoos have to be taught how to breast-feed by their keepers. It is therefore important that breast-feeding should have as high a public profile as possible. Women who have never seen an infant being breast-fed are less likely to want to breast-feed themselves. Education in schools and during pregnancy about the advantages of breast-feeding is advantageous. Advice and support from other women who have breast-fed may be important in dealing with early problems such as engorgement or cracked nipples.

 Newborn infants of mothers planning to breast-feed should ideally not be given any formula feeds.

Formula-feeding

Infants who are not breast-fed require a formulafeed based on cow's milk. Unmodified cow's milk is unsuitable for feeding in infancy as it contains too much protein and electrolytes and inadequate iron and vitamins. Even after considerable modification, differences remain between formula feeds and breastmilk (Table 12.2)

All milks currently available in the UK have been modified to make their mineral content and renal solute load comparable with that of mature human milk. Since these changes were introduced in the UK (in the 1970s), there has been an impressive reduction in the incidence of hypernatraemic dehydration in infants with gastroenteritis. There is no evidence that any one of the many brands is superior to any other.

Introduction of whole, pasteurised cow's milk

Breast-feeding or formula-feeding is recommended until the age of 12 months, and there are advantages in continuing to 18 months of age. Pasteurised cow's milk may be given from 1 year of age but is deficient

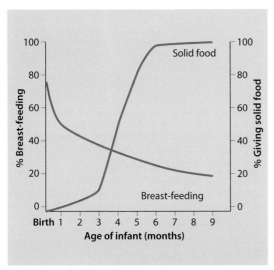

Figure 12.5 Prevalence of breast-feeding and proportion of infants given solid feeds during the first 9 months of life in the UK. Over the last 10 years there has been a marked increase in the prevalence of breast-feeding and delay in weaning onto solid food (Infant Feeding Survey, 2005).

Physiology of breast-feeding

1. **Baby** uses rooting, sucking and swallowing reflexes to locate nipple and feed

2. **Tactile receptors** in nipple activated

3. **Hypothalamus** sends efferent impulses to anterior and posterior pituitary

4. **Anterior pituitary**
Prolactin secretion stimulates milk secretion by cuboidal cells in the acini of the breast

5. **Posterior pituitary**
Oxytocin secretion results in contraction of myoepithelial cells in the alveoli, forcing milk into larger ducts – the so-called 'let-down' reflex

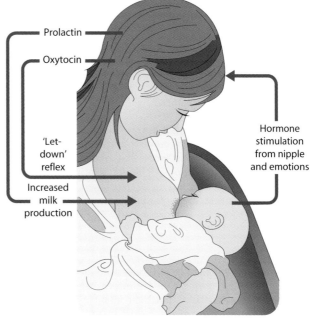

Prolactin

Oxytocin

'Let-down' reflex

Increased milk production

Hormone stimulation from nipple and emotions

Figure 12.6 Physiology of breast-feeding.

Table 12.2 A comparison of human milk, cow's milk and infant formula (per 100 ml)

	Mature breast milk	Cow's milk	Infant formula (modified cow's milk)
Energy (kcal)	62	67	60–65
Protein (g)	1.3	3.5	1.5–1.9
Carbohydrate (g)	6.7	4.9	7.0–8.6
Casein:whey	40:60	63:37	40:60 to 63:37
Fat (g)	3.0	3.6	2.6–3.8
Sodium (mmol)	0.65	2.3	0.65–1.1
Calcium (mmol)	0.88	3.0	0.88–2.1
Phosphorus (mmol)	0.46	3.2	0.9–1.8
Iron (μmol)	1.36	0.9	8–12.5

in vitamins A, C and D and in iron, and supplementation will be required unless the infant is having a good diet of mixed solids. Alternatively, 'follow-on' formulae can be used. They contain more protein and sodium than infant formulae and, in contrast to cow's milk, are fortified with iron and vitamins. Children on cow's milk should receive full fat milk up to the age of 5 years.

 Infant formula, not unmodified cow's milk, should be used in the first year of life.

Specialised infant formula

A specialised formula may be used for cow's milk protein allergy/intolerance, lactose intolerance (primary lactase deficiency or post-gastroenteritis intolerance), cystic fibrosis, neonatal cholestatic liver disease and following neonatal intestinal resection.

In a cow's milk-based formula, the protein is derived from cow's milk protein, the carbohydrate is lactose and the fat mainly long-chain triglycerides. In a specialised formula, the protein is either hydrolysed cow's milk protein, amino acids or from soya, the carbohydrate is glucose polymer and the fat a combination of medium- and long-chain triglycerides. Medium-chain triglycerides are directly absorbed into small intestine and need neither pancreatic enzymes nor bile salts for this process.

A soya formula should not be used below 6 months of age as it has a high aluminium content and contains phytoestrogens (plant substances that mimic the effects of endogenous oestrogens). There is no compelling evidence that the use of a specialised formula prevents the development of atopy (eczema, asthma, etc.).

Weaning

Solid foods are recommended to be introduced after 6 months of age, although they are often introduced earlier as parents often consider that their infant is hungry. It is done gradually, initially with small quantities of pureed fruit, root vegetables, or rice. If weaning takes place before 6 months of age, wheat, eggs and fish should be avoided. Foods high in salt and sugar should also be avoided and honey should not be given until 1 year of age because of risk of infantile botulism. After 6 months of age, breastmilk becomes increasingly nutritionally inadequate as a sole feed, as it does not provide sufficient energy, vitamins or iron.

Failure to thrive

The term 'failure to thrive' is used to describe suboptimal, weight gain in infants and toddlers. It may also be referred to as weight or growth faltering in case parents consider the term critical of their care. Recognition of the entity depends upon demonstration of inadequate weight gain when plotted on a centile chart, mild failure to thrive being a fall across two centile lines and severe being a fall across three centile lines. Between 6 weeks and 1 year of age, only 5% of children will cross two lines, and only 1% will cross three. Most children with 'failure to thrive' have a weight below the 2nd centile. However, the weight of some children with failure to thrive, i.e. they are failing to gain or are losing weight, may still be above the 2nd centile. Repeated observations are therefore essential and are usually available from the child's personal child health record. A single observation of weight is difficult to interpret unless markedly discrepant from the head circumference or length, although the further the weight is below the 2nd centile, the more likely the child is 'failing to thrive'. A weight below the 0.4th centile should always trigger an evaluation.

Differentiating the infant who is failing to thrive from a normal but small or thin baby is often a problem (Fig. 12.7). Normal but short infants have no symptoms, are alert, responsive and happy, and their development is satisfactory. The parents may be short (low midparental height) or the infant may have been extremely preterm or growth-restricted at birth. Any intercurrent illness may be accompanied by a temporary failure to gain weight.

An additional diagnostic problem is 'catch-down' (as opposed to 'catch-up') weight. This is when an infant's weight falls from the birth centile, which is

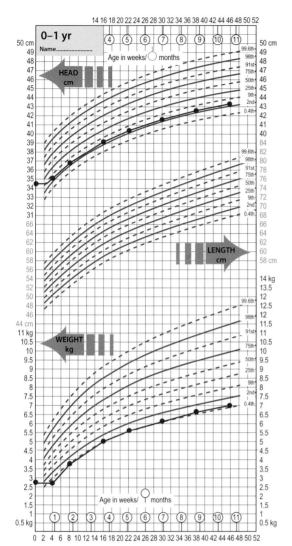

Figure 12.7 Growth chart showing normal weight gain and growth in a constitutionally small infant. The further below the 2nd, and especially the 0.4th, centile, the more likely it is that there will be an organic cause. (Chart © RCPCH, WHO, Department of Health.)

determined by the intrauterine environment, to a lower, genetically determined growth centile. These infants need only close monitoring of their growth over a few months.

While children with recent-onset failure to thrive usually maintain their height, this may become compromised by prolonged, inadequate weight gain. The child's developmental progress may also be adversely affected.

Causes

Failure to thrive is usually classified as organic or non-organic (Fig. 12.8). Traditionally non-organic failure to thrive is believed to be associated with a broad spectrum of psychosocial and environmental deprivation. It is estimated that 5–10% of children with failure to thrive will be on a child protection register or be

subjected to abuse or neglect, while in a larger proportion, socioeconomic deprivation is an important contributing factor.

The mother may be depressed, have an eating disorder herself or have poor understanding of her baby's needs. There may be poor housing, poverty, inadequate social support and lack of an extended family, which make good child care even more difficult. However, some studies suggest that failure to thrive is not more common in deprived than in non-deprived communities, and that identification of deprivation leads to the inappropriate application of that diagnostic label. Undernutrition is the final common pathway for poor weight gain in most cases of organic and non-organic failure to thrive, and in many cases both organic and environmental factors are present.

Organic causes are listed in Figure 12.8. Less than 5% of children with failure to thrive will be found to have an organic cause.

Clinical features and investigation

Studying the growth chart in combination with the history and examination of the child is key to its evaluation. The history should focus on:

- A detailed dietary history, including a food diary over several days
- Feeding, including details of exactly what happens at mealtimes
- Is the child well with lots of energy or does the child have other symptoms such as diarrhoea, vomiting, cough, lethargy?
- Was the child premature or had intrauterine growth restriction at birth or any significant medical problems?
- The growth of other family members and any illnesses in the family
- Is the child's development normal?
- Are there psychosocial problems at home?

Examination should focus on identifying signs of organic disease – dysmorphic features, signs suggestive of malabsorption (distended abdomen, thin buttocks, misery), signs suggestive of chronic respiratory disease (chest deformity,clubbing), signs of heart failure and evidence of nutritional deficiencies.

Further information about the child and family from the health visitor, general practitioner or other professionals involved with the family can be particularly helpful. Investigations to be considered are listed in Box 12.3.

In some children who are failing to thrive, a full blood count and serum ferritin may be helpful to identify iron deficiency anaemia. This is usually secondary to inadequate iron intake and correcting it may improve appetite. In most instances, no investigations are required.

Management

The management of most non-organic failure to thrive is multidisciplinary and is carried out in primary care. The health visitor is well placed to make home visits to

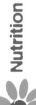

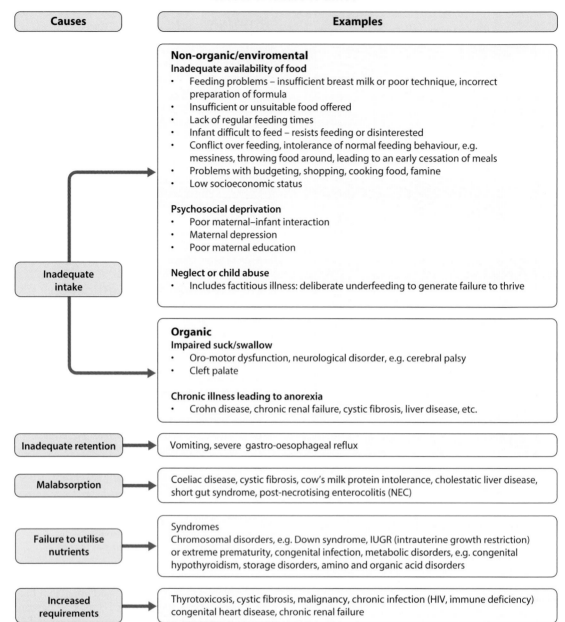

Causes of failure to thrive

Causes	Examples
Inadequate intake	**Non-organic/enviromental**

Non-organic/enviromental
Inadequate availability of food
- Feeding problems – insufficient breast milk or poor technique, incorrect preparation of formula
- Insufficient or unsuitable food offered
- Lack of regular feeding times
- Infant difficult to feed – resists feeding or disinterested
- Conflict over feeding, intolerance of normal feeding behaviour, e.g. messiness, throwing food around, leading to an early cessation of meals
- Problems with budgeting, shopping, cooking food, famine
- Low socioeconomic status

Psychosocial deprivation
- Poor maternal–infant interaction
- Maternal depression
- Poor maternal education

Neglect or child abuse
- Includes factitious illness: deliberate underfeeding to generate failure to thrive

Organic
Impaired suck/swallow
- Oro-motor dysfunction, neurological disorder, e.g. cerebral palsy
- Cleft palate

Chronic illness leading to anorexia
- Crohn disease, chronic renal failure, cystic fibrosis, liver disease, etc.

Inadequate retention → Vomiting, severe gastro-oesophageal reflux

Malabsorption → Coeliac disease, cystic fibrosis, cow's milk protein intolerance, cholestatic liver disease, short gut syndrome, post-necrotising enterocolitis (NEC)

Failure to utilise nutrients → Syndromes
Chromosomal disorders, e.g. Down syndrome, IUGR (intrauterine growth restriction) or extreme prematurity, congenital infection, metabolic disorders, e.g. congenital hypothyroidism, storage disorders, amino and organic acid disorders

Increased requirements → Thyrotoxicosis, cystic fibrosis, malignancy, chronic infection (HIV, immune deficiency) congenital heart disease, chronic renal failure

Figure 12.8 The main causes of failure to thrive.

assess eating behaviour and provide support. Direct practical advice following observation may well be beneficial. A paediatric dietician may be helpful in assessing the quantity and composition of food intake, and recommending strategies for increasing energy intake and a speech and language therapist has specialist skills with feeding disorders. Input from a clinical psychologist and from social services may also be appropriate. Nursery placement may be helpful in alleviating stress at home and assist with feeding.

Hospital admission is usually only necessary in children under 6 months with severe failure to thrive, requiring active refeeding. While hospital admission may offer the opportunity to observe and improve the mother's method and skill in feeding, this rarely transfers from the artificial hospital environment to home. In extreme cases, hospital admission can be used to demonstrate that the child will gain weight when fed appropriately.

Outcome

Follow-up studies suggest that children with non-organic failure to thrive continue to under-eat (see Case History 12.1). Although there is usually a gradual improvement in the preschool years, a lasting deficit is common and these children tend to remain underweight. In contrast, impairment of development is only short term.

Box 12.3 Investigations to be considered in 'failure to thrive'

Investigation	Significance of an abnormality
Full blood count and differential white cell count	Anaemia, neutropenia, lymphopenia (immune deficiency)
Serum creatinine urea, electrolytes, acid–base status, calcium, phosphate	Renal failure, renal tubular acidosis, metabolic disorders, William syndrome
Liver function tests	Liver disease, malabsorption, metabolic disorders
Thyroid function tests	Hypothyroidism or hyperthyroidism
Acute phase reactant, e.g. C-reactive protein	Inflammation
Ferriaztin	Iron deficiency anaemia
Immunoglobulins	Immune deficiency
IgA tissue transglutaminase antibodies	Coeliac disease
Urine microscopy, culture and dipsticks	Urinary tract infection, renal disease
Stool microscopy, culture and elastase	Intestinal infection, parasites, elastase decreased in pancreatic insufficiency
Karyotype in girls	Turner syndrome
Chest X-ray and sweat test	Cystic fibrosis

Summary

Failure to thrive

- is a description, not a diagnosis
- weights of infants are only helpful if accurate and plotted on a centile chart
- is present if an infant's weight falls across two centile lines
- is likely to be present the further the weight is below the 2nd centile
- is mostly due to inadequate food intake
- is accompanied by abnormal symptoms or signs if there is organic disease
- most affected infants and toddlers do not require any investigations and are managed in primary care by increasing energy intake by dietary and behavioural modification and monitoring growth.

Malnutrition

Worldwide, malnutrition is common and is responsible directly or indirectly for about a third of all deaths of children under 5 years of age. Primary malnutrition also continues to occur in developed countries as a result of poverty, parental neglect or poor education. Specific nutritional deficiencies, particularly of iron, remain common in developed countries. Restrictive diets may be iatrogenic as a result of exclusion diets or parental food fads, or may be self-inflicted.

Malnutrition also occurs in 20–40% of children in specialist children's hospitals. At particular risk are those with chronic illness: e.g. the preterm, congenital heart disease, malignant disease during chemotherapy or bone marrow transplantation, chronic gastrointestinal conditions such as short gut syndrome following extensive bowel resection or inflammatory bowel disease, chronic renal failure or cerebral palsy. Malnutrition results from a combination of anorexia, malabsorption and increased energy requirements because of infection or inflammation. Malnutrition in older children and adolescents may also result from eating disorders.

Assessment of nutritional status

Malnutrition must be recognised and accurately defined for rational decisions to be made about refeeding. Evaluation is divided into assessment of past and present dietary intake, anthropometry and laboratory assessments (Fig. 12.10).

Dietary assessment

Parents are asked to record the food the child eats during several days. This gives a guide to food intake.

Anthropometry

In addition to weight and height, skinfold thickness of the triceps reflects subcutaneous fat stores and can be assessed by measuring it. While it is difficult to measure skinfold thickness accurately in young children, mid-upper arm circumference, which is related to skeletal muscle mass, can be measured easily and repeatedly and is independent of age in children 6 months to 6 years. It is especially useful for screening children for malnutrition in the community.

Laboratory investigations

These are useful in the detection of early physiological adaptation to malnutrition, but clinical history, examination and anthropometry are of greater value than any single biochemical or immunological measurement.

Case History

12.1 Non-organic failure to thrive

Jamie, aged 11 months, was causing concern to his health visitor as he was not putting on any weight (Fig. 12.9). She arranged for him to be assessed by his general practitioner, who found that he was otherwise well. His mother was a single parent who left school at 16 years and had Jamie at the age of 18. They lived in a high-rise flat and Jamie's mother received income support. Her own mother lived on the other side of the city.

On visiting the home, the health visitor found Jamie's mother to be tense and anxious. In particular, she was worried about making ends meet. She fed Jamie the same food as she ate herself, together with pasteurised milk, which she had started at 6 months of age. The meals were chaotic. After a few mouthfuls, Jamie stopped eating and his mother did not coax him but became frustrated and angry.

Jamie's health visitor suggested strategies for increasing Jamie's food intake (Box 12.4). She continued to provide support and encouragement to his mother and arranged a nursery placement for Jamie. By 2 years of age, he had caught up by one centile line, but still ate erratically.

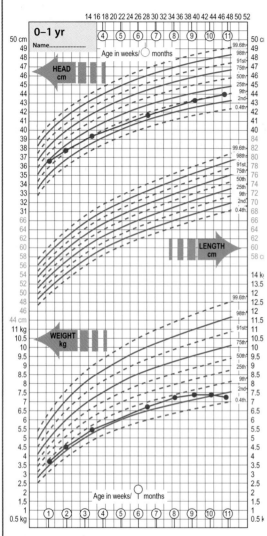

Figure 12.9 Jamie's growth chart. (Chart © RCPCH, WHO, Department of Health.)

Box 12.4 Strategies for increasing energy intake

Dietary

- Three meals and two snacks each day
- Increase number and variety of foods offered
- Increase energy density of usual foods (e.g. add cheese, margarine and cream)
- Decrease fluid intake, particularly squash

Behavioural

- Have meals at regular times, eaten with other family members
- Praise when food is eaten
- Gently encourage child to eat, but avoid conflict
- Never force-feed.

After Wright CM. 2000. Identification and management of failure to thrive: a community perspective. *Archives of Disease in Childhood* 82:5–9.

Consequences of malnutrition

Malnutrition is a multisystem disorder. When severe, immunity is impaired, wound healing is delayed and operative morbidity and mortality increased. Malnutrition worsens the outcome of illness, e.g. respiratory muscle dysfunction may delay a child being weaned from mechanical ventilation. Malnourished children are less active, less exploratory and more apathetic. These behavioural abnormalities are rapidly reversed with proper feeding, but prolonged and profound malnutrition can cause permanent delay in intellectual development.

The role of intensive nutritional support

Children with chronic disorders who are malnourished will grow better if given supplemental nutritional support, which may be provided by the enteral or parenteral route.

Enteral nutrition

Enteral nutrition is used when the digestive tract is functioning, as it maintains gut function, and is safe. Feeds are given nasogastrically, by gastrostomy or

Nutritional assessment

Nutritional assessment

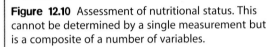

Anthropometry
- Weight
- Height
- Mid-arm circumference
- Skinfold thickness

Laboratory
- Low plasma albumin
- Low concentration of specific minerals and vitamins

Food intake
- Dietary recall
- Dietary diary

Immunodeficiency
- Low lymphocyte count
- Impaired cell-mediated immunity

Figure 12.10 Assessment of nutritional status. This cannot be determined by a single measurement but is a composite of a number of variables.

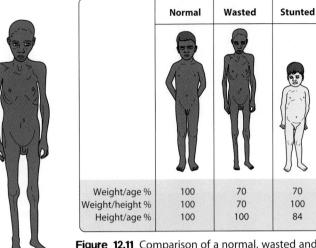

	Normal	Wasted	Stunted
Weight/age %	100	70	70
Weight/height %	100	70	100
Height/age %	100	100	84

Figure 12.11 Comparison of a normal, wasted and stunted child at 1 year. Low weight for height reveals a child of normal height, but who is thin and wasted, whereas low height for age reveals a short, non-wasted child.

occasionally via a feeding tube in the jejunum. Feeds are often given continuously overnight, allowing the child to feed normally during the day. Gastrostomies can either be created endoscopically or surgically. If long-term supplemental enteral nutrition is required, a gastrostomy is prefered as it avoids repeated replacements of nasogastric tubes, which is distressing for the child.

Parenteral nutrition

Parenteral nutrition can be used exclusively or as an adjunct to enteral feeds to maintain and/or enhance nutrition. The aim is to provide a nutritionally complete feed in an appropriate volume of intravenous fluid. It can be delivered at home. However, it is a complex and expensive form of therapy, requiring a multidisciplinary approach incorporating the skills not only of medical and nursing staff but also pharmacists and dieticians. Short term, it is possible to deliver it via peripherally sited canulae; long term, it is delivered via a central venous catheter as this allows infusion of hyperosmolar solutions and does not require repeated resiting of the cannula. It may be inserted surgically or under radiological guidance. Complications include catheter sepsis or blockage, problems of vascular access on repeated line placement and liver disease from the parenteral nitrition itself.

Marasmus and kwashiorkor

Globally, over one-third of childhood deaths are attributable to undernutrition, which leaves the child susceptible and unable to survive common infections.

The World Health Organization recommends that nutritional status is expressed as:

- Weight for height – a measure of wasting and an index of acute malnutrition (Fig. 12.11). Severe malnutrition is defined as a weight for height more than −3 standard deviations below the median plotted on the WHO standard growth chart. This corresponds to a weight for height <70% below the median.
- Mid upper-arm circumference (MUAC) – <115 mm is severe malnutrition
- Height for age – a measure of stunting and an index of chronic malnutrition

Severe protein-energy malnutrition in children usually leads to marasmus, with a weight for height more than −3 standard deviations below the median, corresponding to <70% weight for height, and a wasted, wizened appearance (Fig. 12.12). Oedema is not present. Skinfold thickness and mid-arm circumference are markedly reduced, and affected children are often withdrawn and apathetic.

Kwashiorkor is another manifestation of severe protein malnutrition (Fig. 12.13), in which there is generalised oedema as well as severe wasting. Because of the oedema, the weight may not be as severely reduced. In addition, there may be:

- a 'flaky-paint' skin rash with hyperkeratosis (thickened skin) and desquamation
- a distended abdomen and enlarged liver (usually due to fatty infiltration)
- angular stomatitis
- hair which is sparse and depigmented
- diarrhoea, hypothermia, bradycardia and hypotension

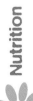

Nutrition

211

Malnutrition

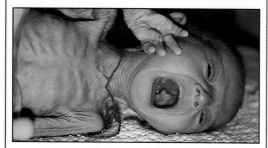

Figure 12.12 Marasmus in a 3-month-old baby who was unable to establish breast-feeding because of a cleft palate.

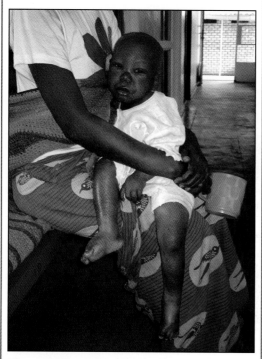

Figure 12.13 Kwashiorkor, a particular manifestation of severe protein-energy malnutrition in some developing countries where infants are weaned late from the breast and the young child's diet is high in starch. There is oedema around the eyes and feet and legs, hyperkeratosis and depigmentation of the skin and redness of the hair.

- low plasma albumin, potassium, glucose and magnesium.

It is unclear why some children with protein-energy malnutrition develop kwashiorkor and others develop marasmus. Kwashiorkor is a feature of children reared in traditional, polygamous societies, where infants are not weaned from the breast until about 12 months of age. The subsequent diet tends to be relatively high in starch. Kwashiorkor often develops after an acute intercurrent infection, such as measles or gastroenteritis.

There is some evidence that kwashiorkor is a manifestation of primary protein deficiency with energy intake relatively well maintained or, alternatively, that it results from excess generation of free radicals.

Management

Severe acute malnutrition has a high mortality; about 30% in children require hospital care. In addition to protein and energy deficiency, there is electrolyte and mineral deficiency (potassium, zinc, magnesium) as well as micronutrient and vitamin deficiency (vitamin A).

Acute management includes:

- Hypoglycaemia – common; correct urgently, particularly if coma or severely ill.
- Hypothermia – wrap, especially at night.
- Dehydration – correct, but avoid being overzealous with intravenous fluids, as may lead to heart failure.
- Electrolytes – correct deficiencies, especially potassium.
- Infection – give antibiotics; fever and other signs may be absent. Treat oral candida if present.
- Micronutrients – give vitamin A and other vitamins
- Initiate feeding – small volumes, frequently, including through the night.

Children with no appetite or medical complications need hospital care. Otherwise care can be community based. Although protein deficient, diet is initially low in protein as high protein feeds are not tolerated. Too rapid feeding may result in diarrhoea. Specialised feeds are widely available. Initially Formula 75 (75 kcal/100 ml), subsequently Formula 100 (100 kcal/100 ml) or Ready-to-Use Therapeutic Food (RUTF). During recovery phase, growth is monitored, sensory stimulation should be provided and discharge preparation undertaken.

Summary

Malnutrition

- Worldwide – contributes to about a third of all childhood deaths; often a consequence of war and social disruption, as well as famine and natural disasters
- In developed countries – results from poverty, parental neglect or poor education, restrictive diets, children with feeding disorders or chronic illness or anorexia nervosa
- Can be identified by anthropometric measurement; laboratory tests are not usually required
- Marasmus – weight for height more than 3 Standard Deviations below the median; wasted, wizened appearance; apathetic
- Kwashiorkor – generalised oedema, sparse and depigmented hair, skin rash, angular stomatitis, distended abdomen and enlarged liver, diarrhoea.

Vitamin D deficiency

Vitamin D deficiency usually results from deficient intake or defective metabolism of vitamin D, causing a low serum calcium (Fig. 12.14). This triggers the secretion of parathyroid hormone and normalises the serum calcium but demineralises the bone. Parathyroid hormone causes renal losses of phosphate and consequently low serum phosphate levels, further reducing the potential for bone calcification.

Vitamin D deficiency usually presents with bony deformity and the classical picture of rickets. It can also present without bone abnormalities but with symptoms of hypocalcaemia, i.e. seizures, neuromuscular irritability (tetany), apnoea, stridor. This presentation is more common before 2 years of age and in adolescence, when a high demand for calcium in rapidly growing bone results in hypocalcaemia before rickets develops.

Rickets

Rickets signifies a failure in mineralisation of the growing bone or osteoid tissue. Failure of mature bone to mineralise is osteomalacia.

Aetiology

The causes of rickets are listed in Box 12.5 The predominant cause of rickets during the early twentieth century was nutritional vitamin D deficiency due to inadequate intake or insufficient exposure to direct sunlight. Nutritional rickets still remains the major cause in developing countries. In developed countries, nutritional rickets has become rare, as formula milk and many foods such as breakfast cereals are supplemented with vitamin D. However, nutritional rickets has re-emerged in developed countries in black or Asian infants totally breast-fed in late infancy. It is also seen in extremely preterm infants from dietary deficiency of phosphorus, together with low stores of calcium and phosphorus.

Children with malabsorptive conditions such as cystic fibrosis, coeliac disease and pancreatic insufficiency can develop rickets due to deficient absorption of vitamin D, calcium or both. Drugs, especially anticonvulsants such as phenobarbital and phenytoin, interfere with the metabolism of vitamin D and may also cause rickets. Rickets may also result from impaired metabolic conversion or activation of vitamin D (hepatic and renal disease).

Clinical manifestations

The earliest sign of rickets is a ping-pong ball sensation of the skull (craniotabes) elicited by pressing firmly over the occipital or posterior parietal bones. The costochondral junctions may be palpable (rachitic rosary), wrists (especially in crawling infants) and ankles (especially in walking infants) may be widened and there may be a horizontal depression on the lower chest corresponding to attachment of the softened ribs and with the diaphragm (Harrison sulcus) (Figs 12.15, 12.16). The legs may become bowed (see Fig. 12.15). The clinical features are listed in Box 12.6 (see also Case History 12.2).

Diagnosis

This is made from:

- Dietary history for vitamin and calcium intake
- Blood tests – serum calcium is low or normal, phosphorus low, plasma alkaline phosphatase activity greatly increased, 25-hydroxyvitamin D may be low and parathyroid hormone elevated.
- X-ray of the wrist joint – shows cupping and fraying of the metaphyses and a widened epiphyseal plate.

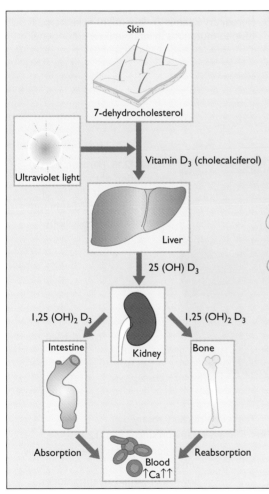

Figure 12.14 Vitamin D metabolism. In most countries, sunlight is the most important source of vitamin D. Vitamin D is not abundant naturally in food, except in fish liver oil, fatty fish and egg yolk. Vitamin D_2 (ergocalciferol) is the form used to fortify food such as margarine. Vitamin D_3 is hydroxylated in the liver and again in the kidney to produce 1,25-dihydroxyvitamin D (1,25(OH)$_2D_3$), the most active form of the vitamin. It is produced following parathyroid hormone secretion in response to a low plasma calcium.

Labels within Figure 12.14: Skin; 7-dehydrocholesterol; Ultraviolet light; Vitamin D_3 (cholecalciferol); Liver; 25 (OH) D_3; 1,25 (OH)$_2$ D_3; Intestine; Kidney; Bone; 1,25 (OH)$_2$ D_3; Absorption; Blood ↑Ca↑↑; Reabsorption

Box 12.5 Causes of rickets

Nutritional (primary) rickets – risk factors

- Living in northern latitudes
- Dark skin
- Decreased exposure to sunlight, e.g. in some Asian children living in the UK
- Maternal vitamin D deficiency
- Diets low in calcium, phosphorus and vitamin D, e.g. exclusive breast-feeding into late infancy or, rarely, toddlers on unsupervised 'dairy-free' diets
- Macrobiotic, strict vegan diets
- Prolonged parenteral nutrition in infancy with an inadequate supply of parenteral calcium and phosphate

Intestinal malabsorption

- Small bowel enteropathy (e.g. coeliac disease)
- Pancreatic insufficiency (e.g. cystic fibrosis)
- Cholestatic liver disease
- High phytic acids in diet (e.g. chapattis)

Defective production of 25(OH)D$_2$

- Chronic liver disease

Increased metabolism of 25(OH)D$_3$

- Enzyme induction by anticonvulsants (e.g. phenobarbital)

Defective production of 1,25(OH)$_2$D$_3$

- Hereditary type I vitamin D-resistant (or dependent) rickets (mutation which abolishes activity of renal hydroxylase)
- Familial (X-linked) hypophosphataemic rickets (renal tubular defect in phosphate transport)
- Chronic renal disease
- Fanconi syndrome (renal loss of phosphate)

Target organ resistance to 1,25(OH)$_2$D$_3$

- Hereditary vitamin D-dependent rickets type II (due to mutations in vitamin D receptor gene).

Rickets

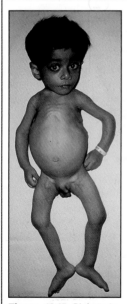

Figure 12.15 Rickets in a 3-year-old boy secondary to coeliac disease. He has frontal bossing, a Harrison sulcus and bow legs.

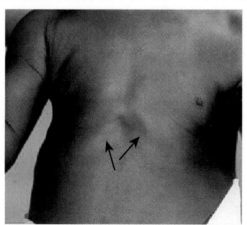

Figure 12.16 Harrison sulcus, indentation of the softened lower ribcage at the site of attachment of the diaphragm. (Courtesy of Dr Nick Shaw.)

Box 12.6 Clinical features of rickets

- Misery
- Failure to thrive/short stature
- Frontal bossing of skull
- Craniotabes
- Delayed closure of anterior fontanelle
- Delayed dentition

- Rickety rosary
- Harrison sulcus (Fig. 12.16)
- Expansion of metaphyses (especially wrist)
- Bowing of weight-bearing bones
- Hypotonia
- Seizures (late).

12.2 Seizures and rickets

Mohammed, a 13-month-old Somalian boy, was admitted to the A&E department with a generalised afebrile seizure. This was initially controlled with per rectum diazepam. Some 20 minutes later he had another generalised seizure and needed intravenous anticonvulsant to control his seizure.

His mother said that he was a healthy child. He was born at term, birthweight 3.1 kg, and was still breast-fed. Some weaning foods were started at 7–8 months, but he preferred feeding at the breast. He had only recently begun to sit without support.

His weight and head circumference were on the 2nd–9th centile. He had marked frontal bossing, widened wrist (Fig. 12.17) and other epiphyses,

Harrison sulci, wide anterior fontanelle, craniotabes and a rachitic rosary. He would not take his weight on standing.

Investigations showed a low calcium and phosphate level, a high alkaline phosphatase and parathyroid hormone level and a very low vitamin D level, confirming rickets. Liver and renal function tests were normal and coeliac screen was negative. His wrist X-ray showed characteristic features (Fig. 12.18). A detailed dietetic history revealed a diet deficient in calcium and vitamin D, confirming nutritional rickets as the cause.

Dietetic input was provided. He was started on oral vitamin D and his solid food intake was increased to ensure that he was receiving sufficient calcium and vitamin D in his diet. His rickets resolved.

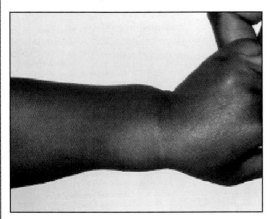

Figure 12.17 Wrist expansion from rickets. (Courtesy of Dr Nick Shaw.)

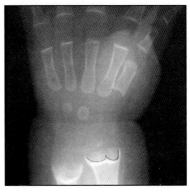

Figure 12.18 X-ray of the child's wrist showing rickets. The ends of the radius and ulna are expanded, rarefied and cup-shaped and the bones are poorly mineralised.

Management

Nutritional rickets is managed by advice about a balanced diet, correction of predisposing risk factors and by the daily administration of vitamin D_3 (cholecalciferol). If compliance is an issue, a single oral high dose of vitamin D_3 can be given, followed by the daily maintenance dose. Healing occurs in 2–4 weeks and can be monitored from the lowering of alkaline phosphatase, increasing vitamin D levels and healing on X-rays, but complete reversal of bony deformities may take years.

Summary

Rickets

- Nutritional – has re-emerged in the UK in Asian and black infants exclusively breast-fed into late infancy
- Diagnosis – serum calcium is low or normal, phosphorus low, plasma alkaline phosphatase greatly increased, 25-hydroxyvitamin D low and parathyroid hormone elevated
- X-ray features – cupping and fraying of the metaphyses and widened epiphyseal plate.

Vitamin A deficiency

In developed countries, vitamin A (retinol) deficiency is seen as a complication of fat malabsorption when supplementation has been inadequate. Clinical manifestations under these circumstances are rare, except for impaired adaptation to dark light. Vitamin A deficiency is the commonest cause of blindness in developing countries. It causes eye damage (xerophthalmia), which may progress from night blindness to corneal ulceration and scarring. It also results in increased susceptibility to infection, especially measles. Prevention in developing countries with high prevalence is by giving young children a dose of vitamin A; in some countries food is fortified. Supplementation is recommended for children with measles.

Obesity

Obesity is the most common nutritional disorder affecting children and adolescents in the developed world. Its importance is in its short- and long-term complications (Box 12.7) and that obese children tend to become obese adults.

Nutrition

Box 12.7 Complications of obesity

- Orthopaedic – slipped upper femoral epiphysis, tibia vara (bow legs), abnormal foot structure and function
- Idiopathic intracranial hypertension (headaches, blurred optic disc margins)
- Hypoventilation syndrome (daytime somnolence; sleep apnoea; snoring; hypercapnia; heart failure)
- Gallbladder disease
- Polycystic ovarian syndrome

- Type 2 diabetes mellitus
- Hypertension
- Abnormal blood lipids
- Other medical sequelae, e.g. asthma, changes in left ventricular mass, increased risk of certain malignancies (endometrial, breast and colonic carcinoma)
- Psychological sequelae – low self-esteem, teasing, depression.

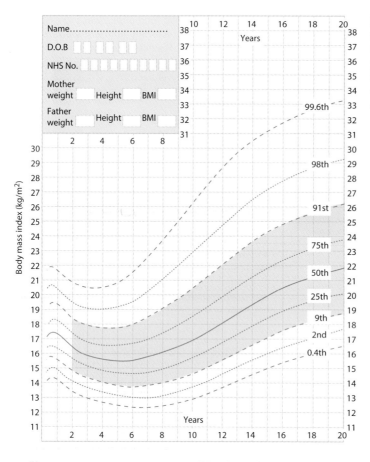

Figure 12.19 Body mass index (BMI) centile chart (Child Growth Foundation, reproduced with permission. Further supplies and information available at: http://www.healthforallchildren.co.uk. Accessed January 2011).

Definitions

In children, the body mass index (BMI = weight in kg/height in metres^2) is expressed as a BMI centile in relation to age and sex-matched population. By convention in the UK, the 1990 chart is used (Fig. 12.19). For clinical use, overweight is a BMI >91st centile, obese is a BMI >98th centile. Very severe obesity is >3.5 standard deviations above the mean; extreme obesity >4 standard deviations. For children over 12 years old, overweight is BMI ≥25, obese ≥30, very severe obesity BMI ≥35 and extreme obesity BMI ≥40 kg/m^2.

In 1995, 11% of males and 12.5% of females aged 2–15 years were obese. By 2006, these figures were 17.5% and 14.5%, respectively.

Aetiology

The reasons for this marked increase in prevalence are unclear but are due to changes in the environment and behaviour relating to diet and activity.

Energy-dense foods are now widely consumed, including high-fat fast foods and processed foods. However, there is no conclusive evidence that obese children eat more than children of normal weight. The National Food Survey showed that UK household energy intake has fallen since the 1970s, the amount of fruit purchased has increased by 75% and the intake of full fat milk decreased by 80%.

Children's energy expenditure has undoubtably decreased. Fewer children walk to school; transport in cars has increased; less time at school is spent doing physical activities; and children spend more time in front of small screens (video-games, mobile phones, computers and television), rather than playing outside.

Children from low socioeconomic homes are more likely to be obese; females from the lowest socioeconomic quintile are 2.5 times more likely to be overweight when compared with the highest quintile.

Prevention

There are few randomised controlled trials and most involve complex packages of interventions. Interventions include decreased fat intake, increased fruit and vegetables, reduction in time spent in front of small screens, increased physical activity, and education. Of these, a reduction in time spent on small screens appears to be the most effective single factor.

Endogenous causes

Overnutrition accelerates linear growth and puberty. Obese children are therefore relatively tall and will usually be above the 50th centile for height. An endogenous cause, i.e. hypothyroidism and Cushing syndrome should be sought in short, obese children, in whom height velocity is decreased as height remains static in these conditions.

In children who are obese with learning disabilities, or who are dysmorphic, a syndrome should be considered. The commonest of these is Prader–Willi (obesity, hyperphagia, poor linear growth, dysmorphic facial features, hypotonia and undescended testes in males; see Chapter 8 and Figure 8.19. In severely obese children under the age of 3 years, gene defects, e.g. leptin deficiency, should be considered.

Management

Most obese children are managed in primary care. Specialist paediatric assessment is indicated in any child with complications (Box 12.7) or if an endogenous cause is suspected.

In the absence of evidence from randomised controlled trials, a pragmatic approach in any individual child based on consensus criteria has to be adopted (Box 12.8). Treatment should be considered where the child is above the 98th centile for BMI and the family are willing to make the necessary difficult lifestyle changes. Weight maintenance is a more realistic goal than weight reduction and will result in a demonstrable fall in BMI on centile chart as height increases. It can only be achieved by sustained changes in lifestyle:

- Healthier eating – no sugar-containing juices or fizzy drinks; decrease food portion size by 10–20%; increase protein- and non-carbohydrate-containing vegetables, discourage snacking and encourage family meals
- An increase in habitual physical activity to 60 min of moderate to vigorous daily physical activity
- Reduce physical inactivity (e.g. small screen time) during leisure time to less than an average of 2 h per day.

Box 12.8 Main messages for patients and parents about obesity

- Incidence of obesity in children is increasing
- Obesity is a health concern in itself and also increases the risk of other serious health problems, such as high blood pressure, diabetes and psychological distress
- An obese child tends to become an obese adult
- Obesity in children may be prevented and treated by increasing physical activity/decreasing physical inactivity (e.g. small screen time) and encouraging a well-balanced and healthy diet
- Lifestyle changes involve making small gradual changes to behaviour
- Family support is necessary for treatment to succeed
- Generally, the aim of treatment is to help children maintain their weight (so that they can 'grow into it')
- Most children are not obese because of an underlying medical problem but as a result of their lifestyle.

Adapted from Scottish Intercollegiate Guidelines Network, SIGN.

Drug treatment and surgery

Drug treatment has a part to play in children over the age of 12 who have extreme obesity (BMI>40 kg/m^2) or have a BMI>35 kg/m^2 and complications of obesity. It is recommended that drug treatment should only be considered after dietary, exercise and behavioural approaches have been started (NICE 2006).

Orlistat is a lipase inhibitor, which reduces the absorption of dietary fat and thus produces steatorrhoea. Fat intake should be reduced to avoid the unpleasant gastrointestinal side-effects. *Metformin* is a biguanide that increases insulin sensitivity, decreases gluconeogenesis and decreases gastrointestinal glucose absorption.

If there is evidence of insulin insensitivity (*Acanthosis nigricans*, see Fig. 25.2), metformin should be considered. Orlistat may be appropriate if fat intake is high.

Bariatric surgery is generally not considered appropriate in children or young people unless they have almost achieved maturity, have very severe or extreme obesity with complications, e.g. type 2 diabetes or hypertension, and all other interventions have failed to achieve or maintain weight loss. American data would suggest that laparoscopic adjustable gastric banding is the most appropriate operation.

Dental caries

Dental caries occurs as a result of exposure to organic acids produced by bacterial fermentation of carbohydrate, particularly sucrose (Fig. 12.20). Prevalence is now rising in young children. It is strongly related to socioeconomic deprivation.

Nutrition

Summary

Obesity

- An increasing major health issue for children, predisposing them to a wide range of medical and psychological problems in childhood and adult life, especially type 2 diabetes mellitus and cardiovascular disease
- Defined as a BMI >98th centile of the UK 1990 reference chart for age and sex; overweight is BMI >91st centile
- Exogenous causes (hypothyroidism and Cushing syndrome) of obesity are rare, and more likely in a child who is also short with falling height velocity; there are also some rare genetic syndromes

- Successful management requires sustained changes in lifestyle, with healthier eating, increased physical activity and reduction in physical inactivity
- Drug treatment and surgical intervention are only appropriate in a small number of children
- Lifestyle changes are difficult to achieve and even harder to maintain
- A cultural change in our society should be considered, e.g. removal of 'tuck shops' and vending machines with unhealthy food and drinks from schools.

Prevention involves:

- A reduction in plaque bacteria (brushing and flossing)
- Less frequent ingestion of carbohydrates
- Regular inspection by a dentist
- An optimal intake of fluoride up to puberty to improve the resistance of the tooth to damage; water fluoridation is one of the most effective ways of achieving this.

Incorporation of fluoride in enamel by ionic substitution leads to replacement of calcium hydroxyapatite with calcium fluorapatite, which is less soluble in organic acids. In areas where drinking water contains a low concentration of fluoride, supplementation with fluoride drops or tablets is needed. Additionally, topical fluoride in toothpaste or mouthwashes is also advisable. Excess fluoride administration, before enamel has formed, may lead to mottled enamel (dental fluorosis).

Infants and children who are put to bed with a bottle containing fermentable liquid (milk or a sucrose-containing fruit juice) are at particular risk of developing severe dental caries. Characteristically, fluid collects around the upper anterior and posterior teeth, which become extensively damaged. Because of reduced salivation and swallowing during sleep, clearance and neutralisation of organic acids are also reduced. So-called 'prop feeding' should therefore be energetically discouraged. Infants fed on specialised formulae are also more at risk of developing dental caries because the carbohydrate in the milk is a glucose polymer.

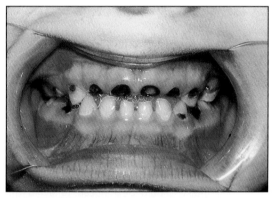

Figure 12.20 Dental caries. Prop-feeding infants when put to sleep with a bottle containing milk or other fermentable liquids places them at high risk of severe dental caries and should be discouraged.

Further reading

Beattie M, Dhawan A, Puntis J: *Paediatric Gastroenterology, Hepatology and Nutrition* (Oxford Specialist Handbooks in Paediatrics), Oxford, 2009, Oxford University Press .

Short handbook.

Websites (Accessed May 2011)

The Baby Friendly Initiative: Available at: http://www.babyfriendly.org.

Practical information on breast-feeding.

World Health Organization: Guidelines for malnutrition in developing countries. Available at: www.who.int.

Infant Feeding Survey: 2005. Available at: http://www.ic.nhs.uk/pubs/ifs2005.

NICE Guideline 43. Obesity: the prevention, identification, assessment and management of overweight and obesity in adults and children. 2006. Available at: http://guidance.nice.org.uk/CG43/Guidance/Section.

Gastroenterology

Features of gastrointestinal disorders in children are:

- Vomiting, abdominal pain and diarrhoea are common and usually transient; serious causes are uncommon but important to identify
- Worldwide, gastroenteritis is responsible for 1.2 million deaths/year, one of the commonest causes of death in children <5 years old
- The number of children and adolescents developing inflammatory bowel disease is increasing
- In contrast to adults, bowel cancer is extremely rare.

Vomiting

Posseting and *regurgitation* are terms used to describe the non-forceful return of milk, but differ in degree. Posseting describes the small amounts of milk which often accompany the return of swallowed air ('wind'), whereas regurgitation describes larger, more frequent losses. Posseting occurs in nearly all babies from time to time, whereas regurgitation may indicate the presence of more significant gastro-oesophageal reflux.

Vomiting is the forceful ejection of gastric contents. It is a common problem in infancy and childhood (Fig. 13.1 and Box 13.1).

Box 13.1 'Red Flag' clinical features in the vomiting child

Bile-stained vomit	Intestinal obstruction
Haematemesis	Oesophagitis, peptic ulceration, oral/nasal bleeding
Projectile vomiting, in first few weeks of life	Pyloric stenosis
Vomiting at the end of paroxysmal coughing	Whooping cough (pertussis)
Abdominal tenderness/abdominal pain on movement	Surgical abdomen
Abdominal distension	Intestinal obstruction, including strangulated inguinal hernia
Hepatosplenomegaly	Chronic liver disease
Blood in the stool	Intussusception, gastroenteritis – salmonella or campylobacter
Severe dehydration, shock	Severe gastroenteritis, systemic infection (urinary tract infection, meningitis), diabetic ketoacidosis
Bulging fontanelle or seizures	Raised intracranial pressure
Failure to thrive	Gasto-oesophageal reflux, coeliac disease and other chronic gastrointestinal conditions

Causes of vomiting

Infants	Preschool children	School-age and adolescents

Infants

Gastro-oesophageal reflux
Feeding problems
Infection
- Gastroenteritis
- Respiratory tract/otitis media
- Whooping cough (pertussis)
- Urinary tract
- Meningitis

Dietary protein intolerances
Intestinal obstruction
- Plyoric stenosis
- Atresia – duodenal, other sites
- Intussusception
- Malrotation
- Volvulus
- Duplication cysts
- Strangulated inguinal hernia
- Hirschsprung disease

Inborn errors of metabolism
Congenital adrenal hyperplasia
Renal failure

Preschool children

Gastroenteritis
Infection
- Respiratory tract/otitis media
- Urinary tract
- Meningitis
- Whooping cough (pertussis)

Appendicitis
Intestinal obstruction
- Intussusception
- Malrotation
- Volvulus
- Adhesions
- Foreign body – bezoar

Raised intracranial pressure
Coeliac disease
Renal failure
Inborn errors of metabolism
Torsion of the testis

School-age and adolescents

Gastroenteritis
Infection – including pyelonephritis, septicaemia, meningitis
Peptic ulceration and *H. pylori* infection
Appendicitis
Migraine
Raised intracranial pressure
Coeliac disease
Renal failure
Diabetic ketoacidosis
Alcohol/drug ingestion or medications
Cyclical vomiting syndrome
Bulimia/anorexia nervosa
Pregnancy
Torsion of the testis

Figure 13.1 Causes of regurgitation/vomiting.

It is usually benign and is often caused by feeding disorders or mild gastro-oesophageal reflux or gastroenteritis. Potentially serious disorders need to be excluded if the vomiting is bilious or prolonged, or if the child is systemically unwell or failing to thrive. In infants, vomiting may be associated with infection outside the gastrointestinal tract, especially in the urinary tract and central nervous system. In intestinal obstruction, the more proximal the obstruction, the more prominent the vomiting and the sooner it becomes bile-stained (unless the obstruction is proximal to the ampulla of Vater). Intestinal obstruction is associated with abdominal distension, more marked in distal obstruction. 'Red Flag' clinical features suggesting significant organic pathology are listed in Box 13.1.

Gastro-oesophageal reflux

Gastro-oesophageal reflux is the involuntary passage of gastric contents into the oesophagus. It is extremely common in infancy. It is caused by inappropriate relaxation of the lower oesophageal sphincter as a result of functional immaturity. A predominantly fluid diet, a mainly horizontal posture and a short intra-abdominal length of oesophagus all contribute. While common in the first year of life, nearly all symptomatic reflux resolves spontaneously by 12 months of age. This is presumably due to a combination of maturation of the lower oesophageal sphincter, assumption of an upright posture and more solids in the diet.

Most infants with gastro-oesophageal reflux have recurrent regurgitation or vomiting but are putting on weight normally and are otherwise well, although the mess, smell and frequent changes of clothes is frustrating for carers.

Complications are listed in Box 13.2.

Summary

Vomiting in infants

- Common chronic causes are gastro-oesophageal reflux and feeding problems, e.g. force-feeding or overfeeding
- If transient, with other symptoms, e.g. fever, diarrhoea or runny nose and cough, most likely to be gastroenteritis or respiratory tract infection, but consider urine infection and meningitis
- If projectile at 2–7 weeks of age, exclude pyloric stenosis
- If bile stained, exclude intestinal obstruction, especially intussusception, malrotation and a strangulated inguinal hernia. Assess for dehydration and shock.

Severe reflux is more common in:

- children with cerebral palsy or other neurodevelopmental disorders, when energetic management, surgical if necessary, may transform the child's quality of life
- preterm infants, especially if coexistent bronchopulmonary dysplasia
- following surgery for oesophageal atresia or diaphragmatic hernia.

Box 13.2 Complications of gastro-oesophageal reflux

- Failure to thrive from severe vomiting
- Oesophagitis – haematemesis, discomfort on feeding or heartburn, iron deficiency anaemia
- Recurrent pulmonary aspiration – recurrent pneumonia, cough or wheeze, apnoea in preterm infants
- Dystonic neck posturing (Sandifer syndrome)
- Apparent life-threatening events (ALTE)

Investigation

Gastro-oesophageal reflux is usually diagnosed clinically and no investigations are required. However, they may be indicated if the history is atypical, complications are present or there is failure to respond to treatment. Investigations include:

- 24-hour oesophageal pH monitoring to quantify the degree of acid reflux (see Case History 13.1).
- 24-hour impedance monitoring. Available in some centres. Weakly acidic or non-acid reflux, which may cause disease, is also measured.
- Endoscopy with oesophageal biopsies to identify oesophagitis and exclude other causes of vomiting.

Case History

13.1 Severe gastro-oesophageal reflux

This infant (Fig. 13.2a) had a history of frequent regurgitation from the first few days of life. He developed two chest infections. Some of the vomits contained altered blood. A 24-hour oesophageal pH study showed severe gastro-oesophageal reflux (Fig. 13.2b,c). Endoscopy showed oesophagitis. He had probably had episodes of aspiration pneumonia. Symptoms resolved on treatment with feed thickeners and omeprazole. His parents also commented on how much better he slept at night. Treatment was reduced from 14 months of age and the symptoms did not recur.

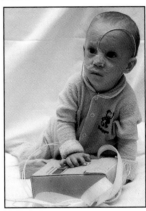

Figure 13.2a A pH sensor has been placed in the lower oesophagus.

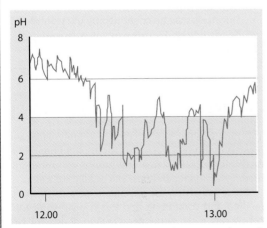

Figure 13.2b A section of the 24-hour oesophageal pH study showing severe reflux, with frequent drops in pH below 4.

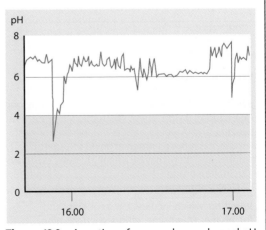

Figure 13.2c A section of a normal oesophageal pH study. The lower oesophageal pH is above 4 for most of the time.

Contrast studies of the upper gastrointestinal tract may support the diagnosis but are neither sensitive nor specific. They may be required to exclude underlying anatomical abnormalities in the oesophagus, stomach and duodenum, and to identify malrotation.

Management

Uncomplicated gastro-oesophageal reflux has an excellent prognosis and can be managed by parental reassurance, adding inert thickening agents to feeds (e.g. Nestargel, Carobel) and positioning in a 30° head-up prone position after feeds.

More significant gastro-oesophageal reflux disease is managed with acid suppression with either H_2 receptor antagonists (e.g. ranitidine) or proton pump inhibitors (e.g. omeprazole). These drugs reduce the volume of gastric contents and treat acid-related oesophagitis. Although the evidence for their use is poor, drugs which enhance gastric emptying (e.g. domperidone) may be tried. If the child fails to respond to these measures, other diagnoses such as cow's milk protein allergy should be considered and further investigations performed.

Surgical management is reserved for children with complications unresponsive to intensive medical treatment or oesophageal stricture. A Nissen fundoplication, in which the fundus of the stomach is wrapped around the intra-abdominal oesophagus, is performed either as an abdominal or laparoscopic procedure.

Summary

Gastro-oesophageal reflux

- . Occurs in otherwise normal infants, but risk is increased if neuromuscular problems or surgery to the oesophagus or diaphragm
- Is treated if troublesome with upright positioning, feed thickening, medication and sometimes fundoplication
- Investigations are performed if diagnosis is unclear or complications occur.

Pyloric stenosis

In pyloric stenosis, there is hypertrophy of the pyloric muscle causing gastric outlet obstruction. It presents at between 2 and 7 weeks of age, irrespective of gestational age. It is more common in boys (4:1), particularly first-borns, and there may be a family history, especially on the maternal side.

Clinical features are:

- Vomiting, which increases in frequency and forcefulness over time, ultimately becoming projectile
- Hunger after vomiting until dehydration leads to loss of interest in feeding
- Weight loss if presentation is delayed.

A hypochloraemic metabolic alkalosis with a low plasma sodium and potassium occurs as a result of vomiting stomach contents.

Diagnosis

Unless immediate fluid resuscitation is required, a test feed is performed. The baby is given a milk feed, which will calm the hungry infant, allowing examination. Gastric peristalsis may be seen as a wave moving from left to right across the abdomen (Fig. 13.3a). The pyloric mass, which feels like an olive, is usually palpable in the right upper quadrant (Fig. 13.3b). If the stomach is overdistended with air, it will need to be emptied by a nasogastric tube to allow palpation. Ultrasound examination is helpful (Fig. 13.3c) if the diagnosis is in doubt.

Management

The initial priority is to correct any fluid and electrolyte disturbance with intravenous fluids (0.45% saline and 5% dextrose with potassium supplements). Once hydration and acid–base and electrolytes are normal, definitive treatment by pyloromyotomy can be performed. This involves division of the hypertrophied muscle down to, but not including, the mucosa (Fig. 13.3d). The operation can be performed either as an open procedure via a periumbilical incision or laparoscopically. Postoperatively, the child can usually be fed within 6 h and discharged within 2 days of surgery.

Summary

Pyloric stenosis

- More common in boys and those with a maternal family history
- Signs are: visible gastric peristalsis, palpable abdominal mass on test feed and possible dehydration
- Associated with hyponatraemia, hypokalaemia and hypochloraemic alkalosis
- Diagnosis may be confirmed by ultrasound
- Treated by surgery after rehydration and correction of electrolyte imbalance.

Crying

The time healthy babies cry for is highly variable. In most, it represents the baby's response to hunger and discomfort. Reassurance and advice on appropriate feeding, wrapping and care will usually suffice.

Some babies cry for prolonged periods in spite of feeding and comforting and this is distressing for all concerned. It can engender a feeling of anxiety, helplessness and depression in the carer, particularly if they are inexperienced or poorly supported. It has also been suggested that the emotional climate within a home may be transmitted to a baby, and that in some

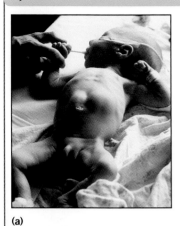
(a)

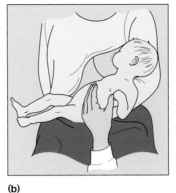
(b)

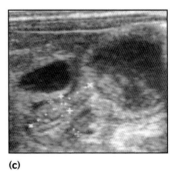
(c)

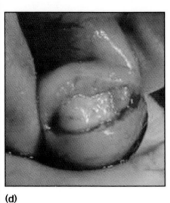
(d)

Figure 13.3 **(a)** Visible gastric peristalsis in an infant with pyloric stenosis. **(b)** Diagram showing a test feed being performed to diagnose pyloric stenosis. The pyloric mass feels like an 'olive' on gentle, deep palpation halfway between the midpoint of the anterior margin of the right ribcage and the umbilicus. **(c)** Ultrasound examination showing pyloric stenosis. **(d)** Pyloric stenosis at operation showing pale, thick pyloric muscle and pyloromyotomy incision.

instances, tense, anxious or irritable caregivers are more likely to have fretful babies. The complaint that a baby is 'always crying' may also be a pointer to potential or actual non-accidental injury.

A significant cause for the crying is identified in a minority of infants. If of sudden onset, it may be due to a urinary tract, middle ear or meningeal infection, to pain from an unrecognised fracture, oesophagitis or torsion of the testis. Severe nappy rash, constipation or coeliac disease may produce a miserable, crying infant. Preterm infants who have spent several weeks in hospital can be difficult to settle, as can infants with a chronic neurological disorder, e.g. cerebral palsy. On the basis of countless reports of parents, eruption of teeth is painful in some infants. However, teething does not cause vomiting, diarrhoea, high fever or seizures.

Infant 'colic'

The term 'colic' is used to describe a common symptom complex which occurs during the first few months of life. Paroxysmal, inconsolable crying or screaming often accompanied by drawing up of the knees and passage of excessive flatus takes place several times a day, particularly in the evening. There is no firm evidence that the cause is gastrointestinal, but this is often suspected. The condition occurs in up to 40% of babies.

It typically occurs in the first few weeks of life and resolves by 4 months of age. The condition is benign but it is very frustrating and worrying for parents and may precipitate non-accidental injury in infants already at risk. Support and reassurance should be given. Gripe water is often recommended but is of unproven benefit. If severe and persistent, it may be due to a cow's milk protein allergy or gastro-oesophageal reflux and an empirical 2-week trial of a whey hydrolysate formula followed by a trial of anti-reflux treatment may be considered.

Acute abdominal pain

Assessment of the child with acute abdominal pain requires considerable skill. The differential diagnosis of acute abdominal pain in children is extremely wide, encompassing non-specific abdominal pain, surgical causes and medical conditions (Fig. 13.4). In nearly half of the children admitted to hospital, the pain resolves undiagnosed. In young children it is essential not to delay the diagnosis and treatment of acute appendicitis, as progression to perforation can be rapid. It is easy to belittle the clinical signs of abdominal tenderness in young children. Of the surgical causes, appendicitis is by far the most common. The testes, hernial orifices

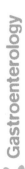

Gastroenterology

223

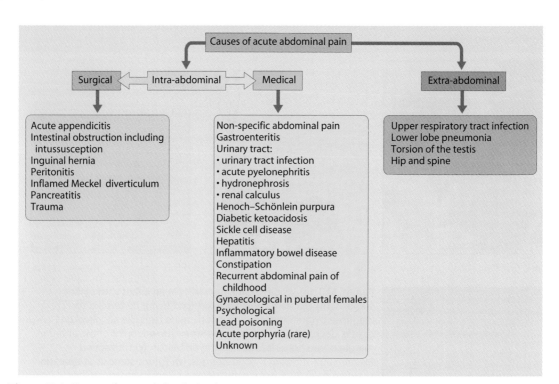

Figure 13.4 Causes of acute abdominal pain.

and hip joints must always be checked. It is noteworthy that:

- Lower lobe pneumonia may cause pain referred to the abdomen
- Primary peritonitis is seen in patients with ascites from nephrotic syndrome or liver disease
- Diabetic ketoacidosis may cause severe abdominal pain
- Urinary tract infection, including acute pyelonephritis, is a relatively uncommon cause of acute abdominal pain, but must not be missed. It is important to test a urine sample, in order to identify not only diabetes mellitus but also conditions affecting the liver and urinary tract.

Acute appendicitis

Acute appendicitis is the commonest cause of abdominal pain in childhood requiring surgical intervention (Fig. 13.5). Although it may occur at any age, it is very uncommon in children <3 years old. The clinical features of acute uncomplicated appendicitis are:

- Symptoms
  - Anorexia
  - Vomiting (usually only a few times)
  - Abdominal pain, initially central and colicky (appendicular midgut colic), but then localising to the right iliac fossa (from localised peritoneal inflammation)
- Signs
  - Flushed face with oral fetor
  - Low-grade fever 37.2–38°C

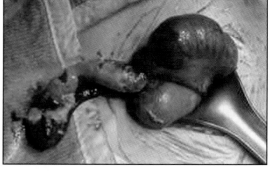

Figure 13.5 Appendicitis at operation showing a perforated acutely inflamed appendix covered in fibrin.

- Abdominal pain aggravated by movement, e.g. on walking, coughing, jumping, bumps on the road during a car journey
- Persistent tenderness with guarding in the right iliac fossa (McBurney's point).

In preschool children:

- The diagnosis is more difficult, particularly early in the disease
- Faecoliths are more common and can be seen on a plain abdominal X-ray
- Perforation may be rapid, as the omentum is less well developed and fails to surround the appendix, and the signs are easy to underestimate at this age.

With a retrocaecal appendix, localised guarding may be absent, and in a pelvic appendix there may be few abdominal signs.

Appendicitis is a progressive condition and so repeated observation and clinical review every few hours are key to making the correct diagnosis, avoiding delay on the one hand and unnecessary laparotomy on the other.

No laboratory investigation or imaging is consistently helpful in making the diagnosis. A neutrophilia is not always present on a full blood count. White blood cells or organisms in the urine are not uncommon in appendicitis as the inflamed appendix may be adjacent to the ureter or bladder. Although ultrasound is no substitute for regular clinical review, it may support the clinical diagnosis (thickened, non-compressible appendix with increased blood flow); demonstrate associated complications such as abscess, perforation or appendix mass; and exclude other pathology causing the symptoms. In some centres, laparoscopy is available to see whether or not the appendix is inflamed.

Appendicectomy is straightforward in uncomplicated appendicitis. Complicated appendicitis includes the presence of an appendix mass, an abscess or perforation. If there is generalised guarding consistent with perforation, fluid resuscitation and intravenous antibiotics are given prior to laparotomy. If there is a palpable mass in the right iliac fossa and there are no signs of generalised peritonitis, it may be reasonable to elect for conservative management with intravenous antibiotics, with appendicectomy being performed after several weeks. If symptoms progress, laparotomy is indicated.

Non-specific abdominal pain and mesenteric adenitis

Non-specific abdominal pain (NSAP) is abdominal pain which resolves in 24–48 h. The pain is less severe than in appendicitis, and tenderness in the right iliac fossa is variable. It is often accompanied by an upper respiratory tract infection with cervical lymphadenopathy. In some of these children, the abdominal signs do not resolve and an appendicectomy is performed. The diagnosis of mesenteric adenitis can only be made definitively in those children in whom large mesenteric nodes are seen at laparotomy or laparoscopy and whose appendix is normal.

Intussusception

Intussusception describes the invagination of proximal bowel into a distal segment. It most commonly involves ileum passing into the caecum through the ileocaecal valve (Fig. 13.6a). Intussusception is the commonest cause of intestinal obstruction in infants after the neonatal period. Although it may occur at any age, the peak age of presentation is between 3 months and 2 years. The most serious complication is stretching and constriction of the mesentery resulting in venous obstruction, causing engorgement and bleeding from the bowel mucosa, fluid loss and subsequently bowel perforation, peritonitis and gut necrosis. Prompt diagnosis, immediate fluid resuscitation and urgent reduction of the intussusception are essential to avoid complications.

Presentation is typically with:

- Paroxysmal, severe colicky pain and pallor – during episodes of pain, the child becomes pale, especially around the mouth, and draws up his legs. He initially recovers between painful episodes, but subsequently becomes increasingly lethargic
- May refuse feeds, may vomit, which may become bile-stained depending on the site of the intussusception
- A sausage-shaped mass – often palpable in the abdomen (Fig. 13.6b)
- Passage of a characteristic redcurrant jelly stool comprising blood-stained mucus – this is a characteristic sign but tends to occur later in the illness and may be first seen after a rectal examination
- Abdominal distension and shock.

Usually, no underlying intestinal cause for the intussusception is found, although there is some evidence that viral infection leading to enlargement of Peyer's patches may form the lead point of the intussusception. An identifiable lead point such as a Meckel diverticulum or polyp is more likely to be present in children over 2 years old. Intravenous fluid resuscitation is likely to be required immediately, as there is often pooling of fluid in the gut, which may lead to hypovolaemic shock.

An X-ray of the abdomen may show distended small bowel and absence of gas in the distal colon or rectum. Sometimes the outline of the intussusception itself can be visualised. Abdominal ultrasound is helpful both to confirm the diagnosis and to check response to treatment. Unless there are signs of peritonitis, reduction of the intussusception by rectal air insufflation is usually attempted by a radiologist (Fig. 13.6c). This procedure should only be carried out once the child has been

Summary

Acute abdominal pain in older children and adolescents

- Exclude medical causes, in particular lower lobe pneumonia, diabetic ketoacidosis, hepatitis, pyelonephritis
- Check for strangulated inguinal hernia or torsion of the testis in boys
- On palpating the abdomen in children with acute appendicitis, guarding and rebound tenderness are often absent or unimpressive, but pain from peritoneal inflammation may be demonstrated on coughing, walking or jumping
- To distinguish between acute appendicitis and non-specific abdominal pain may require close monitoring and repeated evaluation in hospital.

Intussusception

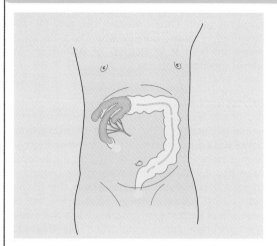

Figure 13.6a Intussusception, showing why the blood supply to the gut rapidly becomes compromised, making relief of this form of obstruction urgent.

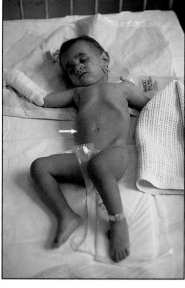

Figure 13.6b A child with an intussusception. The mass can be seen in the upper abdomen. The child has become shocked.

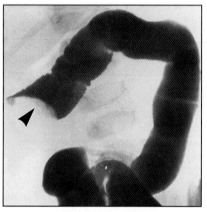

Figure 13.6c An abdominal X-ray demonstrating an intussusception (see arrowhead), taken during reduction by air insufflated per rectum.

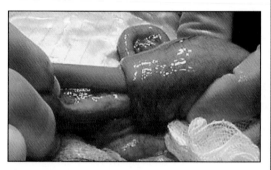

Figure 13.6d Intussusception at operation showing the ileum entering the caecum. The surgeon is squeezing the colon to reduce the intussusception.

Summary

Intussusception

- Usually occurs between 3 months and 2 years of age
- Clinical features are paroxysmal, colicky pain with pallor, abdominal mass, redcurrant jelly stool
- Shock is an important complication and requires urgent treatment
- Reduction is attempted by rectal air insufflation unless peritonitis is present
- Surgery is required if reduction with air is unsuccessful or for peritonitis.

resuscitated and is under the supervision of a paediatric surgeon in case the procedure is unsuccessful or bowel perforation occurs. The success rate of this procedure is about 75%. The remaining 25% require operative reduction (Fig. 13.6d). Recurrence of the intussusception occurs in less than 5% but is more frequent after hydrostatic reduction.

Meckel diverticulum

Around 2% of individuals have an ileal remnant of the vitello-intestinal duct, a Meckel diverticulum, which contains ectopic gastric mucosa or pancreatic tissue. Most are asymptomatic but they may present with severe rectal bleeding, which is classically neither bright red nor true melaena. Other forms of

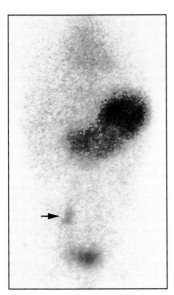

Figure 13.7 Technetium scan showing uptake by ectopic gastric mucosa in a Meckel diverticulum in the right iliac fossa.

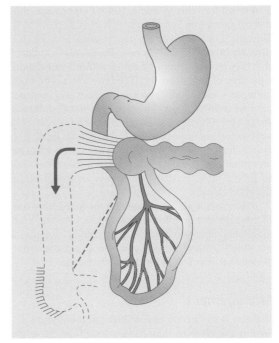

Figure 13.8 The commonest form of malrotation, with the caecum remaining high and fixed to the posterior abdominal wall. There are Ladd bands obstructing the duodenum. Dotted lines show normal anatomy.

presentation include intussusception, volvulus around a band, or diverticulitis which mimics appendicitis. A technetium scan will demonstrate increased uptake by ectopic gastric mucosa in 70% of cases (Fig. 13.7). Treatment is by surgical resection.

Summary

Meckel diverticulum

· Occurs in 2% of individuals.
· Generally asymptomatic, but may present with bleeding (which may be life-threatening), intussusception, volvulus or diverticulitis.
· Treatment is by surgical resection.

Malrotation

During rotation of the small bowel in fetal life, if the mesentery is not fixed at the duodenojejunal flexure or in the ileocaecal region, its base is shorter than normal, and is predisposed to volvulus. Ladd bands may cross the duodenum, contributing to bowel obstruction (Fig. 13.8).

There are two presentations:

● Obstruction
● Obstruction with a compromised blood supply.

Obstruction with bilious vomiting is the usual presentation in the first few days of life but can be seen at a later age. Any child with dark green vomiting needs an urgent upper gastrointestinal contrast study to assess intestinal rotation, unless signs of vascular compromise are present, when an urgent laparotomy is needed.

At operation, the volvulus is untwisted, the duodenum mobilised and the bowel placed in the non-rotated position with the duodenojejunal flexure on the right and the caecum and appendix on the left. The malrotation is not 'corrected', but the mesentery broadened. The appendix is generally removed to avoid diagnostic confusion in the event the child subsequently has symptoms suggestive of appendicitis.

Summary

Malrotation

· Uncommon but important to diagnose
· Usually presents in the first 1–3 days of life with intestinal obstruction from Ladd bands obstructing the duodenum or volvulus
· May present at any age with volvulus causing obstruction and ischaemic bowel
· Clinical features are bilious vomiting, abdominal pain and tenderness from peritonitis or ischaemic bowel
· An urgent upper gastrointestinal contrast study is indicated if there is bilious vomiting
· Treatment is urgent surgical correction.

Recurrent abdominal pain

Recurrent abdominal pain (RAP) is a common childhood problem. It is often defined as pain sufficient to interrupt normal activities and lasts for at least

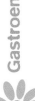

3 months. It occurs in about 10% of school-age children. A cause (see Summary box) is identified in <10%. The pain is characteristically periumbilical and the children are otherwise entirely well. The widely held belief that they have psychogenic pain is without foundation, a number of studies having failed to show a difference between such children and their families and controls. In some children, it may however be a manifestation of stress (see Chapter 23) or it may become part of a vicious cycle of anxiety with escalating pain leading to family distress and demands for increasingly invasive investigations. There is evidence that anxiety may lead to altered bowel motility, which may be perceived by the child as pain.

It is increasingly recognised that many will have one of three distinct symptom constellations resulting from functional abnormalities of gut motility or enteral neurons – irritable bowel syndrome (most common), abdominal migraine or functional dyspepsia.

Management

The aim is to identify any serious cause without subjecting the child to unnecessary investigation, while providing reassurance to the child and parents. To do this, a full history and thorough examination is required, which includes inspection of the perineum for anal fissures. The child's growth should be checked.

A urine microscopy and culture is mandatory as urinary tract infections may cause pain in the absence of other symptoms or signs. An abdominal ultrasound is particularly helpful in excluding gall stones and pelvi-ureteric junction (PUJ) obstruction.

Although there are many potential organic causes, most are rare and further investigations should be performed only if clinically indicated.

With irritable bowel syndrome and functional dyspepsia, it can be helpful to explain to both the child and parents that 'sometimes the insides of the intestine become so sensitive that some children can feel the food going round the bends'. It is also necessary to make a distinction between 'serious' and 'dangerous'. These disorders can be serious, if, for example, they lead to substantial loss of schooling, but they are not dangerous.

The long-term prognosis is that:

- about half of affected children rapidly become free of symptoms
- in one-quarter, the symptoms take some months to resolve
- in one-quarter, symptoms continue or return in adulthood as migraine, irritable bowel syndrome, or functional dyspepsia.

Abdominal migraine

Abdominal migraine is often associated with abdominal pain in addition to headaches, and in some children the abdominal pain predominates. The attacks of abdominal pain are midline associated with vomiting and facial pallor. There is usually a personal or family history of migraine.

Irritable bowel syndrome

This disorder, also common in adults, is associated with altered gastrointestinal motility and an abnormal sensation of intra-abdominal events. Symptoms may occur following a gastrointestinal infection. Studies of pressure changes within the small intestine of children with irritable bowel syndrome suggest that abnormally forceful contractions occur. It has also been shown that affected adults experience pain on inflation of balloons in the intestine at substantially lower volumes than do controls. There is therefore an interplay between these two factors, both of which are modulated by psychosocial factors such as stress and anxiety.

There is often a positive family history and a characteristic set of symptoms, although not all patients experience every symptom:

- Abdominal pain, often worse before or relieved by defecation
- Explosive, loose or mucousy stools
- Bloating
- Feeling of incomplete defecation
- Constipation (often alternating with normal or loose stools).

Peptic ulceration, gastritis and functional dyspepsia

The greater use of endoscopy in children and the identification of the Gram-negative organism *Helicobacter pylori* (*H. pylori*) in association with antral gastritis have focused attention on it as a potential cause of abdominal pain in children. In adults, there is substantial evidence that *H. pylori* is a strong predisposing factor to duodenal ulcers. This association in children is much less clear. Duodenal ulcers are uncommon in children but should be considered in those with epigastric pain, particularly if it wakes them at night, or when there is a history of peptic ulceration in a first-degree relative.

H. pylori causes a nodular antral gastritis which may be associated with abdominal pain and nausea. It is usually identified in gastric antral biopsies. The organism produces urease, which forms the basis for a laboratory test on biopsies, and the ^{13}C breath test following the administration of ^{13}C-labelled urea by mouth. Stool antigen for *H. pylori* may be positive in infected children. Serological tests are unreliable in children.

Children in whom peptic ulceration is suspected should be treated with proton pump inhibitors, e.g. omeprazole, and if investigations suggest they have an *H. pylori* infection, eradication therapy should be given (amoxicillin and metronidazole or clarithromycin). Those that fail to respond to treatment or whose symptoms recur on stopping treatment should have an upper GI endoscopy and, if this is normal, functional dyspepsia is diagnosed.

As well as having symptoms of peptic ulceration, children with functional dyspepsia have rather more non-specific symptoms, including early satiety, bloating and postprandial vomiting and may have delayed gastric emptying as a result of gastric dysmotility. Treatment is difficult but some children respond to a hypoallergenic diet.

Summary

Causes and assessment of the child with recurrent abdominal pain

> >90% no structural cause identified

Gastrointestinal
- Irritable bowel syndrome
- Constipation
- Non-ulcer dyspepsia
- Abdominal migraine
- Gastritis and peptic ulceration
- Inflammatory bowel disease
- Malrotation

Gynaecological
- Dysmenorrhoea
- Ovarian cysts
- Pelvic inflammatory disease

Psychosocial – bullying, abuse, stress, etc. – a small proportion

Hepatobility/pancreatic
- Hepatitis
- Gall stones
- Pancreatitis

Urinary tract
- Urinary tract infection
- Pelvi-ureteric junction (PUJ) obstruction

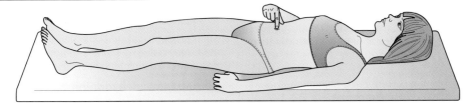

Symptoms and signs that suggest organic disease:
- Epigastric pain at night, haematemesis (duodenal ulcer)
- Diarrhoea, weight loss, growth failure, blood in stools (inflammatory bowel disease)
- Vomiting (pancreatitis)
- Jaundice (liver disease)
- Dysuria, secondary enuresis (urinary tract infection)
- Bilious vomiting and abdominal distension (malrotation)

Gastroenteritis

In developing countries, gastroenteritis remains a major cause of child mortality. In developed countries, it is a cause of significant morbidity, particularly in younger children. In the UK, approximately 10% of under 5 year olds annually present to health services with gastroenteritis and it remains a common reason for hospital admission in young children.

The most frequent cause of gastroenteritis in developed countries is rotavirus infection, which accounts for up to 60% of cases in children <2 years of age, particularly during the winter and early spring. An effective vaccine against rotavirus is now available, but has not been adopted into the national immunisation programme. Other viruses, particularly adenovirus, norovirus, calicivirus, coronavirus and astrovirus, may cause outbreaks.

Bacterial causes are less common in developed countries and are suggested by the presence of blood in the stools. *Campylobacter jejuni* infection, the commonest of the bacterial infections in developed countries, is often associated with severe abdominal pain. *Shigella* and some salmonellae produce a dysenteric type of infection, with blood and pus in the stool, pain and tenesmus. *Shigella* may be accompanied by high fever. Cholera and enterotoxigenic *E. coli* infection are associated with profuse, rapidly

Box 13.3 Conditions which can mimic gastroenteritis

Systemic infection	Septicaemia, meningitis
Local infections	Respiratory tract infection, otitis media, hepatitis A, urinary tract infection
Surgical disorders	Pyloric stenosis, intussusception, acute appendicitis, necrotising enterocolitis, Hirschsprung disease
Metabolic disorder	Diabetic ketoacidosis
Renal disorder	Haemolytic uraemic syndrome
Other	Coeliac disease, cow's milk protein intolerance, adrenal insufficiency

dehydrating diarrhoea. However, clinical features act as a poor guide to the pathogen.

In gastroenteritis there is a sudden change to loose or watery stools often accompanied by vomiting. There may be contact with a person with diarrhoea and/or vomiting or recent travel abroad. A number of disorders may masquerade as gastroenteritis (Box 13.3) and, when in doubt, hospital referral is essential. Dehydration leading to shock is the most serious complication and its prevention or correction is the main aim of treatment.

The following children are at increased risk of dehydration:

- Infants, particularly those under 6 months of age or those born with low birthweight.
- If they have passed ≥6 diarrhoeal stools in the previous 24 h
- If they have vomited three or more times in the previous 24 h
- If they have been unable to tolerate (or not been offered) extra fluids
- If they have malnutrition.

Infants are at particular risk of dehydration because they have a greater surface area to weight ratio than older children, leading to greater insensible water losses (300 ml/m^2 per day, equivalent in infants to 15–17 ml/kg per day). They have higher basal fluid requirements (100–120 ml/kg per day, i.e. 10–12% of bodyweight) and immature renal tubular reabsorption. In addition, they are unable to obtain fluids for themselves when thirsty.

Assessment

Clinical assessment of dehydration is important but difficult. The most accurate measure of dehydration is the degree of weight loss during the diarrhoeal illness. A recent weight measurement is useful but is often not available and may be misleading if the child had clothes on or the different measuring scales are not accurate. The history and examination are used to assess the degree of dehydration as:

- No clinically detectable dehydration (usually <5% loss of body weight)
- Clinical dehydration (usually 5–10%)

- Shock (usually >10%) (Fig. 13.9 and Table 13.1). Shock must be identified without delay.

Isonatraemic and hyponatraemic dehydration

In dehydration, there is a total body deficit of sodium and water. In most instances, the losses of sodium and water are proportional and plasma sodium remains within the normal range (isonatraemic dehydration). When children with diarrhoea drink large quantities of water or other hypotonic solutions, there is a greater net loss of sodium than water, leading to a fall in plasma sodium (hyponatraemic dehydration). This leads to a shift of water from extra- to intracellular compartments. The increase in intracellular volume leads to an increase in brain volume, which may result in convulsions, whereas the marked extracellular depletion leads to a greater degree of shock per unit of water loss. This form of dehydration is more common in poorly nourished infants in developing countries.

Hypernatraemic dehydration

Infrequently, water loss exceeds the relative sodium loss and plasma sodium concentration increases (hypernatraemic dehydration). This usually results from high insensible water losses (high fever or hot, dry environment) or from profuse, low-sodium diarrhoea. The extracellular fluid becomes hypertonic with respect to the intracellular fluid, which leads to a shift of water into the extracellular space from the intracellular compartment. Signs of extracellular fluid depletion are therefore less per unit of fluid loss, and depression of the fontanelle, reduced tissue elasticity and sunken eyes are less obvious. This makes this form of dehydration more difficult to recognise clinically, particularly in an obese infant. It is a particularly dangerous form of dehydration as water is drawn out of the brain and cerebral shrinkage within a rigid skull may lead to jittery movements, increased muscle tone

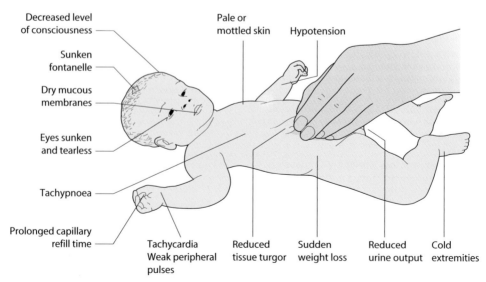

Figure 13.9 Clinical features of shock from dehydration in an infant.

Table 13.1 Clinical assessment of dehydration

	No clinical dehydration	Clinical dehydration	Shock
General appearance	Appears well	Appears unwell or deteriorating 🚩	Appears unwell or deteriorating
Conscious level	Alert and responsive	Altered responsiveness, e.g. irritable, lethargic 🚩	Decreased level of consciousness
Urine output	Normal	Decreased	Decreased
Skin colour	Normal	Normal	Pale or mottled
Extremities	Warm	Warm	Cold
Eyes	Normal	Sunken 🚩	Grossly sunken
Mucous membranes	Moist	Dry	Dry
Heart rate	Normal	Tachycardia 🚩	Tachycardia
Breathing	Normal	Tachypnoea 🚩	Tachypnoea
Peripheral pulses	Normal	Normal	Weak
Capillary refill time	Normal	Normal	Prolonged (>2 s)
Skin turgor	Normal	Reduced 🚩	Reduced
Blood pressure	Normal	Normal	Hypotension (indicates decompensated shock)

🚩, 'Red Flag' sign – helps to identify children at risk of progression to shock.
The more numerous and more pronounced the symptoms and signs, the greater the severity of dehydration.
From NICE Guideline, Diarrhoea and vomiting in children, 2009.

with hyperreflexia, altered consciousness, seizures and multiple, small cerebral haemorrhages. Transient hyperglycaemia occurs in some patients with hypernatraemic dehydration; it is self-correcting and does not require insulin.

Investigation

Usually, no investigations are indicated. Stool culture is required if the child appears septic, if there is blood or mucus in the stools or the child is immunocompromised. It may be indicated following recent foreign travel, if the diarrhoea has not improved by day 7 or the diagnosis is uncertain. Plasma electrolytes, urea, creatinine and glucose should be checked if intravenous fluids are required or there are features suggestive of hypernatraemia. If antibiotics are started, a blood culture should be taken.

Management

This is shown in Figure 13.10.

Hypernatraemic dehydration

The management of hypernatraemic dehydration can be particularly difficult. Oral rehydration solution can be used to rehydrate hypernatraemic children with clinical dehydration. If intravenous fluids are required, a rapid reduction in plasma sodium concentration and osmolality will lead to a shift of water into cerebral cells and may result in seizures and cerebral oedema. The reduction in plasma sodium should therefore be slow. The fluid deficit should be replaced over at least 48 h and the plasma sodium measured regularly, aiming to reduce it at <0.5 mmol/L per hour.

Anti-diarrhoeal drugs (e.g. loperamide, Lomotil) and antiemetics

There is no place for medications for the vomiting or diarrhoea of gastroenteritis as they:

- are ineffective
- may prolong the excretion of bacteria in stools
- can be associated with side-effects
- add unnecessarily to cost
- focus attention away from oral rehydration.

Antibiotics

Antibiotics are not routinely required to treat gastroenteritis, even if there is a bacterial cause. They are only indicated for suspected or confirmed sepsis, extra-intestinal spread of bacterial infection, for salmonella gastroenteritis if <6 months old, in malnourished or immunocompromised children or for specific bacterial or protozoal infections (e.g. *Clostridium difficile*-associated with pseudomembranous colitis, cholera, shigellosis, giardiasis).

Fluid management of dehydration

No clinical dehydration	Clinical dehydration	Shock

Prevent dehydration
Continue breast-feeding and other milk feeds
Encourage fluid intake to compensate for increased gastrointestinal losses
Discourage fruit juices and carbonated drinks
Oral rehydration solution (ORS) as supplemental fluid if at increased risk of dehydration (see list above)

Oral rehydration solution (ORS)
Give fluid deficit replacement fluids (50 ml/kg) over 4 hours as well as maintenance fluid requirement. Give ORS often and in small amounts
Continue breast-feeding
Consider supplementing ORS with usual fluids if inadequate intake of ORS
If inadequate fluid intake or vomits persistently, consider giving ORS via nasogastric tube

Intravenous therapy
Give rapid infusion of 0.9% sodium chloride solution. Repeat if necessary. If remains shocked, consider consulting paediatric intensive care specialist

Deterioration or persistent vomiting

Symptoms/signs of shock improve

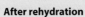

In gastroenteritis, death is from dehydration; its prevention or correction is the mainstay of treatment.

Intravenous therapy for rehydration
Replace fluid deficit and give maintenance fluids
Fluid deficit is 100 ml/kg (10% body weight) if initially shocked, 50 ml/kg (5% body weight) if not shocked
For maintenance fluids see Table 6.1
Give 0.9% sodium chloride solution or 0.9% sodium chloride solution with 5% glucose
Monitor plasma electrolytes, urea, creatinine and glucose. Consider intravenous potassium supplementation
Continue breast-feeding if possible

After rehydration
Give full strength milk and reintroduce usual solid food
Avoid fruit juices and carbonated drinks
Advise parents – diligent hand washing, towels used by infected child not to be shared, do not return to childcare facility or school until 48 hours after last episode

Figure 13.10 Fluid management of dehydration. (Adapted from Diarrhoea and vomiting in children, National Institute for Health and Clinical Excellence, 2009).

Nutrition

In developing countries, multiple episodes of diarrhoea are a major contributing factor to the development of malnutrition. Following diarrhoea, nutritional intake should be increased. Diarrhoea may be associated with zinc deficiency and supplementation may be helpful in both acute diarrhoea and as prophylaxis.

Post-gastroenteritis syndrome

Infrequently, following an episode of gastroenteritis, the introduction of a normal diet results in a return of watery diarrhoea. Temporary lactose intolerance may have developed, which can be confirmed by the presence of non-absorbed sugar in the stools giving a positive 'Clinitest' result. In such circumstances, a return to an oral rehydration solution for 24 h, followed by a further introduction of a normal diet, is usually successful.

Rarely, multiple dietary intolerances may result, such that specialist dietary management is required in the implementation of a diet which excludes cow's milk, disaccharides and gluten. In very severe cases, a period of parenteral nutrition is required to enable the injured small intestinal mucosa to recover sufficiently to absorb luminal nutrients.

Summary

Gastroenteritis

Gastroenteritis in developing countries:

- results in death from dehydration of hundreds of thousands of children worldwide every year
- is mostly bacterial from contaminated drinking water and food
- oral rehydration solution – saves the lives of millions of children worldwide each year.

Gastroenteritis in developed countries:

- is mostly viral, but it can be caused by *Campylobacter*, *Shigella* and *Salmonella*
- infants are particularly susceptible to dehydration
- dehydration is assessed as no clinical dehydration, clinical dehydration or shock according to symptoms and signs, but clinical assessment of severity is problematic
- oral rehydration solution is effective in most, but intravenous fluid is required for shock, ongoing vomiting or clinical deterioration.

Malabsorption

Disorders affecting the digestion or absorption of nutrients manifest as:

- abnormal stools
- failure to thrive or poor growth in most but not all cases
- specific nutrient deficiencies, either singly or in combination.

In general, parents know when their children's stools have become abnormal. The true malabsorption stool is difficult to flush down the toilet and has an odour which pervades the whole house. In general, colour is a poor guide to abnormality. Reliable dietetic assessment is important. It is inappropriate to investigate children for malabsorption as a cause of their failure to thrive when dietary energy intake is demonstrably low and other symptoms are absent. Some disorders affecting the small intestinal mucosa or pancreas may lead to the malabsorption of many nutrients (pan-malabsorption), whereas others are highly specific, e.g. zinc malabsorption in *acrodermatitis enteropathica*.

Coeliac disease

Coeliac disease is an enteropathy in which the gliadin fraction of gluten provokes a damaging immunological response in the proximal small intestinal mucosa. As a result, the rate of migration of absorptive cells moving up the villi (enterocytes) from the crypts is massively increased but is insufficient to compensate for increased cell loss from the villous tips. Villi become progressively shorter and then absent, leaving a flat mucosa.

The incidence of 'classical' coeliac disease, diagnosed in childhood on the basis of characteristic clinical symptoms, has been about 1 in 3000 in Europe, including the UK. The age at presentation is partly influenced by the age of introduction of gluten into the diet.

The classical presentation is of a profound malabsorptive syndrome at 8–24 months of age after the introduction of wheat-containing weaning foods. There is failure to thrive, abdominal distension and buttock wasting abnormal stools and general irritability (see Case History 13.2). However, this is no longer the most common presentation and children are now more likely to present less acutely in later childhood. The clinical features of coeliac disease can be highly variable and include mild, non-specific gastrointestinal symptoms, anaemia (iron and/or folate deficiency) and growth failure. Alternatively, it is identified on screening of children at increased risk (type 1 diabetes mellitus, autoimmune thyroid disease, Down syndrome) and first-degree relatives of individuals with known coeliac disease.

The introduction of highly sensitive and specific serological screening tests (IgA tissue transglutaminase antibodies and endomysial antibodies) has provided evidence that coeliac disease is much more common than previously thought and as many as 1 in 100 UK school-age children may be antibody positive.

Diagnosis

Although the diagnosis is strongly suggested by positive serology, confirmation depends upon the demonstration of mucosal changes (increased intraepithelial lymphocytes and a variable degree of villous atrophy and crypt hypertrophy) on small intestinal biopsy performed endoscopically followed by the resolution of symptoms and catch-up growth upon gluten withdrawal.

There is no place for the empirical use of a gluten-free diet as a diagnostic test for coeliac disease in the absence of a small intestinal biopsy. Serological tests such as IgA tissue transglutaminase antibodies and endomysial antibodies are not currently considered sufficiently sensitive and specific to replace biopsy, particularly as the diet is lifelong.

Management

All products containing wheat, rye and barley are removed from the diet and this results in resolution of symptoms. Supervision by a dietician is essential. In children in whom the initial biopsy or the response to gluten withdrawal is doubtful, or when the disease presents before the age of 2 years, a gluten challenge is required in later childhood to demonstrate continuing susceptibility of the small intestinal mucosa to damage by gluten. This is done by either giving food containing gluten or gluten powder. At the start of the challenge, the serological markers should be negative. The gluten challenge is positive if the serology becomes positive again. Repeat small intestinal biopsy is not required. The gluten-free diet should be adhered to for

Gastroenterology

Case History

13.2 'Classical' coeliac disease

This 2-year-old boy (Fig. 13.11a) had a history of poor growth from 12 months of age (Fig. 13.11b). His parents had noticed that he tended to be crotchety and had three or four foul-smelling stools a day. A jejunal biopsy at 2 years of age showed subtotal villous atrophy (Fig. 13.11c,d) and he was started on a gluten-free diet. Within a few days, his parents commented that his mood had improved and within a month he was a 'different child'. He subsequently exhibited good catch-up growth.

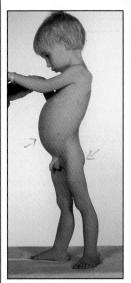

Figure **13.11a** Coeliac disease causing wasting of the buttocks and distended abdomen.

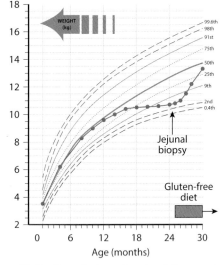

Figure **13.11b** Growth chart showing failure to thrive and response to a gluten-free diet. (Adapted from Chart© RCPCH/WHO/Department of Health.)

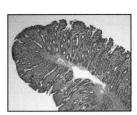

Figure **13.11c** Histology of a jejunal biopsy showing lymphocytic infiltration and villous atrophy confirming coeliac disease. (Courtesy of Dr Marie-Anne Brundler.)

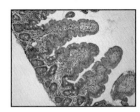

Figure **13.11d** Normal jejunal histology is shown for comparison. (Courtesy of Dr Marie-Anne Brundler.)

Summary

Coeliac disease

- A gluten-sensitive enteropathy
- Classical presentation is at 8–24 months with abnormal stools, failure to thrive, abdominal distension, muscle wasting and irritability
- Other modes of presentation – short stature, anaemia, screening, e.g. children with diabetes mellitus
- Diagnosis – positive serology (IgA tissue transglutaminase and endomysial antibodies), flat mucosa on jejunal biopsy and resolution of symptoms and catch-up growth upon gluten withdrawal
- Treatment – gluten-free diet for life.

life. The incidence of small bowel malignancy in adulthood is increased in coeliac disease, although a gluten-free diet probably reduces the risk to normal.

Food allergy and intolerance

This is described in Chapter 15. Allergy.

Other causes of nutrient malabsorption

These are summarised in Figure 13.12.

Toddler diarrhoea

This condition, also called chronic non-specific diarrhoea, is the commonest cause of persistent loose stools in preschool children. Characteristically, the

Causes of nutrient malabsorption

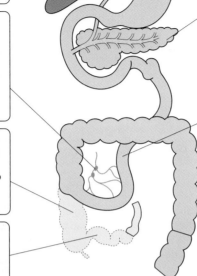

Cholestatic liver disease or biliary atresia
Bile salts no longer enter duodenum in the bile. This leads to defective solubilisation of the products of triglyceride hydrolysis. Fat and fat-soluble malabsorption result

Lymphatic leakage or obstruction
Chylomicrons (containing absorbed lipids) unable to reach thoracic duct and the systemic circulation, e.g intestinal lymphangiectasia (abnormal lymphatics)

Short bowel syndrome
Small-intestinal resection, due to congenital anomalies or necrotising enterocolitis, leads to nutrient, water and electrolyte malabsorption

Loss of terminal ileal function
e.g. resection or Crohn disease
Absent bile acid and vitamin B$_{12}$ absorption

Exocrine pancreatic dysfunction, e.g. cystic fibrosis
Absent lipase, proteases and amylase lead to defective digestion of triglyceride, protein and starch ('pan-nutrient malabsorption')

Small-intestinal mucosal disease
- Loss of absorptive surface area, e.g. coeliac disease
- Specific enzyme defects, e.g. lactase deficiency following gastroenteritis is common in Black and Oriental races
- Specific transport defects, e.g. glucose-galactose malabsorption (severe life-threatening diarrhoea with first milk feed), *acrodermatitis enteropathica* (zinc malabsorption, also erythematous rash of mouth and anus)

Figure 13.12 Causes of nutrient malabsorption. They are uncommon.

stools are of varying consistency, sometimes well formed, sometimes explosive and loose. The presence of undigested vegetables in the stools is common, giving rise to the alternative title 'peas and carrots diarrhoea'. Affected children are well and thriving and there are no precipitating dietary factors.

Toddler diarrhoea probably results from an underlying maturational delay in intestinal motility which leads to intestinal hurry. The loose stools are not due to malabsorption. Most children have grown out of their symptoms by 5 years of age but achieving faecal continence may be significantly delayed. Some relief of

symptoms can be achieved by ensuring that the child's diet contains adequate fat (which slows gut transit) and fibre. Excessive consumption of fresh fruit juice, particularly those high in non-absorbable sorbitol, can exacerbate symptoms.

Inflammatory bowel disease

The incidence of inflammatory bowel disease (IBD) in children has increased markedly in the last two decades. The reason for this is unclear. Approximately a quarter of patients present in childhood or adolescence. Crohn disease can affect any part of the gastrointestinal tract from mouth to anus, whereas in ulcerative colitis the inflammation is confined to the colon. Inflammatory bowel disease results from environmental triggers in a genetically predisposed individual. It may cause poor general health, restrict growth and have an adverse effect on psychological well-being. Management requires a specialist multidisciplinary team.

Crohn disease

The clinical features of Crohn disease are summarised in Figure 13.13. Lethargy and general ill health without gastrointestinal symptoms can be the presenting features, particularly in older children. There may be considerable delay in diagnosis as it may be mistaken for

Summary

Chronic diarrhoea

- In an infant with failure to thrive, consider coeliac disease and cow's milk protein allergy
- Following gastroenteritis, consider post-gastroenteritis syndrome and associated temporary lactose intolerance
- Following bowel resection, cholestatic liver disease or exocrine pancreatic dysfunction, consider malabsorption
- In an otherwise well toddler with undigested vegetables in the stool, consider toddler diarrhoea.

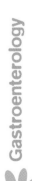

Gastroenterology

235

Presentation of Crohn disease in children and adolescents

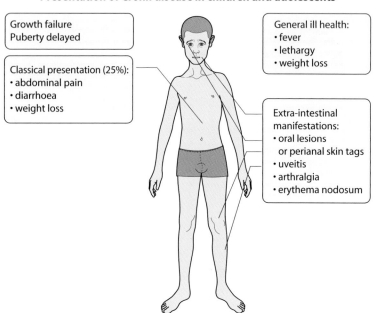

Growth failure
Puberty delayed

Classical presentation (25%):
• abdominal pain
• diarrhoea
• weight loss

General ill health:
• fever
• lethargy
• weight loss

Extra-intestinal
manifestations:
• oral lesions
  or perianal skin tags
• uveitis
• arthralgia
• erythema nodosum

Figure 13.13 Presentation of Crohn disease in children and adolescents.

psychological problems. It may also mimic anorexia nervosa. The presence of raised inflammatory markers (platelet count, ESR and CRP), iron deficiency anaemia and low serum albumin are helpful in both making a diagnosis and confirming a relapse.

Crohn disease is a transmural, focal, subacute or chronic inflammatory disease, most commonly affecting the distal ileum and proximal colon. Initially there are areas of acutely inflamed, thickened bowel. Subsequently, strictures of the bowel and fistulae may develop between adjacent loops of bowel, between bowel and skin or to other organs (e.g. vagina, bladder).

Diagnosis is based on endoscopic and histological findings on biopsy. Upper gastrointestinal endoscopy, ileocolonoscopy and small bowel imaging are required. The histological hallmark is the presence of non-caseating epithelioid cell granulomata, although this is not identified in up to 30% at presentation. Small bowel imaging may reveal narrowing, fissuring, mucosal irregularities and bowel wall thickening.

Remission is induced with nutritional therapy, when the normal diet is replaced by whole protein modular feeds (polymeric diet) for 6–8 weeks. This is effective in 75% of cases. Systemic steroids are required if ineffective.

Relapse is common and immunosuppressant medication (azathioprine, mercaptopurine or methotrexate) may be required to maintain remission. Anti-tumour necrosis factor agents (infliximab or adalimumab) may be needed when conventional treatments have failed. Long-term supplemental enteral nutrition (often with overnight nasogastric or gastrostomy feeds) may be helpful in correcting growth failure. Surgery is necessary for complications of Crohn disease – obstruction, fistulae, abscess formation or severe localised disease unresponsive to medical treatment, often manifesting as growth failure. In general, the long-term prognosis for Crohn disease beginning in childhood is good and most patients lead normal lives, despite occasional relapsing disease.

> **Growth failure and delayed puberty are features of Crohn disease in children.**

Ulcerative colitis

Ulcerative colitis is a recurrent, inflammatory and ulcerating disease involving the mucosa of the colon. Characteristically, the disease presents with rectal bleeding, diarrhoea and colicky pain. Weight loss and growth failure may occur, although this is less frequent than in Crohn disease. Extraintestinal complications include erythema nodosum and arthritis.

The diagnosis is made on endoscopy (upper and ileocolonoscopy) and on the histological features, after exclusion of infective causes of colitis. There is a confluent colitis extending from the rectum proximally for a variable length. In contrast to adults, in whom the colitis is usually confined to the distal colon, 90% of children have a pancolitis. Histology reveals mucosal inflammation, crypt damage (cryptitis, architectural distortion, abscesses and crypt loss) and ulceration. Small bowel imaging is required to check that extra-colonic inflammation suggestive of Crohn disease is not present.

In mild disease, aminosalicylates (balsalazide and mesalazine) are used for induction and maintenance therapy. Disease confined to the rectum and sigmoid colon may be managed with topical steroids. More aggressive or extensive disease requires systemic steroids for acute exacerbations and immunomodulatory therapy, e.g. azathioprine to maintain remission alone or in combination with low-dose corticosteroid therapy.

Severe fulminating disease is a medical emergency and requires treatment with intravenous fluids and steroids. If this fails to induce remission, ciclosporin may be used.

Colectomy with an ileostomy or ileorectal pouch is undertaken for severe fulminating disease which may be complicated by a toxic megacolon, or for chronic poorly controlled disease. There is an increased incidence of adenocarcinoma of the colon in adults (1 in 200 risk for each year of disease between 10 and 20 years from diagnosis). Regular colonoscopic screening is performed after 10 years from diagnosis.

Constipation

Constipation is an extremely common reason for consultation in children. Parents may use the term to describe decreased frequency of defecation; the degree of hardness of the stool and painful defecation. The 'normal' frequency of defecation is highly variable and varies with age. Infants have an average of four stools per day in the first week of life, but this falls to an average of two per day by 1 year of age. Breast-fed infants may not pass stools for several days and be entirely healthy. By 4 years of age, children usually have a stool pattern similar to adults, in whom the normal range varies from three stools per day to three stools per week. A pragmatic definition of constipation is the infrequent passage of dry, hardened faeces often accompanied by straining or pain. There may be abdominal pain which waxes and wanes with passage of stool or overflow soiling (see Chapter 23, Emotions and behaviour).

The cause of constipation is often unclear and multifactorial. In babies, Hirschsprung disease, anorectal abnormalities, hypothyroidism and hypercalcaemia need to be considered. Constipation may be precipitated by dehydration or reduced fluid intake or an anal fissure causing pain. In older children, it may relate to problems with toilet training, unpleasant toilets or stress.

Examination often reveals a palpable abdominal mass in a well-looking child. Digital rectal examination should only be performed by a paediatric specialist and only if a pathological cause is suspected. 'Red Flag' symptoms and signs indicative of more significant pathology are detailed in Box 13.4. Investigations are not usually required to diagnose idiopathic constipation, but are carried out as indicated by history or clinical findings.

Constipation arising acutely in young children, for example after an acute febrile illness, usually resolves spontaneously or with the use of mild laxatives and extra fluids.

In more long-standing constipation, the rectum becomes overdistended, with a subsequent loss of feeling the need to defecate. Involuntary soiling may occur as contractions of the full rectum inhibit the internal sphincter, leading to overflow. Management of these children is likely to be more difficult and protracted (Fig. 13.14). Children of school age are frequently teased as a result and secondary behavioural problems are common.

It should be explained to the child and the parents that the soiling is involuntary and that recovery of normal rectal size and sensation can be achieved but may take a long time. The initial aim is to evacuate the overloaded rectum completely. This can generally be achieved using a disimpaction regimen of stool softeners, initially with a macrogol laxative, e.g. polyethylene

Box 13.4 'Red Flag' symptoms or signs in the child with constipation

'Red Flag' symptom/ signs	Diagnostic concern
Failure to pass meconium within 24 h of life	Hirschsprung disease
Failure to thrive/growth failure	Hypothyroidism, coeliac disease, other causes
Gross abdominal distension	Hirschsprung disease or other gastrointestinal dysmotility
Abnormal lower limb neurology or deformity, e.g. talipes or secondary urinary incontinence	Lumbosacral pathology
Sacral dimple above natal cleft, over the spine – naevus, hairy patch, central pit, or discoloured skin	Spina bifida occulta
Abnormal appearance/ position/patency of anus	Abnormal anorectal anatomy
Perianal bruising or multiple fissures	Sexual abuse
Perianal fistulae, abscesses or fissures	Perianal Crohn disease

glycol + electrolytes (Movicol Paediatric Plain). An escalating dose regimen is administered over 1–2 weeks or until impaction resolves. If this proves unsuccessful, a stimulant laxative, e.g. senna, or sodium picosulphate, may also be required. If the polyethylene glycol + electrolytes is not tolerated, an osmotic laxative can be substituted.

Disimpaction must be followed by maintenance treatment to ensure ongoing regular, pain-free defecation. Polyethylene glycol (with or without a stimulant laxative) is generally the treatment of choice. The dose should be gradually reduced over a period of months in response to improvement in stool consistency and frequency.

Dietary interventions alone are unlikely to be successful in managing constipation in this situation, although the child should receive sufficient fluid and a balanced diet including adequate fibre. The child should be encouraged to sit on the toilet after mealtimes to utilise the physiological gastrocolic reflex and improve the likelihood of success.

The outcome is more likely to be successful if the child is engaged in the treatment process. This requires exploring the child's concerns and motivation to change. Sometimes use of a star chart is helpful to record and reward progress, as well as motivating the child.

Encouragement by family and health professionals is essential, as relapse is common and psychological support is sometimes required. Occasionally, the faecal

Constipation management algorithm

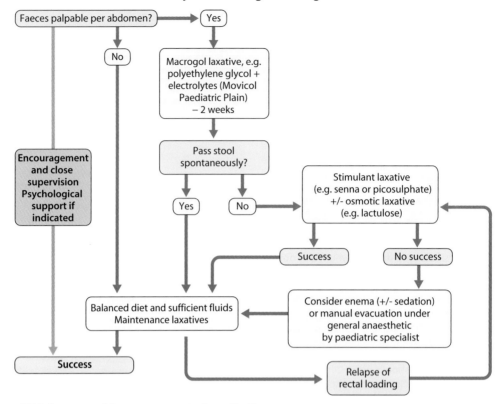

Faeces palpable per abdomen? → Yes

No

Macrogol laxative, e.g. polyethylene glycol + electrolytes (Movicol Paediatric Plain) – 2 weeks

Encouragement and close supervision Psychological support if indicated

Pass stool spontaneously?

Yes   No

Stimulant laxative (e.g. senna or picosulphate) +/- osmotic laxative (e.g. lactulose)

Success   No success

Balanced diet and sufficient fluids Maintenance laxatives

Consider enema (+/- sedation) or manual evacuation under general anaesthetic by paediatric specialist

Success

Relapse of rectal loading

Figure 13.14 Summary of the management of constipation.

retention is so severe that evacuation is only possible using enemas or by manual evacuation under an anaesthetic. They should only be performed under specialist supervision, paying particular attention to avoiding distress and embarrassment for the child.

Hirschsprung disease

The absence of ganglion cells from the myenteric and submucosal plexuses of part of the large bowel results in a narrow, contracted segment. The abnormal bowel extends from the rectum for a variable distance proximally, ending in a normally innervated, dilated colon. In 75% of cases, the lesion is confined to the rectosigmoid, but in 10% the entire colon is involved. Presentation is usually in the neonatal period with intestinal obstruction heralded by failure to pass meconium within the first 24 h of life. Abdominal distension and later bile-stained vomiting develop (Fig. 13.15). Rectal examination may reveal a narrowed segment and withdrawal of the examining finger often releases a gush of liquid stool and flatus. Temporary improvement in the obstruction following the dilatation caused by the rectal examination can lead to a delay in diagnosis.

Occasionally, infants present with severe, life-threatening Hirschsprung enterocolitis during the first few weeks of life, sometimes due to *Clostridium difficile* infection. In later childhood, presentation is with chronic constipation, usually profound, and associated with abdominal distension but usually without soiling. Growth failure may also be present.

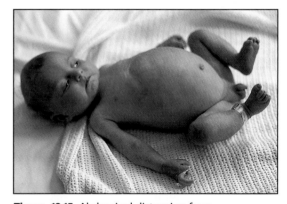

Figure 13.15 Abdominal distension from Hirschsprung disease.

Summary

Hirschsprung disease

- Absence of myenteric plexuses of rectum and variable distance of colon
- Presentation – usually intestinal obstruction in the newborn period following delay in passing meconium. In later childhood – profound chronic constipation, abdominal distension and growth failure
- Diagnosis – suction rectal biopsy.

Diagnosis is made by demonstrating the absence of ganglion cells, together with the presence of large, acetylcholinesterase-positive nerve trunks on a suction rectal biopsy. Anorectal manometry or barium studies may be useful in giving the surgeon an idea of the length of the aganglionic segment but are unreliable for diagnostic purposes. Management is surgical and usually involves an initial colostomy followed by anastomosing normally innervated bowel to the anus.

Further reading

NICE: Guideline. Diarrhoea and vomiting in children under 5, 2009.

NICE: Guideline. Coeliac disease, 2009.

NICE: Guideline. Constipation in children and young people, 2010.

Beattie M, Dhawan A, Puntis J: *Paediatric Gastroenterology, Hepatology and Nutrition* (Oxford Specialist Handbooks in Paediatrics), Oxford, 2009, Oxford University Press.

Short handbook

Kleinman RE, Goulet OJ, Mieli-Vergani G, et al: editors: *Walker's Pediatric Gastrointestinal Disease: Physiology, Diagnosis, Management*, ed 5, Ontario, 2008, Decker.

Comprehensive 2-volume textbook.

Infection and immunity

Infections are the most common cause of acute illness in children.

Worldwide, acute respiratory infections, diarrhoea, neonatal infection, malaria, measles and HIV infection, often accompanied by undernutrition, are responsible for the deaths of more than 4.5 million children <5 years old annually (Fig. 14.1).

In developed countries, morbidity and mortality from infections has declined dramatically, and deaths from infectious diseases are uncommon. However, serious infections still occur, e.g. meningococcal septicaemia, meningitis, and multi-drug resistant pathogens, and some have re-emerged, e.g. tuberculosis and PVL-toxin-secreting *Staphylococcus aureus*, and require early recognition and treatment. Children with immune deficiency are vulnerable to a range of unusual or opportunist pathogens.

With air travel, tropical diseases are encountered in all countries. In addition, epidemics may spread widely, e.g. SARS and H_1N_1, with children (and the elderly) most vulnerable.

The febrile child

Most febrile children have a brief, self-limiting viral infection. Mild localised infections, e.g. otitis media or tonsillitis, may be diagnosed clinically. The clinical problem lies in identifying the relatively few children with a serious infection which needs prompt treatment.

Clinical features

When assessing a febrile child, consider the following.

(i) How is fever identified in children?

Parents usually know if their child has been febrile. In hospital, it is measured at:

- <4 weeks old by an electronic thermometer in the axilla
- 4 weeks to 5 years by an electronic or chemical dot thermometer in the axilla or infrared tympanic thermometer.

In general, axillary temperatures underestimate body temperature by 0.5°C.

(ii) How old is the child?

Febrile infants <3 months old present with non-specific clinical features (see Box 10.2) and often have a bacterial infection, which cannot be identified reliably on clinical examination alone. It is uncommon for them to have the common viral infections of older infants and children because of passive immunity from their mothers (Fig. 14.2). Unless a clear cause for the fever is identified, they require urgent investigation with a septic screen (Box 14.1) and intravenous antibiotic therapy given immediately to avoid the illness becoming more severe and to prevent rapid spread to other sites of the body. This is considered in more detail in the section on neonatal infection (Chapter 10 Neonatal medicine).

(iii) Are there risk factors for infection?

These include:

- Illness of other family members
- If a specific illness is prevalent in the community
- Unimmunised
- Recent travel abroad, e.g. malaria, typhoid

Worldwide causes of death in children < 5 years old

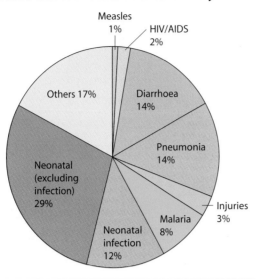

Figure 14.1 Worldwide causes of death in children <5 years old, 2008 (http://www.who.int, Accessed January 2011).

Every year, over half of the 8.8 million deaths of children <5 years old is from infections

---

Malaria
- Deaths mostly from cerebral malaria from *Plasmodium falciparum* in Sub-Saharan Africa
- Deaths have been reduced in many countries by insecticide-treated bed nets and early treatment with artemisinin-based combination therapy

---

Diarrhoea
- Most <2 years old
- Often bacterial, although rotavirus also a major cause globally
- Results in undernutrition, poor growth, death
- Usually treated with oral rehydration solution, continuing to breast-feed
- Antibiotics only for cholera, dysentery, giardiasis, amoebiasis

---

Pneumonia
- Risk factors – low birthweight, young age, not breast-fed, vitamin A deficiency, overcrowding
- Predominantly bacterial
- Strategy to reduce mortality:
  - Prevention – breast feeding and hand hygiene
  - Prevention – immunisation
  - Treatment – effective case management by early diagnosis using WHO guidelines (fever, cough, tachypnoea, chest recession, head nodding) and prompt treatment with antibiotics

---

Measles
- Preventable by immunisation

Neonatal infection
- Remains major cause of death
- Mainly early-onset infection acquired at delivery

- Contact with animals, e.g. brucellosis.
- Increased susceptibility from immunodeficiency. This is usually secondary, e.g. post-autosplenectomy in sickle cell disease or splenectomy or nephrotic syndrome, resulting in increased susceptibility to encapsulated organisms (*Streptococcus pneumoniae*, *Haemophilus influenzae* and salmonella), or rarely, primary immune deficiency.

(iv) How ill is the child?

Red Flag features suggesting serious illness and the need for urgent investigation and treatment are:

- Fever >38°C if <3 months, >39°C if 3–6 months
- Colour – pale, mottled, blue
- Level of consciousness is reduced, neck stiffness, bulging fontanelle, status epilepticus, focal neurological signs or seizures
- Significant respiratory distress
- Bile-stained vomiting
- Severe dehydration or shock.

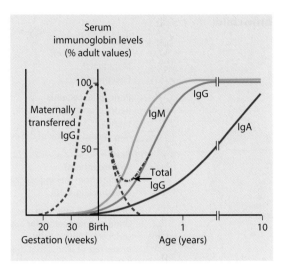

Serum
immunoglobin levels
(% adult values)

Figure 14.2 Serum immunoglobulin levels in the fetus and infant. When maternal immunoglobulin levels decline, infants become susceptible to viral infections.

Box 14.1 Septic screen

- Blood culture
- Full blood count including differential white cell count
- Acute phase reactant, e.g. C-reactive protein (CRP)
- Urine sample

Consider if indicated

- Chest X-ray
- Lumbar puncture (unless contraindicated)
- Rapid antigen screen on blood/CSF/urine
- Meningococcal and pneumococcal PCR on blood/CSF
- PCR for viruses in CSF (especially HSV and enterovirus).

(v) Is there a rash?

Rashes often accompany febrile illnesses. In some, the characteristics of the rash and other clinical features lead to a diagnosis, e.g. meningococcal septicaemia; in many, a specific diagnosis cannot be made clinically.

(vi) Is there a focus for infection?

Examination may identify a focus of infection (Fig. 14.3). If identified, investigations and management will be directed towards its treatment. However, if no focus is identified, this is often because it is the prodromal phase of a viral illness, but may indicate serious bacterial infection, especially urinary tract infection or septicaemia.

Management

Children who are not seriously ill can be managed at home with regular review by the parents, as long as they are given clear instructions (e.g. what clinical features should prompt reassessment by a doctor). Children who are significantly unwell, particularly if there is no focus of infection, will require investigations and observation or treatment in a paediatric assessment unit or A&E department or children's ward. A septic screen will be required (Box 14.1).

Parenteral antibiotics are given immediately to seriously unwell children, e.g. a third-generation cephalosporin such as cefotaxime or ceftriaxone if >3 months old. In infants 1–3 months old, cefotaxime (in case of septicaemia or meningitis) and ampicillin (in case of *Listeria* infection) are usually given. Aciclovir is given if herpes simplex encephalitis is suspected. Supportive care is given as indicated.

The child should not be underdressed. The use of antipyretic agents should be considered in children with fever who appear distressed or unwell. They should not be given if the child is otherwise well. Either paracetamol or ibuprofen can be used. They can be given alternatively if unresponsive to a single agent. Evidence that antipyretics prevent febrile seizures is lacking. There are NICE guidelines for the management of the child with fever.

> **Summary**
>
> ### The febrile child
>
> - Upper respiratory tract infection (URTI) is an extremely common cause
> - Check for otitis media
> - Serious bacterial infection must be considered if there is no focus of infection, especially urinary tract infection or septicaemia, or there are Red Flag features of life-threatening illness
> - The younger the child, the lower the threshold for performing a septic screen and starting antibiotics.

Serious life-threatening infections

Septicaemia

This is considered in Chapter 6 on Paediatric Emergencies.

Meningitis

Meningitis occurs when there is inflammation of the meninges covering the brain. This can be confirmed by finding inflammatory cells in the cerebrospinal fluid (CSF). Viral infections are the most common cause of meningitis, and most are self-resolving. Bacterial meningitis may have severe consequences. Other causes of non-infectious meningitis include malignancy and autoimmune diseases.

The febrile child

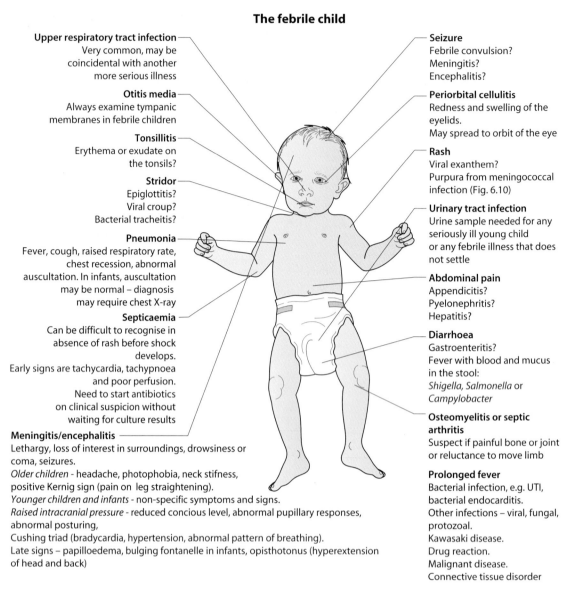

Upper respiratory tract infection
Very common, may be coincidental with another more serious illness

Otitis media
Always examine tympanic membranes in febrile children

Tonsillitis
Erythema or exudate on the tonsils?

Stridor
Epiglottitis?
Viral croup?
Bacterial tracheitis?

Pneumonia
Fever, cough, raised respiratory rate, chest recession, abnormal auscultation. In infants, auscultation may be normal – diagnosis may require chest X-ray

Septicaemia
Can be difficult to recognise in absence of rash before shock develops.
Early signs are tachycardia, tachypnoea and poor perfusion.
Need to start antibiotics on clinical suspicion without waiting for culture results

Meningitis/encephalitis
Lethargy, loss of interest in surroundings, drowsiness or coma, seizures.
Older children - headache, photophobia, neck stifness, positive Kernig sign (pain on leg straightening).
Younger children and infants - non-specific symptoms and signs.
Raised intracranial pressure - reduced concious level, abnormal pupillary responses, abnormal posturing,
Cushing triad (bradycardia, hypertension, abnormal pattern of breathing).
Late signs – papilloedema, bulging fontanelle in infants, opisthotonus (hyperextension of head and back)

Seizure
Febrile convulsion?
Meningitis?
Encephalitis?

Periorbital cellulitis
Redness and swelling of the eyelids.
May spread to orbit of the eye

Rash
Viral exanthem?
Purpura from meningococcal infection (Fig. 6.10)

Urinary tract infection
Urine sample needed for any seriously ill young child or any febrile illness that does not settle

Abdominal pain
Appendicitis?
Pyelonephritis?
Hepatitis?

Diarrhoea
Gastroenteritis?
Fever with blood and mucus in the stool:
Shigella, Salmonella or *Campylobacter*

Osteomyelitis or septic arthritis
Suspect if painful bone or joint or reluctance to move limb

Prolonged fever
Bacterial infection, e.g. UTI, bacterial endocarditis.
Other infections – viral, fungal, protozoal.
Kawasaki disease.
Drug reaction.
Malignant disease.
Connective tissue disorder

Figure 14.3 Some diagnostic clues to evaluating the febrile child.

Bacterial meningitis

Over 80% of patients with bacterial meningitis in the UK are younger than 16 years old. Bacterial meningitis remains a serious infection in children, with a 5–10% mortality. Over 10% of survivors are left with long-term neurological impairment.

Pathophysiology

Bacterial infection of the meninges usually follows bacteraemia. Much of the damage caused by meningeal infection results from the host response to infection and not from the organism itself. The release of inflammatory mediators and activated leucocytes, together with endothelial damage, leads to cerebral oedema, raised intracranial pressure and decreased cerebral blood flow. The inflammatory response below the meninges causes a vasculopathy resulting in cerebral cortical infarction, and fibrin deposits may block the resorption of CSF by the arachnoid villi, resulting in hydrocephalus.

Organisms

The organisms which commonly cause bacterial meningitis vary according to the child's age (Table 14.1).

Table 14.1 Organisms causing bacterial meningitis according to age

Neonatal–3 months	Group B streptococcus
	E. coli and other coliforms
	Listeria monocytogenes
1 month–6 years	*Neisseria meningitidis*
	Streptococcus pneumoniae
	Haemophilus influenzae
>6 years	*Neisseria meningitidis*
	Streptococcus pneumoniae

Presentation

The clinical features are listed in Figure 14.4. The early signs and symptoms of meningitis are non-specific, especially in infants and young children. Only children old enough to talk are likely to describe the classical meningitis symptoms of headache, neck stiffness and photophobia. But neck stiffness may also be seen in some children with tonsillitis and cervical lymphadenopathy. As children with meningitis may also be septicaemic, signs of shock, such as tachycardia, tachypnoea, prolonged capillary refill time, and hypotension, should be sought. Purpura in a febrile child of any age should be assumed to be due to meningococcal sepsis, even if the child does not appear unduly ill at the time; meningitis may or may not be present.

Investigations

The essential investigations are listed in Figure 14.4. A lumbar puncture is performed to obtain CSF to confirm the diagnosis, identify the organism responsible, and its antibiotic sensitivity. If any of the contraindications listed in Figure 14.4 are present, a lumbar puncture should not be performed, as under these circumstances, the procedure carries a risk of coning of the cerebellum through the foramen magnum. In these circumstances, a lumbar puncture can be postponed until the child's condition has stabilised. Even without a lumbar puncture, bacteriological diagnosis can be achieved in at least 50% of cases from the blood by culture or polymerase chain reaction (PCR), and rapid antigen screens can be performed on blood and urine samples. Throat swabs should also be obtained for bacterial and viral cultures. A serological diagnosis can be made on convalescent serum 4–6 weeks after the presenting illness if necessary.

Management

It is imperative that there is no delay in the administration of antibiotics and supportive therapy in a child with meningitis. The choice of antibiotics will depend on the likely pathogen. A third-generation cephalosporin, e.g. cefotaxime or ceftriaxone, is the preferred choice to cover the most common bacterial causes. Although still rare in the UK, pneumococcal resistance to penicillin and cephalosporins is increasing rapidly in certain parts of the world. The length of the course of antibiotics given depends on the causative organism and clinical response. Beyond the neonatal period, dexamethasone administered with the antibiotics reduces the risk of long-term complications such as deafness.

Cerebral complications

These include:

- *Hearing loss*. Inflammatory damage to the cochlear hair cells may lead to deafness. All children who have had meningitis should have an audiological assessment promptly, as children who become deaf may benefit from hearing amplification or a cochlear implant.
- *Local vasculitis*. This may lead to cranial nerve palsies or other focal lesions.
- *Local cerebral infarction*. This may result in focal or multifocal seizures, which may subsequently lead to epilepsy.
- *Subdural effusion*. Particularly associated with *Haemophilus influenzae* and pneumococcal meningitis. This is confirmed by CT scan. Most resolve spontaneously but may require prolonged antibiotic treatment.
- *Hydrocephalus*. May result from impaired resorption of CSF (communicating hydrocephalus) or blockage of the ventricular outlets by fibrin (non-communicating hydrocephalus). A ventricular shunt may be required.
- *Cerebral abscess*. The child's clinical condition deteriorates with the emergence of signs of a space-occupying lesion. The temperature will continue to fluctuate. It is confirmed on CT scan. Drainage of the abscess is required.

Prophylaxis

Prophylactic treatment with rifampicin to eradicate nasopharyngeal carriage is given to all household contacts for meningococcal meningitis and *Haemophilus influenzae* infection. It is not required for the patient if given a third-generation cephalosporin, as this will eradicate nasopharyngeal carriage. Household contacts of patients who have had group C meningococcal meningitis should be vaccinated with the meningococcal group C vaccine.

Partially treated bacterial meningitis

Children are frequently given oral antibiotics for a non-specific febrile illness. If they have early meningitis, this partial treatment with antibiotics may cause diagnostic problems. CSF examination shows a markedly raised number of white cells, but cultures are usually negative. Rapid antigen screens and PCR are helpful in these circumstances. Where the diagnosis is suspected clinically, a full course of antibiotics should be given.

Viral meningitis

Two-thirds of CNS infections are viral. Causes include enteroviruses, Epstein–Barr virus, adenoviruses and mumps. Mumps meningitis is now rare in the UK due to the MMR vaccine. Viral meningitis is usually much less severe than bacterial meningitis and a full recovery

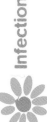

Assessment & investigation of meningitis/encephalitis

History	Examination	Investigations
Fever	Fever	Full blood count and differential count
Headache	Purpuric rash (meningococcal	Blood glucose and blood gas (for acidosis)
Photophobia	disease)	Coagulation screen, C-reactive protein
Lethargy	Neck stiffness (not always	Urea and electrolytes, liver function tests
Poor feeding/vomiting	present in infants)	Culture of blood, throat swab, urine, stool for
Irritability	Bulging fontanelle in infants	bacteria and viruses
Hypotonia	Opisthotonus (arching of back)	Rapid antigen test for meningitis organisms
Drowsiness	Positive Brudzinski/Kernig signs	(can be done on blood, CSF, or urine)
Loss of consciousness	Signs of shock	Lumbar puncture for CSF unless contraindicated
Seizures	Focal neurological signs	(see below for tests on CSF)
	Altered conscious level	Serum for comparison of convalescent titres
	Papilloedema (rare)	PCR of blood and CSF for possible organisms
		If TB suspected: chest X-ray, Mantoux test,
		gastric washings or sputum, early morning
		urines
		Consider CT/MRI brain scan and EEG

Signs associated with neck stiffness

Brudzinski sign – flexion of the neck with the child supine causes flexion of the knees and hips

Kernig sign – with the child lying supine and with the hips and knees flexed, there is back pain on extension of the knee

Contraindications to lumbar puncture:

- Cardiorespiratory instability
- Focal neurological signs
- Signs of raised intracranial pressure, e.g. coma, high BP, low heart rate or papilloedema
- Coagulopathy
- Thrombocytopenia
- Local infection at the site of LP
- If it causes undue delay in starting antibiotics

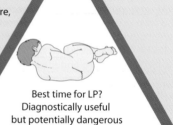

Best time for LP?
Diagnostically useful
but potentially dangerous

Typical changes in the CSF in meningitis or encephalitis, beyond the neonatal period

	Aetiology	Appearance	White blood cells	Protein	Glucose
Normal	—	Clear	0–5/mm^3	0.15–0.4 g/L	≥50% of blood
Meningitis	Bacterial	Turbid	Polymorphs:↑↑	↑↑	↓↓
	Viral	Clear	Lymphocytes:↑ (initially may be polymorphs)	Normal/↑	Normal/↓
	Tuberculosis	Turbid/clear/ viscous	Lymphocytes:↑	↑↑↑	↓↓↓
Encephalitis	Viral/unknown	Clear	Normal/↑ lymphocytes	Normal/↑	Normal/↓

Figure 14.4 Assessment and investigation of meningitis and encephalitis.

can be anticipated. Diagnosis of viral meningitis can be confirmed by culture or PCR of CSF; culture of stool, urine, nasopharyngeal aspirate, throat swabs; and serology.

Uncommon pathogens and other causes

Where the clinical course is atypical or there is failure to respond to antibiotic and supportive therapy, unusual organisms, e.g. *Mycoplasma* or *Borrelia burgdorferi* (Lyme disease), or fungal infections

need to be considered. Uncommon pathogens are particularly likely in children who are immunodeficient. Rarely, recurrent bacterial meningitis may occur in the immunodeficient or in children with structural abnormalities of the skull or meninges which facilitate bacterial access. Aseptic meningitis may be seen in malignancy or autoimmune disorders.

Neonatal meningitis

See Chapter 10.

Summary

Meningitis

- Predominantly a disease of infants and children
- Incidence has been reduced by immunisation
- Clinical features: non-specific in children under 18 months – fever, poor feeding, vomiting, irritability, lethargy, drowsiness, seizures or reduced consciousness; late signs – bulging fontanelle, neck stiffness and arched back (opisthotonos)
- Septicaemia can kill in hours; good outcome requires prompt resuscitation and antibiotics
- Any febrile child with a purpuric rash should be given intramuscular benzylpenicillin immediately and transferred urgently to hospital.

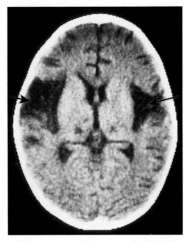

Figure 14.5 Herpes simplex encephalitis. The CT scan shows gross atrophy from loss of neural tissue in the temporoparietal regions (arrows).

Encephalitis/encephalopathy

Whereas in meningitis there is inflammation of the meninges, in encephalitis there is inflammation of the brain substance, although the meninges are often also affected. Encephalitis may be caused by:

- Direct invasion of the cerebrum by a neurotoxic virus (such as herpes simplex virus, HSV)
- Delayed brain swelling following a disordered neuroimmunological response to an antigen, usually a virus (post-infectious encephalopathy), e.g. following chickenpox
- A slow virus infection, such as HIV infection or subacute sclerosing panencephalitis (SSPE) following measles.

In encephalopathy from a non-infectious cause, such as a metabolic abnormality, the clinical features may be similar to an infectious encephalitis.

The clinical features and investigation of encephalitis are described in Figure 14.4. Most children present with fever, altered consciousness and often seizures. Initially, it may not be possible to clinically differentiate encephalitis from meningitis, and treatment for both should be started. The underlying causative organism is only detected in 50% of cases. In the UK, the most frequent causes of encephalitis are enteroviruses, respiratory viruses and herpesviruses (e.g. herpes simplex virus, varicella and HHV6). Worldwide, microorganisms causing encephalitis include *Mycoplasma*, *Borrelia burgdorferi* (Lyme disease), *Bartonella henselae* (cat scratch disease), rickettsial infections (e.g. Rocky Mountain spotted fever) and the arboviruses.

Herpes simplex virus (HSV) is a rare cause of childhood encephalitis but it may have devastating long-term consequences. All children with encephalitis should therefore be treated initially with high-dose intravenous aciclovir, since this is a very safe treatment. Most affected children do not have outward signs of herpes infection, such as cold sores, gingivostomatitis or skin lesions. The PCR of the CSF may be positive for HSV. As HSV encephalitis is a destructive infection, the

EEG and CT/MRI scan may show focal changes, particularly within the temporal lobes (Fig. 14.5). These tests may be normal initially and need to be repeated after a few days if the child is not improving. Later confirmation of the diagnosis may be made from HSV antibody production in the CSF. Proven cases of HSV encephalitis or cases where there is a high index of suspicion should be treated with intravenous aciclovir for 3 weeks, as relapses may occur after shorter courses. Untreated, the mortality rate from HSV encephalitis is over 70% and survivors usually have severe neurological sequelae.

Summary

Encephalitis

- Onset can be insidious and includes behavioural change
- Consider if HSV (herpes simplex virus) could be the cause
- Treat potential HSV with parenteral high-dose aciclovir until diagnosis is excluded.

Toxic shock syndrome

Toxin-producing *Staphylococcus aureus* and group A streptococci can cause this syndrome, which is characterised by:

- Fever >39°C
- Hypotension
- Diffuse erythematous, macular rash.

The toxin can be released from infection at any site, including small abrasions or burns, which may look minor. The toxin acts as a superantigen and, in addition to the features above, causes organ dysfunction, including:

- Mucositis (Fig. 14.6): conjunctivae, oral mucosa, genital mucosa

- Gastrointestinal: vomiting/diarrhoea
- Renal impairment
- Liver impairment
- Clotting abnormalities and thrombocytopenia
- Central nervous system: altered consciousness.

Intensive care support is required to manage the shock. Areas of infection should be surgically debrided. Antibiotics often include a third-generation cephalosporin (such as ceftriaxone) together with clindamycin, which acts on the bacterial ribosome to switch off toxin production. Intravenous immunoglobulin may be given to neutralise circulating toxin. About 1–2 weeks after the onset of the illness, there is desquamation of the palms, soles, fingers and toes.

PVL-producing *Staphylococcus aureus* causes recurrent skin and soft tissue infections, but can also cause necrotising fasciitis and a necrotising haemorrhagic pneumonia following an influenza-like illness; they carry a high mortality. PVL-producing *Staphylococcus aureus* produces a toxin called Panton-Valentine leukocidin (PVL) which has emerged in the UK and other countries. PVL is produced by fewer than 2% of *Staphylococcus aureus* strains (both methicillin-sensitive *Staphylococcus aureus* (MSSA) and methicillin-resistant *Staphylococcus aureus* (MRSA)). In children, the procoagulant state frequently results in venous thrombosis.

Necrotising fasciitis/cellulitis

This is a severe subcutaneous infection, often involving tissue planes from the skin down to fascia and muscle. The area involved may enlarge rapidly, leaving poorly perfused necrotic areas of tissue, usually at the centre. There is severe pain and systemic illness, which may require intensive care. The invading organism may be *Staphylococcus aureus* or a group A streptococcus, with or without another synergistic anaerobic organism. Intravenous antibiotic therapy alone is not sufficient to treat this condition. Without surgical intervention and debridement of necrotic tissue, the infection will continue to spread. Clinical suspicion of necrotising

fasciitis warrants urgent surgical consultation and intervention. Intravenous immunoglobulin (IVIG) may also be given.

Specific bacterial infections

Meningococcal infection

Meningococcal infection is a disease that strikes fear into both parents and doctors, as it can kill previously healthy children within hours (Case History 14.1). However, of the three main causes of bacterial meningitis, meningococcal has the lowest risk of long-term neurological sequelae, with most survivors recovering fully. The septicaemia is usually accompanied by a purpuric rash which may start anywhere on the body and then spread. The rash may or may not be present with meningococcal meningitis. Characteristic lesions are non-blanching on palpation, irregular in size and outline and have a necrotic centre (Fig. 14.8a,b). Any febrile child who develops a purpuric rash should be treated immediately, at home or in the general practitioner's surgery, with systemic antibiotics such as penicillin before urgent admission to hospital. Although there are now polysaccharide conjugate vaccines

---

Case History

14.1 Meningococcal septicaemia

This 7-month-old boy presented with a 12-hour history of lethargy and a spreading purpuric rash. In hospital, he required immediate resuscitation and transfer to a paediatric intensive care unit for multi-organ failure (Fig. 14.7a). The gross oedema is from leak of capillary fluid into the tissues. He required colloid and inotropic support and peritoneal dialysis for renal failure. He made a full recovery (Fig. 14.7b).

 Meningococcal septicaemia can kill children in hours. Optimal outcome requires immediate recognition, prompt resuscitation and antibiotics.

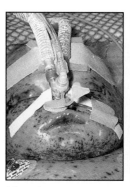 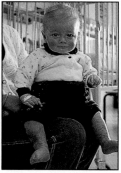

(a)   (b)

Figure 14.7 (a) A boy with meningococcal septicaemia receiving intensive care. **(b)** After full recovery. (Courtesy of Dr Parviz Habibi.)

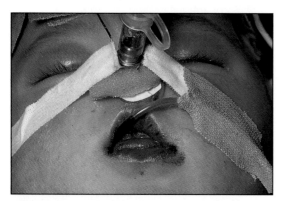

Figure 14.6 A child with toxic shock syndrome receiving intensive care, including artificial ventilation via a nasotracheal tube. The lips are red and the eyelids are oedematous from capillary leak. (Courtesy of Professor Mike Levin.)

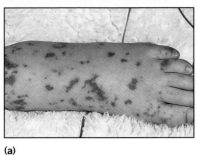
(a)

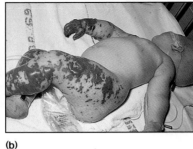
(b)

Figure 14.8 Rash of meningococcal infection. **(a)** Characteristic purpuric skin lesions, irregular in size and outline and with a necrotic centre. **(b)** The lesions may be extensive, when it is called 'purpura fulminans'.

against groups A and C meningococcus, there is still no effective vaccine for group B meningococcus, which accounts for the majority of isolates in the UK.

 Any febrile child with a purpuric rash should be given intramuscular benzylpenicillin immediately and transferred urgently to hospital.

Pneumococcal infections

Streptococcus pneumoniae is often carried in the nasopharynx of healthy children. Asymptomatic carriage is particularly prevalent among young children and may be responsible for the transmission of pneumococcal disease to other individuals by respiratory droplets. The organism may cause pharyngitis, otitis media, conjunctivitis, sinusitis as well as 'invasive' disease (pneumonia, bacterial sepsis and meningitis). Invasive disease, which carries a high burden of morbidity and mortality, mainly occurs in young infants as their immune system responds poorly to encapsulated pathogens such as pneumococcus. With the inclusion of the 13-valent pneumococcal vaccine into the standard immunisation schedule in the UK, the incidence of invasive disease has declined. Children at increased risk, e.g. from hyposplenism, should also be given daily prophylactic penicillin to prevent infection by strains not covered by the vaccine.

Haemophilus infection

H. influenzae type b was an important cause of systemic illness in children, including otitis media, pneumonia, epiglottitis, cellulitis, osteomyelitis and septic arthritis and was the second most common cause of meningitis in the UK. Immunisation has been highly effective and it now rarely causes systemic disease.

Staphylococcal and group A streptococcal infections

Staphylococcal and streptococcal infections are usually caused by direct invasion of the organisms. They may also cause disease by releasing toxins which act as

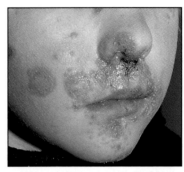

Figure 14.9 Impetigo showing characteristic confluent honey-coloured crusted lesions. (Courtesy of Dr Paul Hutchins.)

Summary

Pneumococcal infection

- Causes not only minor infections such as otitis media but also invasive disease
- Susceptibility is increased in hyposplenism (e.g. sickle cell disease and nephrotic syndrome)
- Vaccination is included in the standard immunisation schedule.

superantigens. Whereas conventional antigens stimulate only a small subset of T cells which have a specific receptor, superantigens bind to a part of the T-cell receptor which is shared by many T cells and therefore stimulates massive T-cell proliferation and cytokine release. Other diseases following staphylococcal and streptococcal infections are immune-mediated.

Impetigo

This is a localised, highly contagious, staphylococcal and/or streptococcal skin infection, most common in infants and young children. It is more common where there is pre-existing skin disease, e.g. atopic eczema. Lesions are usually on the face, neck and hands and begin as erythematous macules which may become vesicular/pustular or even bullous (Fig. 14.9). Rupture

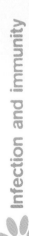
Infection and immunity

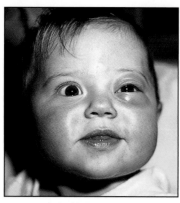

Figure 14.10 Periorbital cellulitis. It should be treated promptly with intravenous antibiotics to prevent spread into the orbit.

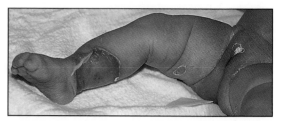

Figure 14.11 Staphylococcal scalded skin syndrome. Its appearance must not be mistaken for a scald from non-accidental injury.

of the vesicles with exudation of fluid leads to the characteristic confluent honey-coloured crusted lesions. Infection is readily spread to adjacent areas and other parts of the body by autoinoculation of the infected exudate. Topical antibiotics (e.g. mupirocin) are sometimes effective for mild cases. Narrow-spectrum systemic antibiotics (e.g. flucloxacillin) are needed for more severe infections, although more broad-spectrum antibiotics such as co-amoxiclav or cefaclor have simpler oral administration regimens, taste better and therefore have better adherence. Affected children should not go to nursery or school until the lesions are dry. Nasal carriage is an important source of infection which can be eradicated with a nasal cream containing mupirocin or chlorhexidine and neomycin.

Boils

These are infections of hair follicles or sweat glands, usually caused by *Staphylococcus aureus*. Treatment is with systemic antibiotics and occasionally surgery. Recurrent boils are usually from persistent nasal carriage in the child or family acting as a reservoir for reinfection. Only rarely are they a manifestation of immune deficiency.

Periorbital cellulitis

In periorbital cellulitis there is fever with erythema, tenderness and oedema of the eyelid (Fig. 14.10). It is almost always unilateral. In young, unimmunised children it may also be caused by *Haemophilus influenzae* type b which may also be accompanied by infection at other sites, e.g. meningitis. It may follow local trauma to the skin. In older children, it may spread from a paranasal sinus infection or dental abscess. Periorbital cellulitis should be treated promptly with intravenous antibiotics to prevent posterior spread of the infection to become an orbital cellulitis. In orbital cellulitis, there is proptosis, painful or limited ocular movement and reduced visual acuity. It may be complicated by abscess formation, meningitis or cavernous sinus thrombosis. Where orbital cellulitis is suspected, a CT scan should be performed to assess the posterior spread of infection and a lumbar puncture may be required to exclude meningitis.

Scalded skin syndrome

This is caused by an exfoliative staphylococcal toxin which causes separation of the epidermal skin through the granular cell layers. It affects infants and young children, who develop fever and malaise and may have a purulent, crusting, localised infection around the eyes, nose and mouth with subsequent widespread erythema and tenderness of the skin. Areas of epidermis separate on gentle pressure (Nikolsky sign), leaving denuded areas of skin (Fig. 14.11), which subsequently dry and heal without scarring. Management is with an intravenous anti-staphylococcal antibiotic, analgesia and monitoring of fluid balance.

> **Summary**
>
> **Staphylococcal and streptococcal infections**
>
> - Symptoms are caused by direct invasion of bacteria or by release of toxins
> - Impetigo is highly contagious
> - Periorbital cellulitis should be treated aggressively to prevent spread to the orbit or brain
> - Scalded skin syndrome is rare but serious.

Common viral infections

Many of the common childhood infections present with fever and a rash (Table 14.2). Incubation periods vary from 24 h for viral gastroenteritis, to about 2 weeks for chickenpox, but for some diseases, such as HIV, the length of time between exposure and the development of symptomatic illness may extend to many years. This is a reflection of host–pathogen interactions; an effective initial host response may result in a prolonged period of clinical latency, whereas an ineffective response permits rapid evolution of disease.

The infectious period characteristically begins a day or two before the rash appears and, for purposes of nursery/school exclusion, is generally considered to last until the rash has resolved or the lesions have dried up. For details about incubation and exclusion periods, see the Health Protection Agency website (http://www.hpa.org.uk).

Table 14.2 Causes of fever and a rash

Maculopapular rash			Vesicular, bullous, pustular		
Viral	HHV6 or 7 (Roseola infantum) – <2 years old		**Viral**	Varicella-zoster virus – chickenpox, shingles	
	Enteroviral rash			Herpes simplex virus	
	Parvovirus ('slapped cheek') – usually school-age			Coxsackie – hand, foot and mouth	
	Measles – uncommon if immunised		**Bacterial**	Impetigo – characteristic crusting	
	Rubella – uncommon if immunised			Boils – infection of hair follicles/sweat glands	
Bacterial	Scarlet fever (group A streptococcus)			Staphylococcal bullous impetigo	
	Erythema marginatum – rheumatic fever			Staphylococcal scalded skin	
	Salmonella typhi (typhoid fever) – classically rose spots			Toxic epidermal necrolysis	
	Lyme disease – erythema migrans		**Other**	Erythema multiforme; Stevens–Johnson syndrome	
Other	Kawasaki disease		**Petechial, purpuric**		
	Juvenile idiopathic arthritis		**Bacterial**	Meningococcal, other bacterial sepsis	
				Infective endocarditis	
			Viral	Enterovirus and other viral infections	
			Other	Henoch–Schönlein purpura (HSP)	
				Thrombocytopenia	
				Vasculitis	
				Malaria	

The human herpesviruses

There are currently eight known human herpesviruses: herpes simplex virus 1 and 2 (HSV1 and HSV2), varicella zoster virus (VZV), cytomegalovirus (CMV), Epstein–Barr virus (EBV), and human herpesviruses 6, 7 and 8 (HHV 6–8). HHV8 is associated with Kaposi sarcoma in HIV-coinfected individuals. The other herpesviruses will be discussed in this section, in order of their prevalence.

The hallmark of the herpesviruses is that, after primary infection, latency is established and there is long-term persistence of the virus within the host, usually in a dormant state. After certain stimuli, reactivation of infection may occur.

Herpes simplex infections

Herpes simplex virus (HSV) usually enters the body through the mucous membranes or skin, and the site of the primary infection may be associated with intense local mucosal damage. HSV1 is usually associated with lip and skin lesions, and HSV2 with genital lesions, but both viruses can cause both types of disease. The wide variety of clinical manifestations are described below. Treatment is with aciclovir, a viral DNA polymerase inhibitor, which may be used to treat severe symptomatic skin, ophthalmic, cerebral and systemic infections.

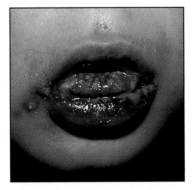

Figure 14.12 Vesicles with ulceration in gingivostomatitis.

Asymptomatic

Herpes simplex infections are very common and are mostly asymptomatic.

Gingivostomatitis

This is the most common form of primary HSV illness in children. It usually occurs from 10 months to 3 years of age. There are vesicular lesions on the lips, gums and anterior surfaces of the tongue and hard palate, which often progress to extensive, painful ulceration with bleeding (Fig. 14.12). There is a high fever and the child

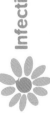

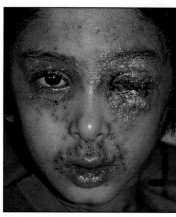

Figure 14.13 Eczema herpeticum.

is very miserable. The illness may persist for up to 2 weeks. Eating and drinking are painful, which may lead to dehydration. Management is symptomatic, but severe disease may necessitate intravenous fluids and aciclovir.

Skin manifestations

Mucocutaneous junctions and damaged skin are particularly prone to infection. 'Cold sores' are recurrent HSV1 lesions on the gingival (lip) margin.

Eczema herpeticum – In this serious condition, widespread vesicular lesions develop on eczematous skin (Fig. 14.13). This may be complicated by secondary bacterial infection, which may result in septicaemia.

Herpetic whitlows – These are painful, erythematous, oedematous white pustules on the site of broken skin on the fingers. Spread is by auto-inoculation from gingivostomatitis and infected adults kissing their children's fingers. In sexually active adolescents, HSV2 may be the cause.

Eye disease

Eye disease may cause a blepharitis or conjunctivitis. It may extend to involve the cornea, producing dendritic ulceration. This can lead to corneal scarring and

ultimately loss of vision. Any child with herpetic lesions near or involving the eye requires ophthalmic investigation of the cornea by slit lamp examination.

Central nervous system infection

Neonatal infection (see Ch. 10) – The infection may be focal, affecting the skin or eyes or encephalitis or may be widely disseminated. Its morbidity and mortality are high.

Infection in the immunocompromised host – Infection may be severe. Cutaneous lesions may spread to involve adjacent sites, e.g. oesophagitis and proctitis. Pneumonia and disseminated infections involving multiple organs are serious complications.

Chickenpox (primary varicella zoster infection)

Clinical features

These are shown in Figure 14.14.

There are a number of rare but serious complications that can occur in previously healthy children:

- *Secondary bacterial infection* with staphylococci, group A streptococcal, or other organisms. May lead to further complications such as toxic shock syndrome or necrotising fasciitis. Secondary bacterial infection should be considered where there is onset of a new fever or persistent high fever after the first few days.
- *Encephalitis*. This may be generalised, usually occurring early during the illness. In contrast to the encephalitis caused by HSV, the prognosis is good. Most characteristic is a VZV-associated cerebellitis. This usually occurs about a week after the onset of rash. The child is ataxic with cerebellar signs. It usually resolves within a month.
- *Purpura fulminans*. This is the consequence of vasculitis in the skin and subcutaneous tissues. It is best known in relation to meningococcal disease and can lead to loss of large areas of skin by necrosis. It may rarely occur after VZV infection due to production of antiviral antibodies which cross-react and inactivate the coagulation factor protein S. There is subsequent dysregulation of fibrinolysis and an increased risk of clotting, most often manifest in the skin.

In the immunocompromised, primary varicella infection may result in severe progressive disseminated disease, which has a mortality of up to 20%. The vesicular eruptions persist and may become haemorrhagic. The disease in the neonatal period is described in Chapter 10.

 Watch for the child with chickenpox whose fever initially settles, but then recurs a few days later – it is likely to be due to secondary bacterial infection.

Treatment and prevention

Oral aciclovir has minimal benefit and is not recommended in the UK. Immunocompromised children should be treated with intravenous aciclovir initially.

Summary

Herpes simplex virus infections

- Most are asymptomatic
- Gingivostomatitis – may necessitate intravenous fluids and aciclovir
- Skin manifestations – mucocutaneous junctions, e.g. lips and damaged skin
- Eczema herpeticum – may result in secondary bacterial infection and septicaemia
- Herpetic whitlows – painful pustules on the fingers
- Eye disease – blepharitis, conjunctivitis, corneal ulceration and scarring
- CNS – aseptic meningitis, encephalitis
- Pneumonia and disseminated infection in the immunocompromised.

Clinical features and complications of chickenpox

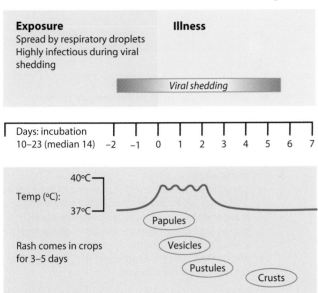

Exposure
Spread by respiratory droplets
Highly infectious during viral shedding

Illness

Viral shedding

Days: incubation
10–23 (median 14)   −2   −1   0   1   2   3   4   5   6   7

Temp (°C):   40°C
             37°C

Papules
Vesicles
Pustules
Crusts

Rash comes in crops
for 3–5 days

Complications

Bacterial superinfection
Staphylococcal
Streptococcal
May lead to toxic shock syndrome or necrotising fasciitis

Central nervous system
Cerebellitis
Generalised encephalitis
Aseptic meningitis

Immunocompromised
Haemorrhagic lesions
Pneumonitis
Progressive and disseminated infection
Disseminated intravascular coagulation

Typical vesicular rash
200–500 lesions start on head and trunk, progress to peripheries. (But may be just a few lesions).
Appear as crops of papules, vesicles with surrounding erythema **(Fig. 14.14)** and pustules at different times for up to one week.
Lesions may occur on the palate.
Itchy and scratching may result in permanent, depigmented scar formation or secondary infection.
If new lesions appear beyond 10 days, suggests defective cellular immunity.

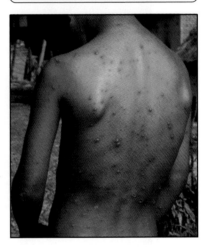

Figure 14.14 Clinical features and complications of chickenpox.

Oral valaciclovir can be substituted if organ dissemination has not occurred. Valaciclovir can be considered for adolescents and adults unlucky enough to develop primary VZV infection, as it is more severe when contracted beyond childhood. Human varicella zoster immunoglobulin (VZIG) is recommended for high-risk immunosuppressed individuals with deficient T-lymphocyte function following contact with chickenpox. Protection from infection with zoster immunoglobulin is not absolute, and depends on how soon after contact with chickenpox it is given.

 Beware of admitting a chickenpox contact to a clinical area with immunocompromised children, in whom it can disseminate and be fatal.

Shingles (herpes zoster)

Shingles is uncommon in children. It is caused by reactivation of latent varicella-zoster virus (VZV), causing a vesicular eruption in the dermatomal distribution of sensory nerves (shingles). It occurs most commonly in the thoracic region, although any dermatome can be affected (Fig. 14.15). Children, unlike adults, rarely suffer neuralgic pain with shingles. Shingles in childhood is more common in those who had primary infection in the first year of life. Recurrent or multidermatomal shingles is strongly associated with underlying immune suppression, e.g. HIV infection. In the immunocompromised, reactivated infection can also disseminate to cause severe disease.

 Recurrent or multidermatomal shingles suggests a T-cell immune defect.

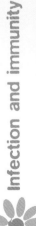

Summary

Chickenpox

- Clinical features – fever and itchy, vesicular rash which crops for up to 7 days
- Complications – secondary bacterial infection, encephalitis; disseminated disease in the immunocompromised
- Human varicella zoster immunoglobulin (VZIG) – if immunosuppressed and in contact with chickenpox or if maternal chickenpox shortly before or after delivery
- Treatment is symptomatic; i.v. aciclovir for severe chickenpox or the immunocompromised.

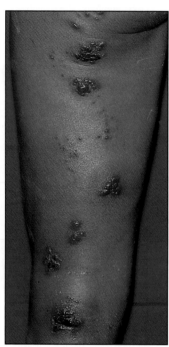

Figure 14.15 Herpes zoster (shingles) in a child. Distribution is along the S1 dermatome. (Courtesy of Dr Sam Walters.)

Epstein–Barr virus: infectious mononucleosis (glandular fever)

Epstein–Barr virus (EBV) is the major cause of the infectious mononucleosis syndrome, but it is also involved in the pathogenesis of Burkitt lymphoma, lymphoproliferative disease in immunocompromised hosts and nasopharyngeal carcinoma. The virus has a particular tropism for B lymphocytes and epithelial cells of the pharynx. Transmission usually occurs by oral contact and the majority of infections are subclinical.

Older children, and occasionally young children, may develop a syndrome with:

- fever
- malaise

- tonsillopharyngitis – often severe, limiting oral ingestion of fluids and food; rarely, breathing may be compromised
- lymphadenopathy – prominent cervical lymph nodes, often with diffuse adenopathy.

Other features include:

- petechiae on the soft palate
- splenomegaly (50%), hepatomegaly (10%)
- a maculopapular rash (5%)
- jaundice.

Diagnosis is supported by:

- atypical lymphocytes (numerous large T cells seen on blood film)
- a positive Monospot test (the presence of heterophile antibodies, i.e. antibodies that agglutinate sheep or horse erythrocytes but which are not absorbed by guinea pig kidney extracts – this test is often negative in young children with the disease)
- seroconversion with production of IgM and IgG to Epstein–Barr virus antigens.

Symptoms may persist for 1–3 months but ultimately resolve. They are caused by the host immune response to the infection, rather than the virus itself.

Treatment is symptomatic. When the airway is severely compromised, corticosteroids may be considered. In 5% of infected individuals, group A streptococcus is grown from the tonsils. This may be treated with penicillin. Ampicillin or amoxicillin may cause a florid maculopapular rash in children infected with EBV and should be avoided.

Cytomegalovirus

Cytomegalovirus (CMV) is usually transmitted via saliva, genital secretions or breast milk, and more rarely via blood products, organ transplants and transplacentally. The virus causes mild or subclinical infection in normal hosts. In developed countries, about half of the adult population show serological evidence of past infection. In developing countries, most children have been infected by 2 years of age, often via breast milk. In the immunocompromised and the fetus, CMV is an important pathogen.

As with EBV, CMV may cause a mononucleosis syndrome. Pharyngitis and lymphadenopathy are not usually as prominent as in EBV infections. Patients may have atypical lymphocytes on the blood film but are heterophile antibody-negative. Maternal CMV infection may result in congenital infection (see Ch. 9), which may be present at birth or develop when older. In the immunocompromised host, CMV can cause retinitis, pneumonitis, bone marrow failure, encephalitis, hepatitis, colitis and oesophagitis. It is a very important pathogen following organ transplantation. Organ recipients are closely monitored for evidence of CMV activation by sensitive tests such as blood polymerase chain reaction (PCR). Interventions used to reduce the risk of transmission of CMV disease are CMV-negative blood for transfusions and anti-CMV drug prophylaxis; also, if possible, CMV-positive organs are not transplanted into CMV-negative recipients.

CMV disease may be treated with ganciclovir or foscarnet, but both have serious side-effects.

Human herpesvirus 6 (HHV6) and HHV7

Human herpesvirus 6 (HHV6) and HHV7 are closely related and have similar presentations, although HHV6 is more prevalent. Most children are infected with HHV6 or HHV7 by the age of 2 years, usually from the oral secretions of a family member. They classically cause exanthem subitum (also known as roseola infantum), characterised by a high fever with malaise lasting a few days, followed by a generalised macular rash, which appears as the fever wanes. Many children have a febrile illness without rash, and many have a subclinical infection. Exanthem subitum is frequently clinically misdiagnosed as measles or rubella; these infections are rare in the UK and if suspected should be confirmed serologically. Another frequent occurrence in primary HHV6 infection is that infants seen by a doctor during the febrile stage are prescribed antibiotics, and when the rash appears, it is erroneously attributed to an 'allergic' reaction to the drug. Primary HHV6/HHV7 infections are a common cause of febrile convulsions. Rarely, they may cause aseptic meningitis, encephalitis, hepatitis, or an infectious mononucleosis-like syndrome.

Parvovirus B19

Parvovirus B19 causes erythema infectiosum or fifth disease (so-named because it was the fifth disease to be described of a group of illnesses with similar rashes), also called slapped-cheek syndrome. Infections can occur at any time of the year, although outbreaks are most common during the spring months. Transmission is via respiratory secretions from viraemic patients, by vertical transmission from mother to fetus and by transfusion of contaminated blood products. Parvovirus B19 infects the erythroblastoid red cell precursors in the bone marrow.

Parvovirus causes a range of clinical syndromes:

- Asymptomatic infection – common; about 5–10% of preschool children and 65% of adults have antibodies
- Erythema infectiosum – the most common illness, with a viraemic phase of fever, malaise, headache and myalgia followed by a characteristic rash a week later on the face ('slapped-cheek'), progressing to a maculopapular, 'lace'-like rash on the trunk and limbs; complications are rare in children, although arthralgia or arthritis is common in adults
- Aplastic crisis – the most serious consequence of parvovirus infection; it occurs in children with chronic haemolytic anaemias, where there is an increased rate of red cell turnover (e.g. sickle cell disease or thalassaemia); and in immunodeficient children (e.g. malignancy) who are unable to produce an antibody response to neutralise the infection
- Fetal disease – transmission of maternal parvovirus infection may lead to fetal hydrops and death due

to severe anaemia, although the majority of infected fetuses will recover.

Summary

Parvovirus

- Usually asymptomatic or erythema infectiosum
- Can cause aplastic crisis in haemolytic anaemias (e.g. sickle cell) or the fetus (causes hydrops).

Enteroviruses

Human enteroviruses, of which there are many (including the coxsackie viruses, echoviruses and polioviruses), are a common cause of childhood infection. Transmission is primarily by the faecal–oral route. Following replication in the pharynx and gut, the virus spreads to infect other organs. Infections occur most commonly in the summer and autumn. Over 90% of infections are asymptomatic or cause a non-specific febrile illness, sometimes with a rash usually over the trunk that is blanching or consists of fine petechiae. A history of loose stools or some vomiting, or a contact history, would be supportive. The child is not usually systemically unwell, but if the rash is non-blanching, admission for observation and 48 h of parenteral antibiotics (such as ceftriaxone) is indicated. It is better to treat a number of enteroviral infections than to send home a child with meningococcal disease, only to have them return moribund 12 h later.

Other characteristic clinical syndromes exist and are listed below. (For polioviruses, see the Immunisation section, below.)

Hand, foot and mouth disease

Painful vesicular lesions on the hands, feet, mouth and tongue, and often on the buttocks. Systemic features are mild. The disease subsides within a few days, with fluids and analgesia.

Herpangina

Vesicular and ulcerated lesions on the soft palate and uvula causing anorexia, pain on swallowing and fever. Resolves with fluids and analgesia.

Meningitis/encephalitis

Aseptic meningitis is caused by many of the enteroviruses. Complete recovery can be expected.

Pleurodynia (Bornholm disease)

An acute illness with fever, pleuritic chest pain and muscle tenderness. There may be a pleural rub but examination is otherwise normal. Recovery is within a few days.

Myocarditis and pericarditis

Rare. Heart failure associated with a febrile illness and ECG evidence of myocarditis.

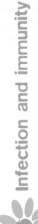

Infection and immunity

255

Summary

Enterovirus infection

- Mostly asymptomatic or self-limiting illness with rash, which may be purpuric
- Can cause hand, foot and mouth disease, herpangina, or meningitis/encephalitis.

Uncommon viral infections

Measles

Health practitioners in the UK need to be aware of measles due to the rise in cases following public anxiety about the MMR vaccination (see the Immunisation section, below), as well as it continuing to be a major cause of morbidity and death worldwide. As with chickenpox and parvovirus, older children and adults tend to have more severe disease than the very young. For epidemiological tracking of infection, virological or serological confirmation of clinical cases of measles should be undertaken by testing either blood or saliva.

Clinical features

These are shown in Figure 14.16. There are a number of serious complications which can occur in previously healthy children:

- *Encephalitis* occurs in about 1 in 5000, about 8 days after the onset of the illness. Initial symptoms are headache, lethargy and irritability, proceeding to convulsions and ultimately coma. Mortality is 15%. Serious long-term sequelae include seizures, deafness, hemiplegia and severe learning difficulties, affecting up to 40% of survivors.
- *Subacute sclerosing panencephalitis* (*SSPE*) is a rare but devastating illness manifesting, on average, 7 years after measles infection in about 1 in 100 000 cases. Most children who develop SSPE had primary measles infection before 2 years of age. SSPE is caused by a variant of the measles virus which persists in the central nervous system. The disorder presents with loss of neurological function, which progresses over several years to dementia and death. The diagnosis is essentially

Clinical features and complications of measles

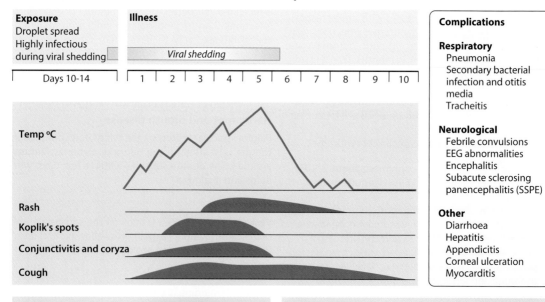

Exposure
Droplet spread
Highly infectious during viral shedding

Days 10-14

Illness

Viral shedding

1 2 3 4 5 6 7 8 9 10

Temp °C

Rash

Koplik's spots

Conjunctivitis and coryza

Cough

Complications

Respiratory
Pneumonia
Secondary bacterial infection and otitis media
Tracheitis

Neurological
Febrile convulsions
EEG abnormalities
Encephalitis
Subacute sclerosing panencephalitis (SSPE)

Other
Diarrhoea
Hepatitis
Appendicitis
Corneal ulceration
Myocarditis

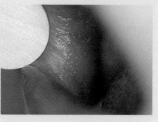

Koplik's spots
White spots on buccal mucosa, seen against bright red background. Pathognomonic, but difficult to see.

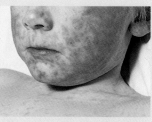

Rash
Spreads downwards, from behind the ears to the whole of the body. Discrete, maculopapular rash initially, becomes blotchy and confluent. May desquamate in the second week.

Figure 14.16 Clinical features and complications of measles.

clinical, supported by finding high levels of measles antibody in both blood and cerebrospinal fluid and by characteristic EEG abnormalities. Since the introduction of measles immunisation, it has become extremely rare.

In developing countries, where malnutrition and vitamin A deficiency lead to impaired cell-mediated immunity, measles often follows a protracted course with severe complications. Impaired cellular immune responses such as in HIV infection may result in a modified or absent rash, with an increased risk of dissemination, including giant-cell pneumonia or encephalitis.

Treatment

Treatment for measles is symptomatic. Children who are admitted to hospital should be isolated. In immunocompromised patients, the antiviral drug ribavirin may be used. Vitamin A, which may modulate the immune response, should be given in developing countries.

Prevention

Prevention by immunisation is the most successful strategy for reducing the morbidity and mortality of measles.

 Measles remains a major cause of death in childhood in developing countries.

Summary

Measles

- Incidence has declined dramatically since immunisation was introduced; a recent small increase has resulted from the fall in immunisation uptake
- Clinical features: fever, cough, runny nose, conjunctivitis, marked malaise, Koplik spots, maculopapular rash
- Complications: common if malnourished or immunocompromised; major cause of death in developing countries.

Mumps

Mumps occurs worldwide, but its incidence has declined dramatically because of the mumps component of the MMR vaccine. Following the decrease in the uptake of the MMR immunisation in the late 1990s, there has been a rise in unimmunised children and unvaccinated young adults. Mumps usually occurs in the winter and spring months. It is spread by droplet infection to the respiratory tract where the virus replicates within epithelial cells. The virus gains access to the parotid glands before further dissemination to other tissues.

Clinical features

The incubation period is 15–24 days. Onset of the illness is with fever, malaise and parotitis, but in up to 30% of cases, the infection is subclinical. Only one side may be swollen initially, but bilateral involvement usually occurs over the next few days. The parotitis is uncomfortable and children may complain of earache or pain on eating or drinking. Examination of the parotid duct may show redness and swelling. Occasionally, parotid swelling may be absent. The fever usually disappears within 3–4 days. Plasma amylase levels are often elevated and, when associated with abdominal pain, may be evidence of pancreatic involvement. Infectivity is for up to 7 days after the onset of parotid swelling. The illness is generally mild and self-limiting. Although hearing loss can follow mumps, it is usually unilateral and transient.

Viral meningitis and encephalitis

Lymphocytes are seen in the CSF in about 50%, meningeal signs are only seen in 10%, and encephalitis in about 1 in 5000. The common clinical features are headache, photophobia, vomiting and neck stiffness.

Orchitis

This is the most feared complication, although it is uncommon in prepubertal males. When it does occur, it is usually unilateral. Although there is some evidence of a reduction in sperm count, infertility is actually extremely unusual. Rarely, oophoritis, mastitis and arthritis may occur.

Rubella (German measles)

Rubella is generally a mild disease in childhood. It occurs in winter and spring. It is an important infection, as it can cause severe damage to the fetus (see Ch. 9). The incubation period is 15–20 days. It is spread by the respiratory route, frequently from a known contact. The prodrome is usually mild with a low-grade fever or none at all. The maculopapular rash is often the first sign of infection, appearing initially on the face and then spreading centrifugally to cover the whole body. It fades in 3–5 days. Unlike in adults, the rash is not itchy. Lymphadenopathy, particularly the suboccipital and postauricular nodes, is prominent. Complications are rare in childhood but include arthritis, encephalitis, thrombocytopenia and myocarditis. Clinical differentiation from other viral infections is unreliable. The diagnosis should be confirmed serologically if there is any risk of exposure of a non-immune pregnant woman. There is no effective antiviral treatment. Prevention therefore lies in immunisation.

Summary

Rubella

Importance – congenital infection.

Prolonged fever

Most childhood infections are acute and resolve in a few days. If not, the child needs to be reassessed for complications of the original illness, e.g. a secondary bacterial infection, or the source of infection may not have been identified, e.g. urinary tract infection. Often, the child has developed another unrelated febrile illness. Assessment of prolonged fever also needs to be made for prompt recognition of Kawasaki disease to avoid complications. Causes of prolonged fever are listed in Box 14.2.

Kawasaki disease

Kawasaki disease (KD) is a systemic vasculitis. Although uncommon, it is an important diagnosis to make because aneurysms of the coronary arteries are a potentially devastating complication. Prompt treatment reduces their incidence.

Kawasaki disease mainly affects children of 6 months to 4 years old, with a peak at the end of the first year. The disease is more common in children of Japanese and, to a lesser extent, Afro-Caribbean ethnicity, than in Caucasians. Young infants tend to be more severely affected than older children and are more likely to have 'incomplete' cases, in which not all the cardinal features are present. Although the specific cause is unknown, it is likely to be the result of immune hyperreactivity to a variety of triggers in a genetically susceptible host (a polymorphism in the *ITPKC* gene, a negative regulator

of T-cell activation on chromosome 19 is strongly associated with susceptibility to the disease).

There is no diagnostic test; instead, the diagnosis is made on clinical findings (Fig. 14.17). In addition to the classic features, affected children are strikingly irritable, have a high fever that is difficult to control, and may also have inflammation of their BCG vaccination site. They have high inflammatory markers (C-reactive protein, ESR, white cell count), with a platelet count that rises typically in the second week of the illness. The coronary arteries are affected in about one-third of affected children within the first 6 weeks of the illness. This can lead to aneurysms which are best visualised on echocardiography (see Case History 14.2). Subsequent narrowing of the vessels from scar formation can result in myocardial ischaemia and sudden death. Mortality is 1–2%.

Prompt treatment with intravenous immunoglobulin (IVIG) given within the first 10 days has been shown to lower the risk of coronary artery aneurysms. Aspirin is used to reduce the risk of thrombosis. It is given at a high anti-inflammatory dose until the fever subsides and inflammatory markers return to normal, and continued at a low antiplatelet dose until echocardiography at 6 weeks reveals the presence or absence of aneurysms. When the platelet count is very high, antiplatelet aggregation agents may also be used to reduce the risk of coronary thrombosis. Children with giant coronary artery aneurysms may require long-term warfarin therapy and close follow-up. Children suspected of having the disease but who do not have all the clinical features should still be considered for treatment. Sometimes, fever recurs despite treatment and these children are given a second dose of IVIG. Persistent inflammation and fever may require treatment with infliximab (a monoclonal antibody against TNF-α), steroids or ciclosporin.

 Prolonged fever – check – is it Kawasaki disease?

Box 14.2 Causes of prolonged fever

Infective:

- Localised infection
- Bacterial infections: e.g. typhoid, *Bartonella henselae* (cat scratch disease), *Brucella*
- Deep abscesses: e.g. intra-abdominal, retroperitoneal, pelvic
- Infective endocarditis
- Tuberculosis
- Non-tuberculous mycobacterial infections: e.g. *Mycobacterium avium* complex
- Viral infections: e.g. EBV, CMV, HIV
- Parasitic infections: e.g. malaria, toxocariasis

Non-infective:

- Systemic juvenile idiopathic arthritis (SJIA)
- Systemic lupus erythematosus (SLE)
- Vasculitis (including Kawasaki disease)
- Inflammatory bowel disease
- Sarcoidosis
- Malignancy: e.g. leukaemia, lymphoma, neuroblastoma
- Macrophage activation syndromes: e.g. HLH (haemophagocytic lymphohistiocytosis)
- Drug fever
- Fabricated or induced illness.

Summary

Kawasaki disease

- Mainly affects infants and young children
- The diagnosis is made on clinical features – fever >5 days and four other features of non-purulent conjunctivitis, red mucous membranes, cervical lymphadenopathy, rash, red and oedematous palms and soles or peeling of fingers and toes
- 'Incomplete' (formerly called 'atypical') cases can occur, especially in infants, so a high index of suspicion should be maintained in a febrile child
- Complications – coronary artery aneurysms and sudden death
- Treatment – intravenous immunoglobulin and aspirin.

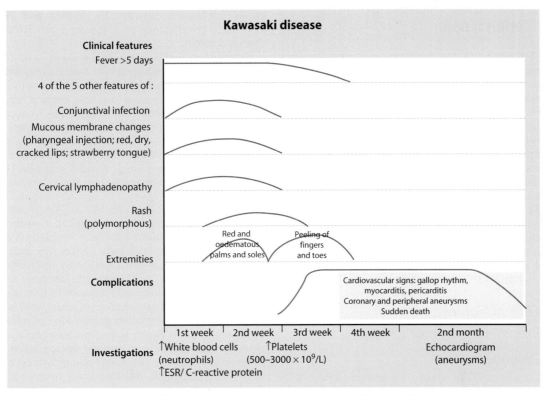

Kawasaki disease

Clinical features
Fever >5 days

4 of the 5 other features of :

Conjunctival infection

Mucous membrane changes
(pharyngeal injection; red, dry,
cracked lips; strawberry tongue)

Cervical lymphadenopathy

Rash
(polymorphous)

Extremities

Red and oedematous palms and soles

Peeling of fingers and toes

Complications

Cardiovascular signs: gallop rhythm,
myocarditis, pericarditis
Coronary and peripheral aneurysms
Sudden death

| 1st week | 2nd week | 3rd week | 4th week | 2nd month |

Investigations
↑White blood cells
(neutrophils)
↑ESR/ C-reactive protein

↑Platelets
(500–3000 × 10⁹/L)

Echocardiogram
(aneurysms)

Figure 14.17 Evolution of clinical features and abnormal investigations in Kawasaki disease.

Case History

14.2 Kawasaki disease

This 2-year-old boy developed a high fever of 2 days' duration. Examination showed a miserable child with mild conjunctivitis, a rash and cervical lymphadenopathy. A viral infection was diagnosed and his mother was reassured. When he presented to hospital 3 days later, he was noted to have cracked red lips (Fig. 14.18a). He was admitted and a full septic screen, including a lumbar puncture, was performed and antibiotics started. The following day, he was still febrile and irritable; his C-reactive protein (CRP) had risen to 135, and ESR (erythrocyte sedimentation rate) to 125. Kawasaki disease was suspected and he was treated with intravenous immunoglobulin and high-dose oral aspirin. His clinical condition improved and he became afebrile the following morning. An echocardiogram at this stage showed no aneurysms of the coronary arteries, which are the most serious complication associated with delayed diagnosis and treatment. On the fifteenth day of the illness there was peeling of the fingers and toes (Fig. 14.18b).

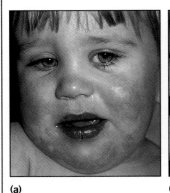
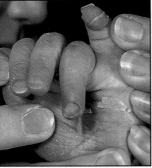

(a)   (b)

Figure 14.18 (a) Red, cracked lips and conjunctival inflammation. **(b)** Peeling of the fingers, which developed on the 15th day of the illness. (Courtesy of Professor Mike Levin.)

Tuberculosis

The decline in the incidence and mortality from tuberculosis (TB) in developed countries was hailed as an example of how public health measures and anti-microbial therapy can dramatically modify a disease. However, TB is again becoming a public health problem, partly through its increasing incidence in patients with HIV infection, and with the emergence of multi-drug resistant strains. Spread of TB is usually by the respiratory route. Close proximity, infectious load and underlying immunodeficiency enhance the risk of transmission. There is an important distinction between TB *infection* (latent TB) and TB *disease*. TB infection is more likely to progress to disease in infants and young children, compared to adults. In contrast to adults, children are generally not infectious, because the disease is paucibacillary. Children usually acquire TB from an infected adult in the household.

Clinical features

These are outlined in Figure 14.19.

Diagnosis

Diagnosis of TB in children is even more difficult than in adults. The clinical features of the disease are non-specific, such as prolonged fever, malaise, anorexia, weight loss or focal signs of infection. Sputum samples are generally unobtainable from children under about 8 years of age, unless specialist induction techniques are used. Children usually swallow sputum, so gastric washings on three consecutive mornings are required to visualise or culture acid-fast bacilli originating from the lung. To obtain these, a nasogastric tube is passed and secretions are rinsed out of the stomach with saline before food. Urine, lymph node excision, CSF and radiological examinations should also be performed where appropriate. Although it is difficult to culture TB from children, the presence of multi-drug resistant strains makes it important to try to grow the organism so that antibiotic sensitivity can be assessed.

If TB is suspected, a Mantoux test is performed – 2 units of purified protein derivative (PPD) of tuberculin (2TU SSI, 0.1 ml intradermal injection, read after 48–72 h as induration measured in mm across the forearm). Because PPD is a mixture of proteins, some of which are common to TB and BCG, the Mantoux test may be positive because of past vaccination rather than TB infection. A history of BCG immunisation therefore needs to be taken into account when interpreting the test. Induration of >10 mm is positive where no BCG has been given, 15 mm where BCG has been given. Heaf tests are no longer used for screening for TB.

A new generation of diagnostic tests is the interferon-gamma release assays (IGRA). These are blood tests that assess the response of T cells to stimulation in vitro with a small number of antigens found in TB but not in BCG. Positive results therefore indicate TB infection rather than BCG vaccination. The sensitivity and specificity of these tests in different settings is being evaluated, but its routine use in clinical practice is increasing. Neither this test nor the Mantoux test can reliably distinguish between TB infection and TB disease, so correlation with clinical signs and symptoms is required.

Co-infection with HIV makes the diagnosis even more difficult. With advanced immune suppression, both skin tests and IGRA are unreactive. Contact history, radiology and possibly tissue diagnosis become even more important. Attention has to be paid to avoiding misdiagnosing TB on chest X-ray appearances alone, as lymphoid interstitial pneumonitis can look similar and occurs in 20% of HIV-infected children. In view of the overlapping epidemiology, all individuals with TB should be tested for HIV, and vice-versa.

Treatment

Triple or quadruple therapy (rifampicin, isoniazid, pyrazinamide, ethambutol) is the recommended initial combination. This is decreased to the two drugs rifampicin and isoniazid after 2 months, by which time antibiotic sensitivities are often known. Treatment for uncomplicated pulmonary or lymph node TB is usually for 6 months; longer treatment courses are required for TB meningitis or disseminated disease. After puberty, pyridoxine is given weekly to prevent the peripheral neuropathy associated with isoniazid therapy, a complication which does not occur in young children. In tuberculous meningitis, dexamethasone is given for the first month at least, to decrease the risk of long-term sequelae.

Asymptomatic children who are Mantoux-positive and therefore latently infected should also be treated (e.g. with rifampicin and isoniazid for 3 months) as this will decrease the risk of reactivation of infection later in life.

Prevention and contact tracing

BCG immunisation has been shown to be helpful in preventing or modifying TB in the UK. However, its use-fulness worldwide in preventing the disease is controversial. In the UK, BCG is recommended at birth for high-risk groups (communities with a relatively high prevalence of TB; i.e. Asian or African origin or TB in a family member in the previous 5 years or if the local area has a high prevalence rate). The UK programme of routine BCG for all tuberculin-negative children between 10 and 14 years has been discontinued. BCG should not be given to HIV-positive or other immuno-suppressed children due to the potential risk of dissemination.

As most children are infected from a household contact, it is essential to screen other family members for the disease. Children who are exposed to smear-positive individuals (where organisms are visualised on sputum) should be assessed for evidence of asymptomatic infection. Mantoux-negative children over 5 years should receive BCG immunisation. Some clinicians suggest that those who are Mantoux-negative and <5 years old should receive chemoprophylaxis (e.g. rifampicin and isoniazid for 3 months). If at the end of this time they remain Mantoux-negative they should also receive BCG immunisation. Again, the aim of treatment is to decrease the risk of reactivation of TB infection later in life.

Clinical features of TB

Primary infection

Asymptomatic

Nearly half of infants and 90% of older children will show minimal signs and symptoms of infection. A local inflammatory reaction limits the progression of infection. However, the disease remains latent and may therefore develop into active disease at a later time. A Mantoux test may become positive and is sufficient evidence to initiate treatment (Fig. 18.19a).

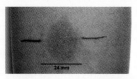

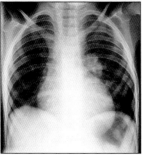

a) Example of a positive Mantoux test (24 mm induration) A Mantoux test (2 units PPD, PurifiedProtein Derivative) is positive if:
> 10 mm induration (no BCG given)
> 15 mm induration (BCG given)
Implies active infection.

b) Chest X-ray of pulmonary TB. There is marked left hilar lymphadenopathy

Symptomatic

In this case the local host response fails to contain the inhaled tubercle bacilli, allowing spread via the lymphatic system to regional lymph nodes. The lung lesion plus the lymph node constitutes the 'Ghon (or primary) complex'.
When the host's cellular immune system responds to the infection (3–6 weeks), mycobacterial replication diminishes but systemic symptoms develop:
- fever
- anorexia and weight loss
- cough
- chest X-ray changes (Fig. 18.19b).

The primary complex usually heals and may calcify. The inflammatory reaction may lead to local enlargement of peribronchial lymph nodes which may cause bronchial obstruction, with collapse and consolidation of the affected lung. Pleural effusions may also be present. Further progression may be halted by the host's immunological response, or there may be local dissemination to other regions of the lung.

Although primary infection most commonly occurs in the lung, it may also involve other organs including gut, skin and superficial lymph nodes. The latter may occasionally caseate forming a 'cold abscess'. Multiple sites may be colonised by metastatic lesions released during the primary infection.

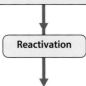

Dormancy and dissemination

Both asymptomatic and symptomatic infections may become dormant but subsequently reactivate and spread by lymphohaematological routes.

Reactivation

Post-primary TB

This may present as local disease or may be widely disseminated, miliary TB to sites such as bones, joints, kidneys, pericardium and CNS. In infants and young children, seeding of the CNS is particularly likely, causing tuberculous meningitis. This was always fatal before antimicrobial therapy was available, and is still associated with significant morbidity and mortality if treatment is not initiated early in the disease.

Figure 14.19 Clinical features of TB.

Non-tuberculous mycobacterial infection

There are numerous non-tuberculous mycobacteria found in the environment. Immunocompetent individuals rarely suffer from diseases caused by these organisms. They occasionally cause persistent lymphadenopathy in young children, which is usually treated surgically by complete node excision, as biopsy or partial excision may result in formation of a chronic fistula. Unlike TB, these organisms are transmitted in soil and water and therefore contact tracing is

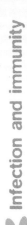

not required following infection. Non-tuberculous mycobacteria may cause disseminated infection in immune deficient individuals. *Mycobacterium avium intracellulare* (MAI) infections are particularly common in patients with advanced HIV disease. These infections do not respond to conventional TB treatment, and require a cocktail of alternative anti-mycobacterial drugs.

Summary

Tuberculosis

- TB affects millions of children worldwide; low but increasing incidence in many developed countries
- Clinical features follow a sequence – primary infection, then dormancy, which may be followed by reactivation to post-primary TB
- Diagnosis is often difficult, so decision to treat is usually based on contact history, Mantoux test, interferon-gamma release assays (IGRA), chest X-ray and clinical features. Young children swallow their sputum, so gastric washings are required
- Adherence to drug therapy can be problematic but is essential for successful treatment
- Contact tracing is important
- TB is more difficult to diagnose and more likely to disseminate in the immunosuppressed.

Tropical infections

Although tropical infections must be considered, children who have been or are in the tropics are still susceptible to the usual range of childhood infections found. The most common or most serious imported infections are outlined in Figure 14.20.

 A febrile child returning from the tropics – commonest causes are non-tropical infections, but consider malaria, typhoid fever and other tropical infections.

HIV infection

Globally, HIV infection affects over 2 million children, mostly in sub-Saharan Africa (Fig. 14.21), and there are still 380 000 children becoming infected each year (Fig. 14.22). The major route of HIV infection in children is mother-to-child transmission (MTCT), which occurs during pregnancy (intrauterine), at delivery (intrapartum) or through breast-feeding (postpartum). The virus may also be transmitted to children by infected blood products, contaminated needles or through child sexual abuse, but this is uncommon.

Diagnosis

In children over 18 months old, HIV infection is diagnosed by detecting antibodies to the virus. Children less than 18 months of age who are born to infected mothers will have transplacental maternal IgG HIV antibodies, and at this age, a positive test confirms HIV exposure but not HIV infection. The most sensitive test for HIV diagnosis before 18 months of age is HIV DNA PCR. All infants born to HIV-infected mothers should be tested for HIV infection, whether or not they are symptomatic. Two negative HIV DNA PCRs within the first 3 months of life, at least 2 weeks after completion of postnatal antiretroviral therapy, indicate the infant is not infected, although this is confirmed by the loss of transplacental maternal HIV antibodies from the infant's circulation after 18 months of age.

Clinical features

A proportion of HIV-infected infants progress rapidly to symptomatic disease and onset of AIDS in the first year of life; however, other infected children remain asymptomatic for months or years before progressing to clinical disease. Some asymptomatic children will only be identified in adolescence at routine screening following diagnosis in another family member. Clinical presentation varies with the degree of immunosuppression. Children with mild immunosuppression may have lymphadenopathy or parotitis; if moderate, they may have recurrent bacterial infections, candidiasis, chronic diarrhoea and lymphocytic interstitial pneumonitis (LIP) (Fig. 14.23). This lymphocytic infiltration of the lungs may be caused by a response to the HIV infection itself, or it may be related to EBV infection. Severe AIDS diagnoses include opportunistic infections, e.g. *Pneumocystis jiroveci (carinii)* pneumonia (PCP), severe failure to thrive, encephalopathy (Fig. 14.24), and malignancy, although this is rare in children. More than one clinical feature is often present. An unusual constellation of symptoms, especially if infectious, should alert one to HIV infection.

 Children with persistent lymphadenopathy, hepatosplenomegaly, recurrent fever, parotid swelling, thrombocytopenia, or any suggestion of SPUR (Serious, Persistent, Unusual, Recurrent) infections should be tested for HIV.

Treatment

A decision to start antiretroviral therapy (ART) is based on a combination of clinical status, HIV viral load and CD4 count, except in infants who should all start ART shortly after diagnosis, because they have a higher risk of disease progression. As in adults, combinations of three (or four) drugs are used. Prophylaxis against *Pneumocystis jiroveci (carinii)* pneumonia (PCP), with co-trimoxazole, is prescribed for infants who are HIV-infected, and for older children with low CD4 counts.

Other aspects of management include:

- Immunisation, which is important because of the higher risk of infections, and should follow

An approach to the febrile child returning from the tropics

History
All places visited and duration of stay. Immunisation, malaria prophylaxis. History of food, drink (infected water), accommodation (exposure to vectors), contacts, swimming (infected rivers and lakes).

↓

Examination
Particular reference to: fever, jaundice, anaemia, enlarged liver or spleen.

↓

Non-tropical causes of fever
Consider non-tropical causes of fever in childhood – upper and lower respiratory tract infections, gastroenteritis, urinary tract infection, septicaemia, meningitis, osteomyelitis, hepatitis, viral infections including the childhood exanthems.

↓

Tropical infections

Malaria

40% of the world's population live in an area where the female *Anopheles* mosquito transmits malaria. Causes over 700,000 child deaths in Africa each year, predominantly from *Plasmodium falciparum* malaria. The clinical features include fever (often not cyclical), diarrhoea, vomiting, flu-like symptoms, jaundice, anaemia and thrombocytopenia.
Whilst typically the onset is 7–10 days after inoculation, infections can present many months later.
Children are particularly susceptible to severe anaemia and the gravest form of the disease, cerebral malaria.
The infection is diagnosed by examination of a thick film. The species (*falciparum, vivax, ovale* or *malariae*) is confirmed on a thin film. Repeated blood films may be necessary.

Quinine is required in most cases of *Plasmodium falciparum* seen in the UK because of the emergence of chloroquine-resistant strains worldwide. Travellers to endemic areas should always seek up-to date information on malaria prevention. Prophylaxis reduces but does not eliminate the risk of infection. Prevention of mosquito bites with repellants and bed nets is also important. In many countries there has been a marked reduction in the incidence of malaria in children from insecticide-treated bed nets, indoor residual spraying of houses with insecticides, destruction of mosquito larvae and breeding areas and prompt treatment with artemisinin-based combination therapy.

Typhoid

A child with worsening fever, headaches, cough, abdominal pain, anorexia, malaise and myalgia may be suffering from infection with *Salmonella typhi* or *paratyphi*. Gastrointestinal symptoms (diarrhoea or constipation) may not appear until the second week. Splenomegaly, bradycardia and rose-coloured spots on the trunk may be present. The serious complications of this disease include gastrointestinal perforation, myocarditis, hepatitis and nephritis.
The recent increase in multi-drug resistant strains, particularly from the Indian subcontinent, means that treatment with cotrimoxazole, chloramphenicol or ampicillin may be inadequate. A third-generation cephalosporin or azithromycin is usually effective.

Dengue fever

This viral infection is widespread in the tropics, and it is transmitted by mosquitoes. The primary infection is characterised by a fine erythematous rash, myalgia, arthralgia and high fever. After resolution of the fever, a secondary rash with desquamation may occur. Dengue haemorrhagic fever, also known as dengue shock syndrome, occurs when a previously infected child has a subsequent infection with a serologically different strain of the virus. Unfortunately, the partially effective host immune response serves to augment the severity of the infection. The child presents with severe capillary leak syndrome leading to hypotension as well as haemorrhagic manifestations. With fluid resuscitation, most children will recover fully. A patient with this condition is not infectious as direct person-to-person spread does not occur.

Gastroenteritis and dysentery

Gastroenteritis frequently accompanies foreign travel. 'Traveller's diarrhoea' is commonly caused by a change in gut flora, viruses including rotavirus and by *E. coli*. It rarely needs more than attention to rehydration. Fever accompanied by loose stools with blood or mucus suggests dysentery caused by *Shigella, Salmonella, Campylobacter* or *Entamoeba histolytica*. Blood cultures and stool cultures should be taken and appropriate antibiotics started, if indicated.

Viral haemorrhagic fevers

Causes include the Lassa, Marburg, Ebola and Crimean–Congo viruses. These rare infections are imported, although Hantavirus has recently been isolated from within the UK. These are highly contagious, often lethal, infections. If suspected, strict isolation procedures should be initiated for any symptomatic patient who has returned from an endemic area within the 21-day incubation period of these infections. Specialist advice should be sought.

Figure 14.20 An approach to the febrile child returning from the tropics.

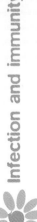

Infection and immunity

263

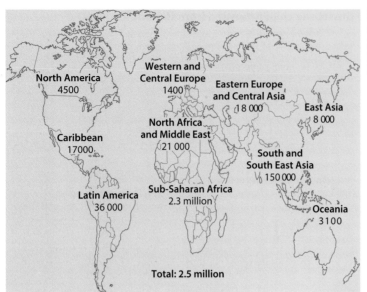

Figure 14.21 Children (<15 years) estimated to be living with HIV, 2009 (UNAIDS, WHO, 2010). Reproduced with the permission of UNICEF.

North America
4500

Western and
Central Europe
1400

Eastern Europe
and Central Asia
18 000

East Asia
8 000

Caribbean
17000

North Africa
and Middle East
21 000

South and
South East Asia
150 000

Latin America
36 000

Sub-Saharan Africa
2.3 million

Oceania
3100

Total: 2.5 million

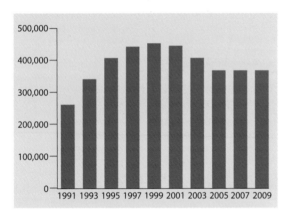

Figure 14.22 New HIV infections among children, 1991–2009, showing recent decline because HIV prevalence in mothers has stabilised and increasing programmes for preventing mother-to-child transmission. (UNAIDS, WHO, 2010; Reproduced with the permission of UNICEF.)

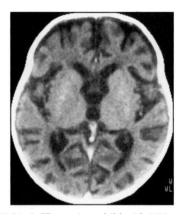

Figure 14.24 A CT scan in a child with HIV encephalopathy showing diffuse increase in CSF spaces from cerebral atrophy and volume loss.

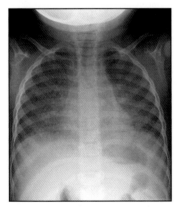

Figure 14.23 Lymphocytic interstitial pneumonitis (LIP) in a child with HIV infection. There is diffuse reticulonodular shadowing with hilar lymphadenopathy.

the routine vaccination schedule, with the exception of BCG which should not be given as it is a live vaccine that can cause disseminated disease. Additional vaccination against influenza, hepatitis A, B and varicella zoster should be considered.

- Multidisciplinary management of children, if possible in a family clinic, where they can be seen together with other members of their family who may be HIV-infected and where the team includes an adult specialist. The team will need to address issues such as adherence to medication, disclosure of HIV diagnosis and planning for the future.
- Regular follow-up, with particular attention paid to weight, neurodevelopment and clinical signs and symptoms of disease. Effective antiretroviral therapy has transformed HIV infection into a chronic disease of childhood. Paediatric HIV clinics increasingly manage adolescents when there may be issues relating to maintaining ART adherence and address maternal issues such as safe sex practices, fertility and pregnancy.

Reduction of vertical transmission

Mothers who are most likely to transmit HIV to their infants are those with a high HIV viral load and more advanced disease. Where mothers breast-feed, 25–40% of infants become infected with HIV and it is known that avoidance of breast-feeding reduces the rate of transmission. In developed countries, perinatal transmission of HIV has been reduced to <1% by using a combination of interventions:

- Use of maternal antenatal, perinatal and postnatal antiretroviral drugs to achieve an undetectable maternal viral load at the time of delivery
- Avoidance of breast-feeding
- Active management of labour and delivery, to avoid prolonged rupture of the membranes or unnecessary instrumentation
- Pre-labour Caesarean section if the mother's viral load is detectable close to the time of delivery.

This effective combination of interventions is not available to all women globally. Avoidance of breast-feeding is not safe in many parts of the world, where use of formula-feeding increases the risk of gastroenteritis and malnutrition. It may be safer for babies in this environment to breast-feed, and antiretroviral drugs may be given to the breast-feeding baby or mother to reduce the ongoing risk of mother-to-child transmission through this route.

 Antenatal antiretroviral drugs, active management of labour and delivery, and avoidance of breast-feeding can reduce vertical transmission of HIV to <1%.

Summary

HIV

- Affects >2 million children worldwide
- Treatment includes combination antiretroviral therapy and prophylaxis against *Pneumocystis jiroveci* pneumonia (PCP)
- The majority of perinatally infected children are surviving into adulthood if ART treatment is available
- Raises complex psychosocial issues for the family and caregivers, including when and what to tell the child and siblings, confidentiality and adherence support.

Lyme disease

This disease, caused by the spirochaete *Borrelia burgdorferi*, was first recognised in 1975 in a cluster of children with arthritis in Lyme, Connecticut. It occurs in the UK. *Borrelia burgdorferi* is transmitted by the hard tick, which has a range of hosts but favours deer and moose. Infections occur most commonly in the summer months in susceptible persons in rural settings.

Clinical features

Following an incubation period of 4–20 days, an erythematous macule at the site of the tick bite enlarges to cause the classical skin lesion known as *erythema migrans,* a painless red expanding lesion with a bright red outer spreading edge. During early disease, the skin lesion is often accompanied by fever, headache, malaise, myalgia, arthralgia and lymphadenopathy. Usually, these features fluctuate over several weeks and then resolve. Dissemination of infection in the early stages is rare, but may lead to cranial nerve palsies, meningitis, arthritis or carditis.

The late stage of Lyme disease occurs after weeks to months with neurological, cardiac and joint manifestations. Neurological disease includes meningoencephalitis and cranial (particularly facial nerve) and peripheral neuropathies. Cardiac disease includes myocarditis and heart block. Joint disease occurs in about 50% and varies from brief migratory arthralgia to acute asymmetric mono- and oligoarthritis of the large joints. Recurrent attacks of arthritis are common. In 10%, chronic erosive joint disease occurs months to years after the initial attack.

Diagnosis

This is based on clinical and epidemiological features and serology. Serology may be negative in early disease, so repeat titres after 2–4 weeks are advised. Isolation of the organism is difficult.

Treatment

The drug of choice for early uncomplicated cases over 12 years of age is doxycycline, and for younger children, amoxicillin. Intravenous treatment with ceftriaxone is required for carditis or neurological disease.

Immunisation

Immunisation is one of the most effective and economic public health measures to improve the health of both children and adults. The most notable success has been the worldwide eradication of smallpox achieved in 1979, but the prevalence of many other diseases has been dramatically reduced.

Differences exist in the composition and scheduling of immunisation programmes in different countries, and schedules change as new vaccines become available. The current UK schedule (Fig. 14.25) is available on the Department of Health website.

Features are:

- In the newborn – BCG is given to infants at high risk of infection
- At 2, 3 and 4 months of age – the '5 in 1' vaccine is given, against diphtheria, tetanus, pertussis, *H. influenzae* type b (Hib) and polio. The oral, live polio vaccine has been replaced by killed-vaccine given by injection, owing to the risk of vaccine-associated polio in unvaccinated family members or immune-deficient people following contact with gastrointestinal excretions of vaccine recipients
- At 2, 4 and 13 months, the pneumococcal conjugate vaccine (PCV13) is given

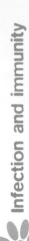

Infection and immunity

Immunisation schedule in the UK (2011)

	Birth	1 month	2 months	3 months	4 months	12-13 months	3 years 4 months +	12-13 years	13-18 years
BCG	BCG if at risk								
Hep B	Hep B if at risk	Hep B if at risk	Hep B if at risk			Hep B if at risk			
Diphtheria, tetanus, pertussis, polio, Haemophilus influenzae type B (DTaP/IPV/Hib)			5 in 1	5 in 1	5 in 1				
Pneumococcal vaccine (PCV)			Pneumo vaccine		Pneumo vaccine	Pneumo vaccine			
Meningococcal group C (MenC)				MenC	MenC				
Hib/MenC						Hib/Men C			
MMR						MMR	MMR		
Diphtheria, tetanus, pertussis, polio, (DTaP/IPV)							DTaP/IPV		
Human papilloma-virus (HPV) Girls only								HPV (3 doses)	
Diphtheria tetanus, polio (Td/IPV)									Td/IPV

Figure 14.25 Immunisation schedule in the UK. (Available at: www.dh.gov.uk, Accessed August 2011.)

- At 3 and 4 months, the conjugate vaccine against group C meningococcus (MenC) is given by separate injection
- At 12–13 months, a booster Hib vaccine is given, MenC and MMR (measles, mumps, rubella) is given
- At 12–13 years of age, the human papillomavirus (HPV) vaccine is given to girls. The rubella vaccine is no longer given to adolescent girls.
- BCG is no longer given to adolescents.

Rationale behind the immunisation programme

Diphtheria – infection causes local disease with membrane formation affecting the nose, pharynx or larynx or systemic disease with myocarditis and neurological manifestations. Immunisation has eradicated the disease in the UK (Fig. 14.26a).

Pertussis – clinical features described in Chapter 16. Huge decline in incidence with immunisation, but epidemics recur when immunisation rates fall (Fig. 14.26b).

Haemophilus influenzae type b – causes invasive disease in young children The number of reports of infection dropped dramatically after the introduction of Hib vaccination (Fig. 14.26c), but a gradual rise from 1988 occurred because protection was not maintained throughout childhood. This was managed with a Hib catch-up programme, and to prevent a further resurgence, a Hib booster dose has been introduced at 12 months of age.

Poliovirus infection – Although most infected children are asymptomatic or have a mild illness, some develop aseptic meningitis and <1% develop paralytic polio. Almost eradicated worldwide (Fig. 14.26d).

Meningococcal C – The marked fall in the number of reports in all age groups is shown in Figure 14.26e.

Pneumococcal vaccination – introduced into the immunisation programme in 2006. Prior to this, about 530 children under 2 years of age developed invasive pneumococcal disease in England and Wales each year. In 2010, a 13-valent conjugate vaccine (PCV, effective against 13 serotypes) was introduced, which protects against about 90% of disease-causing pneumococcal serotypes.

Human papillomavirus (HPV) vaccine – introduced in 2008. Provides protection against the two strains (HPV16 and 18) that cause 70% of cervical cancer. Three doses of vaccine are given over a 6-month period to all girls aged 12–13 years of age.

BCG immunisation – although the number of notifications of TB is rising, it remains uncommon and mainly confined to high-risk populations. BCG immunisation in the neonatal period is therefore targeted to those at increased risk. The main value of BCG is in prevention of disseminated disease (including meningitis) in younger children, hence the rationale for changing the timing of vaccination from early adolescence to the neonatal period.

Hepatitis B and *varicella vaccination* – included in the immunisation programme in the USA and many other countries. In the UK, hepatitis B immunisation is given to babies born to hepatitis B surface antigen positive (HBsAg) mothers at 0, 1, 2 and 12 months of age. Babies born to highly infectious e-antigen positive mothers (HBeAg positive) should additionally receive hepatitis B immunoglobulin at birth. Varicella vaccine is not routinely given in the UK, but may be given to the siblings of 'at-risk' children (e.g. those undergoing chemotherapy).

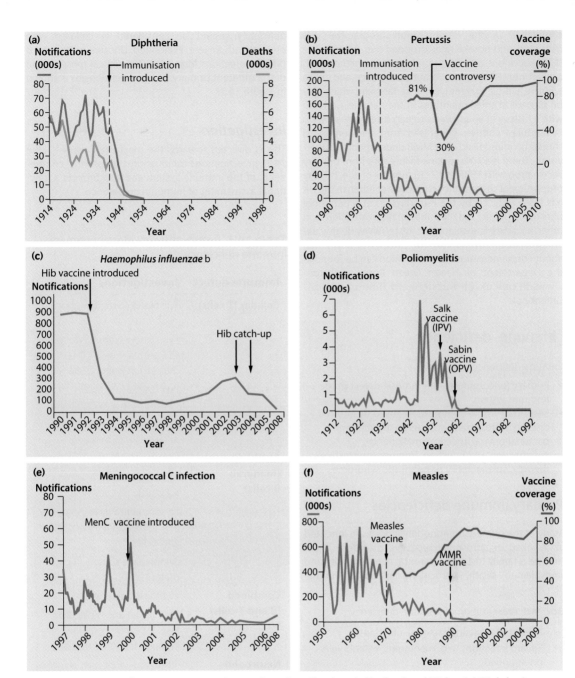

Figure 14.26 Effect of immunisation on the number of notifications in England and Wales. **(a)** Diphtheria. **(b)** Pertussis. **(c)** *Haemophilus influenzae* type b. **(d)** Poliomyelitis. **(e)** Meningococcal disease. **(f)** Measles (Health Protection Agency).

Developing countries – huge effort and funds are devoted to improving immunisation uptake and programmes. The Expanded Programme on Immunization of the WHO is tailored according to healthcare systems. The majority use measles vaccine rather than MMR, for cost–benefit reasons.

Complications and contraindications

Following vaccination, there may be swelling and discomfort at the injection site and a mild fever and malaise. Some vaccines, such as measles and rubella, may be followed by a mild form of the disease 7–10 days later. More serious reactions, including anaphylaxis, may occur but are very rare. Local guidelines about vaccination and its contraindications should be followed. Vaccination should be postponed if the child has an acute illness; however, a minor infection without fever or systemic upset is not a contraindication. Live vaccines should not be given to children with impaired immune responsiveness (except in children with HIV infection in whom MMR vaccine can be given).

The controversy regarding a possible association between MMR vaccination and autism and inflammatory bowel disease has been discredited by a large number of well-conducted studies. However, public confidence in the immunisation programme was damaged, and uptake rates dropped (Fig. 14.26f). The MMR vaccine is only contraindicated in children with proven non-HIV-related immunodeficiency and those who are allergic to neomycin or kanamycin, which may be present in small quantities in the vaccine. Children with a history of anaphylaxis to egg (the virus is grown in fibroblast cultures generated from chick embryos) should be immunised with MMR under medical supervision. There is a 10% vaccine failure rate from primary vaccination with MMR at 12–13 months of age, but the proportion of susceptible school-age children in the UK has been reduced by the introduction of a preschool booster of MMR. Detailed information on MMR and other vaccines is available at: http://www.dh.gov.uk/en/Publichealth/Immunisation; further information about contraindications to vaccination can be found in the Department of Health Green Book, at: http://www.dh.gov.uk/en/Publichealth/Immunisation/Greenbook.

Immune deficiency

Immune deficiency may be:

- Primary (uncommon) – an intrinsic defect in the immune system
- Secondary (more common) – caused by another disease or treatment, such as an intercurrent bacterial or viral infection, malignancy, malnutrition, HIV infection, immunosuppressive therapy, splenectomy or nephrotic syndrome.

Primary immune deficiencies

Many of the primary immunodeficiencies are inherited as X-linked or autosomal recessive disorders. There may be a family history of parental consanguinity and unexplained death, particularly in boys. Immune

Box 14.3 Presentation of immune deficiency

- Recurrent (proven) bacterial infections
- Severe infections (e.g. meningitis, osteomyelitis, pneumonia)
- Infections that present atypically, are unusually severe or chronic or fail regular treatment
- Infections caused by an unexpected or opportunistic pathogen or child has been immunised against
- Severe or long-lasting warts, generalised molluscum contagiosum
- Extensive candidiasis
- Complications of vaccination (disseminated BCG)
- Abscesses of internal organs; recurrent subcutaneous abscesses
- Prolonged or recurrent diarrhoea.

From: de Vries E. 2006. Patient-centred screening for primary immunodeficiency: a multi-stage diagnostic protocol designed for non-immunologists. *Clin Exp Immunol* 145:204–214.

deficiency should be considered in children who present with **S**evere, **P**rolonged, **U**nusual or **R**ecurrent (**SPUR**) infections (Box 14.3). The clinical presentation of the different primary immune deficiencies is shown in Figure 14.27.

Investigation

This is directed towards the most likely cause (Table 14.3). Investigations can quantify the essential components of the immune system and also provide a functional assessment of immunocompetence.

Table 14.3 Investigation to identify primary immune deficiency

Immune defect	Investigations
Cellular (T cells)	Full blood count (lymphocyte count)
	Lymphocyte subsets (to assess CD3+ (total T cell), CD4+ (helper T cell) and CD8+ (cytotoxic T cell) numbers)
	PHA (phytohaemagglutinin)
	Ability of T cells to proliferate in response to mitogen
Antibody (humoral; B cells)	Immunoglobulins
	IgG subclasses (in children >2 years)
	Specific antibody responses (e.g. tetanus, pneumococcal antibodies)
	Lymphocyte subsets (B cells present?)
Combined (B and T cells)	Investigations as above
	Specific genetic/molecular tests for severe combined immunodeficiency (SCID)
Neutrophils	Full blood count (neutropenia)
	Nitroblue tetrazolium (NBT) – abnormal in chronic granulomatous disease
	Tests for leucocyte adhesion deficiency – CD11b/CD18 expression
	Tests of chemotaxis (neutrophil mobility)
Complement/ mannose-binding lectin	Tests of classical and alternative complement pathways (CH50, AP50)
	Assays for individual complement proteins
	Mannose-binding lectin levels

Clinical presentation of primary immune deficiency

| Defect | ⇨ | Presentation | ⇨ | Examples |

T-cell defects ⇨ Severe and/or unusual viral and fungal infections and failure to thrive in first months of life, e.g. severe bronchiolitis, diarrhoea, oral thrush, *Pneumocystis jiroveci (carinii)* pneumonia (PCP). ⇨

Severe combined immunodeficiency (SCID). Heterogeneous group of inherited disorders of profoundly defective cellular and humoral immunity. Fatal without treatment.

HIV infection

Wiskott-Aldrich – triad with thrombocytopenia, and eczema (X-linked).
DiGeorge – with maldevelopment of the 5th branchial arch causing heart defects, palatal and facial defects, absence of thymus and hypocalcaemia (deletion of section of chromosome 22).
Duncan syndrome (X-linked lymphoproliferative disease) – inability to make a normal response to Epstein–Barr virus; either succumb to the initial infection or develop secondary lymphoma (X-linked).
Ataxia telangectasia – defect in DNA repair, also increased risk of lymphoma. Cerebellar ataxia, developmental delay.

B-cell (antibody) defects ⇨ In first 2 years (beyond infancy because of passively acquired maternal antibody) – severe bacterial infections, especially ear, sinus, pulmonary and skin infections; recurrent diarrhoea and failure to thrive. Recurrent pneumonias can lead to bronchiectasis; recurrent ear infections to impaired hearing. ⇨

X-linked (Bruton) agammaglobulinaemia. Abnormal tyrosine kinase gene; essential for B-cell maturation.
Common variable immune deficiency (CVID) – B-cell deficiency. High risk of autoimmune disorders and malignancy. Later onset than Bruton agammaglobulinaemia.
Hyper IgM syndrome – B cells produce IgM but prevented from switching to IgG and IgA.
Selective IgA deficiency – most common primary immune defect. Usually asymptomatic, or recurrent ear, sinus and pulmonary infections.

Neutrophil defects ⇨ Recurrent bacterial infections – abscesses (skin, lymph nodes, lung, liver, spleen, bone), poor wound healing, perianal disease and periodontal infections; invasive fungal infections, such as aspergillosis. Diarrhoea and failure to thrive. Granulomas from chronic inflammation. ⇨

Chronic granulomatous disease – most are X-linked recessive, some autosomal recessive. Defect in phagocytosis as fail to produce superoxide after ingestion of micro-organisms.

Leucocyte function defects ⇨ Delayed separation of umbilical cord, delayed wound healing, chronic skin ulcers and deep-seated infections. ⇨

Leucocyte adhesion deficiency (LAD) – deficiency of neutrophil surface adhesion molecules, CD18, CD11b, leads to inability of neutrophils to migrate to sites of infection/inflammation.

Complement defects ⇨ Recurrent bacterial infections. SLE-like illness. Recurrent meningococcal infections – with deficiency of the terminal complement components (C5b to C9). ⇨

Early complement component deficiency
Terminal complement component deficiency
Mannose-binding lectin (MBL) deficiency.

Figure 14.27 Clinical presentation of primary immune deficiency.

Infection and immunity

Management

Management options include:

- Antimicrobial prophylaxis
  - For T-cell and neutrophil defects – cotrimoxazole to prevent *Pneumocystis jiroveci* infection and itraconazole or fluconazole to prevent other fungal infections
  - For B-cell defects – antibiotic prophylaxis (e.g. azithromycin) to prevent recurrent bacterial (e.g. chest, ear, sinus) infections
- Antibiotic treatment
  - Prompt treatment of infections
  - Appropriate choice of antibiotics to cover likely organisms
  - Generally longer courses, with lower threshold for intravenous therapy
- Screening for end-organ disease
  - e.g. CT scan in children with antibody deficiency to detect bronchiectasis
- Immunoglobulin replacement therapy
  - For children with antibody deficiency
  - Can be given intravenously, which may require central venous (Portacath or Hickman) line insertion or subcutaneously
- Bone marrow transplantation
  - e.g. for SCID (severe combined immuno-deficiency), chronic granulomatous disease
  - Can be matched sibling donor, matched unrelated donor or haploidentical (parental) transplant
- Gene therapy
  - For certain forms of SCID, but associated with a risk of leukaemia.

Further reading

American Academy of Pediatrics: *Report of the Committee on Infectious Diseases. 'Red Book'*, ed 27, Illinois, 2006, AAP.

Useful manual on paediatric infection and immunisation in the USA.

Feigin RD, Cherry JD: *Textbook of Pediatric Infectious Diseases*, ed 5, Philadelphia, PA, 2004, Saunders.

Large comprehensive textbook.

Websites for updates on immunisation and current information on infectious diseases (Accessed May 2011)

Meningitis Research Foundation: Available at: http://www.meningitis.org.

Useful teaching material on meningitis.

American Academy of Pediatrics: Available at: http://www.aap.org.

Centers for Disease Control, Atlanta, USA: Available at: http://www.cdc.gov.

CHIVA: Children's HIV Association of UK and Ireland. Available at: http://www.bhiva.org/chiva.

Guidelines to reduce HIV vertical transmission.

Department of Health Immunisation Information: Available at: http://www.dh.gov.uk/en/Publichealth/Immunisation.

Up-to-date information on the immunisation programme in the UK.

Health Protection Agency: Available at: http://www.hpa.org.uk.

MMR: The facts. Available at: http://www.dh.gov.uk/en/Publicationsandstatistics/Publications/PublicationsPolicyAndGuidance/DH_4002972.

Information about the MMR vaccine.

UNAIDS: Available at: http://www.unaids.org.

Worldwide information on HIV.

World Health Organization: Available at: http://www.who.int.

Allergy

An abnormal immune system may result in:

- Allergic diseases
- Immune deficiencies
- Autoimmune disorders – either organ specific (e.g. type I diabetes mellitus) or systemic (e.g. systemic lupus erythematosus).

Paediatric allergy

Allergic diseases which affect children include food allergy, eczema, allergic rhinitis and conjunctivitis, asthma, urticaria, insect sting hypersensitivity and anaphylaxis. The reasons allergic diseases are important are:

- In the UK up to 40% of children have allergic rhinitis, eczema or asthma and up to 6% develop food allergy
- They are increasing in prevalence in many countries
- They are the commonest chronic diseases of childhood and the commonest cause of school absence and acute hospital admissions
- They cause significant morbidity and can be fatal, with about 20 children dying from asthma and 2 from food anaphylaxis in the UK each year.

Explanations of some of the terms used in 'allergy' are listed in Box 15.1.

Mechanisms of allergic disease

Many genes have been linked to the development of allergic disease. Polymorphisms or mutations in these genes lead to a susceptibility to allergy.

Allergic diseases occur when individuals make an abnormal immune response to harmless environmental stimuli, usually proteins. The developing immune system must be 'sensitised' to an allergen before an allergic immune response develops. However, sensitisation can be 'occult', e.g. sensitisation to egg from exposure to trace quantities of egg in maternal breast milk.

Only a few stimuli account for most allergic disease:

- Inhalant allergens, e.g. house-dust mite, plant pollens, pet dander and moulds in asthma and rhinitis and conjunctivitis
- Ingestant allergens, e.g. nuts, seeds, legumes, cow's milk, egg, seafood and fruits in acute allergic reactions or eczema
- Insect stings/bites, drugs and natural rubber latex.

Proteins with an unstable tertiary structure may be rendered non-allergenic by heat degradation or other forms of processing. For example, some children are allergic to raw apples, but can tolerate eating cooked apples.

Box 15.1 Allergy definitions

- *Hypersensitivity* – objectively reproducible symptoms or signs following exposure to a defined stimulus (e.g. food, drug, pollen) at a dose which is tolerated by normal people.
- *Allergy* – a hypersensitivity reaction initiated by specific immunological mechanisms. This can be IgE mediated (e.g. peanut allergy) or non-IgE mediated (e.g. coeliac disease).
- *Atopy* – a personal and/or familial tendency to produce IgE antibodies in response to ordinary exposures to potential allergens, usually proteins. Strongly associated with asthma, allergic rhinitis and conjunctivitis, eczema and food allergy.
- *Anaphylaxis* – a serious allergic reaction that is rapid in onset and may cause death.

Allergic immune responses are classified as IgE mediated or non-IgE mediated. IgE-mediated allergic reactions have a characteristic clinical course:

- An early phase, occurring within minutes of exposure to the allergen, caused by release of histamine and other mediators from mast cells. Causes urticaria, angioedema, sneezing and bronchospasm
- A late phase response may also occur after 4–6 hours. This causes nasal congestion in the upper airway, and cough and bronchospasm in the lower airway.

The majority of severe life-threatening allergic reactions are IgE mediated.

Non-IgE-mediated allergic immune responses have a delayed onset of symptoms and more varied clinical course.

The hygiene hypothesis

It is not clear why the prevalence of allergic diseases has increased in many countries and the speed of this change suggests an environmental cause. A consistent observation is that the risk is lower in younger children of large families and in children raised on farms. These findings have led to the hygiene hypothesis, which proposes that the increased prevalence is due to altered microbial exposure associated with modern living conditions (Fig. 15.1). Although the hypothesis remains the leading explanation for the increase in allergic disease, it is mainly supported by indirect evidence.

The allergic march

Allergic children develop individual allergic disorders at different ages:

- Eczema and food allergy usually develop in infancy; both are often present

- Allergic rhinitis and conjunctivitis and asthma occur most often in preschool and primary school years
- Rhinitis and conjunctivitis often precede the development of asthma, and in children with asthma, up to 80% have coexistent rhinitis.

The presence of eczema or food allergy in infancy is predictive of asthma and allergic rhinitis in later life. The progression is referred to as the 'allergic march'.

Prevention of allergic diseases

Many interventions have been tried to prevent allergic disease, or interrupt the allergic march. These include exclusive breast-feeding for at least 3–4 months (or if not possible, then use of hydrolysed formula instead of standard formula milk) to reduce the risk of eczema and cow's milk allergy and the use of probiotics for eczema in infancy. Other approaches include altering allergen exposure (avoidance of allergens in early life, or alternatively, exposure to large doses of allergens to induce immune tolerance), prebiotics (non-digestible oligosaccharides naturally present in breast milk), nutritional supplements (e.g. omega-3 fatty acids, vitamin D, antioxidants, trace elements) and medications (e.g. antihistamines, immunotherapy). However, none have been shown, long term, to prevent children from developing allergic diseases.

History and examination

The child and family may not volunteer a history of allergic disease as they have come to consider the symptoms as normal, e.g. the child who coughs most nights or has a blocked nose most of the time may not perceive this as abnormal. As allergic diseases are multisystem, in addition to the signs of individual allergic diseases, examination may reveal:

- Mouth breathing (Fig. 15.2a). Children who habitually breathe with their mouth open may have an obstructed nasal airway from rhinitis, and there may also be a history of snoring or obstructive sleep apnoea
- An allergic salute (Fig. 15.2b), from rubbing an itchy nose
- Pale and swollen inferior nasal turbinates
- Hyperinflated chest or Harrison sulci from chronic undertreated asthma
- Atopic eczema affecting the limb flexures
- Allergic conjunctivitis; may also be prominent creases (Dennie-Morgan folds) and blue-grey discoloration below the lower eyelids.

Growth needs to be checked, especially in those with food allergy, where dietary restrictions or malabsorption can lead to nutritional compromise, and in those treated with high-dose inhaled/nasal/topical corticosteroids.

Management

The individual diseases are managed by general practitioners, general paediatricians or organ-specific specialists, e.g. eczema by dermatologists, asthma by respiratory paediatricians. However, allergic diseases

Hygiene hypothesis

Developed urban environment		Developing rural environment
Small	Family size	Large
Low	Exposure to parasites	High
Few	Infections	Many
High	Antibiotic exposure	Low
Low	Farming exposure	High
Low	Microbiological exposure	High
Allergy and autoimmune disease		No allergy or autoimmune disease

Figure 15.1 Hygiene hypothesis.

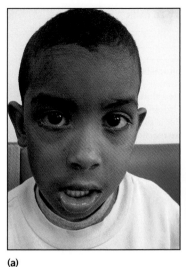
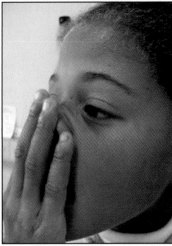

Figure 15.2 Allergic facies. **(a)** There is a habitually open mouth due to mouth breathing. **(b)** An allergic salute, from rubbing an itchy nose. (Courtesy Dr George Du Toit.)

(a)   (b)

coexist and it is therefore helpful to consider allergy as a systemic disease. The role of paediatric allergists is to identify triggers to avoid, and to manage children with multisystem or severe disease.

Management of specific conditions is described below. In addition, specific allergen immunotherapy can be used for treating allergic rhinitis and conjunctivitis, insect stings, anaphylaxis and asthma. During immunotherapy, solutions of an allergen to which the patient is allergic are injected subcutaneously or administered sublingually on a regular basis for 3–5 years, with the aim of developing immune tolerance. It is highly effective in providing protection for many years. However, it must be carried out under specialist supervision due to the risk of inducing severe allergic reactions (anaphylaxis). Allergen immunotherapy is widely used in the USA and some countries in Europe. Sublingual immunotherapy appears to be safer than subcutaneous injections and is used increasingly. Immunotherapy for food allergy is under investigation but has not yet been shown to be safe for use in clinical practice.

Summary

Paediatric allergy

- Includes food allergy, eczema, allergic rhinitis and conjunctivitis, asthma, urticaria, insect sting hypersensitivity and anaphylaxis
- Occurs when a genetically susceptible person reacts abnormally to an environmental antigen
- There is an 'allergic march' of disorders
- Different allergic diseases often coexist – if a child has one, look for others.

Food allergy and food intolerance

A food allergy occurs when a pathological immune response is mounted against a specific food protein. It is usually IgE mediated, but may be non-IgE mediated.

A non-immunological hypersensitivity reaction to a specific food is called food intolerance. An example of each in relation to cow's milk is shown in Figure 15.3.

Food allergy is usually primary, where children have failed to ever develop immune tolerance to the relevant food. Presentation varies with the agent and the child's age:

- In infants, the most common causes are milk, egg and peanut
- In older children, peanut, tree nut and fish and shellfish.

Food allergy can also be secondary, where children initially tolerate a food and then later become allergic to it. Secondary food allergy is usually due to cross-reactivity between proteins present in fresh fruits/vegetables/nuts and those present in pollens, e.g. a child who can eat apples may develop allergy to apples in the future if they develop allergy to birch tree pollen, because the apple and birch pollen share a very similar protein. This is termed the 'oral allergy syndrome' or 'pollen fruit syndrome'. It is very common but generally leads to milder allergic reactions than primary food allergy, often causing an itchy mouth but no systemic symptoms.

Non-IgE food allergy typically occurs hours after ingestion and usually involves the gastrointestinal tract.

Food allergy and intolerance are different from food aversion, where the person refuses the food for psychological or behavioural reasons.

Clinical features

In IgE-mediated food allergy there is a history of allergic symptoms varying from urticaria to facial swelling to anaphylaxis (Fig. 15.3), usually occurring 10–15 min after ingestion of a food. It is often the first occasion the food is knowingly ingested.

Non-IgE-mediated food allergy usually presents with diarrhoea, vomiting, abdominal pain and sometimes failure to thrive. Colic or eczema may also be present. It sometimes presents with blood in the stools in the first few weeks of life from proctitis.

Examples of food allergy and hypersensitivity to milk

Condition	Clinical manifestation	
IgE-mediated food allergy • Immediate cow's milk allergy	This 6-month-old breast-fed infant developed an allergic reaction **(a)**, with widespread urticaria immediately after the first formula feed. Skin-prick test were strongly positive to cow's milk. Widespread urticaria and lip swelling after milk ingestion are shown in **(b)** and **(c)**	**(a) Clinical features of an acute allergic reaction:** **Mild reaction** • Urticaria and itchy skin • Facial swelling **Severe reaction** • Wheeze • Stridor • Abdominal pain, vomiting, diarrhoea • Shock, collapse

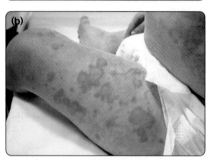 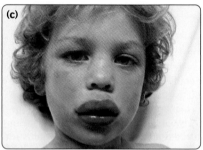

Non-IgE-mediated cow's milk allergy	A 4-month-old infant, formula fed since birth, has loose stools and is failing to thrive. Skin prick test to cow's milk is negative. Elimination of cow's milk results in resolution of symptoms which return on trial re-introduction.
Non-allergic food hypersensitivity • Temporary lactose intolerance	Previously well 12-month-old infant develops diarrhoea and vomiting. The vomiting settles but watery stools continue for several weeks. Stool sample – no pathogens but positive for reducing substances. Diagnosis – temporary lactose intolerance.

Figure 15.3 Examples of food allergy and hypersensitivity to milk. **(a)** Clinical features of an acute allergic reaction. **(b,c)** Widespread urticaria and lip swelling after milk ingestion. (Courtesy Dr Pete Smith.)

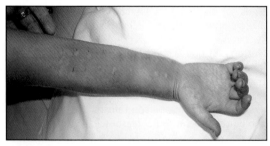

Figure 15.4 Skin-prick testing for IgE-mediated allergy. A drop of the allergen is placed on the skin, the site is marked and pricked with a needle, and any weals measured. Multiple positive results are present. (Courtesy Dr Pete Smith.)

Diagnosis

The most helpful screening tests for IgE-mediated food allergy are skin-prick tests (Fig. 15.4) and measurement of specific IgE antibodies in blood (RAST test). Both tests may yield false-positive results, but the greater the response, the more likely the child is to be allergic. Negative skin test results make IgE-mediated allergy unlikely.

Non-IgE-mediated food allergies are harder to diagnose. Diagnosis relies on clinical history and examination. If indicated, endoscopy and intestinal biopsy may be obtained; the diagnosis is supported by the presence of eosinophilic infiltrates.

For both IgE-mediated and non-IgE-mediated food allergies, the gold standard investigation in cases of doubt is exclusion of the relevant food under a dietitian's supervision, followed by a double-blind placebo-controlled food challenge. This involves the child being given increasing amounts of the food or placebo, starting with a tiny quantity, until a full portion is reached. The test should be performed in hospital with full resuscitation facilities available, and close monitoring for signs of an allergic reaction.

Management

The management of a food-allergic child involves avoidance of the relevant foods. This can be very difficult as the relevant food(s) may be present in small quantities in many foods and food labels are often unclear. Food labelling in the European Union legally requires common food allergens to be clearly disclosed. Food which is packaged or sold elsewhere may be less closely regulated. The advice of a paediatric dietitian is essential to aid patients avoid foods to which they are allergic and avoid nutritional deficiencies.

In addition, the child and family must be able to manage an allergic attack. Written self-management plans and adequate training are essential. Drug management for mild reactions (no cardiorespiratory symptoms) is with antihistamines. If the child has a severe reaction, treatment is with epinephrine (adrenaline) given intramuscularly by auto-injector (e.g. Epipen or Anapen), which the child or parent should carry with them at all times.

Food allergy to cow's milk and egg often resolves in early childhood; food allergy to nuts and seafood usually persists through to adulthood.

Summary

Food allergy

- Affects up to 6% of children
- The most common causes are milk, egg, nuts, seafood, wheat, legumes, seeds and fruits
- Diagnosis of IgE-mediated food allergy is based on a suggestive history supported by skin-prick tests or specific IgE antibodies in blood
- Supervised food challenge is sometimes necessary to clarify the diagnosis
- Those at risk of a severe reaction, e.g. with coexistent asthma, should carry an epinephrine (adrenaline) auto-injector.

Eczema

Eczema is classified as atopic (where there is evidence of IgE antibodies to common allergens) or non-atopic. Atopic eczema is classified as an allergic disease as many affected children will have a family history of allergy, at least 50% develop other allergic diseases and IgE antibodies to common allergens are present. There is a close relationship between eczema and food allergy, particularly in young infants with severe disease; up to 40% of them have an IgE-mediated food allergy, in particular egg allergy. Screening by skin prick or IgE blood testing should be considered. The condition is described in Chapter 24.

Allergic rhinitis and conjunctivitis (rhinoconjunctivitis)

This can be atopic (associated with IgE antibodies to common inhalant allergens) or non-atopic. It is an underestimated cause of childhood morbidity. The

Box 15.2 Range of treatment for allergic rhinoconjunctivitis

- Second-generation non-sedating antihistamines (used topically or systemically)
- Topical corticosteroid nasal or eye preparations (the latter under specialist ophthalmology supervision)
- Cromoglycate eye drops
- Leukotriene receptor antagonists, e.g. montelukast
- Nasal decongestants (use for no more than 7–10 days due to risk of rebound effect)
- Allergen immunotherapy – sublingual or subcutaneous (limited by anaphylaxis risk)
- Systemic corticosteroids should not be used due to the risk of adverse effects.

disease can be classified as intermittent or persistent and mild or severe, although in temperate climates it is often classified as seasonal (related to seasonal grass, weed or tree pollens) and perennial (related to perennial allergens such as house-dust mite and pets). It affects up to 20% of children and can severely disrupt their lives. In addition to its classic presentation of coryza and conjunctivitis, it can also present as 'cough-variant rhinitis' due to a post-nasal drip, and as a chronically blocked nose causing sleep disturbance and impaired daytime behaviour and concentration, or with predominant eye symptoms. It is associated with eczema, sinusitis and adenoidal hypertrophy and is closely associated with asthma. Treatment of allergic rhinitis may improve the control of coexistent asthma. Treatment options are listed in Box 15.2.

Asthma

Allergy is an important component of asthma. Affected children often have IgE antibodies to aeroallergens (house-dust mite; tree, grass and weed pollens; moulds; animal danders). Allergen avoidance is difficult to achieve. Management of asthma is described in Chapter 16 on Respiratory disorders.

Urticaria and angioedema

Acute urticaria usually results from exposure to an allergen or a viral infection, which triggers an urticarial skin reaction. It may also involve deeper tissues to produce swelling of the lips and soft tissues around the eyes (angioedema), and even anaphylaxis.

Chronic urticaria (persisting >6 weeks) is usually non-allergic in origin. It results from a local increase in the permeability of capillaries and venules. These changes are dependent on activation of skin mast cells, which contain a range of mediators including histamine. A classification of urticaria is shown in Box 15.3. Treatment is with second-generation non-sedating antihistamines.

Allergy

Box 15.3 Classification of urticaria/angioedema

- Acute – resolve within 6 weeks; allergy such as food or drug reactions, or infection are common triggers
- Chronic idiopathic – intermittent for at least 6 weeks
- Physical urticarias
  - Cold, delayed pressure, heat contact, solar, vibratory urticaria
- Other causes
  - Water (aquagenic), sweating (cholinergic), exercise-induced
  - Aspirin and other non-steroidal anti-inflammatory agents
  - C1-esterase inhibitor deficiency (angioedema, but no urticaria or pruritus).

Drug allergy

Drug allergies do occur in children, especially to antibiotics, but only a minority who are labelled 'drug allergic' are truly allergic. This is usually because viral illnesses, for which children are often prescribed antibiotics, themselves cause skin rashes. A detailed history is required of the nature and timing of the rash in relation to taking the antibiotics.

Allergy skin and blood tests can be used to support a diagnosis of drug allergy, but a drug challenge may be the only way to conclusively confirm or refute the diagnosis. This is contraindicated after a severe allergic reaction and an alternative drug should be sought.

Insect sting hypersensitivity

This arises mainly from bee and wasp stings, but also from ant species in the USA, Asia and Australia. The severity of the allergic reaction may be:

- mild – local swelling
- moderate – generalised urticaria
- severe – systemic symptoms with wheeze or shock.

Children with a previous mild or moderate reaction are unlikely to develop a severe reaction in the future and the families can be reassured. Those who had a severe reaction should carry an epinephrine (adrenaline) auto-injector, and allergen immunotherapy should be considered.

Summary

Insect sting hypersensitivity

- Mainly to bee and wasp stings
- Following a severe reaction, an epinephrine (adrenaline) auto-injector should be carried
- Immunotherapy is highly effective in children who have had a severe reaction.

Anaphylaxis

This serious and potentially life-threatening allergic reaction is described in Chapter 6 on Paediatric emergencies.

Further reading

Kay AB: Advances in immunology: allergy and allergic disease (first of two parts). *New England Journal of Medicine* 344(1):30–37, 2001.

Lack G: Clinical practice. Food allergy. *New England Journal of Medicine* 359(12):1252–1260, 2008.

Strachan DP: Family size, infection and atopy: the first decade of the 'hygiene hypothesis'. *Thorax* 55(Suppl 1):S2–S10, 2000.

Websites (Accessed April 2011)

Food Allergy and Anaphylaxis Network: Available at http://www.foodallergy.org

A non-profit organisation for people with food allergy.

The UCB Institute of Allergy: Available at http://www.theucbinstituteofallergy.com/healthprofessionals/knowbetterallergy/whatisallergy/index.asp

An industry-supported non-profit organisation for allergy education.

The Anaphylaxis Campaign: Available at: http://www.anaphylaxis.org.uk.

A charity for people at risk from anaphylaxis.

Respiratory disorders

Notable features of respiratory disorders are:

- Worldwide, respiratory disorders are the most common cause of death in children
- In the UK, respiratory disorders account for 50% of consultations with general practitioners for acute illness in young children and a third of consultations in older children
- Respiratory disorders are responsible for about 25% of acute paediatric admissions to hospital, some of which are life-threatening
- Asthma is the most common chronic illness of childhood in the UK
- Cystic fibrosis is the most common inherited life-limiting disorder in Caucasians.

Respiratory infections

These are the most frequent infections of childhood. The preschool child has, on average, 6–8 respiratory infections a year. Most are mild self-limiting illnesses of the upper respiratory tract (ear, nose, throat) but some, such as bronchiolitis or pneumonia, are potentially life-threatening.

Pathogens

Viruses cause 80–90% of childhood respiratory infections. The most important are the respiratory syncytial virus (RSV), rhinoviruses, parainfluenza, influenza, metapneumovirus and adenoviruses. An individual virus can cause several different patterns of illness, e.g. RSV can cause bronchiolitis, croup, pneumonia or a common cold.

The important bacterial pathogens of the respiratory tract are *Streptococcus pneumoniae* (pneumococcus) and other streptococci, *Haemophilus influenzae*, *Moraxella catarrhalis*, *Bordetella pertussis*, which causes whooping cough, and *Mycoplasma pneumoniae*. Dual infections, with two viruses or with a viral and bacterial pathogen, may occur. *Mycobacterium tuberculosis* remains an important pathogen globally. Some pathogens cause predictable epidemics, such as RSV bronchiolitis every winter.

Host and environmental factors

An increased risk of respiratory infection is associated with a range of factors relating to the environment and host:

- Parental smoking, especially maternal
- Poor socioeconomic status – large family size, overcrowded, damp housing
- Poor nutrition
- Underlying lung disease – such as bronchopulmonary dysplasia in infants who were born preterm, cystic fibrosis or asthma
- Male gender
- Haemodynamically significant congenital heart disease
- Immunodeficiency (either primary, see Ch. 14, or secondary, e.g. from HIV infection or chemotherapy).

The child's age influences the prevalence and severity of infections (Fig. 16.1). It is in infancy that serious respiratory illness requiring hospital admission is most common and the risk of death is greatest. There is an increased frequency of infections when the child or older siblings start nursery or school. Repeated upper respiratory tract infection is common and rarely indicates underlying disease.

Classification of respiratory infections

Respiratory infections are classified according to the level of the respiratory tract most involved:

- Upper respiratory tract infection
- Laryngeal/tracheal infection
- Bronchitis
- Bronchiolitis
- Pneumonia.

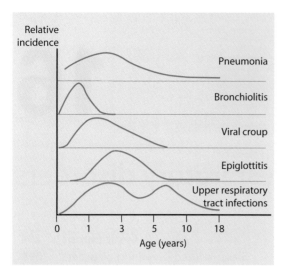

Figure 16.1 Age distribution of acute respiratory infections in children.

Upper respiratory tract infection (URTI)

Approximately 80% of all respiratory infections involve only the nose, throat, ears or sinuses. The term URTI embraces a number of different conditions:

- Common cold (coryza)
- Sore throat (pharyngitis, including tonsillitis)
- Acute otitis media
- Sinusitis (relatively uncommon).

The commonest presentation is a child with a combination of nasal discharge and blockage, fever, painful throat and earache. Cough may be troublesome. URTIs may cause:

- Difficulty in feeding in infants as their noses are blocked and this obstructs breathing
- Febrile convulsions
- Acute exacerbations of asthma.

In infants, hospital admission may be required to exclude a more serious infection, if feeding is inadequate, or for parental reassurance.

The common cold (coryza)

This is the commonest infection of childhood. Classical features include a clear or mucopurulent nasal discharge and nasal blockage. The commonest pathogens are viruses – rhinoviruses (of which there are over 100 different serotypes), coronaviruses and RSV. Health education to advise parents that colds are self-limiting and have no specific curative treatment may reduce anxiety and save unnecessary visits to doctors. Fever and pain are best treated with paracetamol or ibuprofen. Antibiotics are of no benefit as the common cold is viral in origin and secondary bacterial infection is very uncommon.

Sore throat (pharyngitis)

The pharynx and soft palate are inflamed and local lymph nodes are enlarged and tender. Sore throats are usually due to viral infection with respiratory viruses (mostly adenoviruses, enteroviruses and rhinoviruses).

In the older child, group A β-haemolytic streptococcus is a common pathogen.

Tonsillitis

Tonsillitis is a form of pharyngitis where there is intense inflammation of the tonsils, often with a purulent exudate. Common pathogens are group A β-haemolytic streptococci and the Epstein–Barr virus (infectious mononucleosis). Group A β-haemolytic streptococcus can be cultured from many tonsils; however, it is uncertain why it causes recurrent tonsillitis in some children but not in others.

Although the surface exudates seen in infectious mononucleosis are reported to be more membranous in appearance compared to bacterial tonsillitis, in reality it is not possible to distinguish clinically between viral and bacterial causes. Marked constitutional disturbance, such as headache, apathy and abdominal pain, white tonsillar exudate and cervical lymphadenopathy, is more common with bacterial infection.

Antibiotics (often penicillin, or erythromycin if there is penicillin allergy) are often prescribed for severe pharyngitis and tonsillitis even though only a third are caused by bacteria. They may hasten recovery from streptococcal infection. In order to eradicate the organism to prevent rheumatic fever, 10 days of treatment is required, but this is not indicated in the UK where rheumatic fever is now exceedingly rare. In severe cases, children may require hospital admission for intravenous fluid administration and analgesia if they are unable to swallow solids or liquids. Amoxicillin is best avoided as it may cause a widespread maculo-papular rash if the tonsillitis is due to infectious mononucleosis.

 It is not possible to distinguish clinically between viral and bacterial tonsillitis.

Acute infection of the middle ear (acute otitis media)

Most children will have at least one episode of acute otitis media (OM). This is most common at 6–12 months of age. Up to 20% will have three or more episodes. Infants and young children are prone to acute otitis media because their Eustachian tubes are short, horizontal and function poorly. There is pain in the ear and fever. Every child with a fever must have their tympanic membranes examined (Fig. 16.2a–d). In acute otitis media, the tympanic membrane is seen to be bright red and bulging with loss of the normal light reflection (Fig. 16.2b). Occasionally, there is acute perforation of the eardrum with pus visible in the external canal. Pathogens include viruses, especially RSV and rhinovirus, and bacteria including pneumococcus, non-typeable *H. influenzae* and *Moraxella catarrhalis*. Serious complications are mastoiditis and meningitis, but are now uncommon. Pain should be treated with an analgesic such as paracetamol or ibuprofen. Regular analgesia is more effective than intermittent (as required) and may be needed for up to a week until the acute inflammation has resolved. Most cases of acute otitis media resolve spontaneously. Antibiotics marginally shorten the duration of pain but have not been

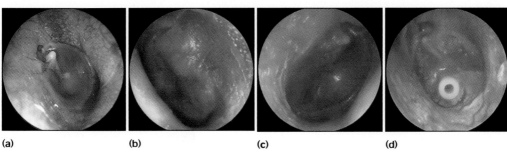

Figure 16.2 Appearance of the eardrum. **(a)** Normal. **(b)** Acute otitis media. **(c)** Otitis media with effusion. **(d)** Grommet. (Courtesy of Mr N Shah & Mr N Tolley.)

shown to reduce the risk of hearing loss (see Ch. 5). It is often useful to give the parents a prescription, but ask them to use it only if the child remains unwell after 2–3 days. Amoxicillin is widely used. Neither decongestants nor antihistamines are beneficial.

Recurrent ear infections can lead to otitis media with effusion (OME or glue ear or serous otitis media). Children are asymptomatic apart from possible decreased hearing. The eardrum is seen to be dull and retracted, often with a fluid level visible (Fig. 16.2c). Confirmation of otitis media with effusion can be gained by a flat trace on tympanometry, in conjunction with evidence of a conductive loss on pure tone audiometry (possible if >4 years old), or reduced hearing on a distraction hearing test in younger children. Otitis media with effusion is very common between the ages of 2 and 7 years, with peak incidence between 2.5 and 5 years. This condition usually resolves spontaneously. Cochrane reviews have shown no evidence of long-term benefit from the use of antibiotics, steroids or decongestants. Otitis media with effusion is the most common cause of conductive hearing loss in children and can interfere with normal speech development and result in learning difficulties in school. In such children insertion of ventilation tubes (grommets, Fig. 16.2d) can be beneficial, but there is evidence, again from Cochrane reviews, that adenoidectomy can offer more long-term benefit. It is believed that the adenoids can harbour organisms within biofilms that contribute to infection spreading up the Eustachian tubes. In addition, grossly hypertrophied adenoids may obstruct and affect the function of the Eustachian tubes, leading to poor ventilation of the middle ear and subsequent recurrent infections. In practice, children with recurrent URTIs and chronic glue ear that do not resolve with conservative measures undergo grommet insertion. If these problems recur

after grommet extrusion, reinsertion of grommets with adjuvant adenoidectomy is usually advocated.

Sinusitis

Infection of the paranasal sinuses may occur with viral URTIs. Occasionally there is secondary bacterial infection, with pain, swelling and tenderness over the cheek from infection of the maxillary sinus. As the frontal sinuses do not develop until late childhood, frontal sinusitis is uncommon in the first decade of life. Antibiotics and analgesia are used for acute sinusitis in addition to topical decongestants. There is some recent evidence that the concurrent use of intranasal corticosteroids or antihistamines together with antibiotics hasten recovery.

Tonsillectomy and adenoidectomy

Children with recurrent tonsillitis are often referred for removal of their tonsils, one of the commonest operations performed in children. Many children have large tonsils but this in itself is not an indication for tonsillectomy, as they shrink spontaneously in late childhood.

The indications for tonsillectomy are controversial, and must be balanced against the risks of surgery, but include:

- Recurrent severe tonsillitis (as opposed to recurrent URTIs) – tonsillectomy reduces the number of episodes of tonsillitis by a third, e.g. from three to two per year, but is unlikely to benefit mild symptoms.
- A peritonsillar abscess (quinsy)
- Obstructive sleep apnoea (the adenoids will also normally be removed).

Like the tonsils, adenoids increase in size until about the age of 8 years and then gradually regress. In young children, the adenoids grow proportionately faster than the airway, so that their effect of narrowing the airway lumen is greatest between 2 and 8 years of age. They may narrow the posterior nasal space sufficiently to justify adenoidectomy. Indications for the removal of both the tonsils and adenoids are controversial but include:

- Recurrent otitis media with effusion with hearing loss, where it gives a significant long-term additional benefit, especially if reinsertion of grommets is considered
- Obstructive sleep apnoea (an absolute indication).

Summary

Acute otitis media
- Can only be diagnosed by examining the tympanic membrane
- Antibiotics marginally shorten the duration of pain but do not reduce hearing loss
- If recurrent, may result in otitis media with effusion, which may cause speech and learning difficulties from hearing loss.

Respiratory disorders

279

Box 16.1 Differential diagnosis of acute upper airways obstruction

Common causes

- Viral laryngotracheobronchitis ('croup' – very common)

Rare causes

- Epiglottitis
- Bacterial tracheitis
- Inhalation of smoke and hot air in fires
- Trauma to the throat
- Retropharyngeal abscess
- Laryngeal foreign body
- Allergic laryngeal angioedema (seen in anaphylaxis and recurrent croup)
- Hypocalcaemia due to poor vitamin D intake
- Infectious mononucleosis causing severe lymph node swelling
- Measles
- Diphtheria

Laryngeal and tracheal infections

The mucosal inflammation and swelling produced by laryngeal and tracheal infections can rapidly cause life-threatening obstruction of the airway in young children. Several conditions can cause acute upper airways obstruction (Box 16.1). They are characterised by:

- Stridor, a rasping sound heard predominantly on inspiration
- Hoarseness due to inflammation of the vocal cords
- A barking cough like a sea lion
- A variable degree of dyspnoea.

The severity of upper airways obstruction is best assessed clinically by the degree of chest retraction (none, only on crying, at rest) and degree of stridor (none, only on crying, at rest or biphasic) (Fig. 16.3).

Severe obstruction leads to increasing respiratory rate, heart rate and agitation. Central cyanosis or drowsiness indicates severe hypoxaemia and the need for urgent intervention – the most reliable objective measure of hypoxaemia is by measuring the oxygen saturation by pulse oximetry.

 Basic management of acute upper airways obstruction

- **Do not examine the throat!**
- **Reduce anxiety by being calm, confident and well organised.**
- **Observe carefully for signs of hypoxia or deterioration.**
- **If severe, administer nebulised epinephrine (adrenaline) and contact an anaesthetist.**
- **If respiratory failure develops from increasing airways obstruction, exhaustion or secretions blocking the airway, urgent tracheal intubation is required.**

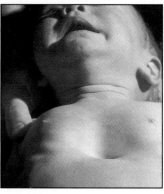

Figure 16.3 The degree of subcostal, intercostal and sternal recession is a more useful indicator of severity of upper airways obstruction than the respiratory rate.

Total obstruction of the upper airway may be precipitated by examination of the throat using a spatula. One must avoid looking at the throat of a child with upper airways obstruction unless full resuscitation equipment and personnel are at hand.

Croup

With laryngotracheobronchitis, usually called croup, there is mucosal inflammation and increased secretions affecting the airway, but it is the oedema of the subglottic area that is potentially dangerous in young children because it may result in critical narrowing of the trachea. Viral croup accounts for over 95% of laryngotracheal infections. Parainfluenza viruses are the commonest cause, but other viruses, such as human metapneumovirus, RSV and influenza, can produce a similar clinical picture. Croup occurs from 6 months to 6 years of age but the peak incidence is in the second year of life. It is commonest in the autumn. The typical features are a barking cough, harsh stridor and hoarseness, usually preceded by fever and coryza. The symptoms often start, and are worse, at night.

When the upper airway obstruction is mild, the stridor and chest recession disappear when the child is at rest. The child can usually be managed at home. The parents need to observe the child closely for the signs of increasing severity. The decision to manage the child at home or in hospital is influenced not only by the severity of the illness but also by the time of day, ease of access to hospital and the child's age (with a low threshold for admission for those <12 months old, due to their narrow airway caliber), and parental understanding and confidence about the disorder.

Inhalation of warm moist air is widely used but is of unproven benefit. Oral dexamethasone, oral prednisolone and nebulised steroids (budesonide) reduce the severity and duration of croup, and the need for hospitalisation.

In severe upper airways obstruction, nebulised epinephrine (adrenaline) with oxygen by facemask provides transient improvement. Close monitoring, along with the advice of an anaesthetist or intensivist, is imperative due to the risk of rebound symptoms once the effects of the epinephrine (adrenaline) diminish after about 2 h. Only a few children with croup require tracheal intubation since the introduction of steroid therapy. Some children have a pattern of recurrent croup, which may be related to atopy.

Bacterial tracheitis (pseudomembranous croup)

This rare but dangerous condition is similar to severe viral croup except that the child has a high fever, appears toxic and has rapidly progressive airways obstruction with copious thick airway secretions. It is caused by infection with *Staphylococcus aureus*. Treatment is by intravenous antibiotics and intubation and ventilation if required.

Acute epiglottitis

Acute epiglottitis is a life-threatening emergency due to the high risk of respiratory obstruction. It is caused by *H. influenzae* type b. In the UK and many other countries, the introduction of universal Hib immunisation in infancy has led to a >99% reduction in the incidence of epiglottitis and other invasive *H. influenzae* type b infections.

There is intense swelling of the epiglottis and surrounding tissues associated with septicaemia. Epiglottitis is most common in children aged 1–6 years but affects all age groups. It is important to distinguish clinically between epiglottitis and croup (Table 16.1), as they require quite different treatment.

The onset of epiglottitis is often very acute (see Case History 16.1), with:

- high fever in an ill, toxic-looking child
- an intensely painful throat that prevents the child from speaking or swallowing; saliva drools down the chin
- soft inspiratory stridor and rapidly increasing respiratory difficulty over hours
- the child sitting immobile, upright, with an open mouth to optimise the airway.

Table 16.1 Clinical features of croup (viral laryngotracheitis) and epiglottitis

	Croup	Epiglottitis
Onset	Over days	Over hours
Preceding coryza	Yes	No
Cough	Severe, barking	Absent or slight
Able to drink	Yes	No
Drooling saliva	No	Yes
Appearance	Unwell	Toxic, very ill
Fever	<38.5°C	>38.5°C
Stridor	Harsh, rasping	Soft, whispering
Voice, cry	Hoarse	Muffled, reluctant to speak

Case History

16.1 Acute epiglottitis

This 5-year-old girl developed a severe sore throat, drooling of saliva, a high fever and increasing difficulty breathing over 8 h (Fig. 16.4a) Epiglottitis was diagnosed and her airway was guaranteed with a nasotracheal tube. Antibiotics were started immediately (Fig. 16.4b,c). She made a full recovery.

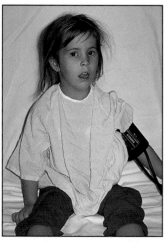 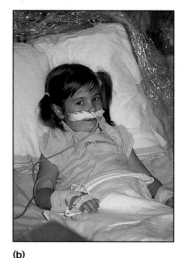 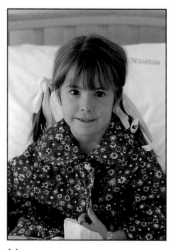

(a) (b) (c)

Figure 16.4 Acute epiglottitis. **(a)** At presentation. **(b)** At 16 h, with nasotracheal and nasogastric tubes and an indwelling cannula for intravenous antibiotics. **(c)** At 36 h, following removal of the nasotracheal and nasogastric tubes.

In contrast to viral croup, cough is minimal or absent. Attempts to lie the child down or examine the throat with a spatula or perform a lateral neck X-ray must not be undertaken as they can precipitate total airway obstruction and death.

If the diagnosis of epiglottitis is suspected, urgent hospital admission and treatment are required. A senior anaesthetist, paediatrician and ENT surgeon should be summoned and treatment initiated without delay. The child should be transferred directly to the intensive care unit or an anaesthetic room, and must be accompanied by senior medical staff in case respiratory obstruction occurs. The child should be intubated under controlled conditions with a general anaesthetic. Rarely, this is impossible and urgent tracheostomy is life-saving. Only after the airway is secured should blood be taken for culture and intravenous antibiotics such as cefuroxime started. The tracheal tube can usually be removed after 24 h and antibiotics given for 3–5 days. With appropriate treatment, most children recover completely within 2–3 days. As with other serious *H. influenzae* infections, prophylaxis with rifampicin is offered to close household contacts.

 Minutes count in acute epiglottitis.

Bronchitis

There is controversy about the term bronchitis in childhood. While some inflammation of the bronchi producing a mixture of wheeze and coarse crackles is often a feature of respiratory infections, bronchitis in children is very different from the chronic bronchitis of adults. In acute bronchitis in children, cough and fever are the main symptoms. The cough may persist for about 2 weeks, or longer with pertussis or *Mycoplasma* infections. There is no evidence that antibiotics, cough suppressants or expectorants speed recovery.

Whooping cough (pertussis)

This is a highly contagious respiratory infection caused by *Bordetella pertussis*. It is endemic, with epidemics every 3–4 years. After a week of coryza (catarrhal phase), the child develops a characteristic paroxysmal or spasmodic cough followed by a characteristic inspiratory whoop (paroxysmal phase). The spasms of cough are often worse at night and may culminate in vomiting. During a paroxysm, the child goes red or blue in the face, and mucus flows from the nose and mouth. The whoop may be absent in infants, but apnoea is a feature at this age. Epistaxis and subconjunctival haemorrhages can occur after vigorous coughing. The paroxysmal phase lasts 3–6 weeks. The symptoms gradually decrease (convalescent phase) but may persist for many months. Complications of pertussis, such as pneumonia, convulsions and bronchiectasis, are uncommon, but there is still a significant mortality, particularly in infants. Infants who have not yet completed their primary vaccination at 4 months are particularly susceptible. Infants and young children suffering severe spasms of cough or cyanotic attacks

should be admitted to hospital and isolated from other children.

The organism can be identified early in the disease from culture of a per-nasal swab, although PCR is more sensitive. Characteristically, there is a marked lymphocytosis ($>15 \times 10^9$/L) on a blood count. Although erythromycin eradicates the organism, it decreases symptoms only if started during the catarrhal phase. Siblings, parents and school contacts may develop a similar cough, and close contacts should receive erythromycin prophylaxis, and unvaccinated infant contacts should be vaccinated. Immunisation reduces the risk of developing pertussis and the severity of disease in those affected, but does not guarantee protection. The level of protection declines steadily during childhood.

> **Summary**
>
> **Pertussis**
> - Caused by *Bordetella pertussis*
> - Paroxysmal cough followed by inspiratory whoop and vomiting; in infants, apnoea rather than whoop, which is potentially dangerous
> - Diagnosis: culture of organism on per-nasal swab, marked lymphocytosis on blood film.

Bronchiolitis

Bronchiolitis is the commonest serious respiratory infection of infancy: 2–3% of all infants are admitted to hospital with the disease each year during annual winter epidemics; 90% are aged 1–9 months (bronchiolitis is rare after 1 year of age). Respiratory syncytial virus (RSV) is the pathogen in 80% of cases. The remainder are accounted for by human metapneumovirus, parainfluenza virus, rhinovirus, adenovirus, influenza virus, and *Mycoplasma pneumoniae*. Dual infection with RSV and human metapneumovirus is associated with severe bronchiolitis.

Clinical features

Coryzal symptoms precede a dry cough and increasing breathlessness. Feeding difficulty associated with increasing dyspnoea is often the reason for admission to hospital. Recurrent apnoea is a serious complication, especially in young infants. Infants born prematurely who develop bronchopulmonary dysplasia or with other underlying lung disease, such as cystic fibrosis or have congenital heart disease, are most at risk from severe bronchiolitis. The characteristic findings on examination (Fig. 16.5) are:

- Sharp, dry cough
- Tachypnoea
- Subcostal and intercostal recession
- Hyperinflation of the chest:
  - Prominent sternum
  - Liver displaced downwards
- Fine end-inspiratory crackles
- High-pitched wheezes – expiratory > inspiratory
- Tachycardia
- Cyanosis or pallor.

Summary

The child with stridor

Clinical features to assess

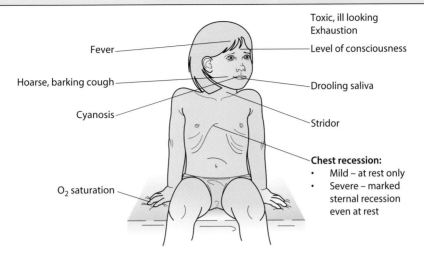

Fever

Hoarse, barking cough

Cyanosis

O_2 saturation

Toxic, ill looking
Exhaustion

Level of consciousness

Drooling saliva

Stridor

Chest recession:
- Mild – at rest only
- Severe – marked sternal recession even at rest

Clinical conditions

Croup
- Mostly viral
- 6 months to 6 years of age
- Harsh, loud stridor
- Coryza and mild fever, hoarse voice

Epiglottitis:
- Caused by *H. influenzae* type b, rare since Hib immunisation
- Mostly aged 1–6 years
- Acute, life-threatening illness
- High fever, ill, toxic-looking
- Painful throat, unable to swallow saliva, which drools down the chin

Bacterial tracheitis:
- High fever, toxic
- Loud, harsh stridor

Inhaled foreign body
- Choking on peanut or toy in mouth
- Sudden onset of cough or respiratory distress

Laryngomalacia or congenital airway abnormality:
- Recurrent or continuous stridor since birth

Other rare causes:
- See Box 16.1

Bronchiolitis

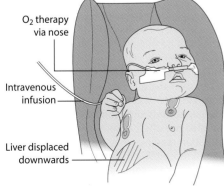

O_2 therapy via nose

Intravenous infusion

Liver displaced downwards

Apnoea in infants <4 months

Sharp, dry cough

Cyanosis or pallor

Hyperinflation of the chest:
- sternum prominent
- liver displaced downwards

Subcostal and intercostal recession

Auscultation:
- fine end-inspiratory crackles
- prolonged expiration

Figure 16.5 Clinical features of severe bronchiolitis in an infant.

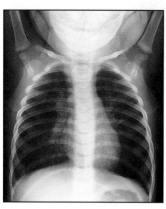

Figure 16.6 In acute bronchiolitis, the chest X-ray shows hyperinflation of the lungs with flattening of the diaphragm, horizontal ribs and increased hilar bronchial markings. However, chest X-ray is rarely helpful in bronchiolitis.

Investigations

Respiratory viruses are now usually identified by PCR analysis of nasopharyngeal secretions. A chest X-ray is unnecessary in straightforward cases, but if performed, typically shows hyperinflation of the lungs due to small airways obstruction, air trapping (Fig. 16.6) and often focal atelectasis. Pulse oximetry is used to measure and monitor arterial oxygen saturation continuously. Blood gas analysis, usually a capillary sample, is only performed in severe disease to identify hypercarbia when additional ventilatory support is considered.

Management

This is supportive. Humidified oxygen is delivered via nasal cannulae; the concentration required is determined by pulse oximetry. The infant is monitored for apnoea. Mist, antibiotics, steroids and nebulised bronchodilators, such as salbutamol or ipratropium, have not been shown to reduce the severity or duration of the illness. Fluids may need to be given by nasogastric tube or intravenously. Assisted ventilation in the form of nasal or facemask CPAP or full ventilation is required in a small percentage of infants admitted to hospital. RSV is highly infectious, and infection control measures, particularly good hand hygiene, are needed to prevent cross-infection to other infants in hospital.

Prognosis

Most infants recover from the acute infection within 2 weeks. However, as many as half will have recurrent episodes of cough and wheeze (see below). Rarely, usually following adenovirus infection, the illness may result in permanent damage to the airways (*bronchiolitis obliterans*).

Prevention

A monoclonal antibody to RSV (palivizumab, given monthly by intramuscular injection) reduces the number of hospital admissions in high-risk preterm infants. Its use is limited by cost and the need for multiple intramuscular injections.

Pneumonia

The incidence of pneumonia peaks in infancy and old age, but is relatively high in childhood. Pneumonia is a major cause of childhood mortality in resource-poor countries. It is caused by a variety of viruses and bacteria, although in over 50% of cases no causative pathogen is identified. Viruses are the most common cause in younger children, while bacteria are commoner in older children. In clinical practice it is difficult to distinguish between viral and bacterial pneumonia.

The pathogens causing pneumonia vary according to the child's age:

- Newborn – organisms from the mother's genital tract, particularly group B streptococcus, but also Gram-negative enterococci
- Infants and young children – respiratory viruses, particularly RSV, are most common, but bacterial infections include *Streptococcus pneumoniae* or *Haemophilus influenzae*. *Bordetella pertussis* and *Chlamydia trachomatis* can also cause pneumonia at this age. An infrequent but serious cause is *Staphylococcus aureus*
- Children over 5 years – *Mycoplasma pneumoniae*, *Streptococcus pneumoniae* and *Chlamydia pneumoniae* are the main causes.
- At all ages *Mycobacterium tuberculosis* should be considered.

A conjugate vaccine (Prevenar), with immunogenicity against thirteen of the most common serotypes of *Streptococcus pneumoniae* responsible for invasive disease, is now included in the routine immunisation schedule in the UK and many countries. There has been a marked reduction in the incidence of pneumonia from *Haemophilus influenzae* type B since the introduction of Hib immunisation.

Clinical features

Fever and difficulty in breathing are the commonest presenting symptoms, usually preceded by an upper respiratory tract infection. Other symptoms include cough, lethargy, poor feeding and an 'unwell' child. Localised chest, abdominal, or neck pain is a feature of pleural irritation and suggests bacterial infection.

Examination reveals tachypnoea, nasal flaring and chest indrawing – the best clinical sign of pneumonia in children is increased respiratory rate, and pneumonia can sometimes be missed if the respiratory rate is not measured in a febrile child (so-called 'silent pneumonia'). There may be end-inspiratory respiratory coarse crackles over the affected area, but the classic signs of consolidation with dullness on percussion, decreased breath sounds and bronchial breathing over the affected area are often absent in young children. Oxygen saturation readings may be decreased; this is an indication for hospital admission.

A chest X-ray may confirm the diagnosis, but with the exception of a classic lobar pneumonia

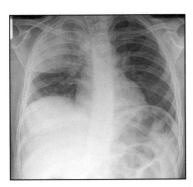

Figure 16.7 Consolidation of the right upper lobe. Lobar consolidation is a feature of pneumococcal pneumonia.

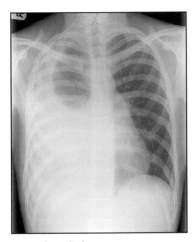

Figure 16.8 Right-sided empyema.

characteristic of *Streptococcus pneumoniae* (Fig. 16.7), a chest X-ray cannot differentiate between bacterial and viral pneumonia. In younger children, a nasopharyngeal aspirate is useful to identify viral causes, but blood tests, including full blood count and acute-phase reactants, are generally unhelpful in differentiating between a viral and bacterial cause. A small proportion of pneumonias are associated with a pleural effusion, where there may be blunting of the costophrenic angle on the chest X-ray. Some of these effusions develop into empyema and fibrin strands may form, leading to septations, which make drainage difficult (Fig. 16.8). The incidence of childhood empyema has risen over the last decade, the precise reason for which remains unclear. Ultrasound of the chest will often distinguish between parapneumonic effusion and empyema.

Management

Evidence-based guidelines for the management of pneumonia in childhood have been published (British Thoracic Society). Most cases can be managed at home, but indications for admission include oxygen saturation <93%, severe tachypnoea and difficulty breathing, grunting, apnoea, not feeding or family unable to provide appropriate care. General supportive care should include oxygen for hypoxia and analgesia if there is pain. Intravenous fluids should be given if necessary, to correct dehydration and maintain adequate hydration and salt balance. Physiotherapy has no role.

The choice of antibiotic is determined by the child's age, severity of illness and appearance on chest X-ray. Newborns require broad-spectrum intravenous antibiotics. Most older infants can be managed with oral amoxicillin, with broader-spectrum antibiotics such as co-amoxiclav being reserved for those who are complicated or unresponsive. For children >5 years of age, either amoxicillin or an oral macrolide such as erythromycin is the treatment of choice.

Parapneumonic effusions usually resolve with appropriate antibiotics, but the small proportion that develop an empyema require drainage of the collection. This may be achieved by either placement of a chest drain with or without the installation of a fibrinolytic agent in the intrapleural space (e.g. urokinase) to break down any septations, or by surgical decortication. Practices vary between different centres.

Prognosis

Follow-up is not generally required for children with simple consolidation on chest X-ray and who recover clinically. Those with evidence of lobar collapse, atelectasis or empyema should have a repeat chest X-ray after 4–6 weeks. Virtually all children with pneumonia, even those with empyema, make a full recovery.

 Consider pneumonia in children with neck stiffness or acute abdominal pain.

Asthma

Asthma is the most common chronic respiratory disorder in childhood, affecting 15–20% of children. Worldwide there has been a significant increase in the incidence of asthma over the last 40 years, although this has now plateaued in many developed countries. Although the symptoms of asthma are readily controlled in most children, it is an important cause of absence from school, restricted activity and anxiety for the child and family. There are still about 20 deaths from asthma in children each year in the UK.

Diagnosing asthma in preschool children is often difficult. Approximately half of all children wheeze at some time during the first 3 years of life. In general, there are two patterns of wheezing (Fig. 16.9):

- Transient early wheezing
- Persistent and recurrent wheezing.

Transient early wheezing

Most wheezy preschool children have *virus-associated wheeze* (also known as *episodic viral wheeze* and *wheezy bronchitis*). Transient early wheezing is thought to result from small airways being more likely to narrow and obstruct due to inflammation and aberrant immune responses to viral infection. This gives the

The infant with tachypnoea or wheeze

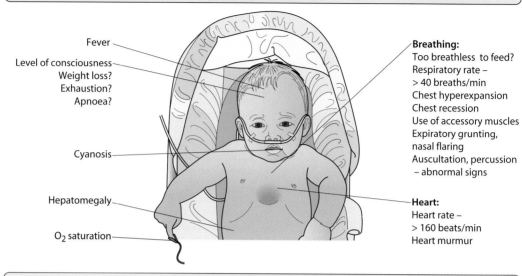

Clinical features to assess

Fever

Level of consciousness
Weight loss?
Exhaustion?
Apnoea?

Cyanosis

Hepatomegaly

O₂ saturation

Breathing:
Too breathless to feed?
Respiratory rate –
> 40 breaths/min
Chest hyperexpansion
Chest recession
Use of accessory muscles
Expiratory grunting,
nasal flaring
Auscultation, percussion
– abnormal signs

Heart:
Heart rate –
> 160 beats/min
Heart murmur

Clinical conditions to consider

Bronchiolitis
- Age 1–9 months
- Poor feeding, apnoea, dry cough
- Laboured breathing – chest recession, hyperinflation of the chest, fine end-inspiratory crackles, wheeze, liver displaced downwards
- Apnoea, cyanosis, respiratory failure
- Increased severity with bronchopulmonary dysplasia in preterm or congenital heart disease

Pneumonia
- Fever, poor feeding, cough, lethargy, cyanosis
- Tachypnoea, nasal flaring, chest recession, wheeze and end-inspiratory coarse crackles over the affected area
- O₂ saturation may be decreased
- Chest X-ray – consolidation, parapneumonic effusion or empyema

Transient early wheezing – with viral infections, risk increased in preterm and maternal smoking

Non-atopic wheezing – following viral lower respiratory infection

Atopic asthma – recurrent wheezing, eczema, positive family history of allergy/atopy

Cardiac failure – respiratory distress, heart murmur, hepatomegaly

Inhaled foreign body – choking on peanut or toy, etc.
Aspiration of feeds – especially with neuromuscular disorder
Other causes – see Box 16.2

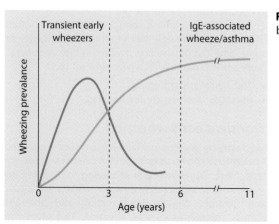

Figure 16.9 Prevalence of wheeze in children caused by the two major phenotypes by age.

condition its episodic nature, being triggered by viruses that cause the common cold. Studies have found that transient early wheezers often have decreased lung function from birth, from small airway diameter. Risk factors include maternal smoking during and/or after pregnancy and prematurity. A family history of asthma or allergy is not a risk factor. Transient early wheezing is more common in males and usually resolves by 5 years of age, presumably from the increase in airway size.

Persistent and recurrent wheezing

Some children, both preschool and school-aged, have frequent wheeze triggered by many stimuli. The presence of IgE to common inhalant allergens, such as house dust mite, pollens or pets, is associated with persistence of wheezing beyond the preschool years. Recurrent wheezing associated with evidence of allergy to one or more inhaled allergens (e.g. by skin-prick test or IgE blood test) is termed 'atopic asthma'. Atopic wheezers have persistent symptoms and decreased lung function. Atopic asthma is strongly associated with other atopic diseases such as eczema, rhinoconjunctivitis and food allergy, and is more common in those with a family history of such diseases.

Box 16.2 Causes of childhood wheeze

- Transient early wheezing
- Atopic asthma (IgE-mediated)
- Non-atopic asthma
- Recurrent aspiration of feeds
- Inhaled foreign body
- Cystic fibrosis
- Recurrent anaphylaxis in a child with food allergies
- Congenital abnormality of lung, airway or heart
- Idiopathic.

A small number of persistent or recurrent wheezing children will have other causes, such as the non-atopic asthmatics. Other causes of recurrent wheeze are listed in Box 16.2.

Pathophysiology of asthma

An outline of the pathophysiology of asthma is shown in Figure 16.10.

Up to 40% of all children are atopic (see Ch. 15). Siblings and parents have an increased risk of allergic diseases. The presence of one allergic condition increases the risk of another, e.g. half of children with allergic asthma have eczema at some time during their lives. The majority of asthma exacerbations are triggered by rhinovirus infection, and there is evidence that those with asthma have specific immune defects which increase their vulnerability to these viruses.

Clinical features

Asthma should be suspected in any child with wheezing on more than one occasion. Wheeze is a polyphonic (multiple pitch) noise coming from the airways believed to represent many airways of different dimensions vibrating from abnormal narrowing. Although it may be clear to most clinicians what 'wheezing' is, patients and parents do not always mean the same thing. It is best to describe the sound to a parent (e.g. 'a whistling in the chest when your child breaths out') and ask if that fits with their child's symptoms. Ideally, the presence of wheeze is confirmed on auscultation by a health professional to distinguish it from transmitted upper respiratory noises. Other key features associated with a high probability of a child having asthma include:

- Symptoms worse at night and in the early morning
- Symptoms that have triggers (e.g. exercise, pets, dust, cold air, emotions, laughter)
- Interval symptoms, i.e. symptoms between acute exacerbations

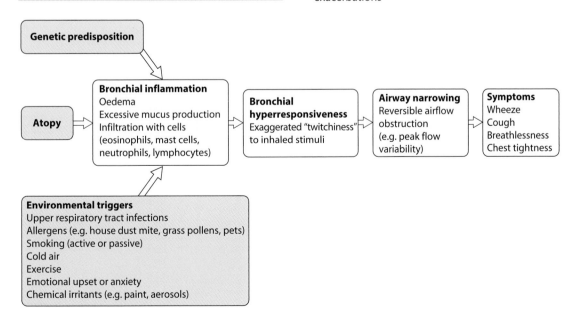

Figure 16.10 Pathophysiology of asthma.

- Personal or family history of an atopic disease
- Positive response to asthma therapy.

Once suspected, the pattern or phenotype should be further explored by asking:

- How frequent are the symptoms?
- What triggers the symptoms? Specifically, are sport and general activities affected by the asthma?
- How often is sleep disturbed by asthma?
- How severe are the interval symptoms between exacerbations?
- How much school has been missed due to asthma?

Examination of the chest is usually normal between attacks. In long-standing asthma there may be hyperinflation of the chest, generalised polyphonic

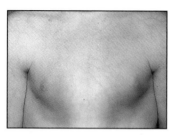

Figure 16.11 The depressions at the base of the thorax associated with the muscular insertion of the diaphragm are called Harrison sulci, and are associated with chronic obstructive airways disease such as asthma during childhood.

expiratory wheeze and a prolonged expiratory phase. Onset of the disease in early childhood may result in Harrison sulci (Fig. 16.11). Evidence of eczema should be sought, as should examination of the nasal mucosa for allergic rhinitis. Growth should be plotted but is normal unless the asthma is extremely severe. The presence of a wet cough or sputum production, finger clubbing, or poor growth suggests a condition characterised by chronic infection such as cystic fibrosis or bronchiectasis.

In practice, the diagnosis is usually made on a history of recurrent wheeze, with exacerbations usually precipitated by viral respiratory infections.

Investigations

Asthma can usually be diagnosed from the history and examination and no investigations are needed. Sometimes, specific investigations are required to confirm the diagnosis, or explore the severity and phenotype in more detail. Skin-prick testing for common allergens is often considered both as an aid to the diagnosis of atopy and to identify allergens which may be acting as triggers. A chest X-ray is usually normal but may help to rule out other conditions. If there is uncertainty, recording peak expiratory flow rate (PEFR) may be useful. Most children over 5 years of age can use a peak flow meter. Uncontrolled asthma leads to increased variability in peak flow, with both diurnal variability (morning PEFR usually lower than evening PEFR) and day-to-day variability (change in PEFR over the course of a week). Often, response to treatment is the most helpful investigation. This can be assessed if

---

Summary

Assessment of the child with chronic asthma

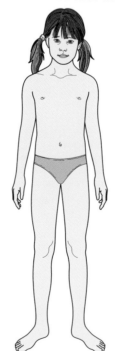

Clinical features to check

Growth and nutrition

Peak flow/spirometry

Chest for:
Hyperinflation
Harrison's sulcus
Wheeze

Are there other allergic disorders?
- Allergic rhinitis
- Eczema, etc.

If there is:
- Sputum
- Finger clubbing
- Growth failure
– If present, other causes should be sought

Monitor:
- Peak flow diary
- Severity and frequency of symptoms
- Exercise tolerance
- Interference with life, time off school
- Is sleep disturbed?
- Use of preventer and reliever medication – are they appropriate?
- Inhaler technique

Consider triggers:
- Allergic rhinitis needing treatment?
- Allergens - animal dander, etc.
- Stress

Table 16.2 Drugs in asthma

Type of drug	Drug
Bronchodilators	
β₂-agonists (relievers)	Salbutamol
	Terbutaline
Anticholinergic bronchodilator	Ipratropium bromide
Preventative/prophylactic treatment	
Inhaled steroids	Budesonide
	Beclometasone
	Fluticasone
	Mometasone
Long-acting β₂-bronchodilators	Salmeterol
	Formoterol
Methylxanthines	Theophylline
Leukotriene inhibitors	Montelukast
Oral steroids	Prednisolone
Anti-IgE injections	Omalizumab

All are given by inhalation, except prednisolone, leukotriene modulators, theophylline preparations, which are by mouth, and omalizumab, which is by injection.

necessary by measuring the PEFR before and after inhaling a bronchodilator; it should increase by more than 10–15%.

Management

The aim of management is to allow the child to lead as normal a life as possible by controlling symptoms and preventing exacerbations, optimising pulmonary function, while minimising treatment and side-effects. It is important to set the aims with the child as they are more likely to comply with their therapy if they are involved in their management. An evidence-based and regularly updated British Guideline on Asthma Management gives guidance on asthma treatment in children and adults.

Medications used to treat children with asthma are shown in Table 16.2.

Bronchodilator therapy

Inhaled β₂-agonists are the most commonly used and most effective bronchodilators. *Short-acting β₂-agonists* (often called *relievers*) such as salbutamol or terbutaline have a rapid onset of action, are effective for 2–4 h and have few side-effects. They are used as required for increased symptoms, and in high doses for acute asthma attacks.

In contrast, *long-acting β₂-agonists* (*LABAs*) such as salmeterol or formoterol are effective for 12 h. They are not used in acute asthma, and should not be used without an inhaled corticosteroid. LABAs are useful in exercise-induced asthma.

Ipratropium bromide, an anticholinergic bronchodilator, is sometimes given to young infants when other bronchodilators are found to be ineffective, or in the treatment of severe acute asthma.

Inhaled corticosteroids

Prophylactic drugs are effective only if taken regularly. *Inhaled corticosteroids* (often called *preventers*) are the most effective inhaled prophylactic therapy. They decrease airway inflammation, resulting in decreased symptoms, asthma exacerbations and bronchial hyperactivity. They are increasingly used in conjunction with an inhaled LABA. They have no clinically significant side-effects when given in conventional licensed doses. They can produce systemic side-effects, including impaired growth, adrenal suppression and altered bone metabolism, when high doses are used.

Add-on therapy

The first choice of add-on therapy in a child over 5 years is a LABA, whereas in children under 5 years, an oral *leukotriene receptor antagonist* such as montelukast is recommended. The latter can also be used in older children when symptoms are not controlled by the addition of a LABA. *Slow-release oral theophylline* is an alternative; however, it has a high incidence of side-effects (vomiting, insomnia, headaches, poor concentration), so it is not commonly used in children.

Other therapies

Oral *prednisolone*, usually given on alternate days to minimise the adverse effect on height, is required only in severe persistent asthma where other treatment has failed. All children on this therapy must be managed by a specialist in childhood asthma. *Anti-IgE therapy (omalizumab)* is an injectable monoclonal antibody that acts against IgE, the natural antibody that mediates allergy. It is used for the treatment of severe atopic asthma, and should only be administered by a specialist in childhood asthma.

Most antibiotics are of no value in the absence of a bacterial infection, although recent data suggest that macrolide antibiotics (e.g. erythromycin) may have a specific role in asthma management, but neither cough medicines nor decongestants are helpful. Antihistamines, e.g. loratadine and nasal steroids, are useful in the treatment of allergic rhinitis.

The British Guideline on Asthma Management uses a stepwise approach, starting treatment with the step most appropriate to the severity of the asthma. Treatment increases from step 1 (mild intermittent asthma) to step 5 (chronic severe asthma requiring continuous or frequent use of oral steroids), stepping down when control is good (Fig. 16.12).

Allergen avoidance and other non-pharmacological measures

Although asthma in many children is precipitated or worsened by specific allergens, complete avoidance of the allergen is difficult to achieve. The value of identifying such triggers by history or allergy testing is controversial. There is currently no conclusive evidence that allergen avoidance measures (such as removal of furry

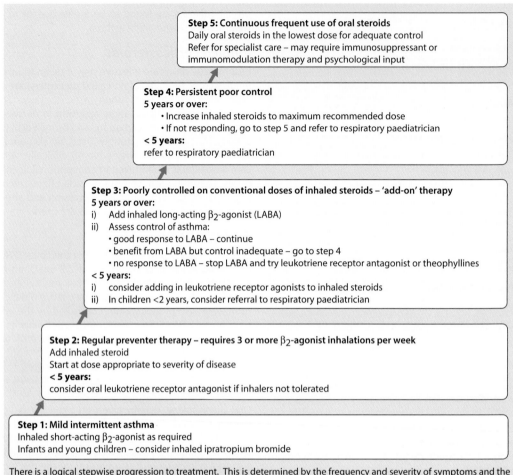

A stepwise approach to the treatment of chronic asthma

Step 5: Continuous frequent use of oral steroids
Daily oral steroids in the lowest dose for adequate control
Refer for specialist care – may require immunosuppressant or
immunomodulation therapy and psychological input

Step 4: Persistent poor control
5 years or over:
   • Increase inhaled steroids to maximum recommended dose
   • If not responding, go to step 5 and refer to respiratory paediatrician
< 5 years:
refer to respiratory paediatrician

Step 3: Poorly controlled on conventional doses of inhaled steroids – 'add-on' therapy
5 years or over:
i)   Add inhaled long-acting β₂-agonist (LABA)
ii)   Assess control of asthma:
   • good response to LABA – continue
   • benefit from LABA but control inadequate – go to step 4
   • no response to LABA – stop LABA and try leukotriene receptor antagonist or theophyllines
< 5 years:
i)   consider adding in leukotriene receptor agonists to inhaled steroids
ii)   In children <2 years, consider referral to respiratory paediatrician

Step 2: Regular preventer therapy – requires 3 or more β₂-agonist inhalations per week
Add inhaled steroid
Start at dose appropriate to severity of disease
< 5 years:
consider oral leukotriene receptor antagonist if inhalers not tolerated

Step 1: Mild intermittent asthma
Inhaled short-acting β₂-agonist as required
Infants and young children – consider inhaled ipratropium bromide

There is a logical stepwise progression to treatment. This is determined by the frequency and severity of symptoms and the response to treatment. The aim is to gain control of symptoms and to then step down treatment over the next few months.

Figure 16.12 A stepwise approach to the treatment of asthma. (From: British Thoracic Society/Scottish Intercollegiate Guideline Network. 2009. The British Guideline on Asthma Management. Reproduced with permission. Available at: http://www.sign.ac.uk/guidelines/ (Accessed January 2011).)

animals or using dust mite impermeable mattress covers) are beneficial, although they may be considered in selected cases. Allergen immunotherapy is effective for treating atopic asthma, but its use is limited by the risk of systemic allergic reactions associated with the treatment (see Ch. 15).

Parents should be advised about the harmful effects of cigarette smoking in the house. Although exercise improves general fitness, there is no evidence that physical training improves asthma itself. Psychological intervention may be useful in chronic severe asthma.

Exercise-induced asthma

Some children's asthma is brought on only by vigorous exercise. With appropriate treatment, asthma should not restrict exercise, and there are many elite athletes with asthma. For most, a short-acting β₂-agonist bronchodilator taken immediately before exercise is sufficient, but if there are more marked symptoms a LABA taken in conjunction with an inhaled steroid will give greater protection. A LABA should not be prescribed without an inhaled steroid.

Acute asthma

Assessment

With each acute attack, the duration of symptoms, the treatment already given and the course of previous attacks should be noted. Clinical features are:

- Wheeze and tachypnoea (respiratory rate >50 breaths/min in children 2–5 years, >30 breaths/min in children ≥5 years) – but poor guide to severity
- Increasing tachycardia (>130 beats/min in children aged 2–5 years, >120 beats/min in children ≥5 years) – better guide to severity
- The use of accessory muscles and chest recession – also better guide to severity
- The presence of marked pulsus paradoxus (the difference between systolic pressure on

Inhaled drugs may be administered via a variety of devices, chosen according to the child's age and preference:

- *Pressurised metered dose inhaler (pMDI) and spacer* (Fig. 16.13).
  - Appropriate for all age groups: 0–2 years, spacer and facemask; >2 years, spacer alone
  - A spacer is recommended for all children as it increases drug deposition to the lungs
  - Useful for acute asthma attacks when poor inspiratory effort may impair the use of inhalers direct to the mouth
- *Breath-actuated metered dose inhalers* (e.g. *Autohaler, Easibreath*): 6+ years. Less coordination needed than a pMDI without spacer. Useful for delivering β-agonists when 'out and about' in older children

- *Dry powder inhaler*: 4+ years (Fig. 16.14). Needs a good inspiratory flow, therefore less good in severe asthma and during an asthma attack. Also easy to use when 'out and about' in older children
- *Nebuliser*: any age (Fig. 16.15). Only used in acute asthma where oxygen is needed in addition to inhaled drugs; occasionally used at home as part of an acute management plan in those with rapid-onset severe asthma (brittle asthma).

Many children fail to gain the benefit of their treatment because they cannot use the inhaler correctly. This must be demonstrated and the child's ability to use it checked. In young children, parents need to be skilled in assisting their child to use the inhaler correctly. Assessing and reassessing inhaler technique is vital to good management and should be a routine part of any review.

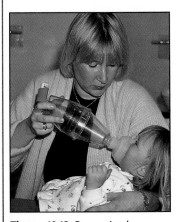

Figure 16.13 Pressurised metered dose inhaler (pMDI) and spacer. Suitable for all ages, with facemask if <2 years old.

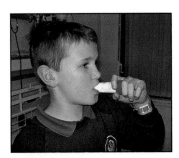

Figure 16.14 Dry powder inhaler, >4 years.

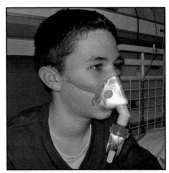

Figure 16.15 Nebuliser: all ages. Only used in acute asthma where oxygen is needed in addition to inhaled drugs.

inspiration and expiration) indicates moderate to severe asthma attack in children but is difficult to measure accurately and is therefore unreliable
- If breathlessness interferes with talking, the attack is severe
- Cyanosis, fatigue and drowsiness are late signs, indicating life-threatening asthma; this may be accompanied by a silent chest on auscultation as little air is being exchanged. This is an emergency as the child may be about to arrest.

However, the severity of an acute asthma attack may be underestimated by clinical examination alone. Therefore:

- Arterial oxygen saturation should be measured with a pulse oximeter in all children presenting to hospital with acute asthma. Oxygen saturation <92% in air implies severe or life-threatening asthma

- Measurement of the peak expiratory flow rate should be routine in school-age children.

The features of a severe and life-threatening acute attack are shown in Figure 16.16.

Criteria for admission to hospital

Children require hospital admission if, after high-dose inhaled bronchodilator therapy, they:

- have not responded adequately clinically; there is persisting breathlessness, tachypnoea
- are exhausted
- still have a marked reduction in their predicted (or usual) peak flow rate
- have a reduced oxygen saturation (<92% in air).

A chest X-ray is indicated only if there are unusual features (e.g. asymmetry of chest signs suggesting pneumothorax, lobar collapse) or signs of severe infection. In children, blood gases are only indicated in life-threatening or refractory cases.

Assessment and management of acute asthma

Assess asthma severity

Moderate
- Oxygen saturation >92%
- Peak flow>50% predicted or best value
- No clinical features of severe asthma

Severe
- Too breathless to talk or feed
- Use of accessory neck muscles
- Oxygen saturation < 92%
- Respirations > 50/min (age 2–5 years) or > 30/min (age over 5 years)
- Pulse > 130/min (age 2–5 years) or > 120/min (age over 5 years)
- Peak flow < 50% predicted or best value

Life threatening
- Silent chest
- Poor respiratory effort
- Altered consciousness
- Cyanosis
- Oxygen saturation < 92%
- Peak flow < 33% predicted or best value

Management

- Short-acting β_2-agonist via spacer, 2–4 puffs, increasing by 2 puffs every 2 min to 10 puffs if required
- Consider oral prednisolone
- Reassess within 1 h

Oxygen via facemask/nasal prongs to achieve normal saturations

- Short-acting β_2-agonist (salbutamol or terbutaline) 10 puffs via spacer or nebulised
- Oral prednisolone or IV hydrocortisone
- Nebulised ipratropium bromide if poor response
- Repeat bronchodilators every 20–30 min as needed

- Nebulised β_2-agonist – salbutamol or terbutaline plus ipratropium bromide
- IV hydrocortisone
- Discuss with senior clinician, PICU team or paediatrician
- Repeat bronchodilators every 20–30 min

Assess response to treatment
Monitor respiratory rate, heart rate, oxygen saturation, peak flow

Responding
- Continue bronchodilators 1–4 h prn
- Discharge when stable on 4-h treatment
- Continue oral prednisolone for up to 3 days

Not responding
- Transfer to HDU (High Dependency Unit) or PICU and consider CXR and blood gases
- Intravenous salbutamol or aminophylline (caution if already receiving theophyllines)
- Consider bolus of IV magnesium sulphate

At discharge
- Review medication and inhaler technique
- Provide personalised asthma action plan
- Arrange follow-up as appropriate

Figure 16.16 Assessment and management of acute asthma. (Adapted from the British Guideline on Asthma Management, 2003.)

Management

Acute breathlessness is frightening for both the child and the parents. Calm and skilful management is the key to their reassurance. High-dose inhaled broncho-dilators, steroids and oxygen form the foundation of therapy of severe acute asthma.

Management is summarised in Figure 16.16. As soon as the diagnosis has been made, the child should be given a β_2-bronchodilator. For severe exacerbations, high-dose therapy should be given and repeated every 20–30 min. For moderate to severe asthma, 10 puffs of β_2-bronchodilator should be given via a pressurised metered dose inhaler (pMDI) and large volume spacer.

This is not only good treatment but also educates the child and parent in using the preferred devices they will have at home. For severe to life-threatening asthma, a β_2-bronchodilator may need to be given via nebuliser driven by high-flow oxygen. The addition of nebulised ipratropium to the initial therapy in severe asthma is beneficial. Oxygen is given when there is any evidence of arterial oxygen desaturation, such as saturations of <92%. A short course (2–5 days) of oral prednisolone expedites the recovery from moderate or severe acute asthma.

Intravenous therapy has a role in the minority of children who fail to respond adequately to inhaled bronchodilator, either aminophylline or intravenous

Summary

Assessment of the child with acute asthma

Determine the severity of the attack
(see Fig 16.16)
- Mild
- Moderate
- Severe
- Life-threatening

Too breathless to talk or eat?

Increased work of breathing
- Tachypnoea – severe if >30 breaths/min

Chest recession:
- Moderate – some intercostal recession
- Severe – use of accessory neck muscles
- Life-threatening – poor respiratory effort

Auscultation:
- Wheeze
- Silent chest – poor air entry in life-threatening

Pulse:
- Severe – >120 beats/min

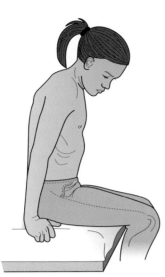

Level of consciousness – altered in life-threatening
Exhaustion

Tongue:
- Cyanosis in life-threatening

Peak flow (% predicted):
- Moderate >50%
- Severe <50%
- Life-threatening <33%

O_2 saturation:
- Moderate >92%
- Severe or life-threatening <92%

Is there a trigger for the attack?:
- URTI or other viral illness
- Pneumonia
- Allergen, e.g. animal dander
- Exercise
- Cold air

salbutamol. For intravenous aminophylline, a loading dose is given over 20 min, followed by continuous infusion. Seizures, severe vomiting and fatal cardiac arrhythmias may follow a rapid infusion. If the child is already on oral theophylline, the loading dose should be omitted. With both aminophylline and salbutamol, the ECG should be monitored and blood electrolytes checked. There is increasing evidence that intravenous magnesium sulphate is helpful in life-threatening asthma. Antibiotics are only given if there are clinical features of bacterial infection. Occasionally, these measures are insufficient and artificial ventilation is required.

Patient education

Prior to discharge from hospital after an acute admission, the following points should be reviewed with the child and family:

- When drugs should be used (regularly or 'as required')
- How to use the drug (inhaler technique)
- What each drug does (relief vs prevention)
- How often and how much can be used (frequency and dosage)
- What to do if asthma worsens (a personal asthma management plan is helpful: see the Appendix for an example).

The child and parents need to know that increasing cough, wheeze and breathlessness, and difficulty in walking, talking and sleeping, or decreasing relief from bronchodilators all indicate poorly-controlled asthma. Some asthmatics find it difficult to identify gradual deterioration – measurement of peak flow rate at home allows earlier recognition. Patients with troublesome asthma are usually given a supply of oral steroids to keep at home, with instructions in the asthma action plan on when to start them.

Recurrent or persistent cough

Cough is the most common symptom of respiratory disease and indicates stimulation of nerve receptors in the pharynx, larynx, trachea or large bronchi. For most children, episodes of cough are due to upper respiratory tract infections caused by the common cold viruses and do not indicate the presence of a long-term or serious underlying respiratory disease. Cough appears persistent because of a series of respiratory tract infections, although some infections, such as pertussis, RSV and *Mycoplasma* infection, can cause a cough that persists for weeks or months. The challenge for the physician is to identify children with other, less common, clinically significant causes of recurrent or persistent cough (Box 16.3).

Asthma is the next most common cause of recurrent cough in childhood. Although there is usually associated wheeze and breathlessness, sometimes the wheezing is not recognised or not described

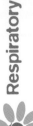

Respiratory disorders

293

Box 16.3 Causes of recurrent or persistent cough

- Recurrent respiratory infections
- Post-specific respiratory infections (e.g. pertussis, RSV, *Mycoplasma*)
- Asthma
- Suppurative lung diseases (e.g. cystic fibrosis, ciliary dyskinesia or immune deficiency)
- Recurrent aspiration (± gastro-oesophageal reflux)
- Persistent endobronchial infection
- Inhaled foreign body
- Cigarette smoking (active or passive)
- Tuberculosis
- Habit cough
- Airway anomalies (e.g. tracheo-bronchomalacia, tracheo-oesophageal fistula).

accurately. Identifying wheeze on auscultation during an acute episode is helpful to make the diagnosis. However, many children with persistent cough without wheeze are treated incorrectly as asthmatics. If the clinical features are not suggestive of asthma or if initial treatment is not beneficial, other diagnoses should be considered or the child referred to a paediatrician with a specialist interest in respiratory disorders.

Persistent cough after an acute infection may indicate cystic fibrosis or unresolved lobar collapse, which will be seen on a chest X-ray. Most children will not expectorate sputum but will swallow their sputum. It is therefore crucial to listen to the quality of the cough. If 'wet' (i.e. sounding like there is excess sputum in the airways) or if the cough is productive, further investigation is required (see below). In any child with a severe, persistent cough, TB should be excluded with a chest X-ray and tuberculin skin (Mantoux) test.

Aspiration of feeds may cause cough and wheeze. This may be caused by gastro-oesophageal reflux or as a result of swallowing disorders, e.g. in children with cerebral palsy. Inhaled foreign body needs to be considered even when there is no clear history.

The significance of parental smoking on children is generally underestimated. If both parents smoke, young children are twice as likely to have recurrent cough and wheeze than in non-smoking households. In the older child, active smoking is common: 10% of 11–15-year-olds and 30% of 16–19-year-olds smoke regularly.

Some older children and adolescents develop a barking, unproductive, habit cough following an infection or an asthma attack. The cough characteristically disappears during sleep and is dry in nature. Reassurance and explanation after a thorough examination are usually effective.

Chronic lung infection

Any child with a persistent cough that sounds 'wet' (i.e. sounds like there is excess sputum in the chest) or is productive should be investigated. The child may have

bronchiectasis, permanent dilatation of the bronchi. Bronchiectasis may be generalised or restricted to a single lobe. Generalised bronchiectasis may be due to cystic fibrosis, primary ciliary dyskinesia, immunodeficiency or chronic aspiration. Cystic fibrosis is considered separately below. Focal bronchiectasis is due to previous severe pneumonia, congenital lung abnormality or obstruction by a foreign body (see Case History 16.2).

In primary ciliary dyskinesia there is congenital abnormality in the structure or function of cilia. This leads to impaired mucociliary clearance. Affected children have recurrent infection of the upper and lower respiratory tract, which if untreated may lead to severe bronchiectasis. They characteristically have a recurrent productive cough, purulent nasal discharge and chronic ear infections; 50% also have dextrocardia and situs inversus (Kartagener syndrome). The diagnosis is made in a specialist laboratory by examination of the structure and function of the cilia of nasal epithelial cells brushed from the nose. The cornerstones of management are daily physiotherapy to clear secretions, proactive treatment of infections with antibiotics and appropriate ENT follow-up.

Children with immunodeficiency may develop severe, unusual or recurrent chest infections. The immune deficiency may be secondary to an illness, e.g. malignant disease or its treatment with chemotherapy. Less commonly it is due to HIV infection or a primary immune deficiency.

Many children with neurodisability will have chronic aspiration, either due to oropharyngeal incoordination or due to gastro-oesophageal reflux.

Tuberculosis remains an important cause of chronic lung infection and all children with a persistent productive cough should have a chest X-ray and tuberculin skin test. Marked hilar or paratracheal lymphadenopathy is highly suggestive of tuberculosis.

Persistent inflammation of the lower airways driven by chronic infection of the lower respiratory tract (persistent endobronchial infection) is increasingly recognised as a cause of chronic wet cough in children. It may be a precursor to bronchiectasis if investigations and treatment are not instituted. Referral to a specialist in paediatric respiratory disorders is indicated. Persistent endobronchial infection is often improved with early access to oral antibiotics or on occasions long-term prophylactic antibiotics.

A plain chest X-ray may show gross bronchiectasis, but will often not identify it. Bronchiectasis is best identified on a CT scan of the chest (Fig. 16.17a,b). To investigate focal disease bronchoscopy is usually indicated to exclude a structural cause.

Cystic fibrosis

Epidemiology, genetics and basic defect

Cystic fibrosis (CF) is the commonest life-limiting autosomal recessive condition in Caucasians with an incidence of 1 in 2500 live births and carrier rate of 1 in 25.

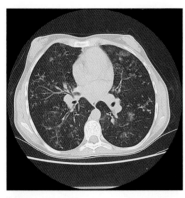

(a)

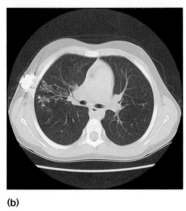

(b)

Figure 16.17 Bronchiectasis on CT scan of the chest. **(a)** Generalised and **(b)** focal, in the right upper lobe.

Case History

16.2 Foreign body inhalation

A previously well 3-year-old boy presented with a 5-day history of severe cough and wheeze. His symptoms developed after choking on some peanuts. A chest X-ray revealed a hyperlucent right lung (Fig. 16.18). Bronchoscopy was performed and revealed a peanut wedged in the right main bronchus.

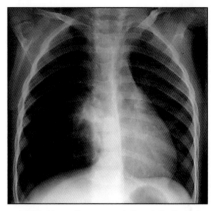

Figure 16.18 Hyperlucency of the right lung and mediastinal shift to the left. (Courtesy of Dr Abbas Khakoo.)

It is well recognised but less common in other ethnic groups. Average life expectancy has increased from a few years to the mid-30s, with a projected life expectancy for current newborns into the 40s.

The fundamental problem in CF is a defective protein called the cystic fibrosis transmembrane conductance regulator (CFTR). CFTR is a cyclic AMP-dependent chloride channel found in the membrane of cells. The gene for CFTR is located on chromosome 7. Over 1000 different gene mutations have been discovered that cause a number of distinct defects in CFTR, but by far the most frequent mutation in the UK is delta F508. The correlation between genotype and phenotype is relatively weak for CF lung disease but stronger for gastrointestinal disease. This suggests that additional factors are important in determining the severity of lung disease, including different microbial pathogens, passive smoking, social deprivation and other 'modifier' genes.

Identification of the gene mutation involved within a family allows prenatal diagnosis and carrier detection in the wider family.

Pathophysiology

CF is a multi-system disorder which results mainly from abnormal ion transport across epithelial cells. In the airways this leads to reduction in the airway surface liquid layer and consequent impaired ciliary function and retention of mucopurulent secretions. Chronic endobronchial infection with specific organisms such as *Pseudomonas aeruginosa* ensues. Defective CFTR also causes dysregulation of inflammation and defence against infection. In the intestine, thick viscid meconium is produced, leading to meconium ileus in 10–20% of infants (see below). The pancreatic ducts also become blocked by thick secretions, leading to pancreatic enzyme deficiency and malabsorption. Abnormal function of the sweat glands results in excessive concentrations of sodium and chloride in the sweat.

Clinical features

In the UK, screening of newborns is now performed as part of the heel-prick bloodspot biochemical screen (Guthrie test). The majority of children with CF are identified by screening; however, children may still present clinically with recurrent chest infections, poor growth or malabsorption (Box 16.4). Chronic infection with specific bacteria – initially *Staphylococcus aureus* and *Haemophilus influenzae* and subsequently with *Pseudomonas aeruginosa* or *Burkholderia* species results from viscid mucus in the smaller airways of the lungs. This leads to damage of the bronchial wall, bronchiectasis and abscess formation (Fig. 16.19). The child has a persistent, loose cough, productive of purulent sputum. On examination there is hyperinflation of the chest due to air trapping, coarse inspiratory crepitations and/or expiratory wheeze. With

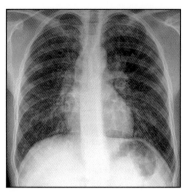

Figure 16.19 A chest X-ray in cystic fibrosis showing hyperinflation, marked peribronchial shadowing, bronchial wall thickening and ring shadows.

Box 16.4 Clinical features of cystic fibrosis

Newborn
- Diagnosed through newborn screening

Infancy
- Meconium ileus in newborn period
- Prolonged neonatal jaundice
- Failure to thrive
- Recurrent chest infections
- Malabsorption, steatorrhoea

Young child
- Bronchiectasis
- Rectal prolapse
- Nasal polyp
- Sinusitis

Older child and adolescent
- Allergic bronchopulmonary aspergillosis (ABPA)
- Diabetes mellitus
- Cirrhosis and portal hypertension
- Distal intestinal obstruction (DIOS, meconium ileus equivalent)
- Pneumothorax or recurrent haemoptysis
- Sterility in males

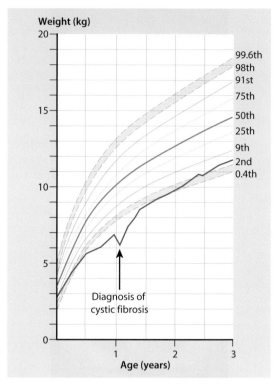

Figure 16.20 Growth chart of a child with cough and recurrent wheeze. Only when the diagnosis of cystic fibrosis was made and appropriate treatment started did he gain weight. (Adapted from growth chart, © RCPCH/WHO/Department of Health.)

the first few days of life. Initial treatment is with Gastrografin enemas, but most cases require surgery.

Diagnosis

The essential diagnostic procedure is the sweat test, to confirm that the concentration of chloride in sweat is markedly elevated (Cl 60–125 mmol/L in cystic fibrosis, 10–40 mmol/L in normal children). Sweating is stimulated by pilocarpine iontophoresis. The sweat is collected into a special capillary tube or absorbed onto a weighed piece of filter paper. Diagnostic errors are common if there is an inadequate volume of sweat collected, so the test must be performed by experienced staff. Confirmation of diagnosis can be made with testing for gene abnormalities in the CFTR protein. If a child is homozygote with two identified mutations then they have cystic fibrosis.

Management

The effective management of CF requires a multi-disciplinary team approach, including paediatricians, physiotherapists, dieticians, specialist nurses, the primary care team, teachers and, most importantly, the child and parents. All patients with CF should be reviewed at least annually in a specialist centre. The aims of therapy are to prevent progression of the lung disease and to maintain adequate nutrition and growth.

established disease, there is finger clubbing. Ultimately, 95% die of respiratory failure.

Over 90% of children with CF have pancreatic exocrine insufficiency (lipase, amylase and proteases), resulting in maldigestion and malabsorption. Untreated, this leads to failure to thrive (Fig. 16.20) and passing frequent large, pale, very offensive and greasy stools (steatorrhoea). Pancreatic insufficiency can be diagnosed by demonstrating low elastase in faeces.

About 10–20% of CF infants present in the neonatal period with meconium ileus, in which inspissated meconium causes intestinal obstruction with vomiting, abdominal distension and failure to pass meconium in

Respiratory management

Recurrent and persistent bacterial chest infection is the major problem. In younger children, respiratory status is monitored on symptoms; older children should have their lung function measured regularly by spirometry. The FEV_1 (forced expiratory volume in 1 second), expressed as a percentage predicted for age, sex and height, is an indicator of clinical severity and declines with disease progression.

With regular treatment, most infants and children with CF should have no respiratory symptoms, and often have no abnormal signs. From diagnosis, children should have physiotherapy at least twice a day, aiming to clear the airways of secretions. In younger children, parents are taught to perform airway clearance at home using chest percussion and postural drainage. Older patients perform controlled deep breathing exercises and use a variety of physiotherapy devices for airway clearance. Physical exercise is beneficial and is encouraged.

Many CF specialists recommend continuous prophylactic oral antibiotics (usually flucloxacillin), with additional rescue oral antibiotics for any increase in respiratory symptoms or decline in lung function. Persisting symptoms or signs require prompt and vigorous intravenous therapy to limit lung damage, usually administered for 14 days via a peripheral venous long line. Increasingly, parents are taught to administer courses of intravenous antibiotics at home, so decreasing disruption of normal activities such as school. Chronic *Pseudomonas* infection is associated with a more rapid decline in lung function, and this is slowed by the use of daily nebulised antipseudomonal antibiotics. Nebulised DNAse or hypertonic saline may be helpful to decrease the viscosity of sputum and so increase its clearance. The macrolide antibiotic azithromycin, given regularly, decreases respiratory exacerbations, probably due to an immunomodulatory effect rather than antibiotic action. Regular, nebulised hypertonic saline may decrease the number of respiratory exacerbations.

More severe CF requires more regular intravenous antibiotic therapy. If venous access becomes troublesome, implantation of a central venous catheter with a subcutaneous port (e.g. Portacath) simplifies venous access, although they require monthly flushing and complications may develop.

Bilateral sequential lung transplantation is the only therapeutic option for end-stage CF lung disease. Fortunately, this is rarely required during childhood. Outcomes following lung transplantation continue to improve with >50% survival at 10 years. Meticulous assessment, for example with regard to comorbidities and microbiology, psychological preparation, optimal timing of transplantation and expert post-transplant care, are all essential parts of the multidisciplinary transplant process.

Nutritional management

Dietary status should be assessed regularly. Pancreatic insufficiency is treated with oral enteric-coated pancreatic replacement therapy taken with all meals and snacks. Dosage is adjusted according to clinical response. A high-calorie diet is essential, and dietary intake is recommended at 150% of normal. To achieve this, overnight feeding via a gastrostomy is increasingly used. Most patients require fat-soluble vitamin supplements.

Teenagers and adults

Most children with CF now survive into adult life. With increasing age come increased complications, most commonly diabetes mellitus due to decreasing pancreatic endocrine function. Up to one-third of patients will have evidence of liver disease with hepatomegaly on liver palpation, abnormal liver function on blood tests or an abnormal ultrasound; regular ursodeoxycholic acid, to improve flow of bile, may be beneficial. Rarely, the liver disease progresses to cirrhosis, portal hypertension and ultimately liver failure. Liver transplant is generally very successful in CF-related liver failure.

In distal intestinal obstruction syndrome (meconium ileus equivalent), viscid mucofaeculent material obstructs the bowel. This is usually cleared by oral Gastrografin.

There may be increasing chest infections, as well as other late respiratory complications including pneumothorax and life-threatening haemoptysis. There is increasing concern over transmission of virulent strains of *Pseudomonas* and *Burkholderia cepacia* between patients, causing rapid decline in lung function. Consequently, patients are often segregated and advised not to socialise with other people with CF.

Females have normal fertility, and unless they have severe lung disease, tolerate pregnancy well. Males are virtually always infertile due to absence of the vas deferens, although they can father children through intracytoplasmic sperm injection (ICSI).

The psychological repercussions on the affected child and family of a chronic and ultimately fatal illness which requires regular physiotherapy and drugs, frequent hospital admissions and absences from school are considerable. The CF team should provide psychological and emotional support. Adolescents have particular needs which must receive special consideration. Older adolescents with CF should transfer to specialist adult CF care.

Gene therapy is currently being assessed but is unlikely to be of practical value in the immediate future.

Screening

All newborn infants born in the UK are screened for CF. Immunoreactive trypsinogen (IRT) is raised in CF patients and can be measured in routine heel-prick blood taken for biochemical screening of all babies (Guthrie test). Those samples with a raised IRT are then screened for common CF gene mutations, and infants with two mutations have a sweat test to confirm the diagnosis.

Early identification of CF allows the early introduction of regular treatment. This leads to better nutrition in childhood and improved neurodevelopmental outcome. It also allows proactive institution of

Summary

Assessment of the adolescent with cystic fibrosis

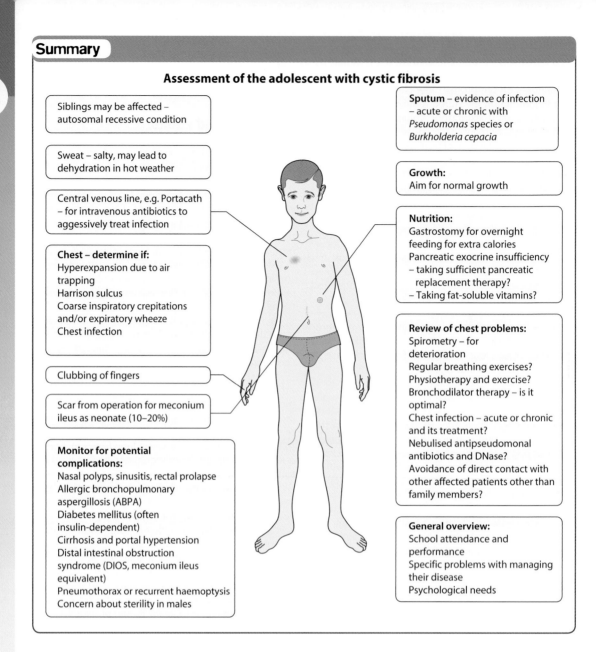

Siblings may be affected – autosomal recessive condition

Sweat – salty, may lead to dehydration in hot weather

Central venous line, e.g. Portacath – for intravenous antibiotics to aggessively treat infection

Chest – determine if:
Hyperexpansion due to air trapping
Harrison sulcus
Coarse inspiratory crepitations and/or expiratory wheeze
Chest infection

Clubbing of fingers

Scar from operation for meconium ileus as neonate (10–20%)

Monitor for potential complications:
Nasal polyps, sinusitis, rectal prolapse
Allergic bronchopulmonary aspergillosis (ABPA)
Diabetes mellitus (often insulin-dependent)
Cirrhosis and portal hypertension
Distal intestinal obstruction syndrome (DIOS, meconium ileus equivalent)
Pneumothorax or recurrent haemoptysis
Concern about sterility in males

Sputum – evidence of infection – acute or chronic with *Pseudomonas* species or *Burkholderia cepacia*

Growth:
Aim for normal growth

Nutrition:
Gastrostomy for overnight feeding for extra calories
Pancreatic exocrine insufficiency – taking sufficient pancreatic replacement therapy?
– Taking fat-soluble vitamins?

Review of chest problems:
Spirometry – for deterioration
Regular breathing exercises?
Physiotherapy and exercise?
Bronchodilator therapy – is it optimal?
Chest infection – acute or chronic and its treatment?
Nebulised antipseudomonal antibiotics and DNase?
Avoidance of direct contact with other affected patients other than family members?

General overview:
School attendance and performance
Specific problems with managing their disease
Psychological needs

---

respiratory management and avoids the morbidity and parental anxiety experienced prior to the clinical diagnosis being established. It also enables early genetic counselling for the parents about the one in four risk of recurrence and the possibility of prenatal diagnosis in future pregnancies.

 Cystic fibrosis should be considered in any child with recurrent infections, loose stools or failure to thrive.

Sleep-related breathing disorders

This is receiving increased recognition. Up to 12% of pre-pubertal school children snore and estimates of the prevalence of obstructive sleep apnoea (OSA)

resulting in gas-exchange abnormalities range from 0.7 to 3%.

Key aspects of the history include loud snoring, witnessed pauses in breathing (apnoeas), restlessness and disturbed sleep. Affected children may be obese, although others may have growth failure. Important consequences of obstructive sleep apnoea include excessive daytime sleepiness, learning and behaviour problems, acute life-threatening cardiorespiratory events and, in severe cases, pulmonary hypertension. In childhood, it is usually due to upper airway obstruction secondary to adenotonsillar hypertrophy. Predisposing causes of sleep-disordered breathing are hypotonia, muscle weakness and anatomical problems, e.g. Down syndrome, achondroplasia, neuromuscular disease, cerebral palsy or craniofacial abnormalities. Such high-risk groups may warrant screening on a regular basis.

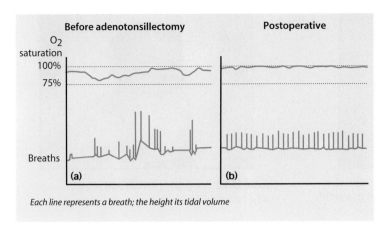

Figure 16.21 Extract from cardiorespiratory monitoring in a child with obstructive sleep apnoea. **(a)** Irregular breathing with periodic pauses associated with oxygen desaturation. **(b)** Post-adenotonsillectomy, the breathing is regular and the desaturation has resolved. (Courtesy of Dr Parviz Habibi.)

The most basic assessment is overnight pulse oximetry, which can be performed in the child's home. The frequency and severity of periods of desaturation (sats <92%) can be quantified. Normal oximetry does not exclude the condition. Limited polysomnography is required in more complex cases; it includes monitoring of heart rate, respiratory effort, airflow, a measure of arterial pCO_2 and video recording. It provides more information about gas exchange and can distinguish between central and obstructive events. Sometimes EEG, electrooculogram and submental EMG is needed to assess neurological arousals and sleep staging.

In cases due to adenotonsillar hypertrophy, adenotonsillectomy is usually curative (Fig. 16.21a,b). Overnight oximetry should be performed prior to surgery for obstructive sleep apnoea to identify severe hypoxaemia, which may increase the risk of perioperative complications. If it persists despite adenotonsillectomy, polysomnography should be performed in a specialist centre. Nasal or facemask continuous positive pressure ventilation (CPAP) or bi-level positive airway pressure (BIPAP) may be required at night.

Congenital central hypoventilation syndrome is a rare congenital condition caused by gene mutations resulting in disordered central control of breathing. In severe cases, life-threatening hypoventilation occurs during sleep, which may result in death in infancy. Long-term ventilation, either continuous or during sleep only, is the mainstay of treatment.

Summary

Sleep disordered breathing

- The majority are due to adenotonsillar hypertrophy, and surgical removal is usually curative

Tracheostomy

The number of children of all ages with a tracheostomy is increasing. Indications are listed in Table 16.3.

Table 16.3 Some indications for tracheostomy in children

Narrow upper airways	Subglottic stenosis
	Laryngeal anomalies (e.g. atresia, haemangiomas, webs)
	Pierre Robin sequence (small jaw and cleft palate)
	Craniofacial anomalies
Lower airway anomalies	Severe tracheo-bronchomalacia
Long-term ventilation	Muscle weakness
	Head or spinal injury
Wean from ventilation	Any prolonged episode of ventilation
Airway protection	Clearance of secretions
	Reduction of aspiration

If a child with a tracheostomy develops sudden and severe breathing difficulties, it may be that the tracheostomy tube is blocked with secretions and needs urgent suction or needs changing immediately. All children with a tracheostomy should have a spare tracheostomy tube with them at all times. If this does not relieve the difficulty in breathing, respiratory support is given via the tracheostomy tube.

Long-term ventilation

An increasing number of children are receiving long-term respiratory support. Preterm infants with severe bronchopulmonary dysplasia (chronic lung disease) may require additional oxygen for many months, and may also require respiratory support with CPAP (continuous positive airway pressure) via nasal prongs or nasal mask. Children with muscle weakness from Duchenne muscular dystrophy, spinal muscular

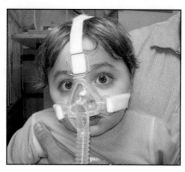

Figure 16.22 Long-term non-invasive respiratory support given overnight via nasal mask to a child with muscle weakness.

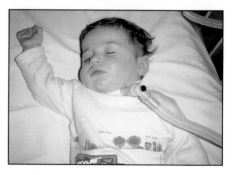

Figure 16.23 Long-term ventilation via a tracheostomy.

atrophy, congenital muscular dystrophy and other rare conditions are increasingly offered long-term ventilatory support. They experience not only hypoxia but also significant hypercapnia due to hypoventilation. This requires bi-level positive airway pressure (BiPAP), which can be delivered non-invasively by a nasal mask or full facemask (Fig. 16.22). In some cases BiPAP may need to be delivered via a tracheostomy (Fig. 16.23). In

Duchenne muscular dystrophy and some other conditions causing muscle weakness, non-invasive ventilation at night provides additional quality years of life. This service can often be provided at home, with considerable specialist community support. With progressive neurological disorders, difficult ethical decisions need to be made about admission for intensive care and initiation of long-term full ventilation.

Further reading

British Thoracic Society: Guidelines for the management of community acquired pneumonia in childhood: Update 2011. Available at: http://www. brit-thoracic.org.uk/clinical-information/pneumonia/ pneumonia-guidelines.aspx (Accessed May 2011).

Primhak R, O'Brien C: Best practice: Sleep apnoea. *Archives of Disease in Childhood – Education and Practice* 90:ep87–ep91, 2005.

Accessible short review of obstructive sleep apnoea in children.

Scottish Intercollegiate Guideline Network: Diagnosis and management of childhood otitis media in primary care. 2003. Available at: http:// www.sign.ac.uk/pdf/sign66.pdf (Accessed May 2011).

Scottish Intercollegiate Guideline Network: Management of sore throat and indications for tonsillectomy. 2010. Available at: http:// www.sign.ac.uk/pdf/sign117.pdf (Accessed May 2011).

Scottish Intercollegiate Guideline Network/British Thoracic Society: The British Guideline on Asthma Management. 2009. Updated May 2011. Available at: http://www.sign.ac.uk/pdf/sign101.pdf (Accessed May 2011).

Taussig LM, Landau LI: *Pediatric Respiratory Medicine*, ed 2, St Louis, MO, 2008, Mosby.

Definitive textbook.

Cardiac disorders

Recent developments in paediatric cardiac disease are:

- Lesions are being increasingly identified on antenatal ultrasound screening
- Most lesions are diagnosed by echocardiography, the mainstay of diagnostic imaging
- MRI allows three-dimensional reconstruction of complex cardiac disorders, assessment of haemodynamics and flow patterns and assists interventional cardiology, reducing the need for cardiac catheterisation
- Most defects can be corrected by definitive surgery at the initial operation
- An increasing number of defects (60%) are treated non-invasively, e.g. persistent ductus arteriosus
- New therapies are available to treat pulmonary hypertension and delay transplantation
- The overall infant cardiac surgical mortality has been reduced from approximately 20% in 1970 to 2% in 2010.

Epidemiology

Heart disease in children is mostly congenital. It is the most common single group of structural malformations in infants:

- 8 per 1000 liveborn infants have significant cardiac malformations
- Some abnormality of the cardiovascular system, e.g. a bicuspid aortic valve, is present in 1–2% of live births

- About 1 in 10 stillborn infants have a cardiac anomaly.

The nine most common anomalies account for 80% of all lesions (Box 17.1), but:

- about 10–15% have complex lesions with more than one cardiac abnormality and
- about 10–15% also have a non-cardiac abnormality.

Box 17.1 The most common congenital heart lesions

Left-to-right shunts (breathless)

- Ventricular septal defect 30%
- Persistent arterial duct 12%
- Atrial septal defect 7%

Right-to-left shunts (blue)

- Tetralogy of Fallot 5%
- Transposition of the great arteries 5%

Common mixing (breathless and blue)

- Atrioventricular septal defect (complete) 2%

Outflow obstruction in a well child (asymptomatic with a murmur)

- Pulmonary stenosis 7%
- Aortic stenosis 5%

Outflow obstruction in a sick neonate (collapsed with shock)

- Coarctation of the aorta 5%.

Aetiology

Genetic causes are increasingly recognised in the aetiology of congenital heart disease, now in more than 10%. These might affect whole chromosomes, point mutations or microdeletions (Table 17.1). Polygenic abnormalities probably explain why having a child with congenital heart disease doubles the risk for subsequent children and the risk is higher still if either parent has congenital heart disease. A small proportion are related to external teratogens.

Circulatory changes at birth

In the fetus, the left atrial pressure is low, as relatively little blood returns from the lungs. The pressure in the right atrium is higher than in the left, as it receives all the systemic venous return including blood from the placenta. The flap valve of the foramen ovale is held open, blood flows across the atrial septum into the left atrium and then into the left ventricle, which in turn pumps it to the upper body (Fig. 17.1).

With the first breaths, resistance to pulmonary blood flow falls and the volume of blood flowing through the lungs increases six-fold. This results in a rise in the left atrial pressure. Meanwhile, the volume of blood returning to the right atrium falls as the placenta is excluded from the circulation. The

change in the pressure difference causes the flap valve of the foramen ovale to be closed. The ductus arteriosus, which connects the pulmonary artery to the aorta in fetal life, will normally close within the first few hours or days. Some babies with congenital heart lesions rely on blood flow through the duct (duct-dependent circulation). Their clinical condition will deteriorate dramatically when the duct closes,

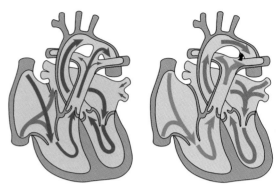

Antenatal circulation   Postnatal circulation

Figure 17.1 Changes in the circulation from the fetus to the newborn. When congenital heart lesions rely on blood flow through the duct (a duct-dependent circulation), there will be a dramatic deterioration in the clinical condition when the duct closes.

Table 17.1 Causes of congenital heart disease

	Cardiac abnormalities	Frequency
Maternal disorders		
Rubella infection	Peripheral pulmonary stenosis, PDA	30–35%
Systemic lupus erythematosus (SLE)	Complete heart block (anti-Ro and anti-La antibody)	35%
Diabetes mellitus	Incidence increased overall	2%
Maternal drugs		
Warfarin therapy	Pulmonary valve stenosis, PDA	5%
Fetal alcohol syndrome	ASD, VSD, tetralogy of Fallot	25%
Chromosomal abnormality		
Down syndrome (trisomy 21)	Atrioventricular septal defect, VSD	30%
Edwards syndrome (trisomy 18)	Complex	60–80%
Patau syndrome (trisomy 13)	Complex	70%
Turner syndrome (45XO)	Aortic valve stenosis, coarctation of the aorta	15%
Chromosome 22q11.2 deletion	Aortic arch anomalies, tetralogy of Fallot, common arterial trunk	80%
Williams syndrome (7q11.23 microdeletion)	Supravalvular aortic stenosis, peripheral pulmonary artery stenosis	85%
Noonan syndrome (PTPN11 mutation and others)	Hypertrophic cardiomyopathy, atrial septal defect, pulmonary valve stenosis	50%

ASD, atrial septal defect; PDA, persistent ductus arteriosus; VSD, ventricular septal defect.

which is usually at 1–2 days of age but occasionally later.

Presentation

Congenital heart disease presents with:

- Antenatal cardiac ultrasound diagnosis
- Detection of a heart murmur
- Heart failure
- Shock.
- Cyanosis.

Antenatal diagnosis

Checking the anatomy of the fetal heart has become a routine part of the fetal anomaly scan performed in developed countries between 18 and 20 weeks' gestation and can lead to 70% of those infants who require surgery in the first 6 months of life being diagnosed antenatally. If an abnormality is detected, detailed fetal echocardiography is performed by a paediatric cardiologist. Any fetus at increased risk, e.g. suspected Down syndrome, where the parents have had a previous child with heart disease or where the mother has congenital heart disease, is also checked. Early diagnosis allows the parents to be counselled. Depending on the diagnosis, some choose termination of pregnancy; the majority continue with the pregnancy and can have their child's management planned antenatally. Mothers of infants with duct-dependent lesions likely to need treatment within the first 2 days of life may be offered delivery at or close to the cardiac centre.

Heart murmurs

The most common presentation of congenital heart disease is with a heart murmur. Even so, the vast majority of children with murmurs have a normal heart. They have an 'innocent murmur', which can be heard at some time in almost 30% of children. It is obviously important to be able to distinguish an innocent murmur from a pathological one.

Hallmarks of an innocent ejection murmur are (all have an 'S', 'innoSent'):

- aSymptomatic patient
- Soft blowing murmur
- Systolic murmur only, not diastolic
- left Sternal edge.

Also:

- Normal heart sounds with no added sounds
- No parasternal thrill
- No radiation.

During a febrile illness or anaemia, innocent or flow murmurs are often heard because of increased cardiac output. Therefore it is important to examine the child when such other illnesses have been corrected.

Differentiating between innocent and pathological murmurs can be difficult. If a murmur is thought to be significant, or if there is uncertainty about whether it is innocent, the child should be seen by an experienced paediatrician to decide about referral to a paediatric cardiologist for echocardiography. A chest radiograph and ECG may help with the diagnosis beyond the neonatal period.

Many newborn infants with potential shunts have neither symptoms nor a murmur at birth, as the pulmonary vascular resistance is still high. Therefore, conditions such as a ventricular septal defect or ductus arteriosus may only become apparent at several weeks of age when the pulmonary vascular resistance falls.

 The features of an innocent murmur can be remembered as the five Ss: 'InnoSent' murmur = Soft, Systolic, aSymptomatic, left Sternal edge.

Heart failure

Symptoms

- Breathlessness (particularly on feeding or exertion)
- Sweating
- Poor feeding
- Recurrent chest infections.

Signs

- Poor weight gain or 'faltering growth'
- Tachypnoea
- Tachycardia
- Heart murmur, gallop rhythm
- Enlarged heart
- Hepatomegaly
- Cool peripheries.

Signs of right heart failure (ankle oedema, sacral oedema and ascites) are rare in developed countries, but may be seen with long-standing rheumatic fever or pulmonary hypertension, with tricuspid regurgitation and right atrial dilatation.

In the first week of life, heart failure (Box 17.2) usually results from left heart obstruction, e.g. coarctation of the aorta. If the obstructive lesion is very severe then

Box **17.2** Causes of heart failure

1. Neonates – obstructed (duct-dependent) systemic circulation

- Hypoplastic left heart syndrome
- Critical aortic valve stenosis
- Severe coarctation of the aorta
- Interruption of the aortic arch

2. Infants (high pulmonary blood flow)

- Ventricular septal defect
- Atrioventricular septal defect
- Large persistent ductus arteriosus

3. Older children and adolescents (right or left heart failure)

- Eisenmenger syndrome (right heart failure only)
- Rheumatic heart disease
- Cardiomyopathy.

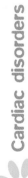

Cardiac disorders

303

arterial perfusion may be predominantly by right-to-left flow of blood via the arterial duct, so-called duct-dependent systemic circulation (Fig. 17.2). Closure of the duct under these circumstances rapidly leads to severe acidosis, collapse and death unless ductal patency is restored (Case History 17.1).

After the first week of life, progressive heart failure is most likely due to a left-to-right shunt (Case History 17.2). During the subsequent weeks, as the pulmonary vascular resistance falls, there is a progressive increase in left-to-right shunt and increasing pulmonary blood flow. This causes pulmonary oedema and breathlessness.

Such symptoms of heart failure will increase up to the age of about 3 months, but may subsequently improve as the pulmonary vascular resistance rises in response to the left-to-right shunt. If left untreated, these children will develop Eisenmenger syndrome, which is irreversibly raised pulmonary vascular

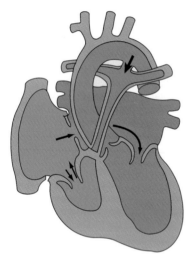

Pulmonary atresia with intact septum

Figure 17.2 The pulmonary circulation is maintained by blood flowing left to right across the duct – an example of a duct-dependent pulmonary circulation.

resistance resulting from chronically raised pulmonary arterial pressure and flow. Now the shunt is from right to left and the teenager is blue. If this develops, the only surgical option is a heart-lung transplant, if available, although medication is now available to palliate the symptoms.

Cyanosis

- Peripheral cyanosis (blueness of the hands and feet) may occur when a child is cold or unwell from any cause or with polycythaemia
- Central cyanosis, seen on the tongue as a slate blue colour, is associated with a fall in arterial blood oxygen tension. It can only be recognised clinically if the concentration of reduced haemoglobin in the blood exceeds 5 g/dl, so it is less pronounced if the child is anaemic
- Check with a pulse oximeter that an infant's oxygen saturation is normal (≥94%). Persistent cyanosis in an otherwise well infant is nearly always a sign of structural heart disease.

Cyanosis in a newborn infant with respiratory distress (respiratory rate >60 breaths/min) may be due to:

- Cardiac disorders – cyanotic congenital heart disease
- Respiratory disorders, e.g. surfactant deficiency, meconium aspiration, pulmonary hypoplasia, etc.
- Persistent pulmonary hypertension of the newborn (PPHN) – failure of the pulmonary vascular resistance to fall after birth
- Infection – septicaemia from group B streptococcus and other organisms
- Metabolic disease – metabolic acidosis and shock.

Whether the presentation of congenital heart disease is with a heart murmur, heart failure, cyanosis or shock depends on the underlying anatomic lesion causing:

- left to right shunt
- right to left shunt
- common mixing
- outflow obstruction in the well or sick child.

This is summarised in Table 17.2.

Table 17.2 Types of presentation with congenital heart disease

Type of lesion	Left-to-right shunt	Right-to-left shunt	Common mixing	Well children with obstruction	Sick neonates with obstruction
Symptoms	Breathless or asymptomatic	Blue	Breathless and blue	Asymptomatic	Collapsed with shock
Examples	ASD	Tetralogy of Fallot	AVSD	AS	Coarctation
	VSD	TGA	Complex congenital heart disease	PS	HLHS
	PDA			Adult-type CoA	

ASD, atrial septal defect; VSD, ventricular septal defect; PDA, patent ductus arteriosus; TGA, transposition of the great arteries; AVSD, atrioventricular; AS, aortic stenosis; PS, pulmonary stenosis; CoA, coarctation of the aorta; HLHS, hypoplastic left heart syndrome.

17.1 Shock

A 2-day-old baby had been discharged home the day after delivery following a normal routine examination. He suddenly collapsed and was rushed to hospital. He was pale, with grey lips. The right brachial pulse could just be felt, the femoral pulses were impalpable and his liver was significantly enlarged. Blood gases showed a severe metabolic acidosis. The differential diagnosis was:

- Congenital heart disease
- Septicaemia
- Inherited disorder of metabolism.

He was ventilated and treated with volume support. Blood cultures were taken and antibiotics started for possible sepsis. Blood and urine samples were taken for an amino acid screen and urine for organic acids. As the femoral pulses remained impalpable, a prostaglandin infusion was started. Within 2 hours, he was pink and well perfused and the acidosis was resolving. Severe coarctation of the aorta (Fig. 17.3) was diagnosed on echocardiography. He had developed shock from a left heart outflow tract obstruction once the arterial duct had closed.

 Maintaining ductal patency is the key to early survival in neonates with a duct-dependent circulation.

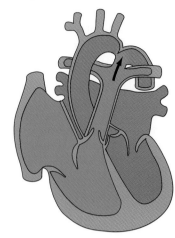

Duct-dependent coarctation

Figure 17.3 The systemic circulation is maintained by blood flowing right to left across the ductus arteriosus – a duct-dependent systemic circulation.

17.2 Heart failure

A 5-week-old female infant was referred to hospital because of wheezing, poor feeding and poor weight gain during the previous 2 weeks. Before this, she had been well. Her routine neonatal examination had been normal. She was tachypnoeic (50–60 breaths/min) and there was some sternal and intercostal recession. The pulses were normal. There was a thrill, a pansystolic murmur at the lower left sternal edge and a slightly accentuated pulmonary component to the second heart sound. There were scattered wheezes. The liver was enlarged, palpable at two fingerbreadths below the costal margin. The ECG was unremarkable. The chest radiograph showed cardiomegaly and increased pulmonary vascular markings. An echocardiogram showed a moderate-sized ventricular septal defect (VSD) (Fig. 17.4). Treatment was medical with diuretics and captopril. The VSD closed spontaneously at 18 months.

This infant developed heart failure from a moderate VSD presenting at several weeks of age when the pulmonary resistance fell, causing increased left-to-right shunting of blood. The defect closed spontaneously.

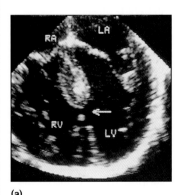

(a)

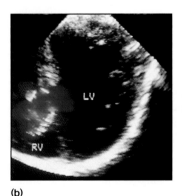

(b)

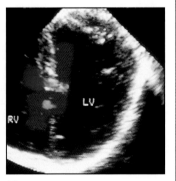

(c)

Figure 17.4 (a) Echocardiogram showing a medium-sized muscular ventricular septal defect (arrow). **(b)** The colour Doppler shows a left-to-right shunt (blue) during systole. **(c)** There is also a small right-to-left shunt (red) during diastole (RA, right atrium; LA, left atrium; RV, right ventricle; LV, left ventricle).

Cardiac disorders

305

Summary

Presentation of congenital heart disease

- Antenatal ultrasound screening – increasing proportion detected
- Detection of a heart murmur – need to differentiate innocent from pathological murmur
- Cyanosis – if duct dependent, prostaglandin to maintain ductal patency is vital for initial survival
- Heart failure – usually from left-to-right shunt when pulmonary vascular resistance falls
- Shock – when duct closes in severe left heart obstruction.

Diagnosis

If congenital heart disease is suspected, a chest radiograph and ECG (Box 17.3) should be performed. Although rarely diagnostic, they may be helpful in establishing that there is an abnormality of the cardiovascular system and as a baseline for assessing future changes. Echocardiography, combined with Doppler ultrasound, enables almost all causes of congenital heart disease to be diagnosed. Even when a paediatric cardiologist is not available locally a specialist echocardiography opinion may be available via telemedicine, or else transfer to the cardiac centre will be necessary. A specialist opinion is required if the child is haemodynamically unstable, if there is heart failure, if there is cyanosis, when the oxygen saturations are <94% due to heart disease and when there are reduced volume pulses.

Nomenclature

The European (as opposed to American) system for naming congenital heart disease is referred to as sequential segmental arrangement. The advantage is

Box 17.3 ECGs in children

Important features
- Arrhythmias
- Superior QRS axis (negative deflection in AVF) (see Fig. 17.5f)
- Right ventricular hypertrophy (upright T wave in V_1, over 1 month of age) (see Fig. 17.6e)
- Left ventricular strain (inverted T wave in V_6) (see Fig. 17.13d)

Pitfalls
- P-wave morphology is rarely helpful in children
- Partial right bundle branch block – most are normal children, although it is common in ASD
- Sinus arrhythmia is a normal finding.

ASD, atrial septal defect.

that it is not necessary to remember the pattern of an eponymous syndrome, e.g. tetralogy of Fallot. The disadvantage is that it is longwinded. The idea is that each component is described in turn, naming the way the atria, then the ventricles and then the great arteries are connected. Hence, a normal heart will be described as situs solitus (i.e. the atria are in the correct orientation), concordant atrioventricular connection and concordant ventriculo–arterial connection. Therefore a heart of any complexity can be described in a logical step-by-step process. This system is not described here, as it is beyond the scope of this book.

Left-to-right shunts

These are:

- Atrial septal defects
- Ventricular septal defects
- Persistent ductus arteriosus.

Atrial septal defect

There are two main types of atrial septal defect (ASD):

- Secundum ASD (80% of ASDs) (Fig. 17.5a)
- Partial atrioventricular septal defect (primum ASD, pAVSD) (Fig 17.5b).

Both present with similar symptoms and signs, but their anatomy is quite different. The secundum ASD is a defect in the centre of the atrial septum involving the foramen ovale.

Partial AVSD is a defect of the atrioventricular septum and is characterised by:

- An inter-atrial communication between the bottom end of the atrial septum and the atrioventricular valves (primum ASD)
- Abnormal atrioventricular valves, with a left atrioventricular valve which has three leaflets and tends to leak (regurgitant valve).

Clinical features

Symptoms

- None (commonly)
- Recurrent chest infections/wheeze
- Arrhythmias (fourth decade onwards).

Physical signs (Fig. 17.5c)

- An ejection systolic murmur best heard at the upper left sternal edge – due to increased flow across the pulmonary valve because of the left-to-right shunt
- A fixed and widely split second heart sound (often difficult to hear) – due to the right ventricular stroke volume being equal in both inspiration and expiration
- With a partial AVSD, an apical pansystolic murmur from atrioventricular valve regurgitation.

Investigations

Chest radiograph (Fig. 17.5d)

Cardiomegaly, enlarged pulmonary arteries and increased pulmonary vascular markings.

(a)

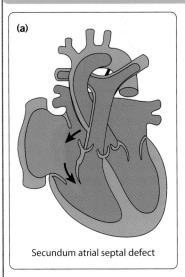

Secundum atrial septal defect

(b)

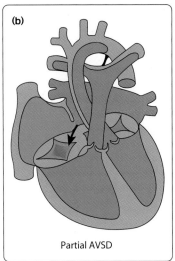

Partial AVSD

(d)

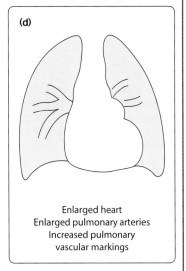

Enlarged heart
Enlarged pulmonary arteries
Increased pulmonary
vascular markings

(c)

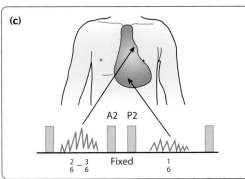

A2 P2

$\frac{2}{6} - \frac{3}{6}$ Fixed $\frac{1}{6}$

(e)   **(f)**

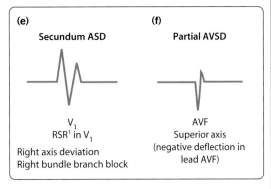

Secundum ASD   Partial AVSD

V_1 AVF
RSR¹ in V_1 Superior axis
                            (negative deflection in
Right axis deviation   lead AVF)
Right bundle branch block

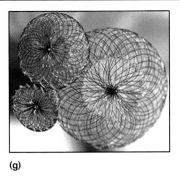

Figure 17.5 Atrial septal defect **(a)** The ostium secundum atrial septal defect (ASD) is a deficiency of the foramen ovale and surrounding atrial septum. **(b)** Partial atrioventricular septal defect (AVSD) is a deficiency of the atrioventricular septum. **(c)** Murmur. **(d)** Chest radiograph. **(e,f)** ECG. **(g)** Examples of an occlusion device used to close secundum atrial septal defects.

(g)

ECG

- Secundum ASD – partial right bundle branch block is common (but may occur in normal children), right axis deviation due to right ventricular enlargement (Fig. 17.5e)
- Partial AVSD – a 'superior' QRS axis (mainly negative in AVF) (Fig 17.5f). This occurs because there is a defect of the middle part of the heart where the atrioventricular node is. The displaced node then conducts to the ventricles superiorly, giving the abnormal axis.

Echocardiography

This will delineate the anatomy and is the mainstay of diagnostic investigations.

Management

Children with significant atrial septal defect (large enough to cause right ventricle dilation) will require treatment. For secundum ASDs, this is by cardiac catheterisation with insertion of an occlusion device (Fig 17.5g), but for partial AVSD, surgical correction is required. Treatment is usually undertaken at about 3–5 years of age in order to prevent right heart failure and arrhythmias in later life.

Ventricular septal defects

Ventricular septal defects (VSDs) are common, accounting for 30% of all cases of congenital heart disease. There is a defect anywhere in the ventricular septum, perimembranous (adjacent to the tricuspid valve) or muscular (completely surrounded by muscle). They can most conveniently be considered according to the size of the lesion.

Small VSDs

These are smaller than the aortic valve in diameter, perhaps up to 3 mm.

Clinical features

Symptoms

- Asymptomatic.

Physical signs

- Loud pansystolic murmur at lower left sternal edge (loud murmur implies smaller defect)
- Quiet pulmonary second sound (P_2).

Investigations

Chest radiograph

- Normal.

ECG

- Normal.

Echocardiography

- Demonstrates the precise anatomy of the defect. It is possible to assess its haemodynamic effects using Doppler echocardiography. There is no pulmonary hypertension.

Management

These lesions will close spontaneously. This is ascertained by the disappearance of the murmur with a normal ECG on follow-up by a paediatrician or paediatric cardiologist and by a normal echocardiogram. While the VSD is present, prevention of bacterial endocarditis is by maintaining good dental hygiene.

Large VSDs

These defects are the same size or bigger than the aortic valve (Fig. 17.6a).

Clinical features

Symptoms

- Heart failure with breathlessness and failure to thrive (faltering growth) after 1 week old
- Recurrent chest infections.

Physical signs (Fig. 17.6b)

- Tachypnoea, tachycardia and enlarged liver from heart failure
- Active precordium
- Soft pansystolic murmur or no murmur (implying large defect)
- Apical mid-diastolic murmur (from increased flow across the mitral valve after the blood has circulated through the lungs)

Summary

Left-to-right shunts

Lesion	Symptoms	Signs	Management
ASD			
Secundum	None	ESM at ULSE	Catheter device closure at 3–5 years
		Fixed split S_2	
Partial AVSD	None	ESM at ULSE	Surgery at 3 years
		Fixed split S_2	
		Pansystolic murmur at apex	
VSD			
Small (80–90% of cases)	None	Pansystolic murmur at LLSE	None
Large (10–20% if cases)	Heart failure	Active precordium, loud P_2, soft murmur, tachypnoea, hepatomegaly	Diuretics, captopril, calories
			Surgery at 3–6 months old
PDA	None	Continuous murmur at ULSE ± bounding pulses	Coil or device closure at cardiac catheter at 1 year, or ligation

ASD, atrial septal defect; AVSD, atrioventricular septal defect; VSD, ventricular septal defect; PDA, persistent ductus arteriosus; ESM, ejection systolic murmur; ULSE, upper left sternal edge; LLSE, lower left sternal edge.

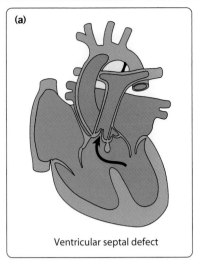

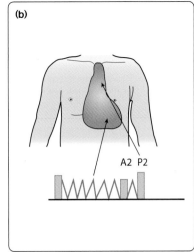

A2 P2

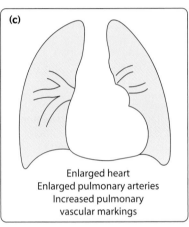

Ventricular septal defect

Enlarged heart
Enlarged pulmonary arteries
Increased pulmonary
vascular markings

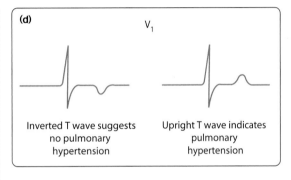

V₁

Inverted T wave suggests
no pulmonary
hypertension

Upright T wave indicates
pulmonary
hypertension

Figure 17.6 Ventricular septal defect. **(a)** Ventricular septal defect showing a left-to-right shunt. **(b)** Murmur. **(c)** Chest radiograph. **(d)** ECG.

- Loud pulmonary second sound (P_2) – from raised pulmonary arterial pressure.

Investigations

Chest radiograph (Fig. 17.6c)

- Cardiomegaly
- Enlarged pulmonary arteries
- Increased pulmonary vascular markings
- Pulmonary oedema.

ECG (Fig. 17.6d)

- Biventricular hypertrophy by 2 months of age.

Echocardiography

- Demonstrates the anatomy of the defect, haemodynamic effects and pulmonary hypertension (due to high flow).

Management

Drug therapy for heart failure is with diuretics, often combined with captopril. Additional calorie input is required. There is always pulmonary hypertension in children with large VSD and left-to-right shunt. This will ultimately lead to irreversible damage of the pulmonary capillary vascular bed (see Eisenmenger syndrome, below). To prevent this, surgery is usually performed at 3–6 months of age in order to:

- Manage heart failure and failure to thrive
- Prevent permanent lung damage from pulmonary hypertension and high blood flow.

Persistent ductus arteriosus (PDA, persistent arterial duct)

The ductus arteriosus connects the pulmonary artery to the descending aorta. In term infants, it normally closes shortly after birth. In persistent ductus arteriosus it has failed to close by 1 month after the expected date of delivery due to a defect in the constrictor mechanism of the duct. The flow of blood across a persistent ductus arteriosus (PDA) is then from the aorta to the pulmonary artery (i.e. left to right), following the fall in pulmonary vascular resistance after birth. In the preterm infant, the presence of a persistent ductus

Cardiac disorders

309

Persistent ductus arteriosus

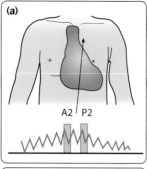

(a)

A2 | P2

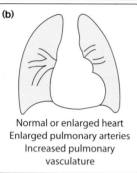

(b)

Normal or enlarged heart
Enlarged pulmonary arteries
Increased pulmonary
vasculature

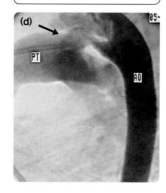

(c) ECG
• Usually normal
• Left ventricular hypertrophy
  with large left-to-right shunt
• Right ventricular hypertrophy
  with pulmonary hypertension

(d)

PT

AO

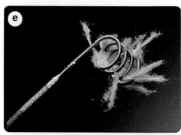

(e)

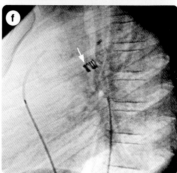

(f)

Figure 17.7 Persistent ductus arteriosus. **(a)** Murmur. **(b)** Chest radiograph. **(c)** ECG. **(d)** A persistent ductus arteriosus visualised on angiography. **(e)** A coil used to close ducts. It is passed through a catheter via the femoral artery or vein. **(f)** Angiogram to show coil in the duct. (PT, pulmonary trunk; AO, aorta.)

arteriosus is not from congenital heart disease but due to prematurity. This is described in Chapter 9.

Clinical features

Most children present with a continuous murmur beneath the left clavicle (Fig. 17.7a). The murmur continues into diastole because the pressure in the pulmonary artery is lower than that in the aorta throughout the cardiac cycle. The pulse pressure is increased, causing a collapsing or bounding pulse. Symptoms are unusual, but when the duct is large there will be increased pulmonary blood flow with heart failure and pulmonary hypertension.

Investigations

The chest radiograph and ECG are usually normal, but if the PDA is large and symptomatic the features on chest radiograph (Fig. 17.7b) and ECG (Fig. 17.7c) are indistinguishable from those seen in a patient with a large VSD. However, the duct is readily identified on echocardiography.

Management

Closure is recommended to abolish the lifelong risk of bacterial endocarditis and of pulmonary vascular disease. Closure is with a coil or occlusion device introduced via a cardiac catheter at about 1 year of age (Fig. 17.7d–f). Occasionally, surgical ligation is required.

Right-to-left shunts

These are:
• Tetralogy of Fallot
• Transposition of the great arteries.

Presentation is with cyanosis (blue, oxygen saturations ≤94% or collapsed), usually in the first week of life.

Hyperoxia (nitrogen washout) test

The test is used to help determine the presence of heart disease in a cyanosed neonate. The infant is placed in 100% oxygen (headbox or ventilator) for 10 min. If the right radial arterial PaO_2 from a blood gas remains low (<15 kPa, 113 mmHg) after this time, a diagnosis of 'cyanotic' congenital heart disease can be made if lung disease and persistent pulmonary hypertension of the newborn (persistent fetal circulation) have been excluded. If the PaO_2 is >20 kPa, it is not cyanotic heart disease. Blood gas analysis must be performed as oxygen saturations are not reliable enough in this range of values.

Management

• Stabilise the airway, breathing and circulation (ABC), with artificial ventilation if necessary

- Start prostaglandin infusion (PGE, 5 ng/kg per min). Most infants with cyanotic heart disease presenting in the first few days of life are duct dependent; i.e. there is reduced mixing between the pink oxygenated blood returning from the lungs and the blue deoxygenated blood from the body. Maintenance of ductal patency is the key to early survival of these children. Observe for potential side-effects – apnoea, jitteriness and seizures, flushing, vasodilatation and hypotension.

Tetralogy of Fallot

This is the most common cause of cyanotic congenital heart disease (Fig. 17.8a).

Clinical features

In tetralogy of Fallot, as implied by the name, there are four cardinal anatomical features:

- A large VSD
- Overriding of the aorta with respect to the ventricular septum
- Subpulmonary stenosis causing right ventricular outflow tract obstruction
- Right ventricular hypertrophy as a result.

Symptoms

Most are diagnosed:

- antenatally *or*
- following the identification of a murmur in the first 2 months of life. Cyanosis at this stage may not be obvious, although a few present with severe cyanosis in the first few days of life.

The classical description of severe cyanosis, hypercyanotic spells and squatting on exercise, developing in late infancy, is now rare in developed countries, but still common where access to the necessary paediatric cardiac services is not available. However, it is important to recognise hypercyanotic spells, as they may lead to myocardial infarction, cerebrovascular accidents and even death if left untreated. They are characterised by a rapid increase in cyanosis, usually associated with irritability or inconsolable crying because of severe hypoxia, and breathlessness and pallor because of tissue acidosis. On auscultation, there is a very short murmur during a spell.

Signs

- Clubbing of the fingers and toes will develop in older children
- A loud harsh ejection systolic murmur at the left sternal edge from day 1 of life (Fig. 17.8b). With

Tetralogy of Fallot

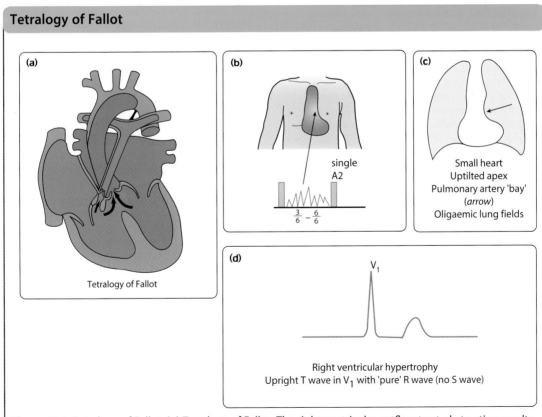

(a) Tetralogy of Fallot

(b) single A2 $\frac{3}{6} - \frac{6}{6}$

(c) Small heart
Uptilted apex
Pulmonary artery 'bay' (*arrow*)
Oligaemic lung fields

(d) V_1
Right ventricular hypertrophy
Upright T wave in V_1 with 'pure' R wave (no S wave)

Figure 17.8 Tetralogy of Fallot. **(a)** Tetralogy of Fallot. The right ventricular outflow tract obstruction results in blood flowing from right to left across the ventricular septal defect **(b)** Murmur. **(c)** Chest radiograph. **(d)** ECG.

increasing right ventricular outflow tract obstruction, which is predominantly muscular and below the pulmonary valve, the murmur will shorten and cyanosis will increase.

Investigations

Chest radiograph (Fig. 17.8c)
A radiograph will show a relatively small heart, possibly with an uptilted apex (boot-shaped) due to right ventricular hypertrophy, more prominent in the older child. There may be a right-sided aortic arch, but characteristically, there is a pulmonary artery 'bay', a concavity on the left heart border where the convex-shaped main pulmonary artery and right ventricular outflow tract would normally be profiled. There may also be decreased pulmonary vascular markings reflecting reduced pulmonary blood flow.

ECG (Fig. 17.8d)
Normal at birth. Right ventricular hypertrophy when older.

Echocardiography
This will demonstrate the cardinal features, but cardiac catheterisation may be required to show the detailed anatomy of the coronary arteries.

Management

- Initial management is medical, with definitive surgery at around 6 months of age. It involves closing the VSD and relieving right ventricular outflow tract obstruction, sometimes with an artificial patch, which extends across the pulmonary valve.
- Infants who are very cyanosed in the neonatal period require a shunt to increase pulmonary blood flow. This is usually done by surgical placement of an artificial tube between the subclavian artery and the pulmonary artery (a modified Blalock–Taussig shunt), or sometimes by balloon dilatation of the right ventricular outflow tract.
- Hypercyanotic spells are usually self-limiting and followed by a period of sleep. If prolonged (beyond about 15 min), they require prompt treatment with:
  - sedation and pain relief (morphine is excellent)
  - intravenous propranolol (or an α adrenoceptor agonist), which probably works both as a peripheral vasoconstrictor and by relieving the subpulmonary muscular obstruction that is the cause of reduced pulmonary blood flow
  - intravenous volume administration
  - bicarbonate to correct acidosis
  - muscle paralysis and artificial ventilation in order to reduce metabolic oxygen demand.

Transposition of the great arteries

The aorta is connected to the right ventricle, and the pulmonary artery is connected to the left ventricle (discordant ventriculo–arterial connection). The blue blood is therefore returned to the body and the pink blood is returned to the lungs (Fig. 17.9a). There are two parallel circulations – unless there is mixing of blood between them this condition is incompatible with life. Fortunately, there are a number of naturally occurring associated anomalies, e.g. VSD, ASD and PDA, as well as therapeutic interventions which can achieve this mixing in the short term.

Clinical features

Symptoms
Cyanosis is the predominant symptom. It may be profound and life-threatening. Presentation is usually on day 2 of life when ductal closure leads to a marked reduction in mixing of the desaturated and saturated blood. Cyanosis will be less severe and presentation delayed if there is more mixing of blood from associated anomalies, e.g. an ASD.

Physical signs (Fig. 17.9b)
- Cyanosis is always present
- The second heart sound is often loud and single
- Usually no murmur, but may be a systolic murmur from increased flow or stenosis within the left ventricular (pulmonary) outflow tract.

Investigations

Chest radiograph (Fig. 17.9c)
This may reveal the classic findings of a narrow upper mediastinum with an 'egg on side' appearance of the cardiac shadow (due to the anteroposterior relationship of the great vessels, narrow vascular pedicle and hypertrophied right ventricle, respectively). Increased pulmonary vascular markings are common due to *increased* pulmonary blood flow.

ECG (Fig. 17.9d)
This is usually normal.

Echocardiography
This is essential to demonstrate the abnormal arterial connections and associated abnormalities.

Management

- In the sick cyanosed neonate, the key is to improve mixing.
- Maintaining the patency of the ductus arteriosus with a prostaglandin infusion is mandatory.
- A balloon atrial septostomy may be a life-saving procedure which may need to be performed in 20% of those with transposition of the great arteries (Fig. 17.9e–g). A catheter, with an inflatable balloon at its tip, is passed through the umbilical or femoral vein and then on through the right atrium and foramen ovale. The balloon is inflated within the left atrium and then pulled back through the atrial septum. This tears the atrial septum, renders the flap valve of the foramen ovale incompetent, and so allows mixing of the systemic and pulmonary venous blood within the atrium.
- All patients with transposition of the great arteries will require surgery, which is usually the arterial switch procedure in the neonatal period. In this operation, performed in the first few days of life, the pulmonary artery and aorta are transected

Transposition of the great arteries

(a)

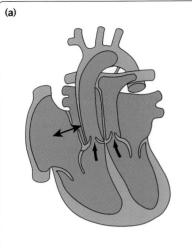

Complete transposition of the great arteries

(b)

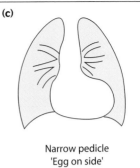

coincident
A2P2 = single
second
sound

Variable
systolic
mumur

(c)

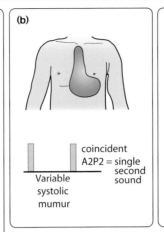

Narrow pedicle
'Egg on side'
cardiac contour
Increased pulmonary
vascular markings

(d) ECG
Usually normal neonatal pattern

(e)

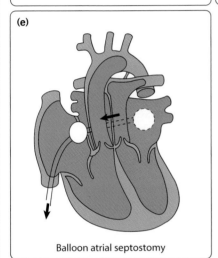

Balloon atrial septostomy

(f)

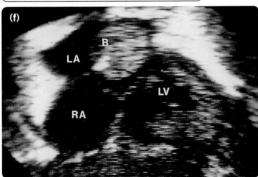

(g)

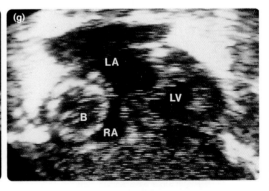

Figure 17.9 Transposition of the great arteries. **(a)** Transposition of the great arteries. There must be mixing of blood between the two circulations for this to be compatible with life. **(b)** Heart sounds. **(c)** Chest radiograph. **(d)** ECG. **(e)** Balloon atrial septostomy. A balloon (about 2 ml) is pulled through the atrial septum from the left atrium to the right atrium in order to increase the size of the atrial defect. This is done with echocardiographic guidance. **(f)** Echocardiogram showing balloon in left atrium. **(g)** Balloon has been pulled through the atrial septum and is now in the right atrium. (B, balloon; LA, left atrium; RA, right atrium; LV, left ventricle)

Cardiac disorders

Summary

Cyanotic congenital heart disease

Lesion	Clinical features	Management
Tetralogy of Fallot	Loud murmur at ULSE Clubbing of fingers and toes (older) Hypercyanotic spells	Surgery at 6–9 months
Transposition of the great arteries	Neonatal cyanosis No murmur	Prostaglandin infusion Balloon atrial septostomy Arterial switch operation in neonatal period
Eisenmenger syndrome	No murmur Right heart failure (late)	Medication to delay transplantation

above the arterial valves and switched over. In addition, the coronary arteries have to be transferred across to the new aorta.

Eisenmenger syndrome

If high pulmonary blood flow due to a large left-to-right shunt or common mixing is not treated at an early stage, then the pulmonary arteries become thick walled and the resistance to flow increases (Fig. 17.10). Gradually, those children that survive, become less symptomatic, as the shunt decreases. Eventually, at about 10–15 years, the shunt reverses and the teenager becomes blue, which is Eisenmenger syndrome. This situation is progressive and the adult will die in right heart failure at a variable age, usually in the fourth or fifth decade of life. Treatment is aimed at prevention of this condition, with early intervention for high pulmonary blood flow. Transplantation is not easily available although there are now medicines to palliate such pulmonary vascular disease (see Pulmonary hypertension, below).

Common mixing (blue and breathless)

These include:

- Atrioventricular septal defect (complete)
- Complex congenital heart disease e.g. tricuspid atresia

Atrioventricular septal defect (complete)

This occurs in:

- Atrioventricular septal defect (complete)
- Complex congenital heart disease

This is most commonly seen in children with Down syndrome (Fig. 17.11). A complete atrioventricular septal defect (cAVSD) is a defect in the middle of the heart with a single five-leaflet (common) valve between

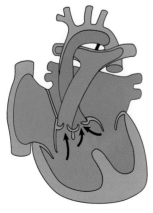

Eisenmenger syndrome

Figure 17.10 Eisenmenger syndrome with right-to-left shunting from pulmonary vascular disease following increased pulmonary blood flow and pulmonary hypertension with large VSD.

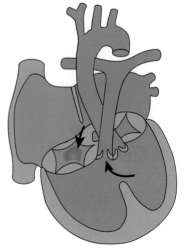

Atrioventricular septal defect

Figure 17.11 Complete atrioventricular septal defect, with a common atrioventricula valve between a large atrial and ventricular component to the AVSD.

Summary

Common mixing

Lesion	Clinical features	Management
Atrioventricular septal defect (complete)	Down syndrome (often) Cyanosis at birth Breathless at 2–3 weeks of life	Treat heart failure medically Surgical repair at 3 months
Complex diseases (e.g. tricuspid atresia)	Cyanosis Breathless	Shunt (Blalock–Taussig) or pulmonary artery banding, then surgery (Fontan operation)

the atria and ventricles which stretches across the entire atrioventricular junction and tends to leak. As there is a large defect there is pulmonary hypertension.

Features of a complete atrioventricular septal defect are:

- Presentation on antenatal ultrasound screening
- Cyanosis at birth or heart failure at 2–3 weeks of life
- No murmur heard, the lesion being detected on routine echocardiography screening in a newborn baby with Down syndrome
- There is always a superior axis on the ECG
- Management is to treat heart failure medically (as for large VSD) and surgical repair at 3–6 months of age.

Complex congenital heart disease

It is difficult to generalise about these conditions, (tricuspid atresia, mitral atresia, double inlet left ventricle, common arterial trunk – truncus arteriosus) since their main presenting feature depends on whether cyanosis or heart failure is more predominant. Tricuspid atresia is the commonest.

Tricuspid atresia

In tricuspid atresia (Fig. 17.12), only the left ventricle is effective, the right being small and non-functional.

Clinical features

There is 'common mixing' of systemic and pulmonary venous return in the left atrium. Presentation is with cyanosis in the newborn period if duct dependent, or the child may be well at birth and become cyanosed or breathless.

Management

Early palliation (as with all the common mixing complex diseases) is performed to maintain a secure supply of blood to the lungs at low pressure, by:

- A Blalock–Taussig shunt insertion (between the subclavian and pulmonary artery) in children who are severely cyanosed
- Pulmonary artery banding operation to reduce pulmonary blood flow if breathless.

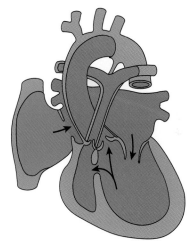

Tricuspid atresia

Figure 17.12 In tricuspid atresia, there is only one effective ventricle because of complete absence of the tricuspid valve.

Completely corrective surgery is not possible with most, as there is often only one effective functioning ventricle. Palliation is performed (Glenn or hemi-Fontan operation connecting the superior vena cava to the pulmonary artery after 6 months of age and a Fontan operation to also connect the inferior vena cava to the pulmonary artery at 3–5 years).

Thus, the left ventricle drives blood around the body and systemic venous pressure supplies blood to the lungs. The Fontan operation results in a less than ideal functional outcome, but has the advantages of relieving cyanosis and removing the long-term volume load on the single functional ventricle.

Outflow obstruction in the well child

These lesions are:

- Aortic stenosis
- Pulmonary stenosis
- Adult-type coarctation of the aorta.

Aortic stenosis

The aortic valve leaflets are partly fused together, giving a restrictive exit from the left ventricle (Fig. 17.13a). There may be one to three aortic leaflets. Aortic stenosis may not be an isolated lesion. It is often associated with mitral valve stenosis and coarctation of the aorta, and their presence should always be excluded.

Clinical features

Most present with an asymptomatic murmur. Those with severe stenosis may present with reduced exercise tolerance, chest pain on exertion or syncope.

In the neonatal period, those with *critical* aortic stenosis and a duct-dependent systemic circulation may present with severe heart failure leading to shock.

Physical signs (Fig. 17.13b)

- Small volume, slow rising pulses
- Carotid thrill (always)
- Ejection systolic murmur maximal at the upper right sternal edge radiating to the neck
- Delayed and soft aortic second sound
- Apical ejection click.

Investigations

Chest radiograph (Fig. 17.13c)
Normal or prominent left ventricle with post-stenotic dilatation of the ascending aorta.

ECG (Fig. 17.13d)
There may be left ventricular hypertrophy.

Management

In children, regular clinical and echocardiographic assessment is required in order to assess when to intervene. Children with symptoms on exercise or who have a high resting pressure gradient (>64 mmHg) across the aortic valve will undergo balloon valvotomy. Balloon dilatation in older children is generally safe and uncomplicated, but in neonates this is much more difficult and dangerous.

Most neonates and children with significant aortic valve stenosis requiring treatment in the first few years of life will eventually require aortic valve replacement. Early treatment is therefore palliative and directed towards delaying this for as long as possible.

Pulmonary stenosis

The pulmonary valve leaflets are partly fused together, giving a restrictive exit from the right ventricle.

Clinical features

Most are asymptomatic (Fig. 17.14a). It is diagnosed clinically. A small number of neonates with *critical* pulmonary stenosis have a duct-dependent pulmonary circulation and present in the first few days of life with cyanosis.

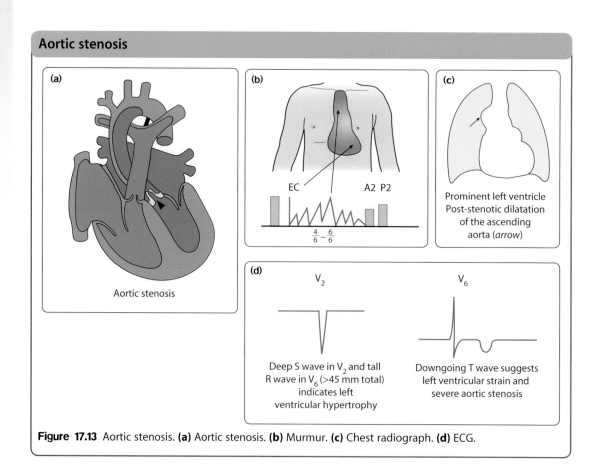

Aortic stenosis

(a) Aortic stenosis

(b) EC   A2 P2 $\frac{4}{6} - \frac{6}{6}$

(c) Prominent left ventricle
Post-stenotic dilatation of the ascending aorta (*arrow*)

(d) V_2 V_6
Deep S wave in V_2 and tall R wave in V_6 (>45 mm total) indicates left ventricular hypertrophy
Downgoing T wave suggests left ventricular strain and severe aortic stenosis

Figure 17.13 Aortic stenosis. **(a)** Aortic stenosis. **(b)** Murmur. **(c)** Chest radiograph. **(d)** ECG.

Physical signs (Fig. 17.14b)

- An ejection systolic murmur best heard at the upper left sternal edge; thrill may be present
- An ejection click best heard at the upper left sternal edge
- When severe, there is a prominent right ventricular impulse (heave).

Investigations

Chest radiograph (Fig. 17.14c)
Normal or post-stenotic dilatation of the pulmonary artery.

ECG (Fig. 17.14d)
Shows evidence of right ventricular hypertrophy (upright T wave in V_1).

Management

Most children are asymptomatic and when the pressure gradient across the pulmonary valve becomes markedly increased (> about 64 mmHg), intervention will be required. Trans-catheter balloon dilatation is the treatment of choice in most children.

Adult-type coarctation of the aorta

This uncommon lesion (Fig. 17.15a) is not duct dependent. It gradually becomes more severe over many years.

Clinical features (Fig 17.15b)

- Asymptomatic
- Systemic hypertension in the right arm
- Ejection systolic murmur at upper sternal edge
- Collaterals heard with continuous murmur at the back
- Radio-femoral delay. This is due to blood bypassing the obstruction via collateral vessels in the chest wall and hence the pulse in the legs is delayed.

Investigations

Chest radiograph (Fig. 17.15c)

- 'Rib notching' due to the development of large collateral intercostal arteries running under the ribs posteriorly to bypass the obstruction
- '3' sign, with visible notch in the descending aorta at site of the coarctation

ECG

- Left ventricular hypertrophy (Fig. 17.15d).

Management

When the condition becomes severe, as assessed by echocardiography, a stent may be inserted at cardiac catheter. Sometimes surgical repair is required.

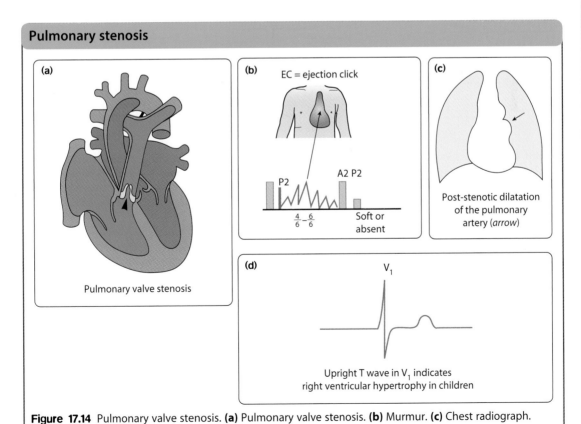

Pulmonary stenosis

(a) Pulmonary valve stenosis

(b) EC = ejection click
P2
A2 P2
$\frac{4}{6} - \frac{6}{6}$
Soft or absent

(c) Post-stenotic dilatation of the pulmonary artery (*arrow*)

(d) V_1
Upright T wave in V_1 indicates right ventricular hypertrophy in children

Figure 17.14 Pulmonary valve stenosis. **(a)** Pulmonary valve stenosis. **(b)** Murmur. **(c)** Chest radiograph. **(d)** ECG.

Summary

Outflow obstruction in the well child

Lesion	Signs	Management
Aortic stenosis	Murmur, upper right sternal edge; carotid thrill	Balloon dilatation
Pulmonary stenosis	Murmur, upper left sternal edge; no carotid thrill	Balloon dilatation
Coarctation (adult type)	Systemic hypertension	Stent insertion or surgery
	Radio-femoral delay	

Coarctation of the aorta

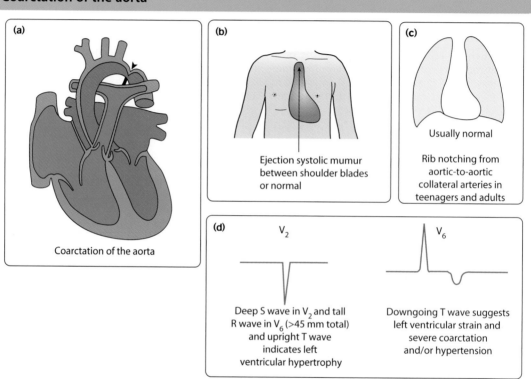

(a) Coarctation of the aorta

(b) Ejection systolic mumur between shoulder blades or normal

(c) Usually normal

Rib notching from aortic-to-aortic collateral arteries in teenagers and adults

(d) V₂ — Deep S wave in V$_2$ and tall R wave in V$_6$ (>45 mm total) and upright T wave indicates left ventricular hypertrophy

V₆ — Downgoing T wave suggests left ventricular strain and severe coarctation and/or hypertension

Figure 17.15 Coarctation of the aorta. **(a)** Coarctation of the aorta. There is narrowing of the aorta distal to the left subclavian artery adjacent to the insertion of the arterial duct. **(b)** Murmur. **(c)** Chest radiograph. **(d)** ECG.

Outflow obstruction in the sick infant

These lesions include:

- Coarctation of the aorta
- Interruption of the aortic arch
- Hypoplastic left heart syndrome.

Clinical features are:

- In all of these children, they usually present sick with heart failure and shock in the neonatal period, unless diagnosed on antenatal ultrasound
- Management is to resuscitate first (ABC)
- Prostaglandin should be commenced at the earliest opportunity

- Referral is made to a cardiac centre for early surgical intervention.

Coarctation of the aorta (Fig. 17.3)

This is due to arterial duct tissue encircling the aorta just at the point of insertion of the duct. When the duct closes, the aorta also constricts, causing severe obstruction to the left ventricular outflow. This is the commonest cause of collapse due to left outflow obstruction.

Clinical features

Examination on the first day of life is usually normal. The neonates usually present with acute circulatory collapse at 2 days of age when the duct closes.

Physical signs
- A sick baby, with severe heart failure
- Absent femoral pulses
- Severe metabolic acidosis.

Investigations
Chest radiograph
Cardiomegaly from heart failure and shock.

ECG
Normal.

Management
As for all the children in this section with an obstructed left outflow tract (see above). Surgical repair is performed soon after diagnosis.

Interruption of the aortic arch

- Uncommon, with *no* connection between the proximal aorta and distal to the arterial duct, so that the cardiac output is dependent on right-to-left shunt via the duct Fig. 17.16

- A VSD is usually present
- Presentation is with shock in the neonatal period as above
- Complete correction with closure of the VSD and repair of the aortic arch is usually performed within the first few days of life.
- Association with other conditions (DiGeorge syndrome – absence of thymus, palatal defects, immunodeficiency and hypocalcaemia and 22q11.2 gene micro-deletion).

Hypoplastic left heart syndrome

In this condition there is underdevelopment of the entire left side of the heart (Fig. 17.17). The mitral valve is small or atretic, the left ventricle is diminutive and there is usually aortic valve atresia. The ascending aorta is very small, and there is almost invariably coarctation of the aorta.

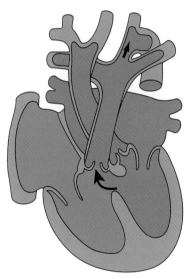

Interrupted aortic arch

Figure 17.16 Interruption of the aortic arch. The lower body circulation is maintained by right-to-left flow of blood across the duct.

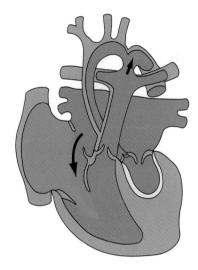

Hypoplastic left heart

Figure 17.17 Hypoplastic left heart syndrome. The entire left side of the heart is underdeveloped.

Summary

Left heart outflow obstruction in the sick infant – duct-dependent lesions

Lesion	Clinical features	Management
Coarctation of the aorta	Circulatory collapse	Maintain ABC
	Absent femoral pulses	Prostaglandin infusion
Interruption of the aortic arch	Circulatory collapse	Maintain ABC
	Absent femoral pulses and absent left brachial pulse	Prostaglandin infusion
Hypoplastic left heart syndrome	Circulatory collapse	Maintain ABC
	All peripheral pulses absent	Prostaglandin infusion

Clinical features

These children may be detected antenatally at ultrasound screening. This allows for effective counselling and prevents the child from becoming sick after birth. If they do present after birth, they are the sickest of all neonates presenting with a duct-dependent systemic circulation. There is no flow through the left side of the heart, so ductal constriction leads to profound acidosis and rapid cardiovascular collapse. There is weakness or absence of all peripheral pulses, in contrast to weak femoral pulses in coarctation of the aorta.

Management

The management of this condition consists of a difficult neonatal operation called the Norwood procedure. This is followed by a further operation (Glenn or hemi-Fontan) at about 6 months and again (Fontan) at about 3 years.

Care following cardiac surgery

Most children recover rapidly following cardiac surgery and are back at nursery or school within a month. Exercise tolerance will be variable and most children can be allowed to find their own limits. Restricted exercise is advised only for children with severe residual aortic stenosis and for ventricular dysfunction.

Most of the children are followed up in specialist cardiac clinics. Most lead normal, unrestricted lives, but any change in symptoms, e.g. decreasing exercise tolerance or palpitations, requires further investigation. An increasing number of adolescents and young adults require revision of surgery performed in early life. The most common reason for this is replacement of artificial valves and relief of post-surgical suture line stenosis, for example re-coarctation or pulmonary artery stenosis.

Cardiac arrhythmias

Sinus arrhythmia is normal in children and is detectable as a cyclical change in heart rate with respiration. There is acceleration during inspiration and slowing on expiration (the heart rate changing by up to 30 beats/min).

Supraventricular tachycardia

This is the most common childhood arrhythmia. The heart rate is rapid, between 250 and 300 beats/min. It can cause poor cardiac output and pulmonary oedema. It typically presents with symptoms of heart failure in the neonate or young infant. It is a cause of *hydrops fetalis* and intrauterine death. The term re-entry tachycardia is used because a circuit of conduction is set up, with premature activation of the atrium via an accessory pathway. There is rarely a structural heart problem, but an echocardiogram should be performed.

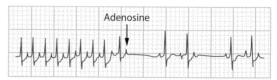

Figure 17.18 Rhythm strip showing supraventricular re-entry tachycardia, in which there is a narrow complex tachycardia (<120 ms or three small squares) of 250–300 beats/min, and response to treatment with adenosine.

Investigation

The ECG will generally show a narrow complex tachycardia of 250–300 beats/min (Fig. 17.18). It may be possible to discern a P wave after the QRS complex due to retrograde activation of the atrium via the accessory pathway. If heart failure is severe, there may be changes suggestive of myocardial ischaemia, with T-wave inversion in the lateral precordial leads. When in sinus rhythm, a short P–R interval may be discernible. In the Wolff–Parkinson–White (WPW) syndrome, the early antegrade activation of the ventricle via the pathway results in a short P–R interval and a delta wave.

Management

In the severely ill child, prompt restoration of sinus rhythm is the key to improvement. This is achieved by:

- Circulatory and respiratory support – tissue acidosis is corrected, positive pressure ventilation if required
- Vagal stimulating manoeuvres, e.g. carotid sinus massage or cold ice pack to face, successful in about 80%
- Intravenous adenosine – the treatment of choice. This is safe and effective, inducing atrioventricular block after rapid bolus injection. It terminates the tachycardia by breaking the re-entry circuit that is set up between the atrioventricular node and accessory pathway. It is given incrementally in increasing doses
- Electrical cardioversion with a synchronised DC shock (0.5–2 J/kg body weight) if adenosine fails.

Once sinus rhythm is restored, maintenance therapy will be required, e.g. with flecainide or sotalol. Digoxin can be used on its own when there is no overt pre-excitation wave (delta wave) on the resting ECG, but propranolol can be added in the presence of pre-excitation. Even though the resting ECG may remain abnormal, 90% of children will have no further attacks after infancy. Treatment is therefore stopped at 1 year of age. Those who have WPW syndrome need to be assessed to ensure they cannot conduct quickly and this may be undertaken in teenage life, with atrial pacing. This will reduce the small chance of sudden death in such patients. Those who relapse or are at risk are usually treated with percutaneous radiofrequency ablation or cryoablation of the accessory pathway.

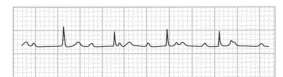

Figure 17.19 ECG of congenital complete heart block. The P waves and QRS complexes are dissociated.

Congenital complete heart block

This is a rare condition (Fig. 17.19) which is usually related to the presence of anti-Ro or anti-La antibodies in maternal serum. These mothers will have either manifest or latent connective tissue disorders. Subsequent pregnancies are often affected. This antibody appears to prevent normal development of the electrical conduction system in the developing heart, with atrophy and fibrosis of the atrioventricular node. It may cause fetal hydrops, death in utero and heart failure in the neonatal period. However, most remain symptom-free for many years, but a few become symptomatic with presyncope or syncope. All children with symptoms require insertion of an endocardial pacemaker. There are other rare causes of complete heart block.

Other arrhythmias

Long QT syndrome may be associated with sudden loss of consciousness during exercise, stress or emotion, usually in late childhood. It may be mistakenly diagnosed as epilepsy. If unrecognised, sudden death from ventricular tachycardia may occur. Inheritance is autosomal dominant; there are several phenotypes. It has been associated with erythromycin therapy, electrolyte disorders and head injury.

It is one of the group of channelopathies caused by specific gene mutations. Abnormalities of the sodium, potassium or calcium channels lead to gain or loss of function. Anyone with a family history of sudden unexplained death, or a history of syncope on exertion should be assessed.

Atrial fibrillation, atrial flutter, ectopic atrial tachycardia, ventricular tachycardia and ventricular fibrillation occur in children, but all are rare. They are most often seen in children who have undergone surgery for complex congenital heart disease.

Syncope

This is a common symptom in teenagers and usually does not represent cardiac disease.

The causes are:

- Neurocardiogenic – prolonged standing and vagal symptoms
- Situational – defecation, urination, cough or swallowing
- Orthostatic – BP fall > 20 mmHg after 3 min
- Ischaemic

- Arrhythmic – heart block, supraventricular tachycardia, ventricular tachycardia.

In most, the cause is non-cardiac. Features suggestive of a cardiac cause are:

- Symptoms on exercise – potentially dangerous
- Family history of sudden unexplained death
- Palpitations.

Check blood pressure and signs of cardiac disease (murmur, femoral pulses, Marfan syndrome).

Investigate with an ECG.

Chest pains

Rarely due to cardiac disease in children. Only those occurring with palpitations or on exertion suggest a possible cardiac origin.

Rheumatic fever

This is now rare in the developed world, but remains the most important cause of heart disease in children worldwide. Improvements in sanitation, social factors, the more liberal use of antibiotics and changes in streptococcal virulence have led to its virtual disappearance in developed countries. In susceptible individuals, there is an abnormal immune response to a preceding infection with group A β-haemolytic streptococcus. The disease mainly affects children aged 5–15 years.

Clinical features

After a latent interval of 2–6 weeks following a pharyngeal infection, polyarthritis, mild fever and malaise develop. The clinical features and diagnostic criteria are shown in Figure 17.20.

Chronic rheumatic heart disease

The most common form of long-term damage from scarring and fibrosis of the valve tissue of the heart is mitral stenosis. If there have been repeated attacks of rheumatic fever with carditis, this may occur as early as the second decade of life, but usually symptoms do not develop until early adult life. Although the mitral valve is the most frequently affected, aortic, tricuspid and, rarely, pulmonary valve disease may occur.

Management

The acute episode is usually treated with bed rest and anti-inflammatory agents. While there is evidence of active myocarditis (echocardiographic changes with a raised ESR), bed rest and limitation of exercise are essential. Aspirin is very effective at suppressing the inflammatory response of the joints and heart. It needs to be given in high dosage and serum levels monitored. If the fever and inflammation do not resolve rapidly, corticosteroids will be required. Symptomatic heart failure is treated with diuretics and ACE inhibitors, and significant pericardial effusions will require pericardiocentesis. Anti-streptococcal antibiotics may be given if there is any evidence of persisting infection.

Jones criteria for diagnosis of rheumatic fever

Required to make the diagnosis

Two major, or one major and two minor, criteria plus supportive evidence of preceding group A streptococcal infection (markedly raised ASO titre or other streptococcal antibodies, or group A streptococcus on throat culture)

Major manifestations

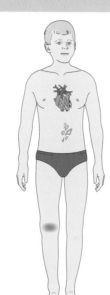

Pancarditis (50%)
Endocarditis
• significant murmur
• valvular dysfunction
Myocarditis
• may lead to heart failure and death
Pericarditis
• pericardial friction rub
• pericardial effusion
• tamponade

Sydenham chorea (10%)
2–6 months after the streptococcal infection
Involuntary movements and emotional lability for 3–6 months

Erythema marginatum (<5%)
Uncommon, early manifestation
Rash on trunk and limbs
Pink macules spread outwards, causing pink border with fading centre. Borders may unite to give a map-like outline

Polyarthritis (80%)
Ankles, knees and wrists
Exquisite tenderness, moderate redness and swelling
'Flitting', lasting <1 week in a joint, but migrating to other joints over 1–2 months

Subcutaneous nodules (rare)
Painless, pea-sized, hard
Mainly on extensor surfaces

Minor manifestations

Fever	Raised acute-phase reactants: ESR, C-reactive protein, leucocytosis
Polyarthralgia	Prolonged P–R interval on ECG
History of rheumatic fever	

Figure 17.20 Jones criteria for diagnosis of rheumatic fever.

Following resolution of the acute episode, recurrence should be prevented. Monthly injections of benzathine penicillin is the most effective prophylaxis. Alternatively, the penicillin can be given orally every day, but compliance may be a problem. Oral erythromycin can be substituted in those sensitive to penicillin. The length of treatment is controversial. Most recommend treatment to the age of 18 or 21 years, but, more recently, lifelong prophylaxis has been advocated. The severity of eventual rheumatic valvular disease relates to the number of childhood episodes of rheumatic fever.

Infective endocarditis

All children of any age with congenital heart disease (except secundum ASD), including neonates, are at risk of infective endocarditis. The risk is highest when there is a turbulent jet of blood, as with a VSD, coarctation of the aorta and persistent ductus arteriosus or if prosthetic material has been inserted at surgery. It may be difficult to diagnose, but should be suspected in any child or adult with a sustained fever, malaise, raised ESR, unexplained anaemia or haematuria. The presence of the classical peripheral stigmata of infective endocarditis should not be relied upon.

Clinical signs

• Fever
• Anaemia and pallor
• Splinter haemorrhages in nailbed
• Clubbing (late)
• Necrotic skin lesions (Fig. 17.21)
• Changing cardiac signs
• Splenomegaly
• Neurological signs from cerebral infarction
• Retinal infarcts
• Arthritis/arthralgia
• Haematuria (microscopic).

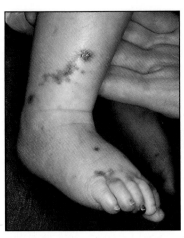

Figure 17.21 Widespread infected emboli and infarcts in a child with bacterial endocarditis. The tip of the third toe is gangrenous.

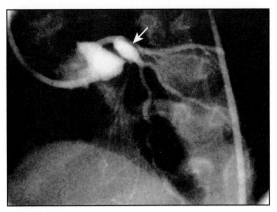

Figure 17.22 Kawasaki disease. Angiogram showing coronary artery aneurysm.

Diagnosis

Multiple blood cultures should be taken before antibiotics are started. Detailed cross-sectional echocardiography may confirm the diagnosis by identification of vegetations but can never exclude it. The vegetations consist of fibrin and platelets and contain infecting organisms. Acute-phase reactants are raised and can be useful to monitor response to treatment.

The most common causative organism is α-haemolytic streptococcus (*Streptococcus viridans*). Bacterial endocarditis is usually treated with high-dose penicillin in combination with an aminoglycoside, giving 6 weeks of intravenous therapy and checking that the serum level of the antibiotic will kill the organism. If there is infected prosthetic material, e.g. prosthetic valves, VSD patches or shunts, there is less chance of complete eradication and surgical removal may be required.

Prophylaxis

The most important factor in prophylaxis against endocarditis is good dental hygiene, and this should be strongly encouraged in all children with congenital heart disease.

Antibiotic prophylaxis is *no longer recommended in the UK*, but may be required in other countries for:

- Dental treatment, however trivial
- Surgery, which is likely to be associated with bacteraemia.

Myocarditis/cardiomyopathy

Dilated cardiomyopathy (a large, poorly contracting heart) may be inherited, secondary to metabolic disease or may result from a direct viral infection of the myocardium. It should be suspected in any child with an enlarged heart and heart failure who has previously been well. The diagnosis is readily made on echocardiography. Treatment is symptomatic with diuretics and ACE inhibitors and carvedilol, a β-adrenoceptor blocking agent. The role of steroids and immunoglobulin infusion is controversial. Myocarditis usually improves spontaneously, but some children ultimately require heart transplantation. Other cardiomyopathies (hypertrophic/restrictive) are rare in childhood and are usually related to a systemic disease (e.g. Hurler, Pompe or Noonan syndromes).

Kawasaki disease

This mainly affects children of 6 months to 5 years. Clinical features are described in Chapter 14. It is uncommon but can cause significant cardiac disease. An echocardiogram is performed at diagnosis which may show a pericardial effusion, myocardial disease (poor contractility), endocardial disease (valve regurgitation) or coronary disease with aneurysm formation, which can be giant (>8 mm in diameter). If the coronary arteries are abnormal, angiography (Fig. 17.22) or MRI will be required.

Pulmonary hypertension

This is of increasing importance in paediatric cardiology, as there is now effective medication for most causes. It can be caused by a number of different diseases (Box 17.4). From the cardiac perspective, most children with pulmonary hypertension (high pulmonary artery pressure, mean >25 mmHg), have a large post-tricuspid shunt with high pulmonary blood flow and low resistance, e.g. VSD, AVSD or PDA. The pressure falls to normal if the defect is corrected by surgery within 6 months of age. If these children are left untreated, however, the high flow and pressure causes irreversible damage to the pulmonary vascular bed (pulmonary vascular disease), which is not correctable other than by heart/lung transplantation.

Many medical therapies are now available, which may act on the pulmonary vasculature on the cyclic

Box 17.4 Causes of pulmonary hypertension

- Pulmonary arterial hypertension
  Idiopathic: sporadic or familial
  Post-tricuspid shunts (e.g. VSD, AVSD, PDA)
  HIV infection
  Persistent pulmonary hypertension of the
    newborn
- Pulmonary venous hypertension
  Left-sided heart disease
  Pulmonary vein stenosis or compression

- Pulmonary hypertension with respiratory disease
  Chronic obstructive or premature lung disease
  Interstitial lung disease
  Obstructive sleep apnoea or upper airway
    obstruction
- Pulmonary thromboembolic disease
- Pulmonary inflammatory or capillary disease.

GMP (guanosine monophosphate) pathway (e.g. inhaled nitric oxide, intravenous magnesium sulphate and oral phosphodiesterase inhibitors including sildenafil) or on the cyclic AMP pathway (intravenous prostacyclin or inhaled iloprost). In addition, endothelin receptor antagonists are valuable but expensive therapy, e.g. oral Bosentan. Anticoagulation is often given with heparin, aspirin or warfarin. These medications allow transplantation to be delayed for many years.

Further reading

Anderson RH, Baker E, Penny D, Redington A, Rigby M, et al: *Paediatric Cardiology,* ed 3. Edinburgh, 2010, Churchill Livingstone.

Website (Accessed May 2011)

Children's Heart Federation: http://www.childrens-heart-fed.org.uk/.

Kidney and urinary tract disorders

The spectrum of renal disease in children differs from that in adults:

- Many structural abnormalities of the kidneys and urinary tract are identified on antenatal ultrasound screening
- Urinary tract infection, vesicoureteric reflux and urinary obstruction have the potential to damage the growing kidney
- Nephrotic syndrome is usually steroid-sensitive and only rarely leads to chronic renal failure
- Chronic renal disorders and the drugs used to treat them may affect growth and development.

Assessment of the kidneys and urinary tract

The glomerular filtration rate (GFR) is low in the newborn infant and is especially low in premature infants; the GFR at 28 weeks' gestation is only 10% of the term infant. In term infants, the corrected GFR (15–20 ml/min per 1.73 m^2) rapidly rises to 1–2 years of age when the adult rate of 80 to 120 ml/min per 1.73 m^2 is achieved (Fig. 18.1). The assessment of renal function in children is listed in Table 18.1 and the radiological investigations of the kidneys and urinary tract in Table 18.2.

Congenital abnormalities

Before antenatal ultrasound scanning became routine, few congenital abnormalities of the kidneys and urinary tract were diagnosed until they caused symptoms in infancy, childhood or, occasionally, adult life. Now the majority are identified in utero and can be managed prospectively. Abnormalities are identified in 1 in 200–400 births. They are potentially important because they may:

- be associated with abnormal renal development or function
- predispose to postnatal infection
- involve urinary obstruction which requires surgical treatment.

The antenatal detection and early treatment of urinary tract anomalies provide an opportunity to minimise or prevent progressive renal damage. A disadvantage is that minor abnormalities are also detected, most commonly mild unilateral pelvic dilatation, which do not require intervention but may lead to over-investigation, unnecessary treatment and unwarranted parental anxiety.

Anomalies detectable on antenatal ultrasound screening

Absence of both kidneys (*renal agenesis*) – as amniotic fluid is mainly derived from fetal urine, there is severe oligohydramnios resulting in Potter syndrome (Fig. 18.2a, 18.2b), which is fatal.

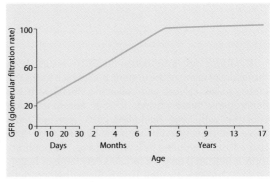

Figure 18.1 Increase in renal function (GFR) with age.

Table 18.1 Assessment of renal function in children

Plasma creatinine concentration (PCr)	Main test of renal function. Rises progressively throughout childhood according to height and muscle bulk. May not be outside laboratory 'normal range' until renal function has fallen to less than half normal
Estimated glomerular filtration rate (eGFR)	The formula eGFR = k × height (cm) ÷ creatinine (μmol/L) provides estimate of GFR. Better measure of renal function than creatinine and useful to monitor renal function serially in children with renal impairment (k is 40 if creatinine measured using Jaffe method or 30 if measured enzymatically)
Inulin or EDTA glomerular filtration rate	More accurate as clearance from the plasma of substances freely filtered at the glomerulus, and is not secreted or reabsorbed by the tubules. Need for repeated blood tests limits use in children
Creatinine clearance	Requires timed urine collection and blood tests. Rarely done in children as inconvenient and inaccurate
Plasma urea concentration	Increased in renal failure, often before creatinine starts rising, and raised levels may be symptomatic. Urea levels also increased by high protein diet and if in a catabolic state.

Table 18.2 Radiological investigation of the kidneys and urinary tract

Ultrasound (US)	Standard imaging procedure of the kidneys and urinary tract, provides anatomical assessment but not function. Excellent at visualising urinary tract dilatation, stones and nephrocalcinosis (small, multiple calcium deposits in renal parenchyma)
	Advantages: non-invasive, mobile
	Disadvantages: operator-dependent, will not detect all renal scars
DMSA scan (^{99m}Tc dimercaptosuccinic acid)	*Static* scan of the renal cortex
	Detects functional defects, such as scars, but very sensitive, so need to wait at least 2 months after a urinary tract infection to avoid diagnosing false 'scars'
Micturating cystourethrogram (MCUG)	Contrast introduced into bladder through urethral catheter.
	Can visualise bladder and urethral anatomy. Detects vesicoureteric reflux (VUR) and urethral obstruction
	Disadvantages: invasive and unpleasant investigation especially beyond infancy, high radiation dose
MAG3 renogram (mercapto-acetyl-triglycine, labelled with ^{99m}Tc)	*Dynamic* scan, isotope-labelled substance MAG3 excreted from the blood into the urine. Measures drainage, best performed with a high urine flow.
	In children old enough to cooperate (usually >4 years), scan during micturition is used to identify VUR
Plain abdominal X-ray	Identifies unsuspected spinal abnormalities
	May identify renal stones, but poor at showing nephrocalcinosis.

Multicystic dysplastic kidney (MCDK) – results from the failure of union of the ureteric bud (which forms the ureter, pelvis, calyces and collecting ducts) with the nephrogenic mesenchyme. It is a non-functioning structure with large fluid-filled cysts with no renal tissue and no connection with the bladder (Fig. 18.3). Half will have involuted by 2 years of age, and nephrectomy is indicated only if it remains very large or hypertension develops, but this is rare. Since they produce no urine, Potter syndrome will result if the lesion is bilateral. Other causes of large cystic kidneys are *autosomal recessive polycystic kidney disease (ARPKD)* (Fig. 18.4), *autosomal dominant polycystic kidney disease (ADPKD)* (Fig. 18.5) and tuberous sclerosis. In contrast to a multicystic dysplastic kidney, in these disorders some or normal renal function is maintained but both kidneys are always affected. Autosomal dominant polycystic kidney disease has an incidence of 1 in 1000; the main symptoms in childhood are hypertension and haematuria and it causes renal failure in late adulthood.

Some congenital abnormalities of the kidneys and urinary tract

Bilateral renal agenesis or bilateral multicystic dysplastic kidneys

↓

Reduced fetal urine excretion

↓

Oligohydramnios causing fetal compression

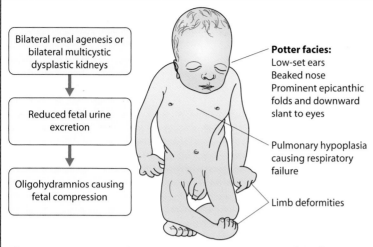

Potter facies:
Low-set ears
Beaked nose
Prominent epicanthic folds and downward slant to eyes

Pulmonary hypoplasia causing respiratory failure

Limb deformities

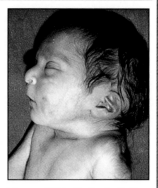

Figure 18.2b Facies in Potter syndrome.

Figure 18.2a Potter syndrome. Intrauterine compression of the fetus from oligohydramnios caused by lack of fetal urine causes a characteristic facies, lung hypoplasia and postural deformities including severe talipes. The infant may be stillborn or die soon after birth from respiratory failure.

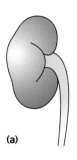
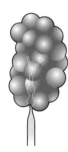

(a)

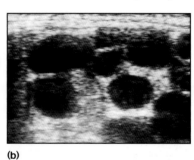

(b)

Figure 18.3 (a) Multicystic renal dysplasia. The kidney is replaced by cysts of variable size, with atresia of the ureter. **(b)** Renal ultrasound showing discrete cysts of variable size.

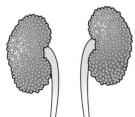

Figure 18.4 Autosomal recessive polycystic kidney disease (ARPKD). There is diffuse bilateral enlargement of both kidneys.

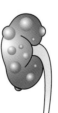
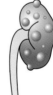

Figure 18.5 Autosomal dominant polycystic kidney disease (ADPKD). There are separate cysts of varying size between normal renal parenchyma. The kidneys are enlarged.

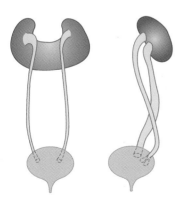

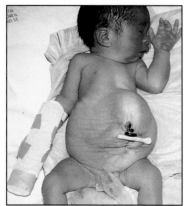

Figure 18.8 Absent musculature syndrome (prune-belly syndrome). The name arises from the wrinkled appearance of the abdomen. It is associated with a large bladder, dilated ureters and cryptorchidism. (Courtesy of Dr Jane Deal.)

Figure 18.6 (left) Horseshoe kidney.
Figure 18.7 (right) Duplex kidney showing ureterocele of upper moiety and reflux into lower pole moiety.

Urinary tract obstruction

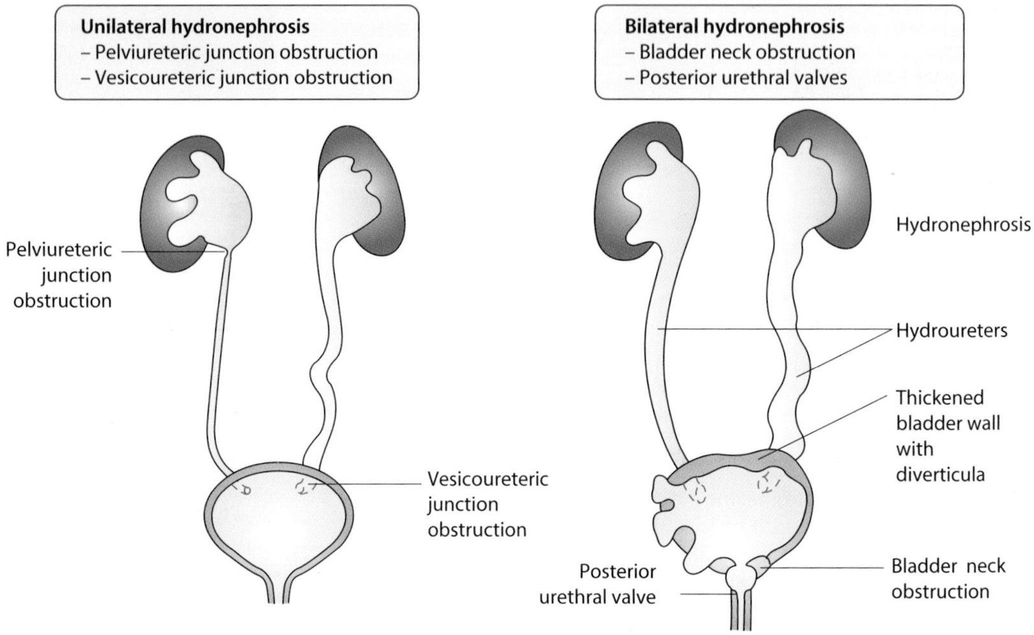

Unilateral hydronephrosis
– Pelviureteric junction obstruction
– Vesicoureteric junction obstruction

Bilateral hydronephrosis
– Bladder neck obstruction
– Posterior urethral valves

Pelviureteric junction obstruction

Hydronephrosis

Hydroureters

Thickened bladder wall with diverticula

Vesicoureteric junction obstruction

Posterior urethral valve

Bladder neck obstruction

Figure 18.9a Obstruction to urine flow results in dilatation of the urinary tract proximal to the site of obstruction. Obstruction may be at the pelviureteric or vesicoureteric junction (left), the bladder neck or urethra (right).

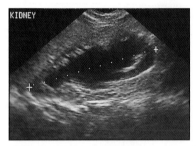

Figure 18.9b An ultrasound showing a dilated renal pelvis from pelviureteric junction obstruction.

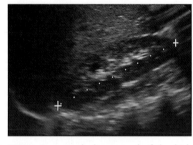

Figure 18.9c A normal ultrasound of the kidney is shown for comparison.

Figure 18.9d Graph from dynamic nuclear medicine scan MAG3 showing delayed excretion from a pelviureteric junction obstruction.

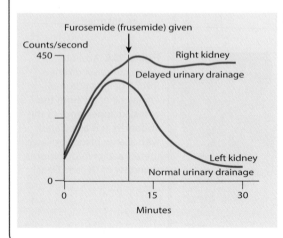

Furosemide (frusemide) given

Counts/second
450

Right kidney

Delayed urinary drainage

Left kidney

Normal urinary drainage

0

0   15   30

Minutes

It is associated with several extra-renal features including cysts in liver and pancreas, cerebral aneurysms and mitral valve prolapse.

Abnormal caudal migration may result in a *pelvic kidney* or a *horseshoe kidney* (Fig. 18.6), when the lower poles are fused in the midline. The abnormal position may predispose to infection or obstruction to urinary drainage.

Premature division of the ureteric bud gives rise to a *duplex system*, which can vary from simply a bifid renal pelvis to complete division with two ureters. These ureters frequently have an abnormal drainage so that the ureter from the lower pole moiety often refluxes, whereas the upper pole ureter may drain ectopically into the urethra or vagina or may prolapse into the bladder (ureterocele) and urine flow may be obstructed (Fig. 18.7).

Failure of fusion of the infraumbilical midline structures results in exposed bladder mucosa (*bladder extrophy*). Absence or severe deficiency of the anterior abdominal wall muscles is frequently associated with a large bladder and dilated ureters (megacystis-megaureters) and cryptorchidism, the *absent musculature syndrome* (*prune-belly syndrome*) (Fig. 18.8).

Obstruction to urine flow may occur at the pelvi-ureteric or vesicoureteric junction, at the *bladder neck* (e.g. due to disruption of the nerve supply, *neuropathic bladder*) or at the *posterior urethra* in a boy due to mucosal folds or a membrane, known as *posterior urethral valves*. The consequences of obstruction to urine flow are shown in Figures 18.9a-18.9d. At worst, this results in a *dysplastic kidney* which is small, poorly functioning and may contain cysts and aberrant embryonic tissue such as cartilage. In the most severe and bilateral cases Potter syndrome is present. Renal dysplasia can also occur in association with severe intrauterine vesicoureteric reflux, in isolation or in certain rare, inherited syndromes affecting multiple systems.

Antenatal treatment

The male fetus with posterior urethral valves may develop severe urinary outflow obstruction resulting in progressive bilateral hydronephrosis, poor renal growth and declining liquor volume with the potential to lead to pulmonary hypoplasia. Intrauterine bladder drainage procedures to prevent severe renal damage have been attempted but results have been disappointing. Early delivery is rarely indicated.

Postnatal management

An example of a protocol for infants with antenatally diagnosed anomalies is shown in Figure 18.10. Prophylactic antibiotics may be started at birth to try to prevent urinary tract infection, although practice varies between centres. As the newborn kidney has a low GFR, urine flow is low and mild outflow obstruction may not be evident in the first few days of life. The ultrasound scan should therefore be delayed for several weeks. However, bilateral hydronephrosis in a male infant warrants an ultrasound shortly after birth to exclude posterior urethral valves, which always requires urological intervention such as cystoscopic ablation (Case History 18.1).

Antenatally diagnosed urinary tract anomalies – a protocol

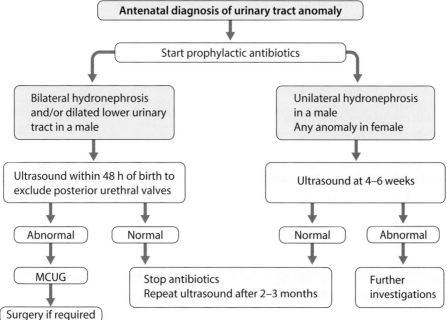

Figure 18.10 An example of a protocol for the management of infants with antenatally diagnosed urinary tract anomalies. (MCUG, micturating cystourethrogram.)

Kidney and urinary tract disorders

Case History

18.1 Posterior urethral valves

Bilateral hydronephrosis was noted on antenatal ultrasound at 20 weeks' gestation in a male fetus. There was poor renal growth, progressive hydronephrosis and decreasing volume of amniotic fluid (Fig. 18.11a) on repeated scans. After birth, prophylactic antibiotics were started. An urgent ultrasound showed bilateral hydronephrosis with small dysplastic kidneys. The bladder and ureters were grossly distended. The plasma creatinine was raised. A micturating cystourethrogram (MCUG) (Fig. 18.11b) showed vesicoureteric reflux, a dilated posterior urethra and posterior urethral valves which was treated endoscopically. Renal function initially improved but then progressed to chronic renal failure. He had a renal transplant at 10 years of age.

 Bilateral hydronephrosis in a male infant requires urgent investigation to exclude posterior urethral valve.

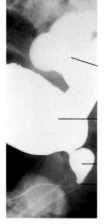

Gross vesicoureteric reflux

Distended bladder with trabeculated wall

Dilated posterior urethra
Posterior urethral valve

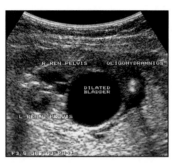

Figure 18.11a Antenatal ultrasound scan in an infant with urinary outflow obstruction from posterior urethral valve. (Courtesy of Mr Karl Murphy.)

Figure 18.11b Micturating cystourethrogram (MCUG) in the same patient.

Urinary tract infection

About 3–7% of girls and 1–2% of boys have at least one symptomatic urinary tract infection (UTI) before the age of 6 years, and 12–30% of them have a recurrence within a year. UTI may involve the kidneys (pyelonephritis), when it is usually associated with fever and systemic involvement, or may be due to cystitis, when there may be no fever. UTI in childhood is important because:

- up to half of patients have a structural abnormality of their urinary tract
- pyelonephritis may damage the growing kidney by forming a scar, predisposing to hypertension and to chronic renal failure if the scarring is bilateral.

There are NICE guidelines on urinary tract infection in children, published in 2007, although they have proved to be controversial.

Clinical features

Presentation of UTI varies with age (Box 18.1). In infants, symptoms are non-specific; fever is usually but not always present, and septicaemia may develop rapidly. The classical symptoms of dysuria, frequency and loin pain become more common with increasing age. Serious illness from septicaemia is described in the child with a fever in Chapter 14. Dysuria alone is usually due to cystitis, or vulvitis in girls or balanitis in uncircumcised boys. Symptoms suggestive of a UTI may also occur following sexual abuse.

Box 18.1 Presentation of UTI in infants and children

Infants	Children
• Fever	• Dysuria and
• Vomiting	frequency
• Lethargy or	• Abdominal pain or
irritability	loin tenderness
• Poor feeding/failure	• Fever with or
to thrive	without rigors
• Jaundice	(exaggerated
• Septicaemia	shivering)
• Offensive urine	• Lethargy and
• Febrile convulsion	anorexia
(>6 months).	• Vomiting, diarrhoea
	• Haematuria
	• Offensive/cloudy
	urine
	• Febrile convulsion
	• Recurrence of
	enuresis.

Collection of samples

The commonest error in the management of UTI in children, and especially in infants, is failure to establish

Table 18.3 Methods and interpretation of dipstick testing in children

Methods of dipstick testing	
Nitrite stick testing	Positive result useful as very likely to indicate a true UTI
	But some children with a UTI are nitrite-negative
Leucocyte esterase stick testing (for WBCs)	May be present in children with UTI but may also be negative
	Present in children with febrile illness without UTIs
	Positive in balanitis and vulvovaginitis
Interpretation of results	
Leucocyte esterase and nitrite positive	Regard as UTI
Leucocyte esterase negative and nitrite positive	Start antibiotic treatment
	Diagnosis depends on urine culture
Leucocyte esterase positive and nitrite negative	Only start antibiotic treatment if clinical evidence of UTI
	Diagnosis depends on urine culture
Leucocyte esterase and nitrite negative	UTI unlikely. Repeat or send urine for culture if clinical history suggests UTI
Blood, protein, and glucose present on stick testing	Useful in any unwell child to identify other diseases, e.g. nephritis, diabetes mellitus, but will not discriminate between children with and without UTIs

the diagnosis properly in the first place. If the diagnosis of a UTI is not made, the opportunity to prevent renal damage may be missed, or, if incorrectly diagnosed, may lead to unnecessary invasive investigations.

For the child in nappies, urine can be collected by:

- A 'clean-catch' sample into a waiting clean pot when the nappy is removed. This is the recommended method
- An adhesive plastic bag applied to the perineum after careful washing, although there may be contamination from the skin
- A urethral catheter if there is urgency in obtaining a sample and no urine has been passed
- Suprapubic aspiration (SPA), when a fine needle attached to a syringe is inserted directly into the bladder just above the symphysis pubis under ultrasound guidance; it may be used in severely ill infants requiring urgent diagnosis and treatment, but it is an invasive procedure, and is increasingly replaced by urethral catheter sampling.

In the older child, urine can be obtained by collecting a midstream sample. Careful cleaning and collection are necessary, as contamination with both white cells and bacteria can occur from under the foreskin in boys, and from reflux of urine into the vagina during voiding in girls.

Ideally, the urine sample should be microscoped to identify organisms and cultured straight away. This is indicated in all infants and children <3 years old with a suspected UTI. If this is not possible, the urine sample should be refrigerated to prevent the overgrowth of contaminating bacteria. Urinary white cells are not a reliable feature of a UTI, as they may lyse during storage and may be present in febrile children without a UTI and in children with balanitis or vulvovaginitis.

Dipsticks can be used as a screening test. Urine culture should still be performed unless both leucocyte esterase and nitrite are negative or if the clinical symptoms and dipstick tests do not correlate (Table 18.3).

A bacterial culture of >10^5 colony-forming units of a single organism per millilitre in a properly collected specimen gives a 90% probability of infection. If the same result is found in a second sample, the probability rises to 95%. A growth of mixed organisms usually represents contamination, but if there is doubt, another sample should be collected. Any bacterial growth of a single organism per millilitre in a catheter sample or suprapubic aspirate is considered diagnostic of infection.

 A urine sample should be tested in all infants with an unexplained fever >38°C.

Bacterial and host factors that predispose to infection

Infecting organism

UTI is usually the result of bowel flora entering the urinary tract via the urethra, except in the newborn when it is more likely to be haematogenous. The commonest organism is *E. coli*, followed by *Klebsiella*, *Proteus* and *Pseudomonas* and *Strep. faecalis*. *Proteus* infection is more commonly diagnosed in boys than in girls, possibly because of its presence under the prepuce. *Proteus* infection predisposes to the formation of phosphate stones by splitting urea to ammonia and thus alkalinising the urine. *Pseudomonas* infection may indicate the presence of some structural abnormality in the urinary tract affecting drainage.

Antenatally diagnosed renal or urinary tract abnormality

Increases risk of infection.

Incomplete bladder emptying

Contributing factors in some children are:

- Infrequent voiding, resulting in bladder enlargement
- Vulvitis
- Incomplete micturition with residual post-micturition bladder volumes
- Obstruction by a loaded rectum from constipation
- Neuropathic bladder
- Vesicoureteric reflux.

Vesicoureteric reflux

Vesicoureteric reflux (VUR) is a developmental anomaly of the vesicoureteric junctions. The ureters are displaced laterally and enter directly into the bladder rather than at an angle, with a shortened or absent intramural course. Severe cases may be associated with renal dysplasia. It is familial, with a 30–50% chance of occurring in first-degree relatives. It may also occur with bladder pathology, e.g. a neuropathic bladder or urethral obstruction, or temporarily after a UTI. Its severity varies from reflux into the lower end of an undilated ureter during micturition to the severest form with reflux during bladder filling and voiding, with a distended ureter, renal pelvis and clubbed calyces (Fig. 18.12). Mild reflux is unlikely to be of significance, but the more severe degrees of VUR may be associated with

intrarenal reflux (IRR), the backflow of urine from the renal pelvis into the papillary collecting ducts; intrarenal reflux is associated with a particularly high risk of renal scarring if UTIs occur. The incidence of renal defects increases with increasing severity of reflux. There is considerable controversy as to whether renal scarring is a congenital abnormality already present in children with reflux and which predisposes to infection or if children with reflux have normal kidneys at birth which are damaged by UTIs and that preventing UTIs in these children prevents scars. Reflux tends to resolve with age especially lower grades of VUR.

Reflux with associated ureteric dilatation is important, as:

- urine returning to the bladder from the ureters after voiding results in incomplete bladder emptying, which encourages infection
- the kidneys may become infected (pyelonephritis), particularly if there is intrarenal reflux
- bladder voiding pressure is transmitted to the renal papillae; this may contribute to renal damage if voiding pressures are high.

Infection may destroy renal tissue, leaving a scar, resulting in a shrunken, poorly functioning segment of kidney (reflux nephropathy). If scarring is bilateral and severe, chronic renal failure may develop. The risk for hypertension in childhood or early adult life is variously estimated to be up to 10%.

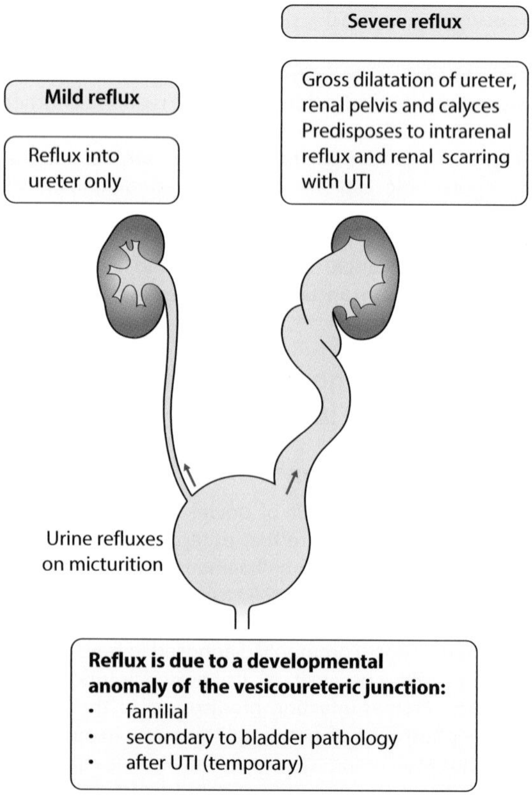

Investigation

The extent to which a child with a UTI should be investigated is controversial. This is not only because of the invasive nature and radiation burden of the tests but also because of the lack of an evidence base to show that outcome is improved (unless urinary obstruction is demonstrated). Mild reflux usually resolves spontaneously, and operative intervention to stop reflux has not been shown to decrease renal damage. Furthermore, there is no evidence that antibiotic prophylaxis is any better than prompt treatment. There has, therefore, been a move away from extensive investigation of all children with UTIs to those who have had atypical or recurrent UTIs. Atypical UTI includes:

- Seriously ill or septicaemia
- Poor urine flow
- Abdominal or bladder mass
- Raised creatinine
- Failure to respond to suitable antibiotics within 48 h
- infection with non-E. coli organism.

An initial ultrasound will identify:

- Serious structural abnormalities and urinary obstruction
- Renal defects (but poor at identifying renal scars).

Subsequent investigations will depend on the results of the ultrasound. The need for any investigations in a child with only bladder symptoms (lower urinary tract infection/cystitis) is also controversial. If urethral obstruction is suspected (abnormal bladder in a boy),

Mild reflux
Reflux into ureter only

Severe reflux
Gross dilatation of ureter, renal pelvis and calyces Predisposes to intrarenal reflux and renal scarring with UTI

Urine refluxes on micturition

Reflux is due to a developmental anomaly of the vesicoureteric junction:
- familial
- secondary to bladder pathology
- after UTI (temporary)

Figure 18.12 Vesicoureteric reflux.

18.2 Urinary tract infection

Jack, a 2-month-old infant, stopped feeding and had a high, intermittent fever. He was referred to hospital, where he had an infection screen. Urine examination showed >100 white blood cells, >10^5 *E. coli*/ml. He was treated with intravenous antibiotics. An ultrasound showed that the left kidney was smaller than the right kidney with dilated ureters. He was started on prophylactic antibiotics. A DMSA scan (Fig. 18.14) performed 3 months later confirmed bilateral renal scarring, with the left kidney contributing 33% of renal function. The MCUG (Fig. 18.15) showed bilateral vesicoureteric reflux. At 4 years of age, the reflux had resolved and antibiotic prophylaxis was stopped. His blood pressure and renal growth and function continue to be monitored.

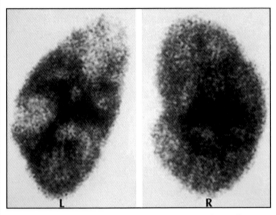

Figure 18.14 DMSA scan showing bilateral renal scarring, more severe on left upper pole.

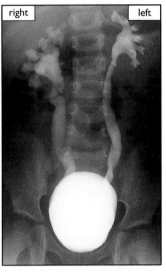

Figure 18.15 Micturating cystourethrogram showing bilateral vesicoureteric reflux with ureteric dilatation and dilated, clubbed calyces on the right.

First urinary tract infection - a protocol for initial management and investigation

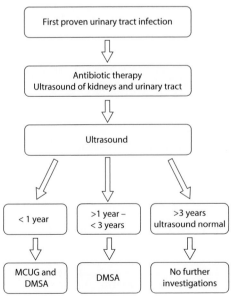

Figure 18.13 An example of a protocol for the initial management and investigation of a first urinary tract infection. This is a controversial area. The UK NICE guidelines, 2007 do not recommend ultrasound examination for first UTI if there was response to antibiotic treatment within 48 h, unless <6 months old or atypical or recurrent, but many paediatric nephrologists consider this approach too conservative and follow protocols like the one shown here.

Kidney and urinary tract disorders

MCUG should be performed promptly. Functional scans should be deferred for 3 months after a UTI, unless the ultrasound is suggestive of obstruction, to avoid missing a newly developed scar and because of false-positive results from transient inflammation. Medical measures for the prevention of UTI should be initiated.

A suggested schema for investigation of the first proven UTI is shown in Figure 18.13, but varies between centres.

Management

All infants <3 months old with suspicion of a UTI or if seriously ill should be referred immediately to a hospital. They require intravenous antibiotic therapy (e.g. cefotaxime) until the temperature has settled, when oral treatment is substituted (see Case History 18.2.)

Infants >3 months and children with acute pyelonephritis/upper urinary tract infection (bacteriuria and fever ≥38°C or bacteriuria and loin pain/tenderness even if fever is <38°C) are usually treated with

oral antibiotics with low resistance patterns (e.g. co-amoxiclav for 7–10 days); or else intravenous antibiotics, e.g. cefotaxime is given for 2–4 days followed by oral antibiotics for a total of 7–10 days. The choice of antibiotic is adjusted according to sensitivity on urine culture.

Children with cystitis/lower urinary tract infection (dysuria but no systemic symptoms or signs) can be treated with oral antibiotics for 3 days.

Medical measures for the prevention of UTI

The aim is to ensure washout of organisms that ascend into the bladder from the perineum; and to reduce the presence of aggressive organisms in the stool, perineum and under the foreskin:

- High fluid intake to produce a high urine output
- Regular voiding
- Ensuring complete bladder emptying by encouraging the child to try a second time to

---

Summary

A child with a first urinary tract infection

Why important?
Up to half have a structural abnormality of their urinary tract
Pyelonephritis may damage the growing kidney by forming a renal scar, which may result in hypertension and chronic renal failure

Diagnosis secure?
- Suggestive clinical features?
- Upper or lower urinary tract infection?
- Urine sample properly collected and processed?
- Culture of single organism >10^5/ml if clean catch or mid-stream urine or else any organisms on suprapubic aspirate or catheter sample?

Predisposing factors?
Incomplete bladder emptying
Constipation
Vesicoureteric reflux

Why investigate?
To identify serious structural abnormalities, urinary obstruction, renal scars, vesicoureteric reflux.

What investigation?
Consider:
- Ultrasound of kidneys and urinary tract
- DMSA to check for renal scars 3 months after UTI
- MAG3 or MCUG to detect obstruction and vesicouretic reflux.

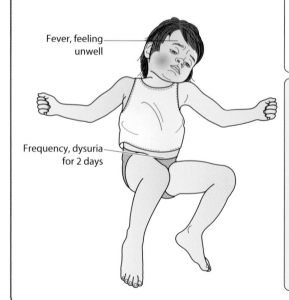

Fever, feeling unwell

Frequency, dysuria for 2 days

Management
Treat infection with antibiotics
Advice about medical preventative measures:
- High fluid intake
- Regular voiding, double micturition
- Prevent or treat constipation
- Good perineal hygiene
- *Lactobacillus acidophilus*
Advise to check urine culture if develops clinical features suggestive of non-specific illness

If renal scarring or reflux on investigation, or develops recurrent UTIs:
- Consider low-dose antibiotic prophylaxis
- Monitor blood pressure, renal growth and function

empty his bladder after a minute or two, commonly known as double micturition; this empties any urine residue or refluxed urine returning to the bladder
- Prevention or treatment of constipation
- Good perineal hygiene
- *Lactobacillus acidophilus*, a probiotic to encourage colonisation of the gut by this organism and reduce the number of pathogenic organisms that might potentially cause invasive disease
- Antibiotic prophylaxis, although this is controversial. It is often used in those under 2 years of age with a congenital abnormality of the kidneys or urinary tract or who have had an upper urinary tract infection and those with severe reflux. Trimethoprim (2 mg/kg at night) is used most often, but nitrofurantoin or cephalexin may be given. Broad-spectrum, poorly absorbed antibiotics such as amoxicillin should be avoided.

Follow-up of children with recurrent UTIs, renal scarring or reflux

In these children:

- Urine culture should be checked with any non-specific illness in case it is caused by a UTI (urine should not be cultured routinely).
- Long-term, low-dose antibiotic prophylaxis can be used. There is no evidence for when antibiotic prophylaxis should be stopped.
- Circumcision in boys may sometimes be considered, as there is evidence that it reduces the incidence of urinary tract infection.
- Anti-reflux surgery may be indicated if there is progression of scarring with ongoing reflux, but it has not been shown to improve outcome.
- Blood pressure should be checked annually if renal defects are present.
- Regular assessment of renal growth and function is necessary if there are bilateral defects because of the risk of chronic renal failure.

If there are further symptomatic UTIs in younger children, investigations are required to determine whether there are new scars or continuing reflux.

Enuresis

Primary nocturnal enuresis

This is considered in Chapter 23.

Daytime enuresis

This is a lack of bladder control during the day in a child old enough to be continent (over the age of 3–5 years). Nocturnal enuresis is also usually present. It may be caused by:

- Lack of attention to bladder sensation: a manifestation of a developmental or psychogenic problem, although it may occur in otherwise normal children who are too preoccupied with what they are doing to respond to the sensation of a full bladder
- Detrusor instability (sudden, urgent urge to void induced by sudden bladder contractions)
- Bladder neck weakness
- A neuropathic bladder (bladder is enlarged and fails to empty properly, irregular thick wall and is associated with spina bifida and other neurological conditions)
- A urinary tract infection (rarely in the absence of other symptoms)
- Constipation
- An ectopic ureter, causes constant dribbling and child is always damp.

Examination may reveal evidence of a neuropathic bladder, i.e. the bladder may be distended, there may be abnormal perineal sensation and anal tone or abnormal leg reflexes and gait. Sensory loss in the distribution of the S2, 3 and 4 dermatomes should be sought. A spinal lesion may be present. Girls who are dry at night but wet on getting up are likely to have pooling of urine from an ectopic ureter opening into the vagina.

A urine sample should be examined for microscopy, culture and sensitivity. Other investigations are performed if indicated. An ultrasound may show bladder pathology, with incomplete bladder emptying or thickening of the bladder wall. Urodynamic studies may be required. An X-ray of the spine may reveal a vertebral anomaly. An MRI scan may be required to confirm or exclude a non-bony spinal defect such as tethering of the cord.

Affected children in whom a neurological cause has been excluded may benefit from star charts, bladder training and pelvic floor exercises. Constipation should be treated. A small portable alarm with a pad in the pants, which is activated by urine, can be used when there is lack of attention to bladder sensation. Anticholinergic drugs, such as oxybutynin, to damp down bladder contractions, may be helpful if other measures fail.

Secondary (onset) enuresis

The loss of previously achieved urinary continence may be due to:

- Emotional upset, the commonest cause
- UTI
- Polyuria from an osmotic diuresis in diabetes mellitus or a renal concentrating disorder, e.g. sickle cell disease or chronic renal failure.

Investigation should include:

- Testing a urine sample for infection, glycosuria and proteinuria
- Assessment of urinary concentrating ability by measuring the osmolality of an early morning urine sample. Rarely, a formal water deprivation test may be needed to exclude a urinary concentrating defect
- Ultrasound of the renal tract.

Summary

Enuresis

Daytime enuresis

- Consider causes – developmental or psychogenic, bladder instability or neuropathy, urinary tract infection, constipation, ectopic ureter.

Secondary (onset) enuresis

- Consider – emotional upset, UTI, polyuria from an osmotic diuresis in diabetes mellitus or a renal concentrating disorder.

Proteinuria

Transient proteinuria may occur during febrile illnesses or after exercise and does not require investigation. Persistent proteinuria is significant and should be quantified by measuring the urine protein/creatinine ratio in an early morning sample (protein should not exceed 20 mg/mmol of creatinine).

A common cause is orthostatic (postural) proteinuria, where proteinuria is only found when the child is upright, i.e. during the day. It can be diagnosed by measuring the urine protein/creatinine ratio in a series of early morning urine specimens. The prognosis is excellent and further investigations are not necessary.

Box 18.2 Causes of proteinuria

- Orthostatic proteinuria
- Glomerular abnormalities
  - Minimal change disease
  - Glomerulonephritis
  - Abnormal glomerular basement membrane (familial nephritides)
- Increased glomerular filtration pressure
- Reduced renal mass
- Hypertension
- Tubular proteinuria.

Other causes of proteinuria, which needs further evaluation, are listed in Box 18.2.

Nephrotic syndrome

In nephrotic syndrome, heavy proteinuria results in a low plasma albumin and oedema. The cause of the condition is unknown, but a few cases are secondary to systemic diseases such as Henoch–Schönlein purpura (HSP) and other vasculitides, e.g. systemic lupus erythematosus (SLE), infections (e.g. malaria) or allergens (e.g. bee sting).

Clinical signs of the nephrotic syndrome are:

- Periorbital oedema (particularly on waking), the earliest sign (Fig. 18.16)
- Scrotal or vulval, leg and ankle oedema (Fig. 18.17)
- Ascites
- Breathlessness due to pleural effusions and abdominal distension.

The initial investigations are listed in Box 18.3.

Steroid-sensitive nephrotic syndrome

In 85–90% of children with nephrotic syndrome, the proteinuria resolves with corticosteroid therapy (steroid-sensitive nephrotic syndrome). These children do not progress to renal failure. It is commoner in boys than in girls, in Asian children than in Caucasians, and there is a weak association with atopy. It is often

Box 18.3 Investigations performed at presentation of nephrotic syndrome

- Urine protein – on test strips ('dipstick')
- Full blood count and ESR
- Urea, electrolytes, creatinine, albumin
- Complement levels – C3, C4
- Antistreptolysin O or anti-DNAse B titres and throat swab
- Urine microscopy and culture
- Urinary sodium concentration
- Hepatitis B and C screen
- Malaria screen if travel abroad.

Nephrotic syndrome

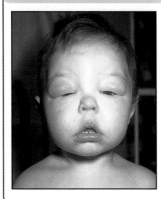

Figure 18.16 Facial oedema in nephrotic syndrome.

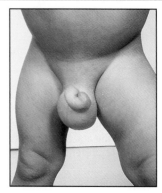

Figure 18.17 Gross oedema of the scrotum and legs as well as abdominal distension from ascites.

precipitated by respiratory infections. Features suggesting steroid-sensitive nephrotic syndrome are:

- Age between 1 and 10 years
- No macroscopic haematuria
- Normal blood pressure
- Normal complement levels
- Normal renal function.

Management

The most widely used protocol is to initially give oral corticosteroids (60 mg/m^2 per day of prednisolone), unless there are atypical features. After 4 weeks, the dose is reduced to 40 mg/m^2 on alternate days for 4 weeks and then stopped. The median time for the urine to become free of protein is 11 days. However, there is now good evidence that extending the initial course of steroids, by gradually tapering the alternate day part of the course, leads to a marked reduction in the proportion of children who develop a frequently relapsing or steroid-dependent course, and this scheme is increasingly being adopted. Children who do not respond to 4–8 weeks of corticosteroid therapy or have atypical features may have a more complex diagnosis and require a renal biopsy. Renal histology in steroid-sensitive nephrotic syndrome is usually normal on light microscopy but fusion of the specialised epithelial cells that invest the glomerular capillaries (podocytes) is seen on electron microscopy. For this reason, it is called minimal change disease.

The child with nephrotic syndrome is susceptible to several serious complications at presentation or relapse:

- *Hypovolaemia*. During the initial phase of oedema formation the intravascular compartment may become volume depleted. The child who becomes hypovolaemic characteristically complains of abdominal pain and may feel faint. There is peripheral vasoconstriction and urinary sodium retention. A low urinary sodium (<20 mmol/L) and a high packed cell volume of red blood cells are indications of hypovolaemia, which requires urgent treatment with intravenous albumin as the child is at risk of vascular thrombosis and shock. Increasing peripheral oedema, assessed clinically and by daily weight, may cause discomfort and respiratory compromise. If severe, this may need treatment with intravenous albumin. Care must be taken with the use of colloid, as it may precipitate pulmonary oedema and hypertension from fluid overload, and also with diuretics, which may cause or worsen hypovolaemia.
- *Thrombosis*. A hypercoagulable state, due to urinary losses of antithrombin, thrombocytosis which may be exacerbated by steroid therapy, increased synthesis of clotting factors and increased blood viscosity from the raised haematocrit, predisposes to thrombosis. This may affect the brain, limbs and splanchnic circulation with potentially catastrophic results.
- *Infection*. Children in relapse are at risk of infection with capsulated bacteria, especially *Pneumococcus*. Spontaneous peritonitis may occur. Pneumococcal and seasonal influenza

vaccination is widely recommended. Chickenpox and shingles should be treated with aciclovir.
- *Hypercholesterolaemia*. This correlates inversely with the serum albumin, but the cause of the hyperlipidaemia is not fully understood.

Prognosis

This is summarised in Figure 18.18. Relapses are identified by parents on urine testing. The side-effects of corticosteroid therapy may be reduced by an alternate-day regimen. If relapses are frequent, or if a high maintenance dose is required, involvement of a paediatric nephrologist is advisable as other drug therapy may be considered to enable reduction in steroid use. Possible steroid-sparing agents include the immunomodulator levamisole, alkylating agents (e.g. cyclophosphamide), calcineurin inhibitors such as tacrolimus and ciclosporin A and the immunosuppressant mycophenolate mofetil.

Steroid-resistant nephrotic syndrome
(Table 18.4)

These children should be referred to a paediatric nephrologist. Management of the oedema is by diuretic therapy, salt restriction, ACE inhibitors and sometimes

---

Summary

Nephrotic syndrome

- Clinical signs – oedema (periorbital, scrotal or vulval, leg and ankle oedema, ascites, pleural effusions)
- Diagnosis – heavy proteinuria and low plasma albumin.

Steroid-sensitive nephrotic syndrome

- Characteristic features – 1 to 10 years old, no macroscopic haematuria, and blood pressure, complement levels and renal function are normal
- Management – oral corticosteroids, renal biopsy if unresponsive or atypical features
- Complications – hypovolaemia, thrombosis, infection (pneumococcal), hypercholesterolaemia
- Prognosis – may resolve or else there may be infrequent or frequent relapse.

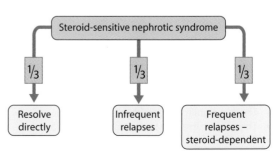

Figure 18.18 Clinical course in steroid-responsive nephrotic syndrome.

Table 18.4 Steroid-resistant nephrotic syndrome

Cause	Specific features	Prognosis
Focal segmental glomerulosclerosis	Most common Familial or idiopathic	30% progress to end-stage renal failure in 5 years; 20% respond to cyclophosphamide, ciclosporin, tacrolimus or rituximab Recurrence post-transplant is common
Mesangiocapillary glomerulonephritis (membranoproliferative glomerulonephritis)	More common in older children Haematuria and low complement level present	Decline in renal function over many years
Membranous nephropathy	Associated with hepatitis B May precede SLE	Most remit spontaneously within 5 years

NSAIDs (non-steroidal anti-inflammatory drugs), which may reduce proteinuria.

Congenital nephrotic syndrome

Congenital nephrotic syndrome presents in the first 3 months of life. It is rare. The commonest kind is recessively inherited and the gene frequency is particularly high in Finns. In the UK, it is more common in consanguineous families. It is associated with a high mortality, usually due to complications of hypoalbuminaemia rather than renal failure. The albuminuria is so severe that unilateral nephrectomy may be necessary for its control, followed by dialysis for renal failure, which is continued until the child is large and fit enough for renal transplantation.

 An oedematous child – test for proteinuria to diagnose nephrotic syndrome.

Haematuria

Urine that is red in colour or tests positive for haemoglobin on urine sticks should be examined under the microscope to confirm haematuria (>10 red blood cells per high-power field). Glomerular haematuria is suggested by brown urine, the presence of deformed red cells (which occurs as they pass through the basement membrane) and casts, and is often accompanied by proteinuria. Lower urinary tract haematuria is usually red, occurs at the beginning or end of the urinary stream, is not accompanied by proteinuria and is unusual in children.

Urinary tract infection is the most common cause of haematuria (Box 18.4), although seldom as the only symptom. The history and examination may suggest the diagnosis, e.g. a family history of stone formation or nephritis or a history of trauma. A plan of investigation is outlined in Box 18.5.

A renal biopsy may be indicated if:

- There is significant persistent proteinuria.
- There is recurrent macroscopic haematuria
- Renal function is abnormal
- The complement levels are persistently abnormal.

Acute nephritis

The causes of acute nephritis in childhood are listed in Box 18.6. Increased glomerular cellularity restricts glomerular blood flow and therefore filtration is decreased. This leads to:

- decreased urine output and volume overload
- hypertension, which may cause seizures
- oedema, characteristically around the eyes
- haematuria and proteinuria.

Management is by attention to both water and electrolyte balance and the use of diuretics when necessary. Rarely, there may be a rapid deterioration in renal function (rapidly progressive glomerulonephritis). This may occur with any cause of acute nephritis, but is uncommon when the cause is post-streptococcal. If left untreated, irreversible renal failure may occur over weeks or months, so renal biopsy and subsequent treatment with immunosuppression and plasma exchange may be necessary.

Post-streptococcal and post-infectious nephritis

Usually follows a streptococcal sore throat or skin infection and is diagnosed by evidence of a recent streptococcal infection (culture of the organism, raised ASO/anti-DNAse B titres) and low complement C3 levels that return to normal after 3–4 weeks. Streptococcal nephritis is a common condition in developing countries, but has become uncommon in developed countries. Long-term prognosis is good.

Henoch–Schönlein purpura

Henoch–Schönlein purpura is the combination of some of the following features:

- Characteristic skin rash
- Arthralgia
- Periarticular oedema
- Abdominal pain
- Glomerulonephritis.

It usually occurs between the ages of 3 and 10 years, is twice as common in boys, peaks during the winter months and is often preceded by an upper respiratory

Box 18.4 Causes of haematuria

Non-glomerular

- Infection (bacterial, viral, TB, schistosomiasis)
- Trauma to genitalia, urinary tract or kidneys
- Stones
- Tumours
- Sickle cell disease
- Bleeding disorders
- Renal vein thrombosis
- Hypercalciuria.

Glomerular

- Acute glomerulonephritis (usually with proteinuria)
- Chronic glomerulonephritis (usually with proteinuria)
- IgA nephropathy
- Familial nephritis, e.g. Alport syndrome
- Thin basement membrane disease.

Box 18.5 Investigation of haematuria

All patients

- Urine microscopy (with phase contrast) and culture
- Protein and calcium excretion
- Kidney and urinary tract ultrasound
- Plasma urea, electrolytes, creatinine, calcium, phosphate, albumin
- Full blood count, platelets, clotting screen, sickle cell screen.

If suggestive of glomerular haematuria

- ESR, complement levels and anti-DNA antibodies
- Throat swab and antistreptolysin O/anti-DNAse B titres
- Hepatitis B and C screen
- Renal biopsy if indicated
- Test mother's urine for blood (if Alport syndrome suspected)
- Hearing test (if Alport syndrome suspected).

Box 18.6 Causes of acute nephritis

- Post-infectious (including streptococcus)
- Vasculitis (Henoch–Schönlein purpura or, rarely, SLE, Wegener granulomatosis, microscopic polyarteritis, polyarteritis nodosa)
- IgA nephropathy and mesangiocapillary glomerulonephritis
- Anti-glomerular basement membrane disease (Goodpasture syndrome) – very rare.

infection. Despite much research, the cause is unknown. It is postulated that genetic predisposition and antigen exposure increase circulating IgA levels and disrupt IgG synthesis. The IgA and IgG interact to produce complexes that activate complement and are deposited in affected organs, precipitating an inflammatory response with vasculitis.

Clinical findings (Fig. 18.19)

At presentation, affected children often have a fever. The *rash* is the most obvious feature. It is symmetrically distributed over the buttocks, the extensor surfaces of the arms and legs, and the ankles. The trunk is spared unless lesions are induced by trauma. The rash may initially be urticarial, rapidly becoming maculopapular and purpuric, is characteristically palpable and may recur over several weeks. The rash is the first clinical feature in about 50% and is the cornerstone of the diagnosis, which is clinical.

Joint pain occurs in two-thirds of patients, particularly of the knees and ankles. There is *periarticular oedema*. Long-term damage to the joints does not occur, and symptoms usually resolve before the rash goes.

Henoch-Schönlein purpura

Rash **(a)**
Buttocks (a)
Extensor surfaces
of legs and arms
Ankles (b)

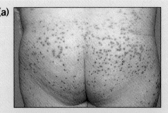

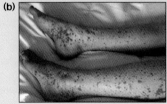

Joint pain and swelling	**Abdominal pain**
Knees and ankles (b)	Haematemesis and melaena Intussusception

Renal
Microscopic/macroscopic haematuria (80%)
Nephrotic syndrome (rare)

Figure 18.19 Main clinical manifestations of Henoch–Schönlein purpura. **(a)** Rash on buttocks. (Courtesy of Dr Michael Markiewicz.) **(b)** Rash around the extensor surfaces of the legs and slight joint swelling. (Courtesy of Professor Tauny Southwood.)

Kidney and urinary tract disorders

Colicky abdominal pain occurs in many children and, if severe, can be treated with corticosteroids. Gastrointestinal petechiae can cause haematemesis and melaena. Intussusception can occur and can be particularly difficult to diagnose under these circumstances. Ileus, protein-losing enteropathy, orchitis and occasionally central nervous system involvement are rare complications.

Renal involvement is common, but is rarely the first symptom. Over 80% have microscopic or macroscopic haematuria or mild proteinuria. These children usually make a complete recovery. If proteinuria is more severe, nephrotic syndrome may result. Risk factors for progressive renal disease are heavy proteinuria, oedema, hypertension and deteriorating renal function, when a renal biopsy will determine if treatment is necessary. All children with renal involvement are followed for a year to detect those with persisting urinary abnormalities (5–10%), who require long-term follow-up. This is necessary as hypertension and declining renal function may develop after an interval of several years.

IgA nephropathy

This may present with episodes of macroscopic haematuria, commonly in association with upper respiratory tract infections. Histological findings and management are as for Henoch–Schönlein purpura, which may be a variant of the same pathological process but not restricted to the kidney. The prognosis in children is better than that in adults.

Familial nephritis

The commonest familial nephritis is Alport syndrome. This is usually an X-linked recessive disorder that progresses to end-stage renal failure by early adult life in males and is associated with nerve deafness and ocular defects. The mother may have haematuria.

Vasculitis

The commonest vasculitis to involve the kidney is Henoch–Schönlein purpura (see above). However, renal involvement may occur in rarer vasculitides such as polyarteritis nodosa, microscopic polyarteritis and Wegener granulomatosis. Characteristic symptoms are fever, malaise, weight loss, skin rash and arthropathy with prominent involvement of the respiratory tract in Wegener disease. ANCA (antineutrophil cytoplasm antibodies) are present and diagnostic in these diseases. Renal arteriography, to demonstrate the presence of aneurysms, will diagnose polyarteritis nodosa. Renal involvement may be severe and rapidly progressive. Treatment is with steroids, plasma exchange and intravenous cyclophosphamide, which may need to be continued for many months.

Systemic lupus erythematosus (SLE)

SLE is a disease that presents mainly in adolescent girls and young women. It is much commoner in Asians and Afro-Caribbeans than Caucasians. It is characterised by the presence of multiple autoantibodies, including antibodies to double-stranded DNA. The C3 and C4 components of complement may be low, particularly during active phases of the disease. Haematuria and proteinuria are indications for renal biopsy, as immunosuppression is always necessary and its intensity will depend on the severity of renal involvement.

Summary

Acute nephritis

- Cause: usually post-infectious or follows a streptococcal infection, but also vasculitis (including Henoch–Schönlein purpura), IgA nephropathy and familial nephritis
- Clinical features: oedema (around the eyes), hypertension, decreased urine output, haematuria and proteinuria
- Management: fluid and electrolyte balance, diuretics, monitor for rapid deterioration in renal function.

Hypertension

Blood pressure in children needs to be measured with a cuff over two-thirds the length of the upper arm (see Ch. 2). Blood pressure increases with age and height and readings should be plotted on a centile chart (see Appendix). Hypertension is blood pressure above 95th percentile for height, age and sex. Symptomatic hypertension in children is usually secondary to renal, cardiac or endocrine causes (Box 18.7).

Presentation includes vomiting, headaches, facial palsy, hypertensive retinopathy, convulsions or proteinuria. Failure to thrive and cardiac failure are the most common features in infants. Phaeochromocytoma may also cause paroxysmal palpitations and sweating.

Some causes are correctable, e.g. nephrectomy for unilateral scarring, angioplasty for renal artery stenosis, surgical repair of coarctation of the aorta, resection of a phaeochromocytoma, but in most cases medical treatment is necessary with antihypertensive drugs.

Box 18.7 Causes of hypertension

- **Renal**
  - Renal parenchymal disease
  - Renovascular, e.g. renal artery stenosis
  - Polycystic kidney disease (ARPKD and ADPKD)
  - Renal tumours
- **Coarctation of the aorta**
- **Catecholamine excess**
  - Phaeochromocytoma
  - Neuroblastoma
- **Endocrine**
  - Congenital adrenal hyperplasia
  - Cushing syndrome or corticosteroid therapy
  - Hyperthyroidism
- **Essential hypertension**
  - A diagnosis of exclusion.

Box **18.8** Causes of palpable kidneys

Unilateral

- Multicystic kidney
- Compensatory hypertrophy
- Obstructed hydronephrosis
- Renal tumour (Wilms tumour)
- Renal vein thrombosis

Bilateral

- Autosomal recessive (infantile) polycystic kidneys
- Autosomal dominant (adult) polycystic kidneys
- Tuberous sclerosis
- Renal vein thrombosis.

Early detection of hypertension is important. Any children with a renal abnormality should have their blood pressure checked annually throughout life. Children with a family history of essential hypertension should be encouraged to restrict their salt intake, avoid obesity and have their blood pressure checked regularly.

Renal masses

An abdominal mass identified on palpating the abdomen should be investigated promptly by ultrasound scan. The causes of palpable kidneys are shown in Box 18.8. Bilaterally enlarged kidneys in early life are most frequently due to autosomal recessive polycystic kidney disease, which is associated with hypertension, hepatic fibrosis and progression to chronic renal failure. This form of polycystic kidney disease must be distinguished from the autosomal dominant adult-type polycystic kidney disease, which has a more benign prognosis in childhood with onset of renal failure in adulthood.

Renal calculi

Renal stones are uncommon in childhood (Fig. 18.20). When they occur, predisposing causes must be sought:

- Urinary tract infection
- Structural anomalies of the urinary tract
- Metabolic abnormalities.

The commonest are phosphate stones associated with infection, especially with *Proteus*. Calcium-containing stones occur in idiopathic hypercalciuria, the most common metabolic abnormality, and with increased urinary urate and oxalate excretion. Deposition of calcium in the parenchyma (nephrocalcinosis) may occur with hypercalciuria, hyperoxaluria and distal renal tubular acidosis. Nephrocalcinosis may be a complication of furosemide therapy in the neonate. Cystine and xanthine stones are rare.

Presentation may be with haematuria, loin or abdominal pain, UTI or passage of a stone.

Stones that are not passed spontaneously should be removed, by either lithotripsy or surgery, and any predisposing structural anomaly repaired. A high

Box **18.9** Causes of Fanconi syndrome

Idiopathic

Secondary to inborn errors of metabolism

- Cystinosis (an autosomal recessive disorder causing intracellular accumulation of cystine)
- Glycogen storage disorders
- Lowe syndrome (oculocerebrorenal dystrophy)
- Galactosaemia
- Fructose intolerance
- Tyrosinaemia
- Wilson disease

Acquired

- Heavy metals
- Drugs and toxins
- Vitamin D deficiency.

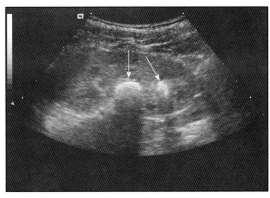

Figure 18.20 Renal ultrasound showing a staghorn calculus.

fluid intake is recommended in all affected children. If the cause is a metabolic abnormality, specific therapy may be possible.

Renal tubular disorders

Abnormalities of renal tubular function may occur at any point along the length of the nephron and affect any of the substances handled by it.

Generalised proximal tubular dysfunction (Fanconi syndrome)

Proximal tubule cells are among the most metabolically active in the body, so are especially vulnerable to cellular damage. The cardinal features are excessive urinary loss of amino acids, glucose, phosphate, bicarbonate, sodium, calcium, potassium and urate. The causes are listed in Box 18.9. Fanconi syndrome should be considered in a child presenting with:

- Polydypsia and polyuria
- Salt depletion and dehydration
- Hyperchloraemic metabolic acidosis
- Rickets
- Failure to thrive/poor growth.

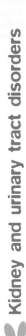

Kidney and urinary tract disorders

341

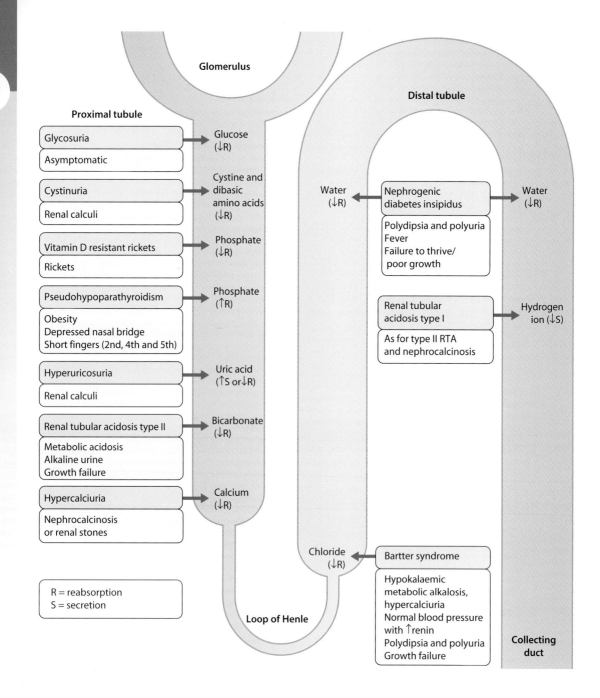

Figure 18.21 Schematic diagram of specific transport defects in some renal tubular disorders.

Specific transport defects

See Figure 18.21.

Acute kidney injury

Acute kidney injury has acute renal failure at the most severe end of the spectrum where there is a sudden, potentially reversible, reduction in renal function.

Oliguria (<0.5 ml/kg per hour) is usually present. It can be classified as (see Box 18.10):

- Prerenal: the commonest cause in children
- Renal: there is salt and water retention; blood, protein and casts are often present in the urine; and there may be symptoms specific to an accompanying disease (e.g. haemolytic uraemic syndrome)
- Postrenal: from urinary obstruction.

Box 18.10 Causes of acute renal failure

Prerenal

- Hypovolaemia:
  - Gastroenteritis
  - Burns
  - Sepsis
  - Haemorrhage
  - Nephrotic syndrome
- Circulatory failure

Renal

- Vascular:
  - Haemolytic uraemic syndrome (HUS)
  - Vasculitis
  - Embolus
  - Renal vein thrombosis
- Tubular:
  - Acute tubular necrosis (ATN)
  - Ischaemic
  - Toxic
  - Obstructive
- Glomerular:
  - Glomerulonephritis
- Interstitial:
  - Interstitial nephritis
  - Pyelonephritis

Postrenal

- Obstruction:
  - Congenital e.g. posterior urethral valves
  - Acquired e.g. blocked urinary catheter

Acute-on-chronic renal failure is suggested by the child having growth failure, anaemia and disordered bone mineralisation (renal osteodystrophy).

Management

Children with acute renal failure should have their circulation and fluid balance meticulously monitored. Investigation by ultrasound scan will identify obstruction of the urinary tract, the small kidneys of chronic renal failure, or large, bright kidneys with loss of cortical medullary differentiation typical of an acute process.

Prerenal failure

This is suggested by hypovolaemia. The fractional excretion of sodium is very low as the body tries to retain fluid. The hypovolaemia needs to be urgently corrected with fluid replacement and circulatory support if acute tubular necrosis is to be avoided.

Renal failure

If there is circulatory overload, restriction of fluid intake and challenge with a diuretic may increase urine output sufficiently to allow gradual correction of sodium and water balance. A high-calorie, normal protein feed will decrease catabolism, uraemia and hyperkalaemia. Emergency management of metabolic acidosis, hyperkalaemia and hyperphosphataemia is shown in Table 18.5. If the cause of renal failure is not obvious, a renal biopsy should be performed to identify rapidly progressive glomerulonephritis, as this may need immediate treatment with immunosuppression. The two commonest renal causes of acute renal failure in children in the UK are the haemolytic uraemic syndrome and acute tubular necrosis, the latter usually in the setting of multisystem failure in the intensive care unit or following cardiac surgery.

Postrenal failure

This requires assessment of the site of obstruction and relief by nephrostomy or bladder catheterisation. Surgery can be performed once fluid volume and electrolyte abnormalities have been corrected.

Table 18.5 Some metabolic abnormalities in acute renal failure and their therapy

Metabolic abnormality	Treatment
Metabolic acidosis	Sodium bicarbonate
Hyperphosphataemia	Calcium carbonate
	Dietary restriction
Hyperkalaemia	Calcium gluconate if ECG changes
	Salbutamol (nebulised or intravenous)
	Calcium exchange resin
	Glucose and insulin
	Dietary restriction
	Dialysis

Dialysis

Dialysis in acute renal failure is indicated when there is:

- Failure of conservative management
- Hyperkalaemia
- Severe hypo- or hypernatraemia
- Pulmonary oedema or hypertension
- Severe acidosis
- Multisystem failure.

Peritoneal dialysis or haemodialysis can be undertaken for acute renal failure. If plasma exchange is part of the treatment, haemodialysis is used. If there is cardiac decompensation or hypercatabolism, continuous arteriovenous or venovenous haemofiltration provides gentle, continuous dialysis and fluid removal. Acute renal failure in childhood generally carries a good prognosis for renal recovery unless complicating a life-threatening condition, e.g. severe infection, following cardiac surgery or multisystem failure.

Kidney and urinary tract disorders

Haemolytic uraemic syndrome

Haemolytic uraemic syndrome (HUS) is a triad of acute renal failure, microangiopathic haemolytic anaemia and thrombocytopenia. Typical HUS is secondary to gastrointestinal infection with verocytotoxin-producing *E. coli* O157:H7, acquired through contact with farm animals or eating uncooked beef, or, less often, *Shigella*. It follows a prodrome of bloody diarrhoea. The toxin from these organisms enters the gastrointestinal mucosa and preferentially localises to the endothelial cells of the kidney where it causes intravascular thrombogenesis. Coagulation cascade is activated and clotting is normal (unlike in disseminated intravascular coagulation, DIC). Platelets are consumed in this process and microangiopathic haemolytic anemia results from damage to red blood cells as they circulate through the microcirculation, which is occluded. Other organs such as the brain, pancreas and heart may also be involved.

With early supportive therapy, including dialysis, the typical diarrhoea-associated HUS usually has a good prognosis, although follow-up is necessary as there may be persistent proteinuria and the development of hypertension and declining renal function in subsequent years. In contrast, atypical HUS has no diarrhoeal prodrome, may be familial and frequently relapses. It has a high risk of hypertension and chronic renal failure and has a high mortality. Children with intracerebral involvement or with atypical HUS may be treated with plasma exchange or plasma infusions, but their efficacy is unproven.

Haemolytic uraemic syndrome (HUS) – the triad of:

- **Acute renal failure**
- **Haemolytic anaemia**
- **Thrombocytopenia.**

Summary

Acute renal failure

- Prerenal: commonest cause in children, from hypovolaemia and circulatory failure
- Renal: most often haemolytic uraemic syndrome or multisystem failure
- Postrenal: from urinary obstruction
- Management: treat underlying cause, metabolic abnormalities, dialysis if necessary.

Chronic kidney disease

Chronic renal failure, with GFR <15 ml/min per 1.73 m^2, is much less common in children than in adults, with an incidence of only 10 per million of the child population each year. Congenital and familial causes are more common in childhood than are acquired diseases (Table 18.6).

Table 18.6 Causes of chronic renal failure

Structural malformations	40%
Glomerulonephritis	25%
Hereditary nephropathies	20%
Systemic diseases	10%
Miscellaneous/unknown	5%

Clinical features

Chronic renal failure presents with:

- Anorexia and lethargy
- Polydipsia and polyuria
- Failure to thrive/growth failure
- Bony deformities from renal osteodystrophy (renal rickets)
- Hypertension
- Acute-on-chronic renal failure (precipitated by infection or dehydration)
- Incidental finding of proteinuria
- Unexplained normochromic, normocytic anaemia.

Many children with chronic renal failure have had their renal disease detected before birth by antenatal ultrasound or have previously identified renal disease. Symptoms rarely develop before renal function falls to less than one-third of normal.

Management

The aims of management are to prevent the symptoms and metabolic abnormalities of chronic renal failure, to allow normal growth and development and to preserve residual renal function. The management of these children should be conducted in a specialist paediatric nephrology centre.

Diet

Anorexia and vomiting are common. Improving nutrition using calorie supplements and nasogastric or gastrostomy feeding is often necessary to optimise growth. Protein intake should be sufficient to maintain growth and a normal albumin, whilst preventing the accumulation of toxic metabolic byproducts.

Prevention of renal osteodystrophy

Phosphate retention and hypocalcaemia due to decreased activation of vitamin D leads to secondary hyperparathyroidism, which results in osteitis fibrosa and osteomalacia. Phosphate restriction by decreasing the dietary intake of milk products, calcium carbonate as a phosphate binder, and activated vitamin D supplements help to prevent renal osteodystrophy.

Control of salt and water balance and acidosis

Many children with chronic renal failure caused by congenital structural malformations and renal dysplasia have an obligatory loss of salt and water. They need salt supplements and free access to water. Treatment with bicarbonate supplements is necessary to prevent acidosis.

Anaemia

Reduced production of erythropoietin and circulation of metabolites that are toxic to the bone marrow result in anaemia. This responds well to the administration of recombinant human erythropoietin.

Hormonal abnormalities

Many hormonal abnormalities occur in chronic renal failure. Most importantly, there is growth hormone resistance with high growth hormone levels but poor growth. Recombinant human growth hormone has been shown to be effective in improving growth for up to 5 years of treatment, but whether it improves final height remains unknown. Many children with chronic renal failure have delayed puberty and a subnormal pubertal growth spurt.

Dialysis and transplantation

It is now possible for all children to enter renal replacement therapy programmes when end-stage renal failure is reached. The optimum management is by renal transplantation. Technically, this is difficult in very small children and a minimum weight, e.g. 10 kg, needs to be reached before transplantation to avoid renal vein thrombosis. Kidneys obtained from living related donors have a higher success rate than deceased donor kidneys, which are matched as far as possible to the recipient's HLA type. Patient survival is high and first-year graft survival is around 97% for living related and 93% for deceased kidneys in the UK. Graft losses from both acute and chronic rejection or recurrent disease mean that the 5-year graft survival is reduced to 91% for living related kidneys and 79% for deceased donor kidney transplants and some children need re-transplantation. Current immunosuppression is mainly with combinations of prednisolone, tacrolimus and azathioprine or mycophenolate mofetil.

Ideally, a child is transplanted before dialysis is required, but if this is not possible, a period of dialysis may be necessary. Peritoneal dialysis, either by cycling overnight using a machine (continuous cycling peritoneal dialysis) or by manual exchanges over 24 h (continuous ambulatory peritoneal dialysis), can be done by the parents at home and is therefore less disruptive to family life and the child's schooling. Haemodialysis is an alternative and is usually done in hospital 3–4 times a week.

Summary

Chronic renal failure

- Causes: congenital (structural malformations and hereditary nephropathies) most common
- Presentation: abnormal antenatal ultrasound, anorexia and lethargy, polydipsia and polyuria, failure to thrive/growth failure, renal rickets, hypertension, proteinuria, anaemia
- Management: diet and nasogastric or gastrostomy feeding, phosphate restriction and activated vitamin D to prevent renal osteodystrophy, salt supplements and free access to water to control salt and water balance, bicarbonate supplements to prevent acidosis, erythropoietin to prevent anaemia, growth hormone and dialysis and transplantation.

Further reading

Avner, ED, Harmon, WE, Niaudet, P, et al: *Pediatric Nephrology*. Philadelphia, 2009, Lippincott Williams & Wilkins.

A comprehensive textbook.

Rees, L, Brogan, P, Webb, N: *Handbook of Paediatric Nephrology*. Oxford, 2007, Oxford University Press.

Websites (Accessed May 2011)

Emedicine: Details about a range of paediatric nephrology conditions. http://emedicine.medscape.com/pediatrics_general#nephrology.

British Association of Paediatric Nephrology: http://www.bapn.org/.

American Society of Pediatric Nephrology: http://www.aspneph.com/patient_info_websites.asp.

Kidney and urinary tract disorders

Genital disorders in boys

Most disorders of the genitalia in childhood are in boys.

Inguinoscrotal disorders

Embryology

The testis is formed from the urogenital ridge on the posterior abdominal wall close to the developing kidney. Gonadal induction to form a testis is regulated by genes on the Y chromosome. During gestation, the testis migrates down towards the inguinal canal, guided by mesenchymal tissue known as the gubernaculum, probably under the influence of anti-Müllerian hormone (Fig. 19.1a).

Inguinoscrotal descent of the testis requires the release of testosterone from the fetal testis. A tongue of peritoneum, the processus vaginalis, precedes the migrating testis through the inguinal canal. This peritoneal extension normally becomes obliterated after birth, but failure of this process may lead to the development of an inguinal hernia or hydrocele (Fig. 19.1b–d).

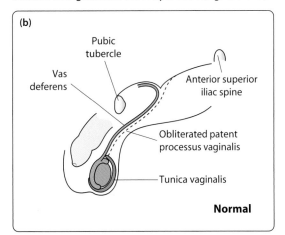

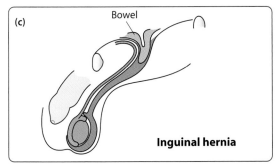

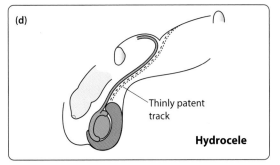

Figure 19.1 **(a)** Embryology of testicular descent. **(b)** The normal testis. **(c)** Inguinal hernia and **(d)** hydrocele are the result of incomplete obliteration of the processus vaginalis.

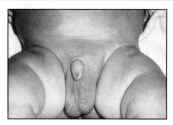

Figure 19.2 Left inguina hernia in an infant. The left groin is only slightly swollen.

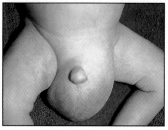

Figure 19.3 Bilateral inguina hernias in a preterm infant. Inguinal hernia is primarily a groin swelling; only when it is large does it extend into the scrotum.

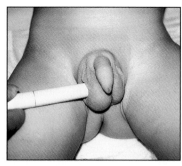

Figure 19.4 Right-sided hydrocele. The scrotal swelling often has a bluish discoloration and will transilluminate in a darkened room.

Inguinal hernia

Inguinal hernias in children are almost always indirect and due to a patent processus vaginalis. They are much more frequent in boys and are particularly common in premature infants. Hernias are more common on the right side. At least 1 in 50 boys will develop an inguinal hernia.

Inguinal hernias usually present as an intermittent swelling in the groin or scrotum on crying or straining. Unless the hernia is observed as an inguinal swelling (Figs 19.2, 19.3), diagnosis relies on the history and the identification of thickening of the spermatic cord (or round ligament in girls). The groin swelling may become visible on raising the intra-abdominal pressure by gently pressing on the abdomen or asking the child to cough.

An inguinal hernia in an infant may present as an irreducible lump in the groin or scrotum. The lump is firm and tender. The infant may be unwell with irritability and vomiting. Most 'irreducible' hernias can be successfully reduced following opioid analgesia and sustained gentle compression. Surgery is delayed for 24–48 hours to allow resolution of oedema. If reduction is impossible, emergency surgery is required because of the risk of strangulation of bowel and damage to the testis. A hernia associated with an undescended testis should be operated early to minimise risks to the testis.

Surgery

The operation is carried out via an inguinal skin crease incision and involves ligation and division of the hernial sac (processus vaginalis). Except in small infants, this can usually be undertaken as a day-case procedure, provided there is appropriate anaesthetic and surgical support.

> **Inguinal hernias in infants should be repaired promptly to avoid the risk of strangulation.**

Hydrocele

A patent processus vaginalis, which is sufficiently narrow to prevent the formation of an inguinal hernia, may still allow peritoneal fluid to track down around the testis to form a hydrocele (Fig. 19.4). Hydroceles are asymptomatic scrotal swellings, often bilateral, and sometimes with a bluish discoloration. They may be tense or lax but are non-tender and transilluminate. Some hydroceles are not evident at birth but present in early childhood after a viral or gastrointestinal illness. The majority resolve spontaneously as the processus continues to obliterate, but surgery is considered if it persists beyond 18–24 months of age. A hydrocele of the cord forms a non-tender mobile swelling in the spermatic cord.

Undescended testis

An undescended testis has been arrested along its normal pathway of descent (Fig. 19.5). At birth, about 4% of full-term male infants will have a unilateral or bilateral undescended testis (cryptorchidism). It is more common in preterm infants because testicular descent through the inguinal canal occurs in the third trimester. Testicular descent may continue during early infancy and by 3 months of age the overall rate of cryptorchidism in boys is 1.5%, with little change thereafter. Contrary to previous teaching, it is now recognised that occasionally a testis which is fully descended at birth can *ascend* to an inguinal position during childhood,

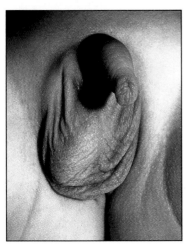

Figure 19.5 A left undescended testis with an empty hemiscrotum.

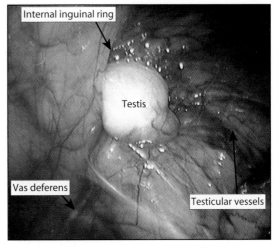

Figure 19.6 Laparoscopic appearance of an intra-abdominal testis.

accounting for some late-presenting 'undescended' or 'ascended' testes. This phenomenon may be due to a relative shortening of cord structures during growth of the child.

Examination

This should be carried out in a warm room, with warm hands and a relaxed child. The testes can then be brought down into a palpable position by gently massaging the contents of the inguinal canal towards the scrotum.

Classification

Retractile

The testis can be manipulated into the bottom of the scrotum without tension, but subsequently retracts into the inguinal region, pulled up by the cremasteric muscle. The testis has usually been found in the scrotum at a neonatal check and been noted by parents on bathing their baby. With age, the testis resides permanently in the scrotum. Follow-up is advisable as, rarely, the testis subsequently ascends into the inguinal canal.

Palpable

The testis can be palpated in the groin but cannot be manipulated into the scrotum. Occasionally, a testis is ectopic, when it lies outside its normal line of descent and may then be found in the perineum or femoral triangle.

Impalpable

No testis can be felt on detailed examination. The testis may be in the inguinal canal, intra-abdominal or absent.

Investigations

Useful investigations include:

- *Ultrasound* – this has a limited role in identifying testes in the inguinal canal in obese boys but cannot reliably distinguish between an intra-abdominal or absent testis. It is performed in children with bilateral impalpable testes to verify internal pelvic organs.
- *Hormonal* – for bilateral impalpable testes, the presence of testicular tissue can be confirmed by recording a rise in serum testosterone in response to intramuscular injections of human chorionic gonadotrophin (HCG); these boys may require specialist endocrine review.
- *Laparoscopy* (Fig. 19.6) – the investigation of choice for the impalpable testis. Under anaesthesia, inguinal examination is first carried out to check that the testis is not in the inguinal canal.

Management

Surgical placement of the testis in the scrotum (*orchidopexy*) is undertaken for several reasons:

- *Fertility* – to optimise spermatogenesis, the testis needs to be in the scrotum below body temperature. The timing of orchidopexy is controversial, but orchidopexy during the second year of life may optimise reproductive potential. After 6 months of age descent of testis is unlikely and referral for paediatric surgical review at that age is recommended. Fertility after orchidopexy for a unilateral undescended testis is close to normal. In contrast, fertility is reduced to around 50% after bilateral orchidopexy for palpable undescended testes, and men with a history of bilaterally impalpable testes are usually sterile.
- *Malignancy* – undescended testes have histological abnormalities and an increased risk of malignancy. The risk is greater for bilateral undescended testes and the greatest risk is for testes which are intra-abdominal. Although the evidence is somewhat contradictory, some studies have suggested that early orchidopexy for a unilateral undescended testis reduces the risk to nearly the same as a normal testis. A scrotal testis can also be more easily self-examined than an inguinal or ectopic one.

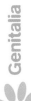

Genitalia

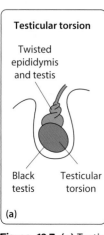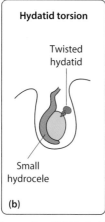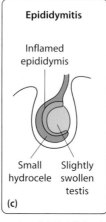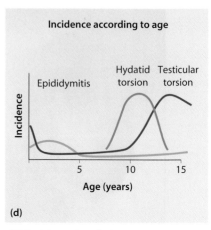

Figure 19.7 (a) Testicular torsion. **(b)** Hydatid torsion. **(c)** Epididymitis. **(d)** Incidence in relation to age.

- *Cosmetic and psychological* – if a testis is absent, a prosthesis can be used but this is best delayed until a larger adult-sized prosthesis can be inserted.

Surgery

Most boys with an undescended testis undergo an orchidopexy via an inguinal incision. The testis is mobilised, preserving the vas deferens and testicular vessels, the associated patent processus vaginalis is ligated and divided, and the testis is placed in the scrotal pouch. The operation is usually performed as a day-case procedure.

Most intra-abdominal testes are amenable to laparoscopic staged orchidopexy. Orchidectomy is considered in rare circumstances of a very high testis in an older child or a unilateral intra-abdominal testis in a postpubertal adolescent with a normal contralateral testis. Before conducting laparoscopy in a peripubertal boy, baseline abdominal ultrasound scan and serum tumour markers are checked. Although intra-abdominal testes have profoundly defective spermatogenesis, they are capable of producing male hormones.

Varicocele

Varicosities of the testicular veins may develop in boys around puberty. They are usually on the left side and there is an association with subfertility. Treatment is indicated for symptoms (dragging, aching), impaired testicular growth and, in later life, for infertility. Obliteration of the testicular veins can be achieved by conventional surgery, laparoscopic techniques or radiological embolisation. The role of such interventions in asymptomatic boys is uncertain.

The acute scrotum

Torsion of the testis

Testicular torsion is most common in adolescents but may occur at any age, including the perinatal period (Fig. 19.7). The pain is not always centred on the scrotum but may be in the groin or lower abdomen.

Atypical presentation is not unusual and the testes must always be examined whenever a boy or young man presents with inguinal or lower abdominal pain of sudden onset (see Case History 19.1). There may be a history of previous self-limiting episodes. Torsion of the testis must be relieved within 6–12 h of the onset of symptoms for there to be a good chance of testicular viability. Surgical exploration is mandatory unless torsion can be excluded. If torsion is confirmed, fixation of the contralateral testis is essential because there may be an anatomical predisposition to torsion, for example the 'bell clapper' testis, where the testis is not anchored properly. An undescended testis is at increased risk of torsion and at increased risk of delayed diagnosis. It may also be confused with an incarcerated hernia. Expert Doppler ultrasound looking at flow in the testicular blood vessels may allow torsion of the testis to be differentiated from epididymitis, but should not be used to diagnose torsion as only early surgical correction may salvage the testis. If there is any doubt about the cause of a painful scrotum, surgery should be performed.

Torsion of testicular appendage

A hydatid of Morgagni is an embryological remnant found on the upper pole of the testis. Torsion of this appendage characteristically affects boys just prior to puberty. This may be because of rapid enlargement of the hydatid in response to gonadotrophins. The pain may increase over 1 or 2 days and occasionally the torted hydatid can be seen or felt (the blue dot sign). Surgical exploration and excision of the appendage leads to rapid resolution of the problem.

Other causes

Viral or bacterial epididymo-orchitis or epididymitis may cause an acute scrotum in infants and toddlers, and scrotal exploration is often necessary to confirm the diagnosis. If an associated urinary tract infection is present, antibiotic treatment and full investigation of the urinary tract will be required. Other conditions which may cause scrotal symptoms and signs are idiopathic scrotal oedema (usually painless, bilateral

19.1 Torsion of the testis

A 13-year-old boy presents to the A&E Department with a 2-hour history of right lower abdominal pain of sudden onset. He has vomited once. Temperature 37.4°C. He indicates that his pain is in the right lower quadrant. Urine dipstick testing was normal. Appendicitis is suspected. However, examination of the abdomen does not reveal any guarding or other signs of peritoneal irritation in the right iliac fossa. When his testes are examined, the right testis is found to be slightly swollen and lying higher in the scrotum than the left testis (Fig. 19.8). Although he has not complained of testicular pain, the testis is tender on palpation. Urgent surgical exploration confirms testicular torsion (Fig. 19.9). After detorsion, the testis appears viable and is conserved. It is fixed with sutures to minimise the risk of further torsion. The left testis is also fixed, as the anatomical variant which predisposes to torsion occurs bilaterally.

This case highlights:

- The clinical features of testicular torsion are variable and can be potentially misleading, with pain predominantly referred to the abdomen or inguinal region and minimal pain felt in the testis itself
- Abdominal examination is never complete without inspection and gentle palpation of both testes
- With torsion, the testis is always tender.

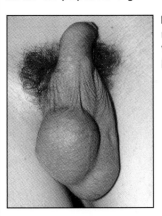

Figure 19.8 Enlarged, raised right testis, which was tender on palpation.

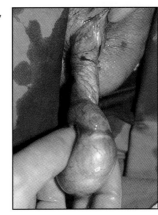

Figure 19.9 Torsion of the testis at surgery.

---

scrotal swelling and redness in a preschool child) or an incarcerated inguinal hernia.

 Torsion of the testis is an emergency.

Abnormalities of the penis

Hypospadias

In the male fetus, urethral tubularisation occurs in a proximal to distal direction under the influence of fetal testosterone. Failure to complete this process leaves the urethral opening proximal to the normal meatus on the glans and this is termed hypospadias (Fig. 19.10). This is a common congenital anomaly, affecting about 1 in every 200 boys. Recent studies suggest that the incidence is increasing.

Hypospadias consists of:

- *A ventral urethral meatus* – in most cases the urethra opens on or adjacent to the glans penis, but in severe cases the opening may be on the penile shaft or in the perineum (Fig. 19.11)
- *A hooded dorsal foreskin* – the foreskin has failed to fuse ventrally

- *Chordee* – a ventral curvature of the shaft of the penis, most apparent on erection. This is only marked in the more severe forms of hypospadias (Fig. 19.12).

Glanular hypospadias may be a solely cosmetic concern, but more proximal varieties may cause functional problems including an inability to micturate in a normal direction and erectile deformity. With more severe varieties of hypospadias, additional genitourinary anomalies should be excluded and sometimes it is necessary to consider disorders of sexual differentiation.

Surgery

Correction is often undertaken before 2 years of age, often as a single-stage operation. The aims of surgery are to produce:

- A terminal urethral meatus so that the boy can micturate in a normal standing position like his peers
- A straight erection
- A penis that looks normal.

 Infants with hypospadias must not be circumcised, as the foreskin is often needed for later reconstructive surgery.

Hypospadias

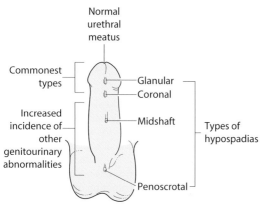

Normal urethral meatus

Commonest types
— Glanular
— Coronal

Increased incidence of other genitourinary abnormalities

— Midshaft

Types of hypospadias

— Penoscrotal

Figure 19.10 Varieties of hypospadias.

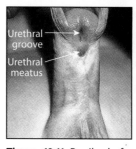

Urethral groove

Urethral meatus

Figure 19.11 Penile shaft hypospadias with dorsal hooded foreskin, showing the urethral groove (arrow) and urethral meatus (arrow).

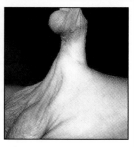

Figure 19.12 In lateral view, the ventral curvature of the penis (chordee) can be seen.

Circumcision

At birth, the foreskin is adherent to the surface of the glans penis. These adhesions separate spontaneously with time, allowing the foreskin to become more mobile and eventually retractile. At 1 year of age, approximately 50% of boys have a *non-retractile fore-skin*, but by 4 years this has declined to 10%, and by 16 years to only 1%. A non-retractile foreskin often leads to ballooning on micturition, which is physiological. Gentle retraction of the foreskin at bathtimes helps to maintain hygiene, but forcible retraction of a healthy non-retractile foreskin should be avoided.

Two conditions that require reassurance are preputial adhesions (when the foreskin remains partially adherent to the glans) and the presence of white 'pearls' under the foreskin due to trapped epithelial squames. Both conditions are usually asymptomatic and resolve spontaneously.

Circumcision is one of the earliest recorded operations and remains an important tradition in the Jewish and Muslim religions. Although routine neonatal circumcision is still common in some Western countries such as the USA, the arguments generally used to justify on medical grounds have been discredited and no national or international medical association currently advocates routine neonatal circumcision. Neonatal circumcision is not without risk of significant morbidity. Nevertheless, the issue is still hotly debated.

There are only a few medical indications for circumcision:

- *Phimosis* (Fig. 19.13). This term is often used to describe the inability to retract the foreskin. As described above, at birth the foreskin is non-retractile and phimosis is physiological. Pathological phimosis is seen as a whitish scarring of the foreskin and is rare before the age of 5 years. The condition is due to a localised skin disease known as balanitis xerotica obliterans (BXO), which also involves the glans penis and can cause urethral meatal stenosis

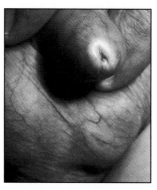

Figure 19.13 Pathological phimosis.

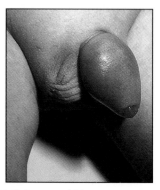

Figure 19.14 Balanoposthitis.

- *Recurrent balanoposthitis* (Fig. 19.14). Single attack of redness and inflammation of the foreskin, sometimes with a purulent discharge, is common and usually responds rapidly to warm baths and a broad-spectrum antibiotic. Recurrent attacks of balanoposthitis (inflammation of the glans and foreskin) are uncommon and circumcision is occasionally indicated.
- *Recurrent urinary tract infections*. Although urinary infection is more common in uncircumcised boys

the overall incidence is low and routine circumcision is not justified as a preventative measure. However, circumcision may be helpful in reducing the risk of urinary tract bacterial colonisation in boys with upper urinary tract anomalies complicated by recurrent urinary infection. It may also be appropriate in boys with spina bifida who need to perform clean intermittent urethral catheterisation.

There is some data from countries with a high prevalence of HIV infection that the risk of transmission is lower in circumcised males.

Surgery

Circumcision for medical indications is performed under a general anaesthetic as a day case. During the procedure, a long-acting local anaesthetic block can be given to reduce postoperative pain. Circumcision is not a trivial operation. Healing can take up to 10 days, with discomfort for several days. Bleeding and infection are well-recognised complications, but more serious hazards, such as damage to the glans, may occur if the procedure is not carried out by appropriately trained personnel. The procedure also carries the risk of psychological trauma.

Preputioplasty can be offered as an effective alternative to circumcision in selected cases. After retraction of the foreskin, the tight preputial ring is incised longitudinally and then sutured transversely. Unlike circumcision, preputioplasty conserves the foreskin and results in less postoperative discomfort and fewer complications. However, regular retraction of the foreskin is required in the first few weeks after surgery and for this reason, preputioplasty is better suited to older boys who are willing to do this.

Topical corticosteroids

Application of a topical steroid ointment to the prepuce has been shown to facilitate retraction of a nonretractile prepuce, with success rates of up to 80%. Different treatment regimens have been described but typically the ointment is applied twice daily for 2–3 months.

Paraphimosis

The foreskin becomes trapped in the retracted position proximal to a swollen glans. The foreskin can usually be reduced, but adequate analgesia (often a general anaesthetic) is needed to achieve this. The problem is not usually recurrent and circumcision is rarely required.

Summary

Genital conditions in male infants and children

Inguinal hernia:
- Presentation – intermittent swelling in the groin or scrotum on crying or as an irreducible lump
- Repair promptly to avoid the risk of strangulation
- If irreducible – sustained gentle compression with analgesia to reduce, followed by delayed surgery

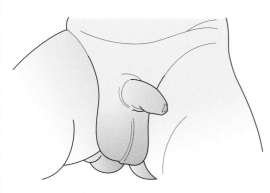

Hypospadias:
- Consists of – ventral urethral meatus, a hooded dorsal foreskin, chordee
- When severe, exclude other genitourinary or endocrine anomalies
- Affected infants must not be circumcised, as the foreskin is often needed for later reconstructive surgery

An undescended testis:
- Is present in about 4% of full-term male infants but only 1.3% at 3 months of age
- May be **retractile**, if it can be brought to bottom of scrotum without tension but subsequently retracts – is usually normal
- Is **palpable** if felt in the groin but cannot be manipulated into the scrotum
- Is **impalpable** if no testis can be felt – may be in the inguinal canal, intra-abdominal or absent
- Orchidopexy – performed to optimise fertility, avoid malignant change, and for cosmetic and psychological reasons

Torsion of the testis:
- Must always be considered in a boy with an acutely painful scrotum
- Must be treated within hours for the testis to be viable

Circumcision:
- Is not recommended routinely, but is a tradition for Jews and Muslims and is still common in the USA
- The only medical indications are – pathological phimosis, recurrent balanoposthitis and possibly some boys with recurrent urinary tract infections
- Complications include pain, bleeding, infection and damage to the glans

Genital disorders in girls

Inguinal hernias

These are much less common than in boys. Sometimes the ovary becomes incarcerated in the hernial sac and can be difficult to reduce. Rarely, androgen insensitivity syndrome (testicular feminisation) can present as a hernia in a phenotypic female who actually has a male genotype.

Labial adhesions

If the labia minora are adherent in the midline, this may give the appearance of absence of the vagina, except there is a characteristic translucent midline raphe partially or totally occluding the vaginal opening. Asymptomatic adhesions can be left alone and will often lyse spontaneously. If there is perineal soreness or urinary irritation, treatment with topical oestrogen treatment applied sparingly twice a day for 1–2 weeks often dissolves the adhesions. Active separation of the adhesions under anaesthesia is sometimes required.

Vulvovaginitis/vaginal discharge

Vulvovaginitis and vaginal discharge are common in young girls. They may result from infection (bacterial or fungal), specific irritants, poor hygiene or sexual abuse, although none of these factors is present in most cases. Vulvovaginitis may rarely be associated with threadworm infestation. Parents should be advised about hygiene, the avoidance of bubble bath and scented soaps and the use of loose-fitting cotton underwear. Swabs should be taken to identify any pathogens, which can then be specifically treated. Salt baths may be helpful. Oestrogen cream applied sparingly to the vulva may relieve the problem in resistant cases by increasing vaginal resistance to infection as prepubertal tissues tend to be atrophic. If there are any concerns about sexual abuse, the child must be seen by a paediatrician (see Ch. 7). Rarely, if the vaginal discharge is persistent or purulent, examination under anaesthesia may be needed to exclude a vaginal foreign body or unusual infections.

Disorders of sexual differentiation are considered in Chapter 11.

Further reading

Gearhart JG, Rink RC, Mouriquand PD, editors: *Pediatric Urology*, Philadelphia, PA, 2009, Saunders.

Thomas D, Duffy PG, Rickwood A: *Essentials of Pediatric Urology*, London, 2008, Informa Healthcare.

Liver disorders

Features of liver disorders in children are:

- Prolonged (persistent) neonatal jaundice is the most common presentation of liver disease in the neonatal period.
- The earlier in life biliary atresia is diagnosed and treated surgically, the better the prognosis.
- Transmission of hepatitis B surface antigen-positive mothers is prevented by immunising their babies.
- Chronic liver disease (Fig. 20.1), cirrhosis and portal hypertension are uncommon and should be managed by, or in conjunction with tertiary or national centres.
- Liver transplantation is an effective therapy for acute or chronic liver failure, with a >80% 5-year survival rate; it is only performed at national centres.

Neonatal liver disease

Many newborn infants become clinically jaundiced. About 5–10% are still jaundiced at >2 weeks of age (3 weeks if preterm), when it is called 'prolonged (or persistent) neonatal jaundice'. This is usually an unconjugated hyperbilirubinaemia, which resolves spontaneously (Box 20.1). Prolonged neonatal jaundice caused by liver disease is characterised by a raised conjugated bilirubin (>20 μmol/L) and is usually accompanied by:

- Pale stools
- Dark urine
- Bleeding tendency
- Failure to thrive.

There is an urgency to diagnose liver disease as early as possible in the neonatal period, because early diagnosis and management improves prognosis.

 In prolonged (persistent) neonatal jaundice, check if it is conjugated hyperbilirubinaemia, as this is due to liver disease.

Bile duct obstruction

Biliary atresia (see Case History 20.1)

This occurs in 1 in 14 000 live births. It is a progressive disease, in which there is destruction or absence of the extrahepatic biliary tree and intrahepatic biliary ducts.

Hepatic dysfunction

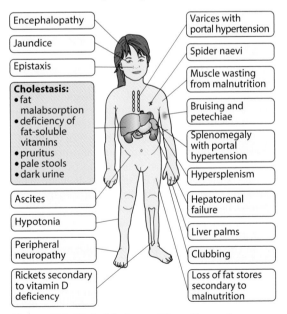

Figure 20.1 Clinical features of liver disease. In addition, these children may have growth failure and developmental delay.

Box 20.1 Causes of prolonged (persistent) neonatal jaundice

Unconjugated

- Breast milk jaundice
- Infection (particularly urinary tract)
- Haemolytic anaemia, e.g. G6PD deficiency
- Hypothyroidism
- High gastrointestinal obstruction
- Crigler–Najjar syndrome

Conjugated (>20 micromol/L)

Bile duct obstruction

- Biliary atresia
- Choledochal cyst

Neonatal hepatitis syndrome

- Congenital infection
- Inborn errors of metabolism
- α_1-Antitrypsin deficiency
- Galactosaemia
- Tyrosinaemia (type 1)
- Errors of bile acid synthesis
- Progressive familial intrahepatic cholestasis (PFIC)
- Cystic fibrosis
- Intestinal failure-associated liver disease – associated with long-term parenteral nutrition

Intrahepatic biliary hypoplasia

- Alagille syndrome.

This leads to chronic liver failure and death unless surgical intervention is performed. Babies with biliary atresia have a normal birthweight but fail to thrive as the disease progresses. They are usually mildly jaundiced and, following passage of meconium, their stools are pale and their urine dark. Although stool colour may fluctuate, pale stools is an important abnormality and warrants investigation, even in the absence of clinical jaundice. Hepatomegaly is often present and splenomegaly will develop secondary to portal hypertension.

Standard liver function tests are of little value in the differential diagnosis. A fasting abdominal ultrasound may demonstrate a contracted or absent gallbladder, though it may be normal. A radioisotope scan with TIBIDA (iminodiacetic acid derivatives) shows good uptake by the liver, but no excretion into the bowel. Liver biopsy demonstrates features of extrahepatic biliary obstruction, although features may overlap with those of neonatal hepatitis, especially if carried out at an early stage of the disease. The diagnosis is confirmed at laparotomy by operative cholangiography which fails to outline a normal biliary tree.

Treatment consists of surgical bypass of the fibrotic ducts, hepatoportoenterostomy (Kasai procedure), in which a loop of jejunum is anastomosed to the cut surface of the porta hepatis, facilitating drainage of bile from any remaining patent ductules. If surgery is performed before the age of 60 days, 80% of children achieve bile drainage. The success rate diminishes with increasing age – hence the need for early diagnosis and treatment. Postoperative complications include cholangitis and malabsorption of fats and fat-soluble vitamins. Even when bile drainage is successful, there is frequently progression to cirrhosis and portal hypertension. If the operation is unsuccessful, liver transplantation has to be considered. Biliary atresia is the single most common indication for liver transplantation in the paediatric age group.

Choledochal cysts

These are cystic dilatations of the extrahepatic biliary system. About 25% present in infancy with cholestasis. In the older age group, choledochal cysts present with abdominal pain, a palpable mass and jaundice or cholangitis. The diagnosis is established by ultrasound or radionuclide scanning. Treatment is by surgical excision of the cyst with the formation of a Roux-en-Y anastomosis to the biliary duct. Future complications include cholangitis and a 2% risk of malignancy, which may develop in any part of the biliary tree.

Neonatal hepatitis syndrome

In neonatal hepatitis syndrome, there is prolonged neonatal jaundice and hepatic inflammation. Its causes are listed in Box 20.1, but often no specific cause is identified. In contrast to biliary atresia, these infants may have intrauterine growth restriction and hepatosplenomegaly at birth. Liver biopsy (Fig. 20.6) is often non-specific, demonstrating a giant cell hepatitis.

α_1-Antitrypsin deficiency A.R

Deficiency of the protease α_1-antitrypsin is associated with liver disease in infancy and childhood and emphysema in adults. It is inherited as an autosomal recessive disorder with an incidence of 1 in 2000–4000 in the UK. There are many phenotypes of the protease inhibitor (Pi) which are coded on chromosome 14. Liver disease is primarily associated with the phenotype PiZZ.

The majority of children who present with α_1-antitrysin deficiency will either have prolonged neonatal jaundice or, less commonly, bleeding due to vitamin K deficiency (haemorrhagic disease of the newborn). Hepatomegaly is present. Splenomegaly develops with cirrhosis and portal hypertension. The diagnosis is confirmed by estimating the level of α_1-antitrypsin in the plasma and identifying the phenotype. Approximately

Case History

20.1 Biliary atresia

A term infant was given oral vitamin K shortly after birth. He was breast-fed. He became mildly jaundiced on the third day of life. At 5 weeks of age, he presented with poor feeding and vomiting and a history of bruising on his forehead and shoulders. His urine had become dark and stools intermittently pale. He was pale, jaundiced, had several bruises and hepatomegaly. Investigations showed:

- Hb 8.8 g/L
- Platelets 465×10^9/L
- Prothrombin time – 28 s (normal range 10–13 s)
- Serum bilirubin 178 micromol/L – 140 micromol/L conjugated.

The investigation of conjugated hyperbilirubinaemia is shown in Figure 20.2. The TIBIDA radionuclide scan showed no excretion at 24 h (Fig. 20.3) and a liver biopsy suggested biliary atresia (Fig. 20.4). A hepatoportoenterostomy was performed at 6 weeks of age (Fig. 20.5).

 In persistent neonatal jaundice, early diagnosis of biliary atresia improves the prognosis.

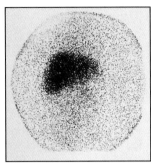

Figure 20.3 Radioisotope scan TIBIDA of liver showing good hepatic uptake of isotope and no excretion into bowel. This scan suggests extrahepatic biliary obstruction or atresia or severe intrahepatic cholestasis.

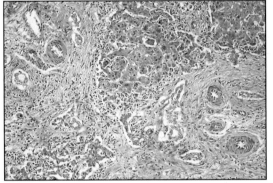

Figure 20.4 Liver biopsy of biliary atresia showing bands of fibrous tissue with bile duct proliferation.

Evaluation of neonatal conjugated hyperbilirubinaemia

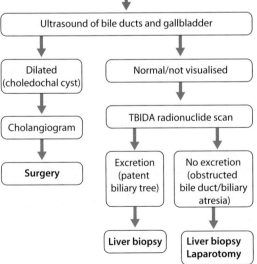

Screen for:
- infection – congenital, hepatitis
- genetic causes – α_1-antitrypsin deficiency, cystic fibrosis, galactosaemia
- metabolic – plasma amino acids and urinary organic acids

Ultrasound of bile ducts and gallbladder

Dilated (choledochal cyst) → Cholangiogram → **Surgery**

Normal/not visualised → TBIDA radionuclide scan

Excretion (patent biliary tree) → **Liver biopsy**

No excretion (obstructed bile duct/biliary atresia) → **Liver biopsy Laparotomy**

Figure 20.2 Evaluation of neonatal conjugated hyperbilirubinaemia.

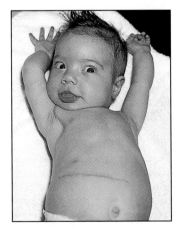

Figure 20.5 Shortly after successful bile drainage by hepatoportoenterostomy (Kasai procedure) for biliary atresia.

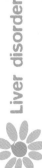

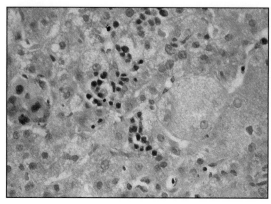

Figure 20.6 Liver biopsy in neonatal hepatitis showing inflammatory infiltrate throughout the liver, and giant cell and rosette formation of liver cells.

50% of children have a good prognosis, but the remainder will develop liver disease and may require transplantation. Pulmonary disease is not significant in childhood, but is likely to develop in adult life. Advice to avoid smoking (both active and passive) should be given. The disorder can be diagnosed antenatally.

Galactosaemia

This very rare disorder has an incidence of 1 in 40 000. The infants develop poor feeding, vomiting, jaundice and hepatomegaly when fed milk. Liver failure, cataracts and developmental delay are inevitable if galactosaemia is untreated. A rapidly fatal course with shock, haemorrhage and disseminated intravascular coagulation, often due to Gram-negative sepsis, may occur.

The condition can be screened for, in prolonged (persistent) jaundice, by detecting galactose, a reducing substance, in the urine. The diagnosis is made by measuring the enzyme galactose-1-phosphate-uridyl transferase in red cells. A recent blood transfusion may mask the diagnosis. A galactose-free diet prevents progression of liver disease, but ovarian failure and learning difficulties may occur later.

Other causes

Neonatal hepatitis may occur following prolonged parenteral nutrition. Rare causes include tyrosinaemia type 1, cystic fibrosis, lipid and glycogen storage disorders, peroxisomal disorders, inborn errors of bile acid synthesis and progressive familial intrahepatic cholestasis (PFIC).

Inborn errors of bile acid synthesis

Patients presenting with neonatal cholestasis of infancy and normal levels of gamma glutamyl transferase (GGT) should be screened for elevated cholenoic bile acids in urine. Diagnosis is confirmed by mass spectrometry of urine for bile acids. Specific treatment is with ursodeoxycholic acid.

Progressive familial intrahepatic cholestasis (PFIC)

This is a heterogeneous group of cholestatic disorders of bile transporter defects caused by recessive mutations in different genes. Children present with jaundice, intense pruritus, diarrhoea with failure to thrive, rickets and a variable progression of liver disease. In two forms of the disorder, the gamma glutamyl transferase (GGT) is low. Prognosis is variable; some children require liver transplantation.

Intrahepatic biliary hypoplasia

Syndromic causes

Alagille syndrome is a rare autosomal dominant condition with widely varying penetrance. Infants may have characteristic triangular facies, skeletal abnormalities, congenital heart disease (classically peripheral pulmonary stenosis), renal tubular disorders, defects in the eye and intrahepatic biliary hypoplasia with severe pruritus and failure to thrive. Prognosis is variable, with 50% of children surviving into adult life without liver transplantation. Intrahepatic biliary hypoplasia also occurs in Down syndrome; there is also a nonsyndromic biliary hypoplasia.

 In persistent jaundice, always look to see if the stools are pale – suggests bile duct obstruction.

Viral hepatitis

The clinical features of viral hepatitis include nausea, vomiting, abdominal pain, lethargy and jaundice; however, 30–50% of children do not develop jaundice. A large tender liver is common and 30% will have splenomegaly. The liver transaminases are usually markedly elevated. Coagulation is usually normal.

Hepatitis A

Hepatitis A virus (HAV) is an RNA virus which is spread by faecal–oral transmission. The incidence of hepatitis A in childhood has fallen as socioeconomic conditions have improved. Many adults are not immune. Vaccination is required for travellers to endemic areas.

The disease may be asymptomatic, but the majority of children have a mild illness and recover both clinically and biochemically within 2–4 weeks. Some may develop prolonged cholestatic hepatitis (which is self-limiting), or fulminant hepatitis. Chronic liver disease does not occur.

The diagnosis can be confirmed by detecting IgM antibody to the virus.

There is no treatment and no evidence that bed rest or change of diet is effective. Close contacts should be given prophylaxis with human normal immunoglobulin (HNIG) or vaccinated within 2 weeks of the onset of the illness.

Hepatitis B

Hepatitis B virus (HBV) is a DNA virus which is an important cause of acute and chronic liver disease worldwide, with high prevalence and carrier rates in the Far

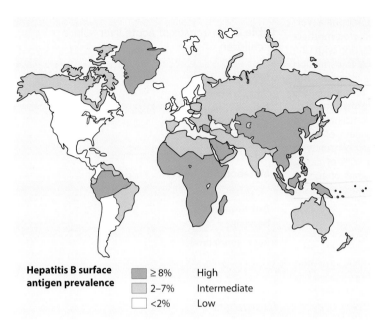

Figure 20.7 Worldwide prevalence of hepatitis B (HBsAg), showing high prevalence in the Far East, sub-Saharan Africa and parts of North and South America (CDC, Centers for Disease Control and Prevention, 2002).

Hepatitis B surface antigen prevalence

≥ 8%	High
2–7%	Intermediate
<2%	Low

East, sub-Saharan Africa and parts of North and South America (Fig. 20.7). HBV is transmitted by:

- Perinatal transmission from carrier mothers
- Transfusion of infected blood or blood products
- Needlestick injuries with infected blood
- Renal dialysis
- Horizontal spread within families.

Among adults it can also be transmitted sexually.

Infants who contract HBV perinatally are asymptomatic, but at least 90% become chronic carriers. Older children who contract HBV may be asymptomatic or have classical features of acute hepatitis. The majority will resolve spontaneously, but 1–2% develop fulminant hepatic failure, while 5–10% become chronic carriers. The diagnosis is made by detecting HBV antigens and antibodies. IgM antibodies to the core antigen (anti-HBc) are positive in acute infection. Positivity to hepatitis B surface antigen (HBsAg) denotes ongoing infectivity. There is no treatment for acute HBV infection.

HBc → acute
HBs → ongoing.

Chronic hepatitis B

Infants infected with HBV by vertical transmission from their mothers usually become asymptomatic carriers. Approximately 30–50% of carrier children will develop chronic HBV liver disease, which may progress to cirrhosis in 10%. There is a long-term risk of hepatocellular carcinoma. Current treatment regimens for chronic HBV have poor efficacy. Interferon treatment for chronic hepatitis B is successful in 50% of children infected horizontally and 30% of children infected perinatally. Oral antiviral therapy such as lamivudine is effective in 23% but is limited by the development of resistance. Newer drugs such as adefovir or long-acting (peg) interferon may be more effective.

Prevention

Prevention of HBV infection is important. All pregnant women should have antenatal screening for HBsAg. Babies of all HBsAg-positive mothers should receive a course of hepatitis B vaccination (given routinely in many countries), with hepatitis B immunoglobulin also being given if the mother is also hepatitis B e antigen (HBeAg)-positive. Antibody response to the vaccination course should be checked in high-risk infants as 5% require further vaccination. Other members of the family should also be vaccinated. There is evidence that effective neonatal vaccination reduces the incidence of HBV-related cancer.

Summary

Hepatitis B virus (HBV)

- Perinatal transmission from carrier mothers should be prevented by maternal screening and giving the infant a course of hepatitis B vaccine with hepatitis B immunoglobulin if indicated
- Infection may result in chronic HBV liver disease, which may progress to cirrhosis and hepatocellular carcinoma.

Hepatitis C

Hepatitis C virus (HCV) is an RNA virus that was responsible for 90% of post-transfusion hepatitis until the screening of donor blood was introduced in 1991. In the UK, about 1 in 2000 donors have HCV antibodies. The prevalence is high among intravenous drug users. Children previously at risk were those who received unscreened blood or blood products, in particular

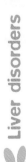

Liver disorders

359

those with haemoglobinopathies or haemophilia. Vertical transmission occurs in 6% from infected mothers but is twice as common if there is co-infection with HIV, and is now the commonest cause of HCV transmission in children. It seldom causes an acute infection, but the majority become chronic carriers, with a 20–25% lifetime risk of progression to cirrhosis or hepatocellular carcinoma. Treatment is with a combination of pegylated interferon and ribavirin. Success of treatment is dependent on virus genotype. In children with genotypes 2/3, it is effective in up to 90% of cases. Treatment is not undertaken before 4 years of age, as it may resolve spontaneously following vertically acquired infections.

Hepatitis D virus

Hepatitis D virus (HDV) is a defective RNA virus that depends on hepatitis B virus for replication. It occurs as a co-infection with hepatitis B virus or as a superinfection causing an acute exacerbation of chronic hepatitis B virus infection. Cirrhosis develops in 50–70% of those who develop chronic HDV infection.

Hepatitis E virus

This is an RNA virus that is enterally transmitted, usually by contaminated water. Epidemics occur in some developing countries.

Non-A to G hepatitis

Clinical presentation is similar to hepatitis A. When a viral aetiology of hepatitis is suspected but not identified, it is known as non-A to G hepatitis.

Epstein–Barr virus

Children with Epstein–Barr virus (EBV) infection are usually asymptomatic. Some 40% have hepatitis that may become fulminant. Less than 5% are jaundiced.

Acute liver failure (fulminant hepatitis)

Acute liver failure in children is the development of massive hepatic necrosis with subsequent loss of liver function, with or without hepatic encephalopathy. The disease is uncommon, but has a high mortality. Most of the cases in childhood are attributed to paracetamol overdosage, non-A to G viral hepatitis and metabolic conditions (Table 20.1). The child may present within hours or weeks with jaundice, encephalopathy, coagulopathy, hypoglycaemia and electrolyte disturbance. Early signs of encephalopathy include alternate periods of irritability and confusion with drowsiness. Older children may be aggressive and unusually difficult. Complications include cerebral oedema, haemorrhage from gastritis or coagulopathy, sepsis and pancreatitis.

Table 20.1 Causes of acute liver failure in children

Infection	Viral hepatitis A, B, C, non-A to G
Poisons/drugs	Paracetamol, isoniazid, halothane, *Amanita phalloides* (poisonous mushroom)
Metabolic	Wilson disease, tyrosinaemia
Autoimmune hepatitis	
Reye syndrome	

Diagnosis

Bilirubin may be normal in the early stages, particularly with metabolic disease. Transaminases are greatly elevated (10–100 times normal), alkaline phosphatase is increased, coagulation is very abnormal and plasma ammonia is elevated. It is essential to monitor the acid–base balance, blood glucose and coagulation times. An EEG will show acute hepatic encephalopathy and a CT scan may demonstrate cerebral oedema.

Management

This includes:

- Maintaining the blood glucose (>4 mmol/L) with intravenous dextrose
- Preventing sepsis with broad-spectrum antibiotics and antifungals
- Preventing haemorrhage, particularly from the gastrointestinal tract with intravenous vitamin K, fresh frozen plasma or cryoprecipitate and H_2-blocking drugs or proton pump inhibitors (PPIs)
- Treating cerebral oedema by fluid restriction and mannitol diuresis
- Urgent transfer to a specialist liver unit.

Features suggestive of a poor prognosis are a shrinking liver, rising bilirubin with falling transaminases, a worsening coagulopathy or progression to coma. Without liver transplantation, 70% of children who progress to coma will die.

Reye syndrome and Reye-like syndrome

Reye syndrome is an acute non-inflammatory encephalopathy with microvesicular fatty infiltration of the liver. Although the aetiology is unknown, there is a close association with aspirin therapy. Since stopping giving aspirin to children aged under 12 years, Reye syndrome has virtually disappeared. With the introduction of tandem mass spectroscopy in the neonatal screening programme, the commonest beta oxidation defect, medium-chain acyl-CoA dehydrogenase (MCAD) deficiency, is diagnosed early in many regions of the UK.

Many of these patients would have presented with a Reye-like syndrome later in life.

Chronic liver disease

The causes of chronic liver disease are given in Box 20.2. The clinical presentation varies from an apparent acute hepatitis to the insidious development of hepatosplenomegaly, cirrhosis and portal hypertension with lethargy and malnutrition. The commonest causes of chronic hepatitis are hepatitis viruses (B or C) and autoimmune hepatitis, but Wilson disease should always be excluded. Histology may demonstrate varying degrees of hepatitis, with an inflammatory infiltrate in the portal tracts that spreads into the liver lobules.

Autoimmune hepatitis

The mean age of presentation is 7–10 years. It is more common in girls. It may present as an acute hepatitis, as fulminant hepatic failure or chronic liver disease with autoimmune features such as skin rash, lupus erythematosus, arthritis, haemolytic anaemia or nephritis. Diagnosis is based on elevated total protein, hypergammaglobulinaemia (IgG >20 g/L); positive autoantibodies, a low serum complement (C4); and typical histology. Autoimmune hepatitis may occur in isolation or in association with inflammatory bowel disease, coeliac disease or other autoimmune diseases. Some 90% of children will respond to prednisolone and azathioprine.

Cystic fibrosis

Liver disease is the second commonest cause of death after respiratory disease in cystic fibrosis. The most common liver abnormality is hepatic steatosis (fatty liver). It may be associated with protein energy malnutrition or micronutrient deficiencies. Steatosis does not generally progress and treatment involves ensuring optimal nutritional support. More significant liver disease arises from thick tenacious bile with abnormal bile acid concentration leading to progressive biliary fibrosis. Cirrhosis and portal hypertension develop in 20% of children by mid-adolescence. Early liver disease is difficult to detect by biochemistry, ultrasound or radioisotope scanning. Liver histology includes fatty liver, focal biliary fibrosis or focal nodular cirrhosis. Therapy includes standard supportive and nutritional therapy and treatment with ursodeoxycholic acid. Liver transplantation may be considered for those with end-stage liver disease, either alone or in combination with a heart–lung transplant.

Wilson disease A R.

Wilson disease is an autosomal recessive disorder with an incidence of 1 in 200 000. Many mutations have now been identified (on chromosome 13). The basic genetic defect is a combination of reduced synthesis of caeruloplasmin (the copper-binding protein) and defective excretion of copper in the bile, which leads to an accumulation of copper in the liver, brain, kidney and cornea. Wilson disease rarely presents in children under the age of 3 years. In those presenting in childhood, a hepatic presentation is more likely. They may present with almost any form of liver disease, including acute hepatitis, fulminant hepatitis, cirrhosis and portal hypertension. Neuropsychiatric features are more common in those presenting from the second decade onwards and include deterioration in school performance, mood and behaviour change, and extrapyramidal signs such as incoordination, tremor and dysarthria. Renal tubular dysfunction, with vitamin D-resistant rickets, and haemolytic anaemia also occur. Copper accumulation in the cornea (Kayser–Fleischer rings) (Fig. 20.8) is not seen before 7 years of age.

Diagnosis can be problematic. A low serum caeruloplasmin and copper is characteristic, but not universal. Urinary copper excretion is increased and this further increases after administering the chelating agent penicillamine. However, the diagnosis is confirmed by the finding of elevated hepatic copper on liver biopsy or identification of the gene mutation.

Treatment is with penicillamine or trientine. Both promote urinary copper excretion, reducing hepatic and central nervous system copper. Zinc is given to

Box 20.2 Causes of chronic liver disease in children

Chronic hepatitis
- Post-viral hepatitis B, C
- Autoimmune hepatitis
- Drugs (nitrofurantoin, non-steroidal anti-inflammatory)
- Inflammatory bowel disease
- Primary sclerosing cholangitis (± ulcerative colitis)

Wilson disease (>3 years)

α_1-Antitrypsin deficiency

Cystic fibrosis

Neonatal liver disease

Bile duct lesions.

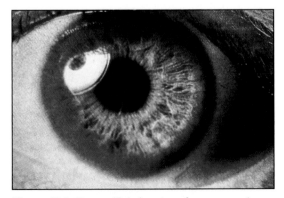

Figure 20.8 Kayser–Fleischer rings from copper in the cornea in a child with Wilson disease.

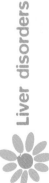

reduce copper absorption. Pyridoxine is given to prevent peripheral neuropathy. Neurological improvement may take up to 12 months of therapy. About 30% of children with Wilson disease will die from hepatic complications if untreated. Liver transplantation is considered for children with acute liver failure or severe end-stage liver disease.

Fibropolycystic liver disease

This is a range of inherited conditions affecting the development of the intrahepatic biliary tree. Presentation is with liver and renal disease. The liver disease may include cystic disease of the liver or biliary tree or congenital hepatic fibrosis.

Congenital hepatic fibrosis (CHF) presents in children over 2 years old with hepatosplenomegaly, abdominal distension and portal hypertension. It differs from cirrhosis in that liver function tests are normal in the early stage. Liver histology shows large bands of hepatic fibrosis containing abnormal bile ductules. The consequent portal hypertension causes bleeding from varices. Cystic renal disease may coexist and may cause hypertension or renal dysfunction.

Non-alcoholic fatty liver disease

Non-alcoholic fatty liver disease (NAFLD) is the single most common cause of chronic liver disease in the developed world. It is a spectrum of disease, ranging from simple fatty deposition (steatosis) through to inflammation (steatohepatitis), fibrosis, cirrhosis and end-stage liver failure. The prognosis in childhood is uncertain; very few develop cirrhosis in childhood in contrast to 8–17% of adults. Most affected children are obese. They are usually asymptomatic, although some complain of vague right upper quadrant abdominal pain or lethargy. The diagnosis is often suspected following the incidental finding of an echogenic liver on ultrasound or mildly elevated transaminases carried out for some other reason. Liver biopsy demonstrates marked steatosis with or without inflammation or fibrosis. The pathogenesis is not fully understood but may be linked to insulin resistance. Treatment is targeted at weight loss, which may lead to liver function tests returning to normal.

Cirrhosis and portal hypertension

Cirrhosis is the end result of many forms of liver disease. It is defined pathologically as extensive fibrosis with regenerative nodules. It may be secondary to hepatocellular disease or to chronic bile duct obstruction (biliary cirrhosis). The main pathophysiological effects of cirrhosis are diminished hepatic function and portal hypertension with splenomegaly, varices and ascites (see Fig. 20.1). Hepatocellular carcinoma may develop.

Children with compensated cirrhosis may be asymptomatic if liver function is adequate. They will not be jaundiced and may have normal liver function tests. As the cirrhosis increases, however, the results of

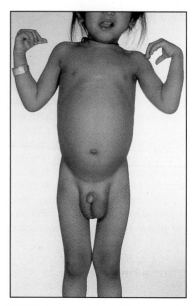

Figure 20.9 Cirrhosis and portal hypertension. (i) Malnutrition with loss of fat and muscle bulk; (ii) distended abdomen from hepatosplenomegaly and ascites; (iii) scrotal swelling from ascites; and (iv) no jaundice, despite advanced liver disease.

deteriorating liver function and portal hypertension become obvious (Fig. 20.9). Physical signs include palmar and plantar erythema and spider naevi, malnutrition and hypotonia. Dilated abdominal veins and splenomegaly suggest portal hypertension, although the liver may be impalpable.

Investigations include:

- Screening for the known causes of chronic liver disease (see Box 20.2)
- Upper gastrointestinal endoscopy to detect the presence of oesophageal varices and/or erosive gastritis
- Abdominal ultrasound – may show a shrunken liver and splenomegaly with gastric and oesophageal varices
- Liver biopsy – may be difficult because of increased fibrosis but may indicate the aetiology (e.g. typical changes in congenital hepatic fibrosis, copper storage).

As cirrhosis decompensates, biochemical tests may demonstrate an elevation of aminotransferases and alkaline phosphatase. The plasma albumin falls and the prothrombin time becomes increasingly prolonged.

Oesophageal varices

These are an inevitable consequence of portal hypertension and may develop rapidly in children. They are best diagnosed by upper gastrointestinal endoscopy, as a barium swallow may miss small varices. Acute bleeding is treated conservatively with blood transfusions and H_2-blockers (e.g. ranitidine) or omeprazole. If bleeding persists, octreotide infusion, vasopressin analogues, sclerotherapy or band ligation may be effective.

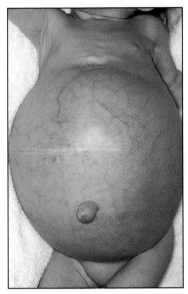

Figure 20.10 This infant has a grossly distended abdomen from ascites. There are dilated abdominal veins secondary to portal hypertension and an umbilical hernia from increased abdominal pressure. There is a surgical scar.

Portacaval shunts may preclude liver transplantation, but radiological placement of a stent between the hepatic and portal veins can be used as a temporary measure if transplantation is being considered.

Ascites

Ascites is a major problem (Fig. 20.10). The pathophysiology of ascites is uncertain, but contributory factors include hypoalbuminaemia, sodium retention, renal impairment and fluid redistribution. It is treated by sodium and fluid restriction and diuretics. Additional therapy for refractory ascites includes albumin infusions or paracentesis.

Spontaneous bacterial peritonitis

This should always be considered if there is undiagnosed fever, abdominal pain, tenderness or an unexplained deterioration in hepatic or renal function. A diagnostic paracentesis should be performed and the fluid sent for white cell count and differential and culture. Treatment is with broad-spectrum antibiotics.

Encephalopathy

This occurs in end-stage liver disease and may be precipitated by gastrointestinal haemorrhage, sepsis, sedatives, renal failure or electrolyte imbalance. It is difficult to diagnose in children as the level of consciousness may vary throughout the day. Infants present with irritability and sleepiness, while older children present with abnormalities in mood, sleep rhythm, intellectual performance and behaviour.

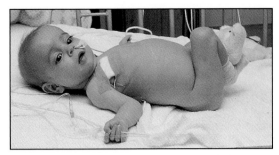

Figure 20.11 Many infants and children with liver disease need intensive nutritional supplementation. This malnourished infant is having both parenteral nutrition via a central line and continuous nasogastric feeding.

Plasma ammonia may be elevated and an EEG is always abnormal.

Renal failure

This may be secondary to renal tubular acidosis, acute tubular necrosis or functional renal failure (hepatorenal syndrome).

Management of children with liver disease

Although certain diseases may require specific treatment, the management of the sequelae of chronic liver disease is supportive, with the emphasis on correction of nutritional abnormalities, prevention of complications and intensive family support.

Nutrition

Malnutrition may be due to protein malnutrition, fat malabsorption, anorexia or fat-soluble vitamin deficiency (vitamins A, D, E and K).

Treatment is to provide a high-protein, high-carbohydrate diet with 50% more calories than the recommended dietary allowance. In children with cholestasis, medium-chain triglycerides, which are absorbed by the portal circulation, will provide fat, but 20–40% long-chain triglycerides are required to prevent essential fatty acid deficiency. Many children will require nasogastric tube feeding or parenteral nutrition (Fig. 20.11).

Fat-soluble vitamins

Vitamin K deficiency in liver disease may be due to malabsorption or diminished synthesis. Water-soluble forms of vitamin K are available.

Vitamin A deficiency causes night blindness in adults and retinal changes in infants. It is easily prevented with oral vitamin A.

Vitamin E deficiency causes peripheral neuropathy, haemolysis and ataxia. It is very poorly absorbed in cholestatic conditions and high oral doses are required.

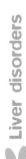

Vitamin D deficiency causes rickets and pathological fractures. It is prevented by using a water-soluble form of vitamin D. Vitamin D-resistant rickets indicates renal tubular acidosis.

Pruritus

Many children with cholestasis have severe pruritus. Management is problematic but may include:

- Loose cotton clothing, avoiding overheating
- Emollients or evening primrose oil
- Phenobarbital to stimulate bile flow; cholestyramine which is a bile salt resin; ursodeoxycholic acid, an oral bile acid.

Encephalopathy

In children, encephalopathy is managed by treating the precipitating factor (sepsis, gastrointestinal haemorrhage) by protein restriction or by using oral lactulose to reduce ammonia reabsorption by lowering colonic pH and increasing colonic transit.

Liver transplantation

Liver transplantation is an accepted therapy for acute or chronic end-stage liver failure and has revolutionised the prognosis for these children. Transplantation is also considered for some hepatic malignancy.

The indications for transplantation in chronic liver failure are:

- Severe malnutrition unresponsive to intensive nutritional therapy
- Recurrent complications (bleeding varices, resistant ascites)
- Failure of growth and development
- Poor quality of life.

Liver transplant evaluation includes assessment of the vascular anatomy of the liver and exclusion of irreversible disease in other systems. Absolute contraindications include sepsis, untreatable cardiopulmonary disease or cerebrovascular disease.

There is considerable difficulty in obtaining small organs for children. Most children receive part of an adult's liver, either a cadaveric graft or more recently from a living related donor. A cadaveric organ may either be reduced to fit the child's abdomen (reduction hepatectomy) or split (shared between an adult and child).

Complications post-transplantation include:

- Primary non-function of the liver (5%)
- Hepatic artery thrombosis (10–20%)
- Biliary leaks and strictures (20%)
- Rejection (30–60%)
- Sepsis, the main cause of death.

In large national centres, the overall 1-year survival is approximately 90%, and the overall 5-year survival is >80%. Most deaths occur in the first 3 months. Children who survive the initial postoperative period usually do well. Long-term studies indicate normal psychosocial development and quality of life in survivors.

Further reading

Beattie M, Dhawan A, Puntis J: *Paediatric Gastroenterology, Hepatology and Nutrition*, Oxford Specialist Handbooks in Paediatrics, Oxford, 2009, Oxford University Press.

Short handbook.

Kelly DA: *Diseases of the Liver and Biliary System in Childhood*, ed 3. Oxford, 2008, Blackwell Science.

Comprehensive textbook.

Malignant disease

Cancer in children is not common.

- Around 1 child in 500 develops cancer by 15 years of age.
- Each year, in Western countries, there are 120–140 new cases per million children aged under 15 years, equivalent to about 1500 new cases each year in the UK.

The types of disease seen (Fig. 21.1) are very different from those in adults, where carcinomas of the lung, breast, gut and skin predominate. The age at presentation varies with the different types of disease:

- Leukaemia affects children at all ages (although there is an early childhood peak).
- Neuroblastoma and Wilms tumour are almost always seen in the first 6 years of life.
- Hodgkin lymphoma and bone tumours have their peak incidence in adolescence and early adult life.

Despite significant improvements in survival over the last four decades (Fig. 21.2), cancer is the commonest

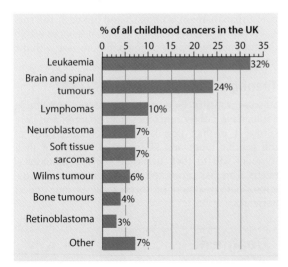

Figure 21.1 Relative frequency of different types of cancer in children in the UK.

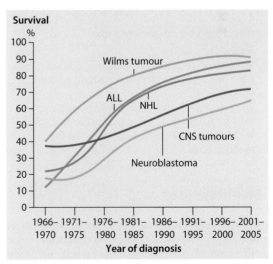

Figure 21.2 Five-year survival rates showing the considerable improvement over the last 50 years. (ALL, acute lymphoblastic leukaemia; NHL, non-Hodgkin lymphoma.) (Sources: 1971–2000. Stiller C (Editor) *Childhood Cancer in Britain – Incidence, Survival, Mortality*, Oxford, 2007, Oxford University Press; and 1966–1970 & 2001–2005, National Registry of Childhood Tumours, unpublished data.)

disease causing death in childhood (beyond the neonatal period). Overall, the 5-year survival of children with all forms of cancer is about 75%, most of whom can be considered cured, although cure rates vary considerably for different diagnoses. This improved life expectancy can be attributed mainly to the introduction of multi-agent chemotherapy, supportive care and specialist multidisciplinary management. However, for some children, the price of survival is long-term medical or psychosocial difficulties.

 In children, leukaemia is the most common malignancy followed by brain tumours.

Aetiology

In most cases, the precise aetiology of childhood cancer is unclear, but it is likely to involve an interaction between environmental factors (e.g. viral infection) and host genetic susceptibility. In fact, there are very few established environmental risk factors, and although cancer occurs as a result of mutations in cellular growth controlling genes, which are usually sporadic but may be inherited, in most cases a specific gene mutation is unknown. One example of an inherited cancer is bilateral retinoblastoma, which is associated with a mutation within the RB gene located on chromosome 13. There is a wide range of syndromes associated with an increased risk of cancer in childhood, e.g. associations exist between Down syndrome and leukaemia, and neurofibromatosis and glioma. In time, the further identification of biological characteristics of specific tumour cells may also help elucidate the basic pathogenetic mechanisms behind their origin.

Clinical presentation

Cancer in children can present with:

- A localised mass
- The consequences of disseminated disease, e.g. bone marrow infiltration, causing systemic ill-health
- The consequences of pressure from a mass on local structures or tissue, e.g. airway obstruction secondary to enlarged lymph nodes in the mediastinum.

Investigations

Initial symptoms can be very non-specific and this can often lead to significant delays in diagnosis. Once a diagnosis of malignancy is suspected, the child should be referred to a specialist centre for further investigation.

Radiology

The location of solid tumours and evidence of any metastases are identified and localised, using a combination of ultrasound, plain X-rays, CT and MRI scans.

Nuclear medicine imaging (e.g. radiolabelled technetium bone scan) may be useful to identify bone or bone marrow disease or, using special markers (MIBG scan), localise tumours of neural crest origin, e.g. neuroblastoma.

Tumour marker studies

Increased urinary catecholamine excretion (e.g. VMA, vanillylmandelic acid) is useful in confirming the diagnosis of neuroblastoma. High α-fetoprotein (αFP) production is often observed in germ cell tumours and liver tumours and can be used to monitor treatment response.

Pathology

All diagnoses must be confirmed histologically, either by bone marrow aspiration for cases of leukaemia or by biopsy for most solid tumours, although this may not always be possible for brain tumours. Histological techniques such as immunohistochemistry are routinely used to differentiate tumour types. Molecular and genetic techniques are also used to confirm diagnosis (e.g. translocation of chromosomes 11 and 22 in Ewing sarcoma) and to predict prognosis (e.g. amplification of the 'N-*myc*' oncogene associated with a poor prognosis in neuroblastoma).

Management

Once malignancy has been diagnosed, the parents and child need to be seen and the diagnosis explained to them in a realistic, yet positive way. Detailed investigation to define the extent of the disease (staging) is paramount to planning treatment. Children are usually treated as part of national and international collaborative studies that offer consistency in care and have contributed to improvements in outcome.

In the UK, children with cancer are initially investigated and treated in specialist centres where experienced multidisciplinary teams can provide the intensive medical and psychosocial support required. Subsequent management is often shared between the specialist centre, referral hospital and local services within the community, to provide the optimum care with the least disruption to the family.

Teenagers and young adults (TYA)

Survival statistics suggest that teenagers and young adults have poorer outcomes than children and constitute a distinct population. This relates both to the specific types and biological behaviour of their tumours and to their particular social/psychological needs. This has prompted the development of age-appropriate treatment protocols, facilities and support networks.

Treatment

Treatment may involve chemotherapy, surgery or radiotherapy, alone or in combination.

Chemotherapy

This is used:

- as primary curative treatment, e.g. in acute lymphoblastic leukaemia
- to control primary or metastatic disease before definitive local treatment with surgery and/or radiotherapy, e.g. in sarcoma or neuroblastoma
- as adjuvant treatment to deal with residual disease and to eliminate presumed micrometastases, e.g. after initial local treatment with surgery in Wilms tumour

The use of biologically targeted therapies and their role in combination with conventional treatment modalities is an area of active research that is likely to increase in importance in the near future.

Radiotherapy

This retains a role in the treatment of some tumours, but the risk of damage to growth and function of normal tissue is greater in a child than in an adult. The need for adequate protection of normal tissues and for careful positioning and immobilisation of the patient during treatment raises practical difficulties, particularly in young children.

Surgery

Initial surgery is frequently restricted to biopsy to establish the diagnosis, and more extensive operations are usually undertaken to remove residual tumour after chemotherapy and/or radiotherapy.

High-dose therapy with bone marrow rescue

The limitation of both chemotherapy and radiotherapy is the risk of irreversible damage to normal tissues, particularly bone marrow. Transplantation of bone marrow stem cells can be used as a strategy to intensify the treatment of patients with the administration of potentially lethal doses of chemotherapy and/or radiation. The source of the marrow stem cells may be allogeneic (from a compatible donor) or autologous (from the patient him/herself, harvested beforehand, while the marrow is uninvolved or in remission). Allogeneic transplantation is principally used in the management of high-risk or relapsed leukaemia and autologous stem cell support is used most commonly in the treatment of children with solid tumours whose prognosis is poor using conventional chemotherapy, e.g. advanced neuroblastoma.

Supportive care and side-effects of treatment

Cancer treatment produces frequent, predictable and often severe multisystem side-effects (Fig. 21.3). Supportive care is an important part of management and improvements in this aspect of cancer care have contributed to the increasing survival rates.

Short-term side-effects of chemotherapy

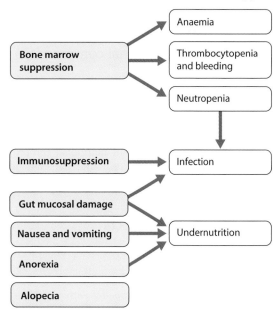

Figure 21.3 Short-term side-effects of chemotherapy.

Infection from immunosuppression

Due to both treatment (chemotherapy or wide-field radiation) and underlying disease, children with cancer are immunocompromised and at risk of serious infection. Children with fever and neutropenia must be admitted promptly to hospital for cultures and treatment with broad-spectrum antibiotics. Some important opportunistic infections associated with therapy for cancer include *Pneumocystis jiroveci* (*carinii*) pneumonia (especially in children with leukaemia), disseminated fungal infection (e.g. aspergillosis and candidiasis) and coagulase-negative staphylococcal infections of central venous catheters.

Most common viral infections are no worse in children with cancer than in other children, but measles and varicella zoster (chickenpox) may have atypical presentation and can be life-threatening. If non-immune, immunocompromised children are at risk from contact with measles or varicella, some protection can be afforded by prompt administration of immunoglobulin or zoster immune globulin. Aciclovir is used to treat established varicella infection, but no treatment is available for measles. During chemotherapy and from 6 months to a year subsequently, the use of live vaccines is contraindicated due to depressed immunity. After this period, re-immunisation against common childhood infections is recommended.

Bone marrow suppression

Anaemia may require blood transfusions. Thrombocytopaenia presents the hazard of bleeding, and considerable blood product support may be required, particularly for children with leukaemia, those undergoing intensive therapy requiring bone marrow transplantation and in the more intensive solid tumour protocols.

Gastrointestinal damage, nausea and vomiting and nutritional compromise

Mouth ulcers are common, painful and, when severe, can prevent a child eating adequately. Many chemotherapy agents are nauseating and induce vomiting, which may be only partially prevented by the routine use of antiemetic drugs. These two complications can result in significant nutritional compromise. Chemotherapy-induced gut mucosal damage also causes diarrhoea and may predispose to Gram-negative infection.

Drug-specific side-effects

Many individual drugs have very specific side-effects: e.g. cardiotoxicity with doxorubicin; renal failure and deafness with cisplatin; haemorrhagic cystitis with cyclophosphamide; and neuropathy with vincristine. The extent of these side-effects is not always predictable and patients require careful monitoring during, and in some cases, after treatment is complete.

Other supportive care issues

Fertility preservation

Some patients may be at risk of infertility as a result of their cancer treatment. Appropriate fertility preservation techniques may involve surgically moving a testis or ovary out of the radiotherapy field; sperm banking (which should be offered to boys mature enough to achieve this); and consideration of newer techniques such as cryopreservation of ovarian cortical tissue, although the long-term efficacy of this is still uncertain.

Venous access

The discomfort of multiple venepunctures for blood sampling and intravenous infusions can be avoided with central venous catheters, although these do carry a risk of infection (Fig. 21.4).

 Fever with neutropenia requires hospital admission, cultures and intravenous antibiotics.

Psychosocial support

The diagnosis of a potentially fatal illness has an enormous and long-lasting impact on the whole family. They need the opportunity to discuss the implications of the diagnosis and its treatment and their anxiety, fear, guilt and sadness. Most will benefit from the counselling and practical support provided by health professionals. Help with practical issues, including transport, finances, accommodation and care of siblings, is an early priority. The provision of detailed written material for parents will help them understand their child's disease and treatment. The children themselves, and their siblings, need an age-appropriate explanation of the disease. Once treatment is

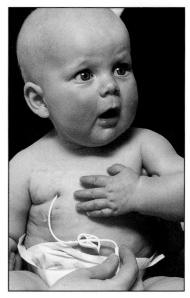

Figure 21.4 The central venous catheter allows pain-free blood tests and injections for this child on chemotherapy, which has caused the alopecia.

established and the disease appears to be under control, families should be encouraged to return to as normal a lifestyle as possible. Early return to school is important and children with cancer should not be allowed to under-achieve the expectations previously held for them. It is easy to underestimate the severe stress that persists within families in relation to the uncertainty of the long-term outcome. This often manifests itself as marital problems in parents and behavioural difficulties in both the child and siblings.

Summary

Malignant disease in children

- Uncommon, but affects 1 in 500 by 15 years of age
- The overall 5-year survival rate is 75%
- Presents with a localised mass or its pressure effects or disseminated disease
- Treatment may involve chemotherapy, surgery, radiotherapy or high-dose therapy with bone marrow rescue
- Fever with neutropenia must be investigated and treated urgently
- Measles and varicella zoster infection are potentially life-threatening
- Requires a multidisciplinary team to provide supportive care and psychosocial support
- Supportive care – includes not only management of side-effects but also pain management and fertility preservation
- Psychosocial support – includes not only the patient and parents but also siblings and other family and community members.

Leukaemia

Acute lymphoblastic leukaemia (ALL) accounts for 80% of leukaemia in children. Most of the remainder is acute myeloid/acute non-lymphocytic leukaemia (AML/ANLL). Chronic myeloid leukaemia and other myeloproliferative disorders are rare.

Clinical presentation

Presentation of acute lymphoblastic leukaemia peaks at 2–5 years. Clinical symptoms and signs result from disseminated disease and systemic ill-health from infiltration of the bone marrow or other organs with leukaemic blast cells (Fig. 21.5). In most children, leukaemia presents insidiously over several weeks (see Case History 21.1) but in some children the illness presents and progresses very rapidly.

Investigations

Full blood count – in most but not all children, the blood count is abnormal, with low haemoglobin, thrombocytopenia and evidence of circulating leukaemic blast cells. Bone marrow examination is essential to confirm the diagnosis and to identify immunological and cytogenetic characteristics which give useful prognostic information. Chest X ray is required to identify a mediastinal mass characteristic of T-cell disease.

Both ALL and AML are classified by morphology. Immunological phenotyping further subclassifies ALL; the common (75%) and T-cell (15%) subtypes are the most common. Prognosis and some aspects of clinical presentation vary according to different subtypes, and treatment intensity is adjusted accordingly.

Management of acute lymphoblastic leukaemia

A number of factors contribute to prognosis in ALL and dictate the intensity of therapy (Table 21.1).

A typical treatment schema is shown in Figure 21.7.

Remission induction

Before starting treatment of the disease, anaemia may require correction with blood transfusion, the risk of bleeding minimised by transfusion of platelets, and infection must be treated. Additional hydration and allopurinol (or urate oxidase when the white cell count is high and the risk is greater) are given to protect renal function against the effects of rapid cell lysis. Remission implies eradication of the leukaemic blasts and restoration of normal marrow function. Four weeks of

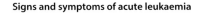

Signs and symptoms of acute leukaemia

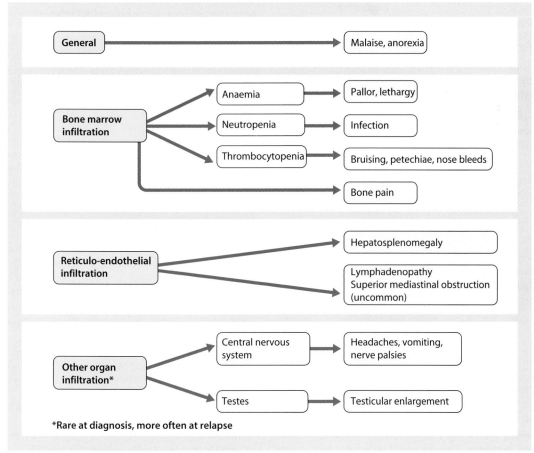

*Rare at diagnosis, more often at relapse

Figure 21.5 Signs and symptoms of acute leukaemia.

Case History

21.1 Disseminated disease, e.g. bone marrow infiltration, causing systemic ill-health

A 4-year-old girl was generally unwell, lethargic, looking pale and occasionally febrile over a period of 9 weeks. Two courses of antibiotics for recurrent sore throat failed to result in any benefit. Her parents returned to their general practitioner when she developed a rash. Examination showed pallor, petechiae, modest generalised lymphadenopathy and mild hepatosplenomegaly. A full blood count showed:

- Hb 8.3 g/dl
- WBC 15.6×10^9/L
- Platelets 44×10^9/L.

Blast cells were seen on the peripheral blood film. Cerebrospinal fluid (CSF) examination was normal. Bone marrow examination confirmed acute lymphoblastic leukaemia (Fig. 21.6).

Diagnosis: Acute lymphoblastic leukaemia.

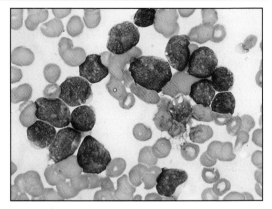

Figure 21.6 Leukaemic blast cells on a bone marrow smear.

Table 21.1 Prognostic factors in acute lymphatic leukaemia

Prognostic factor	High-risk features
Age	<1 year or >10 years
Tumour load (measured by the white cell count, WBC)	$>50 \times 10^9$/L
Cytogenetic/molecular genetic abnormalities in tumour cells	e.g. MLL rearrangement, t(4;11), hypodiploidy (<44 chromosomes)
Speed of response to initial chemotherapy	Persistence of leukaemic blasts in the bone marrow
Minimal residual disease assessment (MRD) (submicroscopic levels of leukaemia detected by PCR)	High

combination chemotherapy is given and current induction treatment schedules achieve remission rates of 95%.

Intensification

A block of intensive chemotherapy is given to consolidate remission. This improves cure rates but at the expense of increased toxicity.

Central nervous system

Cytotoxic drugs penetrate poorly into the CNS. As leukaemic cells in this site may survive effective systemic treatment, additional treatment with intrathecal chemotherapy is used to prevent CNS relapse.

Continuing therapy

Chemotherapy of modest intensity is continued over a relatively long period of time, up to 3 years from diagnosis. Co-trimoxazole prophylaxis is given routinely to prevent *Pneumocystis carinii* pneumonia.

Treatment of relapse

High-dose chemotherapy, usually with total body irradiation (TBI) and bone marrow transplantation, is used as an alternative to conventional chemotherapy after a relapse.

Brain tumours

In contrast to adults, brain tumours in children are almost always primary and 60% are infratentorial. They are the most common solid tumour in children and are the leading cause of childhood cancer deaths in the UK. The types of brain tumour are:

- Astrocytoma (~40%) – varies from benign to highly malignant (*glioblastoma multiforme*)
- Medulloblastoma (~20%) – arises in the midline of the posterior fossa. May seed through the CNS via the CSF and up to 20% have spinal metastases at diagnosis
- Ependymoma (~8%) – mostly in posterior fossa where it behaves like medulloblastoma
- Brainstem glioma (6%)
- Craniopharyngioma (4%) – a developmental tumour arising from the squamous remnant of

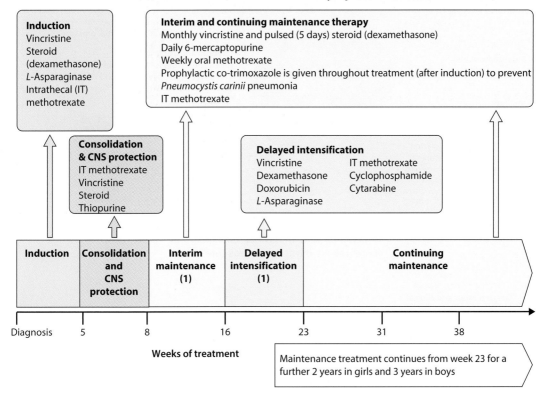

Treatment schema for standard-risk acute lymphoblastic leukaemia

Induction
Vincristine
Steroid
(dexamethasone)
L-Asparaginase
Intrathecal (IT)
methotrexate

Interim and continuing maintenance therapy
Monthly vincristine and pulsed (5 days) steroid (dexamethasone)
Daily 6-mercaptopurine
Weekly oral methotrexate
Prophylactic co-trimoxazole is given throughout treatment (after induction) to prevent
Pneumocystis carinii pneumonia
IT methotrexate

**Consolidation
& CNS protection**
IT methotrexate
Vincristine
Steroid
Thiopurine

Delayed intensification
Vincristine   IT methotrexate
Dexamethasone   Cyclophosphamide
Doxorubicin   Cytarabine
L-Asparaginase

Induction	Consolidation and CNS protection	Interim maintenance (1)	Delayed intensification (1)	Continuing maintenance

Diagnosis   5   8   16   23   31   38

Weeks of treatment

Maintenance treatment continues from week 23 for a
further 2 years in girls and 3 years in boys

Figure 21.7 Treatment schema for standard-risk acute lymphoblastic leukaemia.

Rathke pouch. It is not truly malignant but is locally invasive and grows slowly in the suprasellar region.

Clinical features

Signs and symptoms are often related to evidence of raised intracranial pressure but focal neurological signs may be detected depending on the site of the tumour (see below). Spinal tumours, primary or metastatic, can present with back pain, peripheral weakness of arms or legs or bladder/bowel dysfunction, depending on the level of the lesion.

 Persistent back pain in children warrants investigation with MRI scan.

Investigations

Brain tumours are best characterised on MRI scan. Magnetic resonance spectroscopy can be used to examine the biological activity of a tumour. Lumbar puncture must not be performed without neurosurgical advice if there is any suspicion of raised intracranial pressure.

Management

Surgery is usually the first treatment and is aimed at treating hydrocephalus, providing a tissue diagnosis and attempting maximum resection. In some cases the anatomical position of the tumour means biopsy is not safe, e.g. tumours in the brainstem. Even tumours

which are histologically 'benign' can cause major challenges to survival. The use of radiotherapy and/or chemotherapy varies with tumour type and the age of the patient.

Late effects

The functional implications of the site of the tumour, the potential hazards of surgery and the importance of radiotherapy in treatment all combine to place children with brain tumours at particular risk of neurological disability and of growth, endocrine, neuropsychological and educational problems. Survivors may present complex combinations of these problems.

Lymphomas

Lymphomas are malignancies of the cells of the immune system and can be divided into Hodgkin and non-Hodgkin lymphoma (NHL). NHL is more common in childhood, while Hodgkin lymphoma is seen more frequently in adolescence.

Hodgkin lymphoma

Clinical features

Classically presents with painless lymphadenopathy, most frequently in the neck. Lymph nodes are much larger and firmer than the benign lymphadenopathy

Malignant disease

371

Brain tumours – clinical features

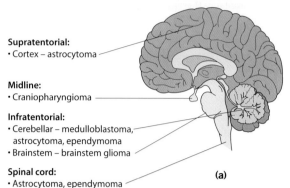

Supratentorial:
• Cortex – astrocytoma

Midline:
• Craniopharyngioma

Infratentorial:
• Cerebellar – medulloblastoma, astrocytoma, ependymoma
• Brainstem – brainstem glioma

Spinal cord:
• Astrocytoma, ependymoma

(a)

> **Raised intracranial pressure**
>
> **Children and adolescents**
> Headache – worse in the morning
> Vomiting – especially on waking in the morning
> Behaviour/personality change
> Visual disturbance
> Papilloedema
>
> **Infants**
> Vomiting
> Separation of sutures/tense fontanelle
> Increased head circumference
> Head tilt/posturing
> Developmental delay/regression

 Headaches and behaviour changes – is there raised intracranial pressure?

Site of tumour and clinical features specific to anatomical postition	MRI Scans	Typical case history
Supratentorial – cortex Seizures Hemiplegia Focal neurological signs (b)		14 year old. Aggressive behaviour at school, headaches, seizure MRI scan – **(Fig 21.8b)** Diagnosis – **astrocytoma – glioblastoma multiforme** Management – surgery, radiotherapy +/- chemotherapy, but prognosis poor (<30% survival) Astrocytomas – commonly found in the cerebral hemispheres, thalamus and hypothalamus. For posterior fossa tumours, see below.
Midline Visual field loss – bitemporal hemianopia Pituitary failure – growth failure, diabetes insipidus, weight gain (c)		10 year old complaining of headaches, vomiting, poor growth, struggling to see the board at school. MRI scan – **(Fig 21.8c)** Diagnosis – **craniopharyngioma** Management – surgical excision +/- radiotherapy Prognosis – good survival but risk of long-term visual Impairment and lifelong, complex pituitary insufficiency
Cerebellar and IVth ventricle Truncal ataxia Coordination difficulties Abnormal eye movements (d)		3 year old vomiting in the mornings, unsteady on his feet, new-onset convergent squint. MRI scan – **(Fig 21.8d)** Diagnosis – **medulloblastoma** Management – surgery, chemotherapy, radiotherapy. Prognosis – survival rates are improving with 5-year survival about 50% Other posterior fossa tumours: Astrocytoma – cystic, slow growing. Good prognosis following surgery. Ependymoma – behaves like medulloblastoma
Brainstem Cranial nerve defects Pyramidal tract signs Cerebellar signs – ataxia Often no raised intracranial pressure (e)		4 year old. Refuses to walk, unable to climb stairs, squint, facial asymmetry and drooling. MRI scan – **(Fig 21.8e)** Diagnosis – **brainstem glioma.** But not for biopsy as too hazardous. Management – palliative radiotherapy Prognosis – very poor (<10% survival)

Figure 21.8 Location and clinical features of brain tumours. (a) Location of brain tumours. MRI scans showing (b) fronto-parietal mass, (c) large midline suprasellar mass, (d) cerebellar mass and (e) brainstem mass.

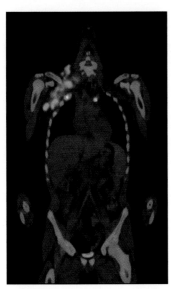

Figure 21.9 PET scan showing active disease in the right cervical and axillary nodes by uptake of FDG (an analogue of glucose).

commonly seen in young children. The lymph nodes may cause airways obstruction (see Case History 21.2). The clinical history is often long (several months) and systemic symptoms (sweating, pruritus, weight loss and fever – the so-called 'B' symptoms) are uncommon, even in more advanced disease.

Investigations

Lymph node biopsy, radiological assessment of all nodal sites and bone marrow biopsy is used to stage disease and determine treatment.

Management

Combination chemotherapy with or without radiotherapy. Positron emission tomography (PET) scanning is used in the UK to monitor treatment response and guide further management (Figure 21.9).

Overall, about 80% of all patients can be cured. Even with disseminated disease, about 60% can be cured.

Non-Hodgkin lymphoma

T-cell malignancies may present as acute lympho-blastic leukaemia or non-Hodgkin lymphoma, with both being characterised by a mediastinal mass with varying degrees of bone marrow infiltration. The mediastinal mass may cause superior vena caval obstruction. B-cell malignancies present more commonly as non-Hodgkin lymphoma, with localised lymph node disease usually in the head and neck or abdomen. Abdominal disease presents with pain from intestinal obstruction, a palpable mass or even intussusception in cases with involvement of the ileum.

Investigations

Biopsy, radiological assessment of all nodal sites (CT or MRI) and examination of the bone marrow and CSF.

Case History

21.2 Pressure from a mass on local structures or tissue, e.g. airway obstruction secondary to enlarged lymph nodes

A 14-year-old girl complained of a cough for 2 weeks which was non-productive and worse at night. She had seen her general practitioner and her chest was clear. She returned 2 weeks later, as she had noticed a swelling in her neck. On examination, she had a large anterior cervical lymph node which was non-tender. On referral to hospital, she had a chest X-ray, which showed a large mediastinal mass (Fig. 21.10).

Differential diagnosis

- T-cell non-Hodgkin lymphoma/acute lymphatic leukaemia
- Hodgkin lymphoma

Her full blood count was normal. A biopsy of the mass was consistent with a diagnosis of Hodgkin lymphoma.
Diagnosis: Hodgkin lymphoma.

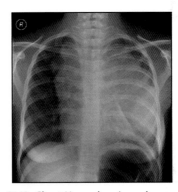

Figure 21.10 Chest X-ray showing a large mediastinal mass.

Management

Multi-agent chemotherapy. The majority of patients now do well and survival rates of over 80% are expected for both T- and B-cell disease.

Neuroblastoma

Neuroblastoma and related tumours arise from neural crest tissue in the adrenal medulla and sympathetic nervous system. It is a biologically unusual tumour in that spontaneous regression sometimes occurs in very young infants. There is a spectrum of disease from the benign (ganglioneuroma) to the highly malignant (neuroblastoma). Neuroblastoma is most common before the age of 5 years.

Clinical features

At presentation (Box 21.1), most children have an abdominal mass, but the primary tumour can lie anywhere along the sympathetic chain from the neck to the pelvis. Classically, the abdominal primary is of adrenal origin, but at presentation the tumour mass is often large and complex, crossing the midline and enveloping major blood vessels and lymph nodes. Paravertebral tumours may invade through the adjacent intervertebral foramen and cause spinal cord compression. Over the age of 2 years, clinical symptoms are mostly from metastatic disease, particularly bone pain, bone marrow suppression causing weight loss and malaise (see Case History 21.3).

Box 21.1 Presentation of neuroblastoma

Common	Less common
Pallor	Paraplegia
Weight loss	Cervical
Abdominal mass	lymphadenopathy
Hepatomegaly	Proptosis
Bone pain	Periorbital bruising
Limp	Skin nodules

Case History

21.3 Neuroblastoma

Jack, a 3-year-old boy, was taken to his general practitioner by his mother because he was not eating as well as usual and had a distended abdomen. Recently, he appeared reluctant to walk and sometimes cried when he was picked up. His grandmother thought he had lost weight. On examination, the general practitioner confirmed that he seemed generally miserable and pale. He was concerned to note a large abdominal mass. Urgent referral to his local hospital was made and, on arrival, he was also noted to be hypertensive.

Differential diagnosis and specific investigations

An initial ultrasound examination confirmed the abdominal mass and an MRI scan characterised a very large upper abdominal mass in complex relationship with the left kidney and the major vessels but extending towards the midline, suggestive of neuroblastoma (Fig. 21.11). Subsequent investigations confirmed bone marrow infiltration by tumour cells and a positive MIBG scan showing uptake at the primary and distant sites consistent with metastatic disease (Fig 21.12).

Diagnosis: Metastatic neuroblastoma.

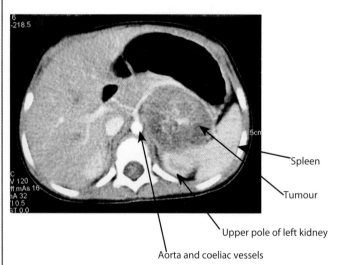

6
-218.5

5cm

C
V 120
ff.mAs 16
nA 32
T 0.5
GT 0.0

Spleen

Tumour

Upper pole of left kidney

Aorta and coeliac vessels

Figure 21.11 Transverse MRI image showing a large left-sided primary neuroblastoma arising from the adrenal region and distorting coeliac and mesenteric blood vessels.

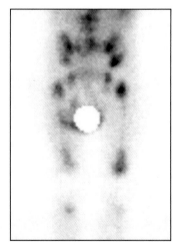

Figure 21.12 The MIBG scan 'maps' metastatic tumour marrow. This image shows the lower half of the abdomen, pelvis and legs. The dark areas are evidence of high isotope uptake and the pattern is consistent with widespread metastatic disease. (Normal uptake from excretion of isotope into urine in the bladder has been blocked in this exposure.)

Investigations

Characteristic clinical and radiological features with raised urinary catecholamine levels suggest neuroblastoma. Confirmatory biopsy is usually obtained and evidence of metastatic disease detected with bone marrow sampling, MIBG (metaiodobenzylguanidine) scan (as in Fig. 21.12) with or without a bone scan.

Age and stage of disease at diagnosis are the major factors which influence prognosis. Unfortunately, the majority of children over 1 year present with advanced disease and have a poor prognosis. Increasingly, information about the biological characteristics of neuroblastoma is being used to guide therapy and prognosis. Overexpression of the N-*myc* oncogene, evidence of deletion of material on chromosome 1 (del 1p) and gain of genetic material on chromosome 17q in tumour cells are all associated with a poorer prognosis.

Management

Localised primaries without metastatic disease can often be cured with surgery alone.

Metastatic disease is treated with chemotherapy, including high-dose therapy with autologous stem cell rescue, surgery and radiotherapy. Risk of relapse is high and the prospect of cure for children with metastatic disease is still little better than 30%. Immunotherapy and the use of long-term 'maintenance' treatment with differentiating agents (retinoic acid) are now establishing a role in those with high-risk disease.

Wilms tumour (nephroblastoma)

Wilms tumour originates from embryonal renal tissue and is the commonest renal tumour of childhood. Over 80% of patients present before 5 years of age and it is very rarely seen after 10 years of age.

Clinical features

Most children present with a large abdominal mass, often found incidentally in an otherwise well child. Other clinical features are listed in Box 21.2.

Investigations

Ultrasound and/or CT/MRI (Fig. 21.13) is usually characteristic, showing an intrinsic renal mass distorting the normal structure. Staging is to assess for distant metastases (usually in the lung), initial tumour resectability and function of the contralateral kidney.

Management

In the UK, children receive initial chemotherapy followed by delayed nephrectomy, after which the tumour is staged histologically and subsequent treatment is planned according to the surgical and pathological findings. Radiotherapy is restricted to those with more advanced disease.

Prognosis is good, with more than 80% of all patients cured. Cure rate for patients with metastatic disease at presentation (~15%) is over 60%, but relapse carries a poor prognosis.

Soft tissue sarcomas

Rhabdomyosarcoma is the most common form of soft tissue sarcoma in childhood. The tumour is thought to originate from primitive mesenchymal tissue and there are a wide variety of primary sites, resulting in varying presentations and prognosis.

Box 21.2 Presentation of Wilms tumour

Common	Uncommon
Abdominal mass	Abdominal pain
	Anorexia
	Anaemia (haemorrhage into mass)
	Haematuria
	Hypertension

About 5% have bilateral disease at diagnosis.

Wilms tumour

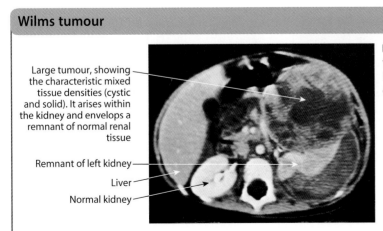

Large tumour, showing the characteristic mixed tissue densities (cystic and solid). It arises within the kidney and envelops a remnant of normal renal tissue

Remnant of left kidney

Liver

Normal kidney

Figure 21.13 Large Wilms tumour arising within the left kidney, showing characteristic cystic and solid tissue densities.

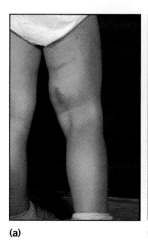

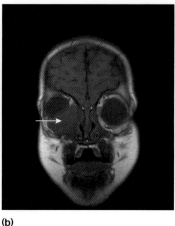

(a)   (b)

Figure 21.14 Rhabdomyosarcoma. **(a)** Soft tissue mass of lower limb. The scar is from a biopsy. **(b)** MRI scan of a child presenting with proptosis of the right eye. It shows a right periorbital soft tissue mass displacing the globe and compressing other orbital structures. Histology confirmed the diagnosis of rhabdomyosarcoma.

Clinical features

Head and neck are the most common sites of disease (40%), causing, e.g. proptosis, nasal obstruction or bloodstained nasal discharge.

Genitourinary tumours may involve the bladder, paratesticular structures or the female genitourinary tract. Symptoms include dysuria and urinary obstruction, scrotal mass or bloodstained vaginal discharge.

Metastatic disease (lung, liver, bone or bone marrow) is present in approximately 15% of patients at diagnosis and is associated with a particularly poor prognosis.

Investigations

Biopsy and full radiological assessment of primary disease and any evidence of metastasis (Fig. 21.14).

Management

Multimodality treatment (chemotherapy, surgery and radiotherapy) is used, dependent on the age of the patient and the site, size and extent of disease. The tumour margins are deceptively ill-defined, and attempts at primary surgical excision are often unsuccessful and are not attempted unless this can be achieved without mutilation or irreversible organ damage. Overall cure rates are about 65%.

Bone tumours

Malignant bone tumours are uncommon before puberty. Osteogenic sarcoma is more common than Ewing sarcoma, but Ewing sarcoma is seen more often in younger children. Both have a male predominance.

Clinical features

The limbs are the most common site. Persistent localised bone pain is the characteristic symptom, usually preceding the detection of a mass, and is an indication for early X-ray. At diagnosis, most patients are otherwise well.

Investigations

Plain X-ray is followed by MRI and bone scan (Fig. 21.15a–c). A bone X-ray shows destruction and variable periosteal new bone formation. In Ewing sarcoma, there is often a substantial soft tissue mass. Chest CT is used to assess for lung metastases and bone marrow sampling to exclude marrow involvement.

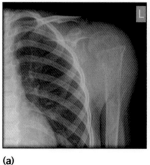
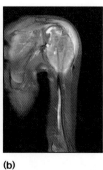
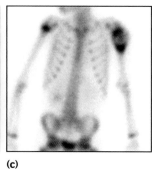
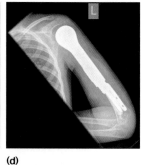

(a)   (b)   (c)   (d)

Figure 21.15 Ewing sarcoma of the humerus. **(a)** Plain X-ray shows a destructive bone lesion within the proximal humeral metaphysis. **(b)** MRI shows a large destructive soft tissue mass arising from the proximal metadiaphysis of the left humerus. **(c)** Bone scan shows prominent abnormal tracer uptake in the proximal left humerus. **(d)** Post-surgery, most of the humerus has been resected and replaced by a metallic prosthesis.

Management

In both tumours, treatment involves the use of combination chemotherapy given before surgery. Whenever possible, amputation is avoided by using *en bloc* resection of tumours with endoprosthetic resection (Fig. 21.15d). In Ewing sarcoma, radiotherapy is also used in the management of local disease, especially when surgical resection is impossible or incomplete, e.g. in the pelvis or axial skeleton.

Retinoblastoma

Retinoblastoma is a malignant tumour of retinal cells and, although rare, it accounts for about 5% of severe visual impairment in children. It may affect one or both eyes. All bilateral tumours are hereditary, as are about 20% of unilateral cases. The retinoblastoma susceptibility gene is on chromosome 13, and the pattern of inheritance is dominant, but with incomplete penetrance. Most cases present within the first 3 years of life. Children from families with the hereditary form of the disease should be screened regularly from birth.

Clinical features

The most common presentation of unsuspected disease is when a white pupillary reflex is noted to replace the normal red one (Fig. 21.16) or with a squint.

Investigations

MRI and examination under anaesthetic. Tumours are frequently multifocal.

Treatment

The aim is to cure, yet preserve vision. Biopsy is not undertaken and treatment is based on the ophthalmological findings. Enucleation of the eye may be necessary for more advanced disease. Chemotherapy is used, particularly in bilateral disease, to shrink the tumour(s), followed by local laser treatment to the retina. Radiotherapy may be used in advanced disease, but it is more often reserved for the treatment of recurrence. Most patients are cured, although many are visually impaired. There is a significant risk of second malignancy (especially sarcoma) among survivors of hereditary retinoblastoma.

Rare tumours

Liver tumours

Primary malignant liver tumours are mostly hepatoblastoma (65%) or hepatocellular carcinoma (25%). Presentation is usually with abdominal distension or with a mass. Pain and jaundice are rare. Elevated serum α-fetoprotein (αFP) is detected in nearly all cases of hepatoblastoma and in some cases of hepatocellular carcinoma. Management includes chemotherapy, surgery and, in inoperable cases, liver transplantation is required. The majority of children with hepatoblastoma can now be cured, but the prognosis for children with hepatocellular carcinoma is less satisfactory.

Germ cell tumours

Germ cell tumours (GCTs) may be benign or malignant. They arise from the primitive germ cells which migrate from yolk sac endoderm to form gonads in the embryo. Benign tumours are most common in the sacrococcygeal region, and most malignant germ cell tumours are found in the gonads. Serum markers (αFP and β-HCG) are invaluable in confirming the diagnosis and in monitoring response to treatment. Malignant germ cell tumours are very sensitive to chemotherapy, and a very good outcome can be expected for disease at most sites, including the brain.

Langerhans cell histiocytosis

Langerhans cell histiocytosis (LCH) is a rare disorder characterised by an abnormal proliferation of histiocytes. It is no longer believed to be a truly malignant condition and is classified as a disorder of dendritic (antigen presenting) cells. However, its sometimes aggressive behaviour and its response to chemotherapy place it within the practice of oncologists. Clinically, its manifestations include:

- Bone lesions – present at any age with pain, swelling or even fracture. X-ray reveals a characteristic lytic lesion with a well-defined border, often involving the skull (Fig. 21.17).

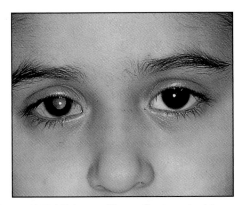

Figure 21.16 White pupillary reflex in retinoblastoma.

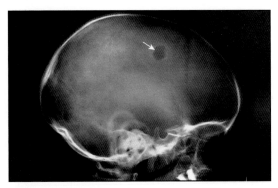

Figure 21.17 Lytic bone lesions on a skull X-ray in Langerhans cell histiocytosis.

Malignant disease

377

- Diabetes insipidus – may be associated with skull disease with proptosis and hypothalamic infiltration
- Systemic LCH – the most aggressive form which tends to present in infancy with a seborrhoeic rash (Fig. 21.18) and soft tissue involvement of the gums, ears, lungs, liver, spleen, lymph nodes and bone marrow. This form of LCH is usually progressive and requires chemotherapy, although spontaneous regression may occur.

The prognosis is variable, but most patients are cured.

Long-term survivors

Improved survival rates means an ever-increasing population of adult survivors of childhood cancer. Over half have at least one residual problem as a consequence of either the disease or its treatment (Table 21.2).

All survivors need regular long-term follow-up to provide appropriate treatment or advice. This need for specialist multidisciplinary follow-up continues into adulthood, and its provision presents a challenge within adult healthcare services. Until recently, the

majority of survivors have remained under the care of paediatric oncologists, although specialist adult clinics are being established. Some survivors will require specific counselling for problems such as poor or asymmetric growth, infertility and sexual dysfunction, and advances in the use of adult growth hormone. Assisted conception techniques have enhanced the lives of many patients. The risk of second cancer is small, but nevertheless survivors are at increased risk and this may rise with increasing survival rates. When new treatment protocols for childhood cancers are developed, there is a need to reduce, whenever possible, the toxicity of treatment to spare the children adverse short- and long-term effects.

Palliative care

When a child relapses, further treatment may be considered. A reasonable number can still be cured and others may have a further significant remission with good-quality life. However, for some children, a time comes when death is inevitable and the staff and family must make the decision to concentrate on palliative care.

Most parents prefer to care for their terminally ill child at home, but will need practical help and emotional support. Pain control and symptom relief are a serious source of anxiety for parents, but they can often be achieved successfully at home. Health professionals with experience in palliative care for children work together with the family and local healthcare workers. After the child's death, families should be offered continuing contact with an appropriate member of the team who looked after their child, and be given support through their bereavement.

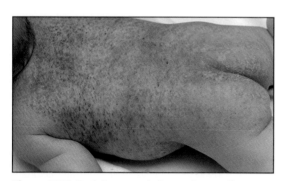

Figure 21.18 Rash in systemic Langerhans cell histiocytosis. It is often mistaken for seborrhoeic dermatitis or eczema.

 With adequate support from health professionals, palliative care for children can usually be provided at home.

Table 21.2 Some problems that may occur following cure of childhood cancer

Problem	Cause
Specific organ dysfunction	Nephrectomy for Wilms tumour
	Toxicity from chemotherapy, e.g. renal from cisplatin or ifosfamide, cardiac from doxorubicin or mediastinal radiotherapy
Growth/endocrine problems	Growth hormone deficiency from pituitary irradiation
	Bone growth retardation at sites of irradiation
Infertility	Gonadal irradiation
	Alkylating agent chemotherapy (cyclophosphamide, ifosfamide)
Neuropsychological problems	Cranial irradiation (particularly at age <5 years)
	Brain surgery
Second malignancy	Irradiation
	Alkylating agent chemotherapy
Social/educational disadvantage	Chronic ill health
	Absence from school

Summary

Presentation of malignant disease in children

Brain tumours:
- Raised intracranial pressure
- Neurological signs – depends on anatomical position

Retinoblastoma:
- Screening if positive family history
- White pupillary reflex or squint

Lymphomas:
- Enlarged lymph nodes in the head and neck or abdomen
- Mediastinal mass – may cause superior vena caval obstruction.

Wilms tumour:
- Large abdominal mass in a well child
- Occasionally anorexia, abdominal pain, haematuria

Langerhans cell histiocytosis:
- Seborrhoeic rash
- Widespread soft tissue infiltration
- Bone pain, swelling or fracture
- Diabetes insipidus

Soft tissue sarcomas:
- Mass any site

Neuroblastoma:
- Abdominal mass, crosses the midline
- Spinal cord compression
- Weight loss and malaise
- Pallor, bruising
- Bone pain

Acute lymphoblastic leukaemia (ALL):
- Malaise, anorexia
- Pallor, lethargy
- Infections
- Bruising, petichiae, nose bleeds
- Lymphadenopathy
- Hepatosplenomegaly
- Bone pain

Malignant bone tumours:
- Localised bone pain

Pre-school (<5 years old)	School-aged	Adolescence
Acute lymphoblastic leukaemia (ALL) – peak incidence Non-Hodgkin lymphoma	Acute lymphoblastic leukaemia (ALL)	Acute lymphoblastic leukaemia (ALL) Hodgkin lymphoma
Neuroblastoma	Brain tumours	Malignant bone tumours
Wilm tumour		Soft tissue sarcomas
Retinoblastoma		

Further reading

Bailey S, Skinner R, editors: *2009 Paediatric Haematology and Oncology.* Oxford Specialist Handbooks in Paediatrics. Oxford University Press, Oxford.

Short textbook

Carroll WL, Finlay JL, editors: *Cancer in Children and Adolescents,* Sudbury, MA, 2009, Jones and Bartlett Publishers.

Comprehensive textbook

Pizzo PA, Poplack DG, editors: *Principles and Practice of Pediatric Oncology,* ed 6, Lippincott, 2010, Williams and Wilkins.

Comprehensive textbook

Stevens MCG, Caron HN, Biondi A, editors: *Cancer in Children: Clinical Management,* ed 6, Oxford, 2011, Oxford University Press.

Short textbook

Stiller C, editor: *2007 Childhood Cancer in Britain: Incidence, Survival, Mortality,* Oxford, 2007, Oxford University Press.

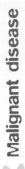

Malignant disease

Websites (Accessed May 2011)

CCLG (Children Cancer and Leukaemia Group):
Available at: http://www.cclg.org.uk/index.php
Association of healthcare professionals involved in the treatment and care of children and younger teenagers with cancer, underpins all the activity in paediatric oncology in the UK.

Cure4Kids. Available at: http://www.cure4kids.org
Dedicated to improving healthcare for children with cancer and other catastrophic diseases around the globe. Provides continuing medical education and communication tools to healthcare professionals and scientists worldwide.

Haematological disorders

Haemopoiesis is the process which maintains lifelong production of haemopoietic (blood) cells. The main site of haemopoiesis in fetal life is the liver, whereas throughout postnatal life, it is the bone marrow. All haemopoietic cells are derived from *pluripotent haemopoietic stem cells*, which are crucial for normal blood production; deficiency causes bone marrow failure because stem cells are required for the ongoing replacement of dying cells. Haemopoietic stem cells can also be used for treatment, e.g. cells from healthy donors can be transplanted into children with bone marrow failure (*stem cell transplantation*).

Haemoglobin production in the fetus and newborn

The most important difference between haemopoiesis in the fetus compared with postnatal life is the changing pattern of haemoglobin (Hb) production at each stage of development. The composition and names of these haemoglobins are shown in Table 22.1. Understanding the developmental changes in haemoglobin helps to explain the patterns of abnormal haemoglobin production in some inherited childhood anaemias. Embryonic haemoglobins (Hb Gower 1, Hb Gower 2 and Hb Portland) are produced between 4 and 8 weeks' gestation, after which haemoglobin production switches to fetal haemoglobin (HbF). HbF is made up of 2 α chains and 2 γ chains ($\alpha_2\gamma_2$) and is the main Hb during fetal life. HbF has a higher affinity for oxygen than adult Hb (HbA), and is therefore better able to hold on to oxygen, an advantage in the relatively hypoxic environment of the fetus (Fig. 22.1). At birth, the types of Hb are: HbF, HbA and HbA$_2$. HbF is gradually replaced by HbA and HbA$_2$ during the first year of life. By 1 year of age, the percentage of HbF is very low in healthy children and increased proportions of HbF are a sensitive indicator of some inherited disorders of haemoglobin production (haemoglobinopathies) .

Haematological values at birth and the first few weeks of life

Features are:

- At birth, the Hb in term infants is high, 14–21.5 g/dl, to compensate for the low oxygen concentration in the fetus. The Hb falls over the first few weeks, mainly due to reduced red cell production, reaching a nadir of around 10 g/dl at 2 months of age (Fig. 22.2). Normal haematological

Table 22.1 Embryonic, fetal and adult haemoglobins

Haemoglobin type	Globin chains	
	α-gene cluster	β-gene cluster
Embryonic		
Hb Gower 1	ξ_2	ε_2
Hb Gower 2	α_2	ε_2
Hb Portland	ξ_2	γ_2
Fetal		
HbF	α_2	γ_2
Adult		
HbA	α_2	β_2
HbA$_2$	α_2	δ_2
Haemoglobin types in newborns and adults		
Newborn	HbF 74%, HbA 25%, HbA$_2$ 1%	
Children >1 year old and adults	HbA 97%, HbA$_2$ 2%	

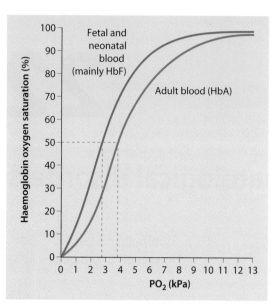

Figure 22.1 Oxygen dissociation curve showing the left shift of HbF compared with HbA. HbF-containing red cells have a higher affinity for oxygen and hold on to oxygen, delivering less to the tissues.

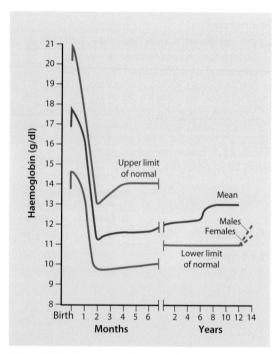

Figure 22.2 Changes in haemoglobin concentration with age, showing that the haemoglobin is high at birth, falling to its lowest concentration at 2–3 months of age.

values at birth and during childhood are shown in the Appendix.
- Preterm babies have a steeper fall in Hb to a mean of 6.5–9 g/dl at 4–8 weeks chronological age.
- Normal blood volume at birth varies with gestational age. In healthy term infants the

average blood volume is 80 ml/kg; in preterm infants the average blood volume is 100 ml/kg.
- Stores of iron, folic acid and vitamin B_{12} in term and preterm babies are adequate at birth. However, in preterm infants, stores of iron and folic acid are lower and are depleted more quickly, leading to deficiency after 2–4 months if the recommended daily intakes are not maintained by supplements.
- White blood cell counts in neonates are higher than in older children (10–25×10^9/L).
- Platelet counts at birth are within the normal adult range (150–400×10^9/L).

Summary

Haemoglobin at birth

- The Hb concentration is high at birth (>14 g/dl) but falls to its lowest level at 2 months of age.
- Fetal Hb (HbF) is gradually replaced by adult Hb (HbA + HbA_2) during infancy.

Anaemia

Anaemia is defined as an Hb level below the normal range. The normal range varies with age, so anaemia can be defined as:

- Neonate: Hb <14 g/dl
- 1–12 months: Hb <10 g/dl
- 1–12 years: Hb <11 g/dl.

Anaemia results from one or more of the following mechanisms:

- Reduced red cell production – either due to ineffective erythropoiesis (e.g. iron deficiency, the commonest cause of anaemia) or due to red cell *aplasia*
- Increased red cell destruction (*haemolysis*)
- Blood loss – relatively uncommon cause in children.

There may be a combination of these three mechanisms, e.g. *anaemia of prematurity*.

Using this approach, the principal causes of anaemia are shown in Figure 22.3 and a diagnostic approach to identifying their causes is shown in Figure 22.4.

 The definition of anaemia varies with age: Hb <10 g/dl in infants (post-neonatal), Hb <11 g/dl from 1 to 12 years old.

Anaemia due to reduced red cell production

Reduced red cell production may be due to:

- 'Ineffective erythropoiesis': here red cell production occurs at a normal or increased rate but differentiation or survival of the red cells is defective (e.g. iron deficiency).
- Complete absence of red cell production (red cell aplasia).

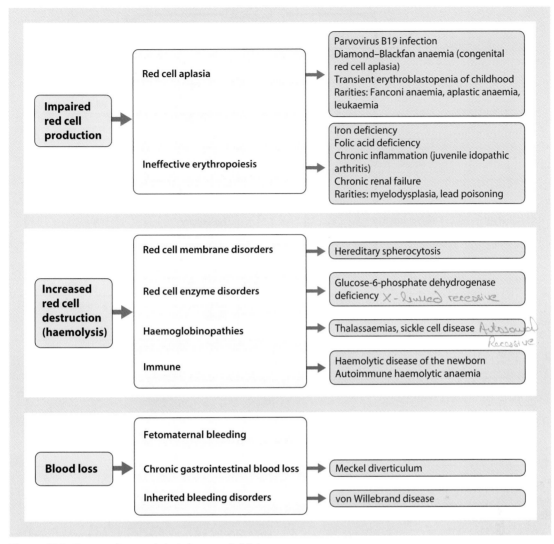

Figure 22.3 Causes of anaemia in infants and children.

Causes of anaemia in infants and children

Diagnostic clues to ineffective erythropoiesis are:

- Normal reticulocyte count
- Abnormal mean cell volume (MCV) of the red cells: low in iron deficiency and raised in folic acid deficiency.

Iron deficiency

The main causes of iron deficiency are:

- Inadequate intake
- Malabsorption
- Blood loss.

Inadequate intake of iron is common in infants because additional iron is required for the increase in blood volume accompanying growth and to build up the child's iron stores (Fig. 22.5). A 1-year-old infant requires an intake of iron of about 8 mg/day, which is about the same as his father (9 mg/day) but only half that of his mother (15 mg/day).

Iron may come from:

- Breast milk (low iron content but 50% of the iron is absorbed)
- Infant formula (supplemented with adequate amounts of iron)
- Cow's milk (higher iron content than breast milk but only 10% is absorbed)
- Solids introduced at weaning, e.g. cereals (cereals are supplemented with iron but only 1% is absorbed).

Iron deficiency may develop because of a delay in the introduction of mixed feeding beyond 6 months of age or to a diet with insufficient iron-rich foods, especially if it contains a large amount of cow's milk (Box 22.1). Iron absorption is markedly increased when eaten with food rich in vitamin C (fresh fruit and vegetables) and is inhibited by tannin in tea.

Haematological disorders

383

Simple diagnostic approach to anaemia in children

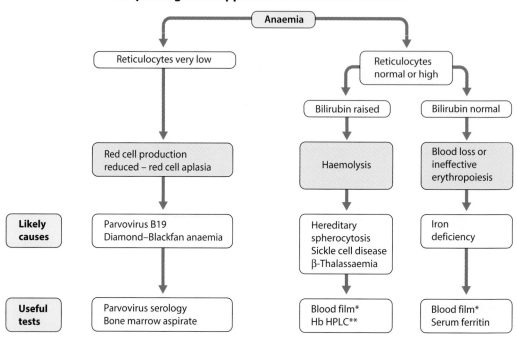

Figure 22.4 Diagnostic approach to anaemia.

Box 22.1 Dietary sources of iron

High in iron

- Red meat – beef, lamb
- Liver, kidney
- Oily fish – pilchards, sardines, etc.

Average iron

- Pulses, beans and peas
- Fortified breakfast cereals with added vitamin C
- Wholemeal products
- Dark green vegetables – broccoli, spinach, etc.
- Dried fruit – raisins, sultanas
- Nuts and seeds – cashews, peanut butter, etc.

Foods to avoid in excess in toddlers

- Cow's milk
- Tea: tannin inhibits iron uptake
- High-fibre foods: phytates inhibit iron absorption.

 Infants should not be fed unmodified cow's milk as its iron content is low and poorly absorbed.

Clinical features

Most infants and children are asymptomatic until the Hb drops below 6–7 g/dl. As the anaemia worsens, children tire easily and young infants feed more slowly than usual. The history should include asking about blood loss and symptoms or signs suggesting malabsorption. They may appear pale but pallor is an unreliable sign unless confirmed by pallor of the conjunctivae, tongue or palmar creases. Some children have 'pica', a term which describes the inappropriate eating of non-food materials such as soil, chalk, gravel or foam rubber (see Case History 22.1). There is evidence that iron deficiency anaemia may be detrimental to behaviour and intellectual function.

Iron requirements during childhood

Diagnosis

The diagnostic clues are:

- Microcytic, hypochromic anaemia (low MCV and MCH)
- Low serum ferritin.

The other main causes of microcytic anaemia are:

- β-thalassaemia trait (usually children of Asian, Arabic or Mediterranean origin)

Iron requirements during childhood

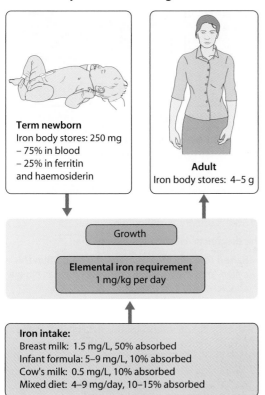

Term newborn
Iron body stores: 250 mg
– 75% in blood
– 25% in ferritin
and haemosiderin

Adult
Iron body stores: 4–5 g

Growth

Elemental iron requirement
1 mg/kg per day

Iron intake:
Breast milk: 1.5 mg/L, 50% absorbed
Infant formula: 5–9 mg/L, 10% absorbed
Cow's milk: 0.5 mg/L, 10% absorbed
Mixed diet: 4–9 mg/day, 10–15% absorbed

Figure 22.5 Iron requirements during childhood.

Case History

22.1 Iron deficiency anaemia

Ayesha, aged 2 years, was noted to look pale when she attended her general practitioner for an upper respiratory tract infection. A blood count showed Hb 5.0 g/dl, MCV 54 fl (normal 72–85 fl) and MCH 16 (normal 24–39 pg). She was drinking 3 pints of cow's milk per day and was a very fussy eater, refusing meat. She had started eating soil when playing in the garden.

Because of the inappropriately large volume of milk she was drinking, she was not sufficiently hungry to eat solid food. Replacing some of the milk with iron-rich food and treatment with oral iron produced a rise in the Hb to 7.5 g/dl within 4 weeks. Her pica (eating non-food materials) stopped. Oral iron was continued until her Hb had been normal for 3 months.

- α-thalassaemia trait (usually children of African or Far Eastern origin)
- Anaemia of chronic disease (e.g. due to renal failure).

Management

For most children, management involves *dietary advice* and supplementation with *oral iron*. The best tolerated preparations are Sytron (sodium iron edetate) or Niferex (polysaccharide iron complex) – unlike some other preparations these do not stain the teeth. Iron supplementation should be continued until the Hb is normal and then for a minimum of a further 3 months to replenish the iron stores. With good compliance, the Hb will rise by about 1 g/dl per week. Failure to respond to oral iron usually means the child is not getting the treatment. However, investigation for other causes, in particular malabsorption (e.g. due to coeliac disease) or chronic blood loss (e.g. due to Meckel diverticulum) is advisable if the history or examination suggests a non-dietary cause or if there is failure to respond to therapy in compliant patients. Blood transfusion should never be necessary for dietary iron deficiency. Even children with an Hb as low as 2–3 g/dl due to iron deficiency have arrived at this low level over a prolonged period and can tolerate it.

Treatment of iron deficiency with normal Hb

Some children have biochemical evidence of iron deficiency (e.g. low serum ferritin) but have not yet developed anaemia. Whether these children should be treated with oral iron is controversial. In favour of treatment is the knowledge that iron is required for normal brain development and there is evidence that iron deficiency anaemia is associated with behavioural and intellectual deficiencies, which may be reversible with iron therapy. However, it is not yet clear whether treatment of subclinical iron deficiency confers significant benefit. Treatment also carries a risk of accidental poisoning with oral iron, which is very toxic. A simple strategy is to provide dietary advice to increase oral iron and its absorption in all children with subclinical deficiency and to offer parents the option of additional treatment with oral iron supplements.

 Treatment of iron deficiency anaemia is with dietary advice and oral iron therapy for several months.

Red cell aplasia

There are three main causes of red cell aplasia in children:

- Congenital red cell aplasia ('Diamond–Blackfan anaemia')
- Transient erythroblastopenia of childhood
- Parvovirus B19 infection (this infection only causes red cell aplasia in children with inherited haemolytic anaemias and not in healthy children).

The diagnostic clues to red cell aplasia are:

- Low reticulocyte count despite low Hb
- Normal bilirubin
- Negative direct antiglobulin test (Coombs test)
- Absent red cell precursors on bone marrow examination.

Diamond–Blackfan anaemia (DBA) is a rare disease (5–7 cases/million live births). There is a family history in 20% of cases; the remaining 80% are sporadic. Specific

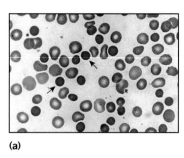
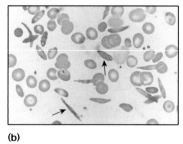
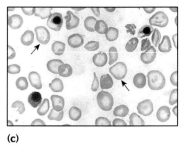

(a) (b) (c)

Figure 22.6 Abnormally shaped red blood cells help make the diagnosis in haemolytic anaemias. **(a)** Spherocytes (arrows) in hereditary spherocytosis. **(b)** Sickle cells (arrows) in sickle cell disease. **(c)** Hypochromic cells (arrows) in thalassaemia.

gene mutations in ribosomal protein (RPS) genes are implicated in some cases. Most cases present at 2–3 months of age, but 25% present at birth. Affected infants have symptoms of anaemia; some have other congenital anomalies, such as short stature or abnormal thumbs. Treatment is by oral steroids; monthly red blood cell transfusions are given to children who are steroid unresponsive and some may also be offered stem cell transplantation.

Transient erythroblastopenia of childhood (TEC) is usually triggered by viral infections and has the same haematological features as Diamond–Blackfan anaemia. The main differences between them is that, unlike Diamond–Blackfan anaemia, transient erythroblastopenia of childhood always recovers, usually within several weeks, there is no family history or RPS gene mutations and there are no congenital anomalies.

Increased red cell destruction (haemolytic anaemia)

Haemolytic anaemia is characterised by reduced red cell lifespan due to increased red cell destruction in the circulation (intravascular haemolysis) or liver or spleen (extravascular haemolysis). The lifespan of a normal red cell is 120 days and the bone marrow produces 173 000 million red cells per day. In haemolysis, red cell survival may be reduced to a few days but bone marrow production can increase about eight-fold, so haemolysis only leads to anaemia when the bone marrow is no longer able to compensate for the premature destruction of red cells.

In children, unlike neonates, immune haemolytic anaemias are uncommon. The main cause of haemolysis in children is *intrinsic* abnormalities of the red blood cells:

- Red cell membrane disorders (e.g. hereditary spherocytosis)
- Red cell enzyme disorders (e.g. glucose-6-phosphate dehydrogenase deficiency)
- Haemoglobinopathies (abnormal haemoglobins, e.g. β-thalassaemia major, sickle cell disease).

Haemolysis from increased red cell breakdown leads to:

- Anaemia
- Hepatomegaly and splenomegaly

- Increased blood levels of unconjugated bilirubin
- Excess urinary urobilinogen.

The diagnostic clues to haemolysis are:

- Raised reticulocyte count (on the blood film this is called 'polychromasia' as the reticulocytes have a characteristic lilac colour)
- Unconjugated bilirubinaemia and increased urinary urobilinogen
- Abnormal appearance of the red cells on a blood film (e.g. spherocytes, sickle shaped or very hypochromic) (Fig. 22.6)
- Positive direct antiglobulin test (only if an immune cause, as this test identifies antibody-coated red blood cells)
- Increased red blood cell precursors in the bone marrow.

Hereditary spherocytosis

HS occurs in 1 in 5000 births in Caucasians. It usually has an autosomal dominant inheritance, but in 25% there is no family history and it is caused by new mutations. The disease is caused by mutations in genes for proteins of the red cell membrane (mainly spectrin, ankyrin or band 3). This results in the red cell losing part of its membrane when it passes through the spleen. This reduction in its surface-to-volume ratio causes the cells to become spheroidal, making them less deformable than normal red blood cells and leads to their destruction in the microvasculature of the spleen.

Clinical features

The disorder is often suspected because of the family history. The clinical manifestations are highly variable. Although hereditary spherocytosis-affected individuals may be completely asymptomatic, the clinical features include:

- Jaundice – usually develops during childhood but may be intermittent; may cause severe haemolytic jaundice in the first few days of life
- Anaemia – presents in childhood with mild anaemia (haemoglobin 9–11 g/dl), but the haemoglobin level may transiently fall during infections
- Mild to moderate splenomegaly – depends on the rate of haemolysis
- Aplastic crisis – uncommon, transient (2–4 weeks), caused by parvovirus B19 infection
- Gallstones – due to increased bilirubin excretion.

Diagnosis

The blood film is usually diagnostic but more specific tests are available (e.g. osmotic fragility, dye binding tests), although seldom required. Autoimmune haemolytic anaemia is also associated with spherocytes and this should be excluded with a direct antibody test in the absence of a family history of hereditary spherocytosis.

Management

Most children have mild chronic haemolytic anaemia and the only treatment they require is oral folic acid as they have a raised folic acid requirement secondary to their increased red blood cell production. Splenectomy is beneficial but is only indicated for poor growth or troublesome symptoms of anaemia (e.g. severe tiredness, loss of vigour) and is usually deferred until after 7 years of age because of the risks of post-splenectomy sepsis. Prior to splenectomy all patients should be checked that they have been vaccinated against *Haemophilus influenzae* (Hib), meningitis C and *Streptococcus pneumoniae* and lifelong daily oral penicillin prophylaxis is advised. Aplastic crisis from parvovirus B19 infection usually requires one or two blood transfusions over 3–4 weeks when no red blood cells are produced. If gallstones are symptomatic, cholecystectomy may be necessary.

Glucose-6-phosphate dehydrogenase (G6PD) deficiency

G6PD deficiency is the commonest red cell enzymopathy affecting over 100 million people worldwide. It has a high prevalence (10–20%) in individuals originating from central Africa, the Mediterranean, the Middle East and the Far East. Many different mutations of the gene have been described, leading to different clinical features in different populations.

G6PD is the rate-limiting enzyme in the pentose phosphate pathway and is essential for preventing oxidative damage to red cells. Red cells lacking G6PD are susceptible to oxidant-induced haemolysis. G6PD deficiency is X-linked and therefore predominantly affects males. Females who are heterozygotes are usually clinically normal as they have about half the normal G6PD activity. Females may be affected either if they are homozygous or, more commonly, when by chance more of the normal than the abnormal X chromosomes have been inactivated (extreme Lyonisation – the Lyon hypothesis is that, in every XX cell, one of the X chromosomes is inactivated and that this is random). In Mediterranean, Middle Eastern and Oriental populations, affected males have very low or absent enzyme activity in their red cells. Affected Afro-Caribbeans have 10–15% normal enzyme activity.

Clinical manifestations

Children usually present clinically with:

- *Neonatal jaundice* – onset is usually in the first 3 days of life. Worldwide it is the most common cause of severe neonatal jaundice requiring exchange transfusion

- *Acute haemolysis* – precipitated by:
  - infection, the most common precipitating factor
  - certain drugs (see Box 22.2)
  - fava beans (broad beans)
  - naphthalene in mothballs.

Haemolysis due to G6PD deficiency is predominantly intravascular. This is associated with fever, malaise and the passage of dark urine, as it contains haemoglobin as well as urobilinogen. The haemoglobin level falls rapidly and may drop below 5 g/dl over 24–48 h.

Diagnosis

Between episodes, almost all patients have a completely normal blood picture and no jaundice or anaemia. The diagnosis is made by measuring G6PD activity in red blood cells. During a haemolytic crisis, G6PD levels may be misleadingly elevated due to the higher enzyme concentration in reticulocytes, which are produced in increased numbers in response to the destruction of mature red cells. A repeat assay is then required in the steady state to confirm the diagnosis.

Management

The parents should be given advice about the signs of acute haemolysis (jaundice, pallor and dark urine) and provided with a list of drugs, chemicals and food to avoid (Box 22.2). Transfusions are rarely required, even for acute episodes.

Haemoglobinopathies

These are red blood cell disorders which cause haemolytic anaemia because of reduced or absent production of HbA (α- and β-thalassaemias) or because of the production of an abnormal Hb (e.g. sickle cell disease). α-Thalassaemias are caused by deletions (occasionally mutations) in the α-globin gene. β-Thalassaemia and

Table 22.2 Haemoglobins in haemoglobinopathies

	HbA	HbA$_2$	HbF	HbS
Newborn	25%	1%	74%	–
Adult	97%	2%	–	–
β-Thalassaemia trait	>90%	↑	+ ↑	–
β-Thalassaemia major	–	↑	↑	–
Sickle cell trait	✓	✓	+ ↑	✓
Sickle cell disease	–	✓	+ ↑	✓

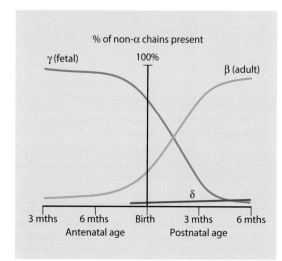

Figure 22.7 Changes in haemoglobin chains in the fetus and infancy.

sickle cell disease are caused by mutations in the β-globin gene. Clinical manifestations of the haemoglobinopathies affecting the β-chain are delayed until after 6 months of age when most of the HbF present at birth has been replaced by adult HbA (Fig. 22.7, Table 22.2).

Sickle cell disease

This is now the commonest genetic disorder in children in many European countries, including the UK (prevalence 1 in 2000 live births). Sickle cell disease is the collective name given to haemoglobinopathies in which HbS is inherited. HbS forms as a result of a point mutation in codon 6 of the β-globin gene, which causes a change in the amino acid encoded from glutamine to valine. Sickle cell disease is most common in patients whose parents are black and originate from tropical Africa or the Caribbean but it is also found in the Middle East and in low prevalence in most other parts of the world except for northern Europeans.

There are three main forms of sickle cell disease and the sickle trait:

- *Sickle cell anaemia* (*HbSS*) – patients are homozygous for HbS, i.e. virtually all their Hb is HbS; they have small amounts of HbF and *no* HbA because they have the sickle mutation in both β-globin genes.
- *HbSC disease* (*HbSC*) – affected children inherit HbS from one parent and HbC from the other parent (HbC is formed as a result of a different point mutation in β-globin), so they also have *no* HbA because they have no normal β-globin genes.
- *Sickle β-thalassaemia* – affected children inherit HbS from one parent and β-thalassaemia trait from the other. They have no normal β-globin genes and most patients can make no HbA and therefore have similar symptoms to those with sickle cell anaemia.
- *Sickle trait* – inheritance of HbS from one parent and a normal β-globin gene from the other parent, so approximately 40% of the haemoglobin is HbS. They do not have sickle cell disease but are carriers of HbS, so can transmit HbS to their offspring. They are asymptomatic and are only identified as a result of blood tests.

Pathogenesis

In all forms of sickle cell disease, HbS polymerises within red blood cells forming rigid tubular spiral bodies which deform the red cells into a sickle shape. Irreversibly sickled red cells have a reduced lifespan and may be trapped in the microcirculation, resulting in blood vessel occlusion (vaso-occlusion) and therefore ischaemia in an organ or bone. This is exacerbated by low oxygen tension, dehydration and cold.

The clinical manifestations of sickle cell disease vary widely between different individuals. Disease severity also varies with different forms of sickle cell disease; in general, HbSS is the most severe form of the disease. Some patients produce more HbF (e.g. 10–15% of their Hb may be HbF, while most patients with sickle cell disease have HbF levels of 1%) and this results in a marked reduction in disease severity.

Clinical features

These are listed in Figure 22.8.

Management

Prophylaxis – Because of increased susceptibility to infection, especially encapsulated organisms, e.g. *Streptococcus pneumoniae* and *Haemophilus influenzae* type B because of functional asplenia, children should be fully immunised, including against pneumococcal, *Haemophilus influenzae* type B and meningococcus infection. To ensure full coverage of all pneumococcal subgroups, daily oral penicillin throughout childhood should be given. Patients should receive once-daily oral folic acid because of the increased demand for folic acid caused by the chronic haemolytic anaemia. Vaso-occlusive crises should be minimised by avoiding exposure to cold, dehydration, excessive exercise, undue stress or hypoxia. This requires practical measures such as dressing children warmly, giving drinks especially before exercise and taking extra care to keep children warm after swimming or when playing outside in the winter.

Clinical manifestations of sickle cell disease

Anaemia → All have moderate anaemia (usually Hb 6–10 g/dl) with clinically detectable jaundice from chronic haemolysis

Infection → All have marked increase in susceptibility to infection from encapsulated organisms such as pneumococci and *Haemophilus influenzae*. There is also an increased incidence of osteomyelitis caused by *Salmonella* and other organisms. This susceptibility to infection is due to **hyposplenism** secondary to chronic sickling and **microinfarction** in the spleen in infancy. The risk of overwhelming sepsis is greatest in early childhood

Painful crises → **Vaso-occlusive crises** causing pain affect many organs of the body with varying frequency and severity. A common mode of presentation in late infancy is the hand-foot syndrome, in which there is dactylitis with swelling and pain of the fingers and/or feet from vaso-occlusion (Fig. 22.9).
The bones of the limbs and spine are the most common sites. The most serious type of painful crisis is acute chest syndrome, which can lead to severe hypoxia and the need for mechanical ventilation and emergency transfusion. Avascular necrosis of the femoral heads may also occur. Acute vaso-occlusive crises may be precipitated by exposure to cold, dehydration, excessive exercise or stress, hypoxia or infection

Acute anaemia → Sudden drop in haemoglobin from:
Haemolytic crises – sometimes associated with infection
Aplastic crises – haemoglobin may fall precipitously. Parvovirus infection causes complete, though temporary, cessation of red blood cell production
Sequestration crises – sudden splenic or hepatic enlargement, abdominal pain and circulatory collapse from accumulation of sickled cells in spleen

Priapism → Needs to be treated promptly with exchange transfusion as it may lead to fibrosis of the corpora cavernosa and subsequent erectile impotence

Splenomegaly → Common in young children, but becomes much less frequent in older children

Long-term problems → **Short stature and delayed puberty**
Stroke and cognitive problems – although 1 in 10 children with sickle cell disease have a stroke, twice that number develop more subtle neurological damage (Fig. 22.10), often manifest with poor concentration and school performance
Adenotonsillar hypertrophy – causing sleep apnoea syndrome leading to nocturnal hypoxaemia, which can cause vaso-occlusive crises and/or stroke
Cardiac enlargement – from chronic anaemia
Heart failure – from uncorrected anaemia
Renal dysfunction – may exacerbate enuresis because of inability to concentrate urine
Pigment gallstones – due to increased bile pigment production
Leg ulcers – uncommon in children
Psychosocial problems – difficulties with education and behaviour exacerbated by time off school may occur

Figure 22.8 Clinical manifestations of sickle cell disease.

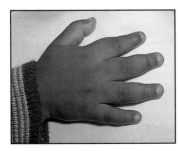

Figure 22.9 Dactylitis in sickle cell disease.

Treatment of acute crises – Painful crises should be treated with oral or intravenous analgesia according to need (may require opiates) and good hydration (oral or intravenous as required); infection should be treated with antibiotics; oxygen should be given if the oxygen saturation is reduced. Exchange transfusion is indicated for acute chest syndrome, stroke and priapism.

Treatment of chronic problems – Children who have recurrent hospital admissions for painful vaso-occlusive crises or acute chest syndrome (see Case History 22.2)

Haematological disorders

389

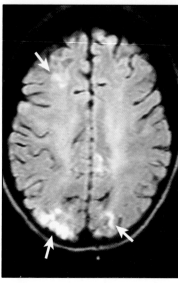

Figure 22.10 MRI of the brain in sickle cell disease showing multiple cerebral infarcts.

may benefit from hydroxyurea, a drug which increases their HbF production and helps protect against further crises. It requires monitoring for side-effects, especially white blood cell suppression. The most severely affected children (1–5%) who have had a stroke or who do not respond to hydroxyurea may be offered a bone marrow transplant. This is the only cure for sickle cell disease but can only be safely carried out if the child has an HLA-identical sibling who can donate their bone marrow – the cure rate is 90% but there is a 5% risk of fatal transplant-related complications.

Prognosis

Sickle cell disease is a cause of premature death due to one or more of these severe complications; around 50% of patients with the most severe form of sickle cell disease die before the age of 40 years. However, the mortality rate during childhood is around 3%, usually from bacterial infection.

Prenatal diagnosis and screening

Many countries with a high prevalence of haemoglobinopathies, including the UK, perform neonatal screening on dried blood spots (Guthrie test) collected in the first week of life. Early diagnosis of sickle cell disease allows penicillin prophylaxis to be started in early infancy instead of awaiting clinical presentation, possibly due to a severe infection. Prenatal diagnosis can be carried out by chorionic villus sampling at the end of the first trimester if parents wish to choose this option to prevent the birth of an affected child.

SC disease

Children with SC disease usually have a nearly normal haemoglobin level and fewer painful crises than those with HbSS, but they may develop proliferative retinopathy in adolescence. Their eyes should be checked periodically. They are also prone to develop osteonecrosis of the hips and shoulders.

Case History

22.2 Acute sickle chest syndrome

Princess, a 9-year-old girl with known sickle cell anaemia (HbSS), presented with increasing chest pain for 6 h. She had a non-productive cough. On examination, she had a fever of 39.7°C. Her breathing was laboured, respiratory rate increased and there was reduced air entry at both bases.

Investigations

- Haemoglobin 6 g/dl, WBC 14×10^9/L, platelets 350×10^9/L
- Chest X-ray (see Fig. 22.11)
- Oxygen saturation – 89% in air
- Arterial PO_2 – 9.3 kPa (70 mmHg) breathing face-mask oxygen
- Blood cultures were taken and viral titres performed.

A diagnosis of acute sickle chest syndrome was made, a potentially fatal condition. She was given oxygen by CPAP (continuous positive airways pressure). An exchange transfusion was performed. Broad-spectrum antibiotics were commenced. She responded well to treatment.

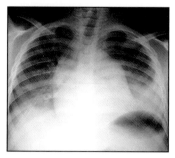

Figure 22.11 Chest X-ray in acute sickle chest syndrome showing bilateral lower zone consolidation. (Courtesy of Dr Parviz Habibi.)

Sickle cell trait (AS)

This is asymptomatic and rarely causes problems except under conditions of low oxygen tension. General anaesthesia does not constitute a risk in this population as long as they have been identified and hypoxia avoided.

β-Thalassaemias

The β-thalassaemias occur most often in people from the Indian subcontinent, Mediterranean and Middle East (Fig. 22.12). In the UK, most affected children are born to parents from the Indian subcontinent; in the past, many were born to Greek Cypriots, but this has become uncommon through active genetic counselling within their community.

There are two main types of β thalassaemia – both of which are characterised by a severe reduction in the production of β-globin (and thereby reduction in HbA production). All affected individuals have a

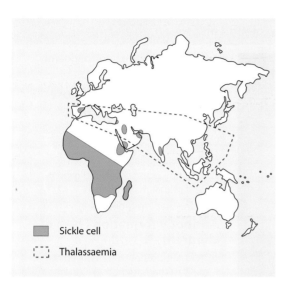

Sickle cell

Thalassaemia

Figure 22.12 Ethnic origin of most families with sickle cell disease and thalassaemia.

severe reduction in β-globin and disease severity depends on the amount of residual HbA and HbF production.

- *β-Thalassaemia major* – This is the most severe form of the disease. HbA ($\alpha_2\beta_2$) cannot be produced because of the abnormal β-globin gene.
- *β-Thalassaemia intermedia* – This form of the disease is milder and of variable severity. The β-globin mutations allow a small amount of HbA and/or a large amount of HbF to be produced.

Clinical features (Fig. 22.13)

These are:

- Severe anaemia, which is transfusion dependent, from 3–6 months of age and jaundice
- Failure to thrive/growth failure
- Extramedullary haemopoiesis, prevented by regular blood transfusions. In the absence of regular blood transfusion, develop hepatosplenomegaly and bone marrow expansion; the latter leads to the classical facies with maxillary overgrowth and skull bossing (very rare in the UK and developed countries).

Management

The condition is uniformly fatal without regular blood transfusions, so all patients are given lifelong monthly transfusions of red blood cells. The aim is to maintain the haemoglobin concentration above 10 g/dl in order to reduce growth failure and prevent bone deformation. Repeated blood transfusion causes chronic iron overload, which causes cardiac failure, liver cirrhosis, diabetes, infertility and growth failure. For this reason, all patients are treated with iron chelation with subcutaneous desferrioxamine, or with an oral iron chelator drug, such as deferasirox, starting from 2 to 3 years of age. Patients who comply well with transfusion and chelation have a 90% chance of living into their forties and beyond. However, compliance is difficult. Those who cannot comply have a high mortality in early

adulthood from iron overload. The complications of multiple transfusions are shown in Box 22.3. An alternative treatment for β-thalassaemia major is bone marrow transplantation, which is currently the only cure. It is generally reserved for children with an HLA-identical sibling as there is then a 90–95% chance of success (i.e. transfusion independence and long-term cure) but a 5% chance of transplant-related mortality.

Prenatal diagnosis

For parents who are both heterozygous for β-thalassaemia, there is a 1 in 4 risk of having an affected child. Prenatal diagnosis of β-thalassaemia (DNA analysis of a chorionic villus sample) should be offered together with genetic counselling to help parents to make informed decisions about whether or not to continue the pregnancy.

β-Thalassaemia trait

Heterozygotes are usually asymptomatic. The red cells are hypochromic and microcytic. Anaemia is mild or absent, with a disproportionate reduction in MCH (18–22 fl) and MCV (60–70 fl). The red blood cell count is therefore usually increased (>5.5×10^{12}/L). The most important diagnostic feature is a raised HbA$_2$, usually about 5% , and in about half there is a mild elevation of HbF level of 1–3%. β-Thalassaemia trait can cause confusion with mild iron deficiency because of the hypochromic/microcytic red cells but can be distinguished by measuring serum ferritin, which is low in iron deficiency but not β-thalassaemia trait.

To avoid unnecessary iron therapy, serum ferritin levels should be measured in patients with mild anaemia and microcytosis prior to starting iron supplements.

α-Thalassaemias

Healthy individuals have four α-globin genes. The manifestation of α-thalassaemia syndromes depends on the number of functional α-globin genes.

The most severe α-thalassaemia, *α-thalassaemia major* (also known as Hb Barts hydrops fetalis) is caused by deletion of all four α-globin genes, so no HbA ($\alpha_2\beta_2$) can be produced. It occurs mainly in families of Southeast Asian origin and presents in mid-trimester with fetal hydrops (oedema and ascites) from fetal anaemia, which is always fatal in utero or within hours of delivery. The only long-term survivors of α-thalassaemia major are those who have received monthly intrauterine transfusions until delivery followed by lifelong monthly transfusions after birth. The diagnosis is made by Hb electrophoresis or Hb HPLC (high-performance liquid chromatography), which shows only Hb Barts.

When only three of the α-globin genes are deleted (*HbH disease*), affected children have mild–moderate anaemia but occasional patients are transfusion-dependent.

Deletion of one or two α-globin genes (known as α-thalassaemia trait) is usually asymptomatic and anaemia is mild or absent. The red cells may be hypochromic and microcytic, which may cause confusion with iron deficiency.

391

Clinical features and complications of β-thalassaemia major

Pallor

Jaundice

Bossing of the skull
Maxillary overgrowth

Splenomegaly and
hepatomegaly

**Need for repeated
blood transfusions**
Complications shown in
Box 22.3

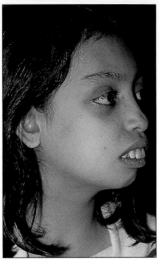

Figure 22.13 Facies in β-thalassaemia showing maxillary overgrowth and skull bossing in a child who has not been adequately transfused. This is now very rare in the UK and developed countries.

Box 22.3 Complications of long-term blood transfusion in children

Iron deposition – the most important (all patients)

- Heart – cardiomyopathy
- Liver – cirrhosis
- Pancreas – diabetes
- Pituitary gland – delayed growth and sexual maturation
- Skin – hyperpigmentation

Antibody formation (10% of children)

- Allo-antibodies to transfused red cells in the patient make finding compatible blood very difficult

Infection – now uncommon (<10% of children)

- Hepatitis A, B, C
- HIV
- Malaria
- Prions (e.g. new variant CJD)

Venous access (common problem)

- Often traumatic in young children
- Central venous access device (e.g. Portacath) may be required; these predispose to infection.

Anaemia in the newborn

Reduced red blood cell production

There are two main but rare causes in the newborn and both cause red cell aplasia:

- Congenital infection with parvovirus B19
- Congenital red cell aplasia (Diamond–Blackfan anaemia).

In this situation, the Hb is low and the red blood cells look normal. The diagnostic clue is that the reticulocyte count is low and the bilirubin is normal.

Increased red cell destruction (haemolytic anaemia)

This occurs either because of an antibody destroying the red blood cells (i.e. an extrinsic cause) or because there is an intrinsic abnormality of the surface or intracellular contents of the red blood cell. The main causes of haemolytic anaemia in neonates are:

- Immune (e.g. haemolytic disease of the newborn)
- Red cell membrane disorders (e.g. hereditary spherocytosis)
- Red cell enzyme disorders (e.g. glucose-6-phosphate dehydrogenase deficiency)

- Abnormal haemoglobins (e.g. α-thalassaemia major).

The diagnostic clues to a haemolytic anaemia are an increased reticulocyte count (due to increased red cell production to compensate for the anaemia) and increased unconjugated bilirubin (due to increased red cell destruction with release of this bile pigment into the plasma).

Haemolytic disease of the newborn (immune haemolytic anaemia of the newborn) is due to antibodies against blood group antigens. The most important are: anti-D (a 'rhesus' antigen), anti-A or anti-B (ABO blood group antigens) and anti-Kell. The mother is always negative for the relevant antigen (e.g. rhesus D-negative) and the baby is always positive; the mother then makes antibodies against the baby's blood group and these antibodies cross the placenta into the baby's circulation causing fetal or neonatal haemolytic anaemia. The diagnostic clue to this type of haemolytic anaemia is a positive direct anti-globulin test (Coombs test). This test is only positive in antibody-mediated anaemias and so is negative in all the other types of haemolytic anaemia. (These conditions are considered further in Chapter 10.)

The most common causes of non-immune haemolytic anaemia in neonates are: G6PD (glucose-6-

Anaemia

```
┌──────────────────────┐                              ┌──────────────────────┐
│  Reduced red cell    │ ◄──────┐       ┌─────► │  Increased red cell  │
│     production       │        │       │        │     destruction      │
└──────────────────────┘        │       │        │     (haemolysis)     │
                          ┌──────────────────┐   └──────────────────────┘
                          │ Causes of anaemia│
┌──────────────────────┐  └──────────────────┘   ┌──────────────────────┐
│ Combination of causes,│ ◄─────┘       └─────► │     Blood loss       │
│ e.g. anaemia of       │                         │     (uncommon)       │
│ prematurity           │                         └──────────────────────┘
└──────────────────────┘
```

Reduced red cell production

Iron deficiency anaemia
- Common in infants and toddlers, especially if of Indian subcontinent origin
- Usually dietary in origin
- Occurs because of high iron requirement (1 mg/kg/day) for growth and body stores
- Will occur if infants are weaned at 6 months of age on to a mixed diet including iron-rich food
- Is diagnosed from a hypochromic microcytic anaemia and low serum ferritin
- Is treated with dietary advice and oral iron therapy for at least 3 months

Red cell aplasia
- Congenital red cell aplasia ('Diamond–Blackfan anaemia')
- Transient erythroblastopenia of childhood (TEC)
- Parvovirus B19 infection

Increased red cell production (haemolysis)

Hereditary spherocytosis
- Inheritance is autosomal dominant, but in 25% of cases there is no family history
- May cause early, severe jaundice in newborn infants
- Is often asymptomatic, but it may cause anaemia, jaundice, splenomegaly, aplastic crisis and gallstones
- Can usually be diagnosed from the blood film
- Treatment is with folic acid, splenectomy if symptomatic

β-Thalassaemia major
- Mutation of the β-globin gene results in an inability to produce HbA ($\alpha_2\beta_2$)
- Clinical features: severe anaemia, failure to thrive/growth failure and hepatosplenomegaly
- Condition is fatal without regular blood transfusions, but blood transfusions cause iron overload
- Iron chelation therapy with desferrioxamine or oral iron chelation is essential in all patients to minimise iron overload

β-Thalassaemia trait and α-thalassaemia trait
- Can cause diagnostic confusion with mild iron deficiency

α-Thalassaemia major
- Deletion of all 4 α-globin genes, α-thalassaemia major is fatal in utero (Hb Barts) or within hours of birth

Isoimmune
- Haemolytic disease of the newborn
Immune haemolytic anaemia

G6PD deficiency
- Affects over 100 million people worldwide, usually of Mediterranean, Middle East, Far East and Central African ethnicity
- Is X-linked and therefore predominantly affects males, but females may be affected
- May present with neonatal jaundice
- Causes acute intermittent haemolysis precipitated by infection, certain drugs, fava beans (broad beans) and naphthalene in mothballs
- Parents should be given a list of drugs, chemicals and food to avoid

Sickle cell disease
- Family usually originates from tropical Africa or the Caribbean
- Autosomal recessive
- Sickled red cells result in ischaemia in organs or bones
- Main clinical features are: anaemia, infection, painful crises, sequestration crises, splenomegaly in some young children, growth failure, gallstones, behaviour and learning problems
- The most serious clinical complications are bacterial infection, acute chest syndrome, strokes and priapism
- Management: prophylactic penicillin and immunisation; folic acid; maintain good hydration
  Treat crises: analgesia, hydration, antibiotics, exchange or blood transfusion as indicated
  Long-term: hydroxyurea or occasionally bone marrow transplant

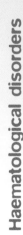

Haematological disorders

393

phosphate dehydrogenase) deficiency and hereditary spherocytosis. Haemoglobinopathies, apart from α-thalassaemia, rarely present with clinical features in the neonatal period but are detected on neonatal haemoglobinopathy screening (Guthrie test).

Blood loss

The main causes are:

- Feto-maternal haemorrhage (occult bleeding into the mother)
- Twin-to-twin transfusion (bleeding from one twin into the other one)
- Blood loss around the time of delivery (e.g. placental abruption).

The main diagnostic clue is severe anaemia with a raised reticulocyte count and normal bilirubin.

Anaemia of prematurity

The main causes are:

- Inadequate erythropoietin production
- Reduced red cell lifespan
- Frequent blood sampling whilst in hospital
- Iron and folic acid deficiency (after 2–3 months).

Bone marrow failure syndromes

Bone marrow failure (also known as aplastic anaemia) is a rare condition characterised by a reduction or absence of all three main lineages in the bone marrow leading to peripheral blood pancytopenia. It may be inherited or acquired. The acquired cases may be due to viruses (especially hepatitis viruses), drugs (such as sulphonamides, chemotherapy) or toxins (such as benzene, glue); however, many cases are labelled as 'idiopathic' because a specific cause cannot be identified.

The condition may be partial or complete. It may start as failure of a single lineage but progress to involve all three cell lines.

The clinical presentation is with:

- Anaemia due to reduced red cell numbers
- Infection due to reduced white cell numbers (especially neutrophils)
- Bruising and bleeding due to thrombocytopenia.

Inherited aplastic anaemia

These disorders are all rare.

Fanconi anaemia

This is the most common inherited form of aplastic anaemia. It is an autosomal recessive condition. The majority of children have congenital anomalies, including short stature, abnormal radii and thumbs, renal malformations, microphthalmia and pigmented skin lesions. Children may present with one or more of these anomalies or with signs of bone marrow failure which do not usually become apparent until the age of 5 or 6 years. Neonates with Fanconi anaemia nearly always have a normal blood count but it can be diagnosed by demonstrating increased chromosomal breakage of peripheral blood lymphocytes. This test can be used to identify affected family members or for prenatal diagnosis. Affected children are at high risk of death from bone marrow failure or transformation to acute leukaemia. The recommended treatment is bone marrow transplantation using normal donor marrow from an unaffected sibling or matched unrelated marrow donor.

Shwachman–Diamond syndrome

This rare autosomal recessive disorder is characterised by bone marrow failure, together with signs of pancreatic exocrine failure and skeletal abnormalities. Most are caused by mutations in the SBDS gene, which can be used for identifying unusual cases or prenatal diagnosis. The most common haematological problem is an isolated neutropenia or mild pancytopenia. Like Fanconi anaemia, there is an increased risk of transforming to acute leukaemia.

Bleeding disorders

Normal haemostasis

Haemostasis describes the normal process of blood clotting. It takes place via a series of tightly regulated interactions involving cellular and plasma factors.

There are five main components:

1. *Coagulation factors* – are produced (mainly by the liver) in an inactive form and are activated when coagulation is initiated (usually by tissue factor (TF), which is released by vessel injury; see Fig. 22.14)
2. *Coagulation inhibitors* – these either circulate in plasma or are bound to endothelium and are necessary to prevent widespread coagulation throughout the body once coagulation has been initiated
3. *Fibrinolysis* – this process limits fibrin deposition at the site of injury due to activity of the key enzyme plasmin
4. *Platelets* – are vital for haemostasis as they aggregate at sites of vessel injury to form the primary haemostatic plug which is then stabilised by fibrin
5. *Blood vessels* – both initiate and limit coagulation. Intact vascular endothelium secretes prostaglandin I_2 and nitric oxide (which promote vasodilatation and inhibit platelet aggregation). Damaged endothelium releases TF and procoagulants (e.g. collagen and von Willebrand factor) and there are inhibitors of coagulation on the endothelial surface (thrombomodulin, antithrombin and protein S) to modulate coagulation.

The endpoint of the coagulation cascade is generation of thrombin. A simplified model is shown in Figure 22.14. The two main pathways for thrombin generation were identified many years ago as the intrinsic and extrinsic pathways. Important components of these pathways are still being discovered. In recent years, the crucial role of tissue factor (TF) in haemostasis has been recognised and it is now thought that the extrinsic pathway is the one primarily responsible for initiating both normal haemostasis and thrombotic disease.

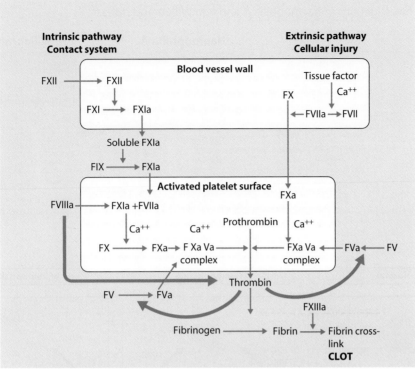

Figure 22.14 Schematic representation of the coagulation pathway.

Box 22.4 Helpful clinical features in evaluating bleeding disorders

Age of onset

- Neonate – in 20% of haemophilias, bleeding occurs in the neonatal period, usually with intracranial haemorrhage or bleeding after circumcision
- Toddler – haemophilias may present when starting to walk
- Adolescent – von Willebrand disease may present with menorrhagia

Family history

- Family tree – detailed family tree required
- Gender of affected relatives (if all boys, suggests haemophilia)

Bleeding history

- Previous surgical procedures and dental extractions – if uncomplicated, suggests bleeding tendency is acquired rather then inherited

- Presence of systemic disorders
- Drug history, e.g. anticoagulants
- Unusual pattern or inconsistent history – consider non-accidental injury

Pattern of bleeding

- Mucous membrane bleeding and skin haemorrhage – characteristic of platelet disorders or von Willebrand disease
- Bleeding into muscles or into joints – characteristic of haemophilia
- Scarring and delayed haemorrhage – suggestive of disorders of connective tissue, e.g. Marfan syndrome, osteogenesis imperfecta or factor XIII deficiency.

Diagnostic approach

Defects in the coagulation factors, in platelet number or function or in the fibrinolytic pathway are associated with an increased risk of bleeding. In contrast, defects in the naturally occurring inhibitors of coagulation (e.g. antithrombin) or in the vessel wall (e.g. damage from vascular catheters) are associated with thrombosis. In some cases, both pro- and anticoagulant abnormalities can occur at the same time, as seen in disseminated intravascular coagulation (DIC).

The diagnostic evaluation of an infant or child for a possible bleeding disorder includes:

- Identifying features in the clinical presentation that suggest the underlying diagnosis, as indicated in Box 22.4
- Initial laboratory screening tests to determine the most likely diagnosis (Table 22.3)

Table 22.3 Investigations in haemophilia A and von Willebrand disease

	Haemophilia A	von Willebrand disease
PT	Normal	Normal
APTT	↑↑	↑ or normal
Factor VIII:C	↓↓	↓ or normal
vWF Antigen	Normal	↓
RiCoF (activity)	Normal	↓
Ristocetin-induced platelet aggregation	Normal	Abnormal
vWF multimers	Normal	Variable

PT, prothrombin time; APTT, activated partial thromboplastin time; RiCoF, ristocetin co-factor, measures vWD activity.

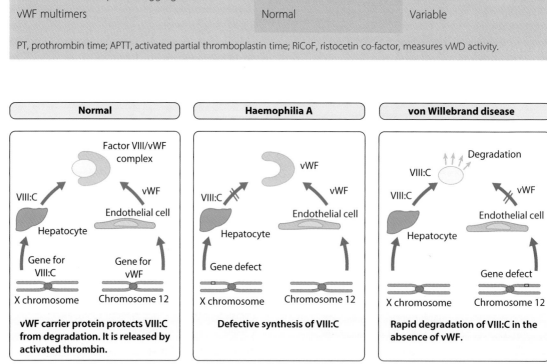

Figure 22.15 Factor VIII synthesis: normal, haemophilia A and von Willebrand disease.

- Specialist investigation to characterise a deficiency or exclude important conditions that can present with normal initial investigations, e.g. mild von Willebrand disease, factor XIII deficiency and platelet function disorders.

The most useful initial screening tests are:

- Full blood count and blood film
- Prothrombin time (PT) – measures the activity of factors II, V, VII and X
- Activated partial thromboplastin time (APTT) – measures the activity of factors II, V, VIII, IX, X, XI and XII
- If PT or APTT is prolonged, a 50:50 mix with normal plasma will distinguish between possible factor deficiency or presence of inhibitor
- Thrombin time – tests for deficiency or dysfunction of fibrinogen
- Quantitative fibrinogen assay
- D-dimers – to test for fibrin degradation products
- Biochemical screen, including renal and liver function tests.

The 'bleeding time' is no longer used to investigate platelet disorders, as it is unreliable. It has been replaced by in vitro tests of platelet function on a platelet function analyser, which can be performed on a peripheral blood sample.

In the neonate, the levels of all clotting factors except factor VIII (FVIII) and fibrinogen are lower; preterm infants have even lower levels. Therefore the results have to be compared with normal values in infants of a similar gestational and postnatal age. In view of this, and since it is often difficult to obtain good-quality neonatal samples, it is sometimes necessary to exclude an inherited coagulation factor deficiency by testing the coagulation of both parents.

Haemophilia

The commonest severe inherited coagulation disorders are haemophilia A and haemophilia B. Both have X-linked recessive inheritance. In haemophilia A, there is FVIII deficiency (Fig. 22.15); it has a frequency of 1 in 5000 male births. Haemophilia B (FIX deficiency)

Table 22.4 Severity of haemophilia

Factor VIII:C	Severity	Bleeding tendency
<1%	Severe	Spontaneous joint/muscle bleeds
1–5%	Moderate	Bleed after minor trauma
>5–40%	Mild	Bleed after surgery

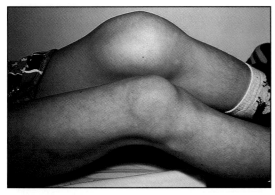

Figure 22.16 Severe arthropathy from recurrent joint bleeds in haemophilia. The aim of modern management is to prevent this from occurring.

has a frequency of 1 in 30 000 male births. Two-thirds of newly diagnosed infants have a family history of haemophilia, whereas one-third are sporadic. Identifying female carriers requires a detailed family history, analysis of coagulation factors and DNA analysis. Prenatal diagnosis is available using DNA analysis.

Clinical features

The disorder is graded as severe, moderate or mild, depending on the FVIII:C (or IX:C in haemophilia B) level (Table 22.4). The hallmark of severe disease is recurrent spontaneous bleeding into joints and muscles, which can lead to crippling arthritis if not properly treated (Fig. 22.16). Most children present towards the end of the first year of life, when they start to crawl or walk (and fall over). Bleeding episodes are most frequent in joints and muscles. Where there is no family history, non-accidental injury may initially be suspected. Almost 40% of cases present in the neonatal period, particularly with intracranial haemorrhage, bleeding post-circumcision or prolonged oozing from heel stick and venepuncture sites. The severity usually remains constant within a family.

Management

Recombinant FVIII concentrate for haemophilia A or recombinant FIX concentrate for haemophilia B is given by prompt intravenous infusion whenever there is any bleeding. If recombinant products are unavailable, highly purified, virally inactivated plasma-derived products should be used. The quantity required

Box 22.5 Complications of treatment of haemophilia

Inhibitors, i.e. antibodies to FVIII or FIX
- Develop in 5–20%
- Reduce or completely inhibit the effect of treatment
- Require the use of very high doses of factor VIII or bypassing agents (e.g. FVIIa) for treating bleeding
- May be amenable to immune tolerance induction

Transfusion-transmitted infections
- Hepatitis A, B and C
- HIV
- ?Prions

Vascular access
- Peripheral veins – may be difficult to cannulate
- Central venous access devices may become infected or thrombosed.

depends on the site and nature of the bleed. In general, raising the circulating level to 30% of normal is sufficient to treat minor bleeds and simple joint bleeds. Major surgery or life-threatening bleeds require the level to be raised to 100% and then maintained at 30–50% for up to 2 weeks to prevent secondary haemorrhage. This can only be achieved by regular infusion of factor concentrate (usually 8–12-hourly for FVIII, 12–24-hourly for FIX, or by continuous infusion) and by closely monitoring plasma levels. *Intramuscular injections, aspirin and non-steroidal anti-inflammatory drugs should be avoided in all patients with haemophilia.*

Complications are listed in Box 22.5.

Home treatment is encouraged to avoid delay in treatment, which increases the risk of permanent damage, e.g. progressive arthropathy. Parents are usually taught to give replacement therapy at home when the child is 2–3 years of age and many children are able to administer their own treatment from 7–8 years of age.

Prophylactic FVIII is given to all children with severe haemophilia A to further reduce the risk of chronic joint damage by raising the baseline level above 2%. Primary prophylaxis usually begins at age 2–3 years, and is given two to three times per week. If peripheral venous access is poor, a central venous access device (e.g. Portacath) may be required. Prophylaxis has been shown to result in better joint function in adult life. Similarly, patients with severe haemophilia B are usually given prophylactic FIX.

Desmopressin (DDAVP) may allow mild haemophilia A to be managed without the use of blood products. It is given by infusion and stimulates endogenous release of FVIII:C and von Willebrand factor (vWF). Adequate levels can be achieved to enable minor surgery and dental extraction to be undertaken. DDAVP is ineffective in haemophilia B.

Haemophilia centres should supervise the management of children with bleeding disorders. They provide a multidisciplinary approach with expert medical, nursing and laboratory input. Specialised physiotherapy is needed to preserve muscle strength and avoid damage from immobilisation. Psychosocial support is an integral part of maintaining compliance.

Self-help groups such as the Haemophilia Society may provide families with helpful information and support.

von Willebrand disease (vWD)

Von Willebrand factor (vWF) has two major roles:

- It facilitates platelet adhesion to damaged endothelium
- It acts as the carrier protein for FVIII:C, protecting it from inactivation and clearance.

Von Willebrand disease (vWD) results from either a quantitative or qualitative deficiency of von Willebrand factor (vWF). This causes defective platelet plug formation and, since vWF is a carrier protein for FVIII:C, patients with vWD also are deficient in FVIII:C (see Fig. 22.15).

There are many different mutations in the vWF gene and many different types of vWD. The inheritance is usually autosomal dominant. The commonest subtype, type 1 (60–80%), is usually fairly mild and is often not diagnosed until puberty or adulthood.

Clinical features

These are:

- Bruising
- Excessive, prolonged bleeding after surgery
- Mucosal bleeding such as epistaxis and menorrhagia.

In contrast to haemophilia, spontaneous soft tissue bleeding such as large haematomas and haemarthroses are uncommon.

Management

Treatment depends on the type and severity of the disorder. Type 1 vWD can usually be treated with DDAVP, which causes secretion of both FVIII and vWF into plasma. DDAVP should be used with caution in children <1 year of age as it can cause hyponatraemia due to water retention and may cause seizures, particularly after repeated doses, and if fluid intake is not strictly regulated. More severe types of vWD have to be treated with *plasma-derived* FVIII concentrate, as DDAVP is ineffective and recombinant FVIII concentrate contains no vWF. Cryoprecipitate is no longer used to treat vWD as it has not undergone viral inactivation. *Intramuscular injections, aspirin and nonsteroidal anti-inflammatory drugs should be avoided in all patients with vWD.*

Summary

The child with abnormal bleeding
– into soft tissues, mucocutaneous or following surgery

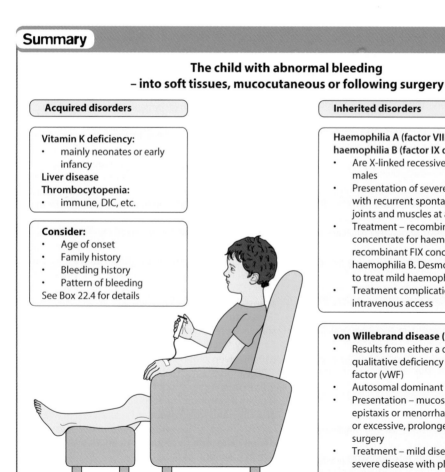

Acquired disorders

Vitamin K deficiency:
- mainly neonates or early infancy

Liver disease

Thrombocytopenia:
- immune, DIC, etc.

Consider:
- Age of onset
- Family history
- Bleeding history
- Pattern of bleeding

See Box 22.4 for details

Inherited disorders

Haemophilia A (factor VIII deficiency) and haemophilia B (factor IX deficiency):
- Are X-linked recessive disorders affecting males
- Presentation of severe disease – usually with recurrent spontaneous bleeding into joints and muscles at about 1 year of age
- Treatment – recombinant FVIII concentrate for haemophilia A or recombinant FIX concentrate for haemophilia B. Desmopressin (DDAVP) to treat mild haemophilia A
- Treatment complications – inhibitors and intravenous access

von Willebrand disease (vWD):
- Results from either a quantitative or qualitative deficiency of von Willebrand factor (vWF)
- Autosomal dominant
- Presentation – mucosal bleeding, e.g. epistaxis or menorrhagia in adolescence or excessive, prolonged bleeding after surgery
- Treatment – mild disease with DDAVP, severe disease with plasma-derived FVIII concentrate

Acquired disorders of coagulation

The main acquired disorders of coagulation affecting children are those secondary to:

- Haemorrhagic disease of the newborn due to vitamin K deficiency (see Ch. 10)
- Liver disease
- ITP (immune thrombocytopenia)
- DIC (disseminated intravascular coagulation).

Vitamin K is essential for the production of active forms of factors II, VII, IX, X and for the production of naturally occurring anticoagulants such as proteins C and S. Vitamin K deficiency therefore causes reduced levels of all of these factors. The main clinical consequence of this is a prolonged prothrombin time and an increased risk of bleeding. Children may become deficient in vitamin K due to:

- Inadequate intake (e.g. neonates, long-term chronic illness with poor intake)
- Malabsorption (e.g. coeliac disease, cystic fibrosis, obstructive jaundice)
- Vitamin K antagonists (e.g. warfarin).

Thrombocytopenia

Thrombocytopenia is a platelet count $<150 \times 10^9/L$. The risk of bleeding depends on the level of the platelet count:

- Severe thrombocytopenia (platelets $<20 \times 10^9/L$) – risk of spontaneous bleeding
- Moderate thrombocytopenia (platelets $20–50 \times 10^9/L$) – at risk of excess bleeding during operations or trauma but low risk of spontaneous bleeding
- Mild thrombocytopenia (platelets $50–150 \times 10^9/L$) – low risk of bleeding unless there is a major operation or severe trauma.

Table 22.5 Causes of purpura or easy bruising

Platelet count reduced, i.e. thrombocytopenia	
Increased platelet destruction or consumption	
Immune	ITP (immune thrombocytopenia)
	SLE (systemic lupus erythematosus)
	Alloimmune neonatal thrombocytopenia
Non-immune	Haemolytic uraemic syndrome
	Thrombotic thrombocytopenic purpura
	DIC (disseminated intravascular coagulation)
	Congenital heart disease
	Giant haemangiomas (Kasabach–Merritt syndrome)
	Hypersplenism
Impaired platelet production	
Congenital	Fanconi anaemia
	Wiskott–Aldrich syndrome
	Bernard–Soulier syndrome
Acquired	Aplastic anaemia
	Marrow infiltration (e.g. leukaemia)
	Drug-induced
Platelet count normal	
Platelet dysfunction	
Congenital	Rare disorders, e.g. Glanzmann thromboasthenia
Acquired	Uraemia, cardiopulmonary bypass
Vascular disorders	
Congenital	Rare disorders, e.g. Ehlers–Danlos, Marfan syndrome, hereditary haemorrhagic telangiectasia
Acquired	Meningococcal and other severe infections
	Vasculitis, e.g. Henoch–Schönlein purpura, SLE
	Scurvy

Thrombocytopenia may result in bruising, petechiae, purpura and mucosal bleeding (e.g. epistaxis, bleeding from gums when brushing teeth). Major haemorrhage in the form of severe gastrointestinal haemorrhage, haematuria and intracranial bleeding is much less common. The causes of easy bruising and purpura are listed in Table 22.5. While purpura may signify thrombocytopenia, it also occurs with a normal platelet count from platelet dysfunction and vascular disorders.

Immune thrombocytopenia (ITP)

Immune thrombocytopenia is the commonest cause of thrombocytopenia in childhood. It has an incidence of around 4 per 100 000 children per year. It is usually caused by destruction of circulating platelets by anti-platelet IgG autoantibodies. The reduced platelet count may be accompanied by a compensatory increase of megakaryocytes in the bone marrow.

Clinical features

Most children present between the ages of 2 and 10 years, with onset often 1–2 weeks after a viral infection. In the majority of children, there is a short history of days or weeks. Affected children develop petechiae, purpura and/or superficial bruising (see Case History 22.3). It can cause epistaxis and other mucosal bleeding but profuse bleeding is uncommon, despite the fact that the platelet count often falls to $<10\times10^9$/L. Intracranial bleeding is a serious but rare complication, occurring in 0.1–0.5%, mainly in those with a long period of severe thrombocytopenia.

Diagnosis

ITP is a diagnosis of exclusion, so careful attention must be paid to the history, clinical features and blood film to ensure that another more sinister diagnosis is not missed. In the younger child, a congenital cause (such as Wiskott–Aldrich or Bernard–Soulier syndromes) should be considered. Any atypical clinical features, such as the presence of anaemia, neutropenia, hepatosplenomegaly or marked lymphadenopathy, should prompt a bone marrow examination to exclude acute leukaemia or aplastic anaemia. A bone marrow examination should also be performed if the child is going to be treated with steroids, since this treatment may temporarily mask the diagnosis of acute lymphoblastic leukaemia (ALL). Inadvertent steroid therapy in undiagnosed ALL mimicking ITP will compromise the long-term outcome of such patients. Systemic lupus erythematosus (SLE) should also be considered. However, if the clinical features are characteristic, with no abnormality in the blood other than a low platelet count and no intention to treat, there is no need to examine the bone marrow.

Management

In about 80% of children, the disease is acute, benign and self-limiting, usually remitting spontaneously within 6–8 weeks. Most children can be managed at home and do not require hospital admission. Treatment is controversial. Most children do not need any therapy even if their platelet count is $<10\times10^9$/L but treatment should be given if there is evidence of major

---

Case History

22.3 Immune thrombocytopenic purpura (ITP)

Sian, aged 5 years, developed bruising and a skin rash over 24 h. She had had an upper respiratory tract infection the previous week. On examination she appeared well but had a purpuric skin rash with some bruises on the trunk and legs (Fig. 22.17). There were three blood blisters on her tongue and buccal mucosa, but no fundal haemorrhages, lymphadenopathy or hepatosplenomegaly. Urine was normal on dipsticks testing. A full blood count showed Hb 11.5 g/dl with normal indices, WBC and differential normal, platelet count 17×10^9/L. The platelets on the blood film were large; the film was otherwise normal. A diagnosis of ITP was made and she was discharged home. Her parents were counselled and given emergency contact names and telephone numbers. They were also given literature on the condition and advised that she should avoid contact sports but should continue to attend school. Over the next 2 weeks she continued to develop bruising and purpura but was asymptomatic. By the third week, she had no new bruises, and her platelet count was 25×10^9/L; the blood count and film showed no new abnormalities. The following week, the platelet count was 74×10^9/L and a week later it was 200×10^9/L. She was discharged from follow-up.

 In immune thrombocytopenic purpura, in spite of impressive cutaneous manifestations and extremely low platelet count, the outlook is good and most will remit quickly without any intervention.

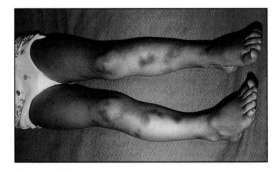

Figure 22.17 Bruising and purpura from immune thrombocytopenic purpura.

bleeding (e.g. intracranial or gastrointestinal haemorrhage) or persistent minor bleeding that affects daily lives such as excessive epistaxis or menstrual bleeding. The treatment options include oral prednisolone, intravenous anti-D or intravenous immunoglobulin and all have significant side-effects. Platelet transfusions are reserved for life-threatening haemorrhage as they raise the platelet count only for a few hours. The parents need immediate 24-hour access to hospital treatment, and the child should avoid trauma, as far as possible, and contact sports while the platelet count is very low.

Chronic ITP

In 20% of children, the platelet count remains low 6 months after diagnosis; this is known as chronic ITP. In the majority of children, treatment is mainly supportive; drug treatment is only offered to children with chronic persistent bleeding that affects daily activities or impairs quality of life. Children with significant bleeding are rare and require specialist care. A variety of treatment modalities are available, including rituximab, a monoclonal antibody directed against B lymphocytes. Newer agents such as thrombopoietic growth factors have shown clinical response in adults and may be used in children with severe non-responsive disease. Splenectomy can be effective for this group but is mainly reserved for children who fail drug therapy as it significantly increases the risk of infections and patients require lifelong antibiotic prophylaxis. If ITP in a child becomes chronic, regular screening for SLE should be performed, as the thrombocytopenia may predate the development of autoantibodies.

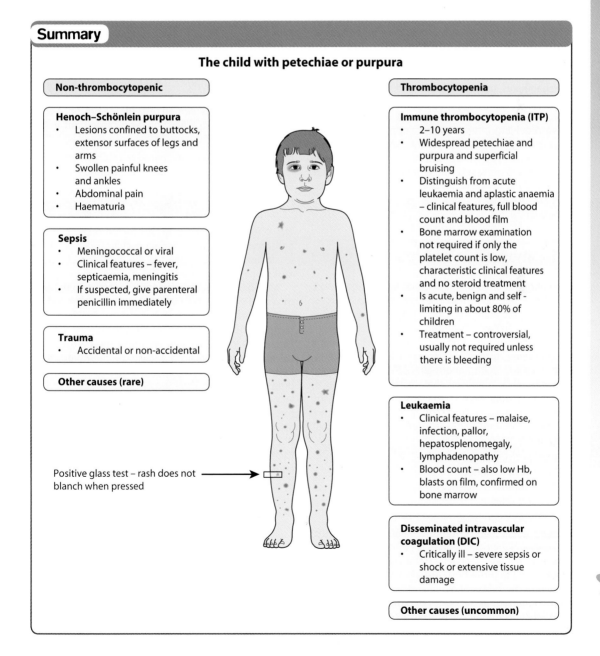

Summary

The child with petechiae or purpura

Non-thrombocytopenic

Henoch–Schönlein purpura
- Lesions confined to buttocks, extensor surfaces of legs and arms
- Swollen painful knees and ankles
- Abdominal pain
- Haematuria

Sepsis
- Meningococcal or viral
- Clinical features – fever, septicaemia, meningitis
- If suspected, give parenteral penicillin immediately

Trauma
- Accidental or non-accidental

Other causes (rare)

Positive glass test – rash does not blanch when pressed

Thrombocytopenia

Immune thrombocytopenia (ITP)
- 2–10 years
- Widespread petechiae and purpura and superficial bruising
- Distinguish from acute leukaemia and aplastic anaemia – clinical features, full blood count and blood film
- Bone marrow examination not required if only the platelet count is low, characteristic clinical features and no steroid treatment
- Is acute, benign and self-limiting in about 80% of children
- Treatment – controversial, usually not required unless there is bleeding

Leukaemia
- Clinical features – malaise, infection, pallor, hepatosplenomegaly, lymphadenopathy
- Blood count – also low Hb, blasts on film, confirmed on bone marrow

Disseminated intravascular coagulation (DIC)
- Critically ill – severe sepsis or shock or extensive tissue damage

Other causes (uncommon)

Disseminated intravascular coagulation

Disseminated intravascular coagulation (DIC) describes a disorder characterised by coagulation pathway activation leading to diffuse fibrin deposition in the microvasculature and consumption of coagulation factors and platelets.

The commonest causes of activation of coagulation are severe sepsis or shock due to circulatory collapse, e.g. in meningococcal septicaemia, or extensive tissue damage from trauma or burns. DIC may be acute or chronic and is likely to be initiated through the tissue factor pathway. The predominant clinical feature is bruising, purpura and haemorrhage. However, the pathophysiological process is characterised by microvascular thrombosis and purpura fulminans may occur.

No single test reliably diagnoses DIC. However, DIC should be suspected when the following abnormalities coexist – thrombocytopenia, prolonged prothrombin time (PT), prolonged APTT, low fibrinogen, raised fibrinogen degradation products and D-dimers and microangiopathic haemolytic anaemia. There is also usually a marked reduction in the naturally occurring anticoagulants, proteins C and S and antithrombin.

The most important aspect of management is to treat the underlying cause of the DIC (usually sepsis) while providing intensive care. Supportive care may be provided with fresh frozen plasma (to replace clotting factors), cryoprecipitate and platelets. Antithrombin and protein C concentrates have been used, particularly in severe meningococcal septicaemia with purpura fulminans. The use of heparin remains controversial.

Thrombosis in children

Thrombosis is uncommon in children and about 95% of venous thromboembolic events are secondary to underlying disorders associated with hypercoagulable states (see below). Thrombosis of cerebral vessels usually presents with signs of a stroke. (The condition is considered further in Chapters 10 and 27.) Rarely, children may inherit abnormalities in the coagulation and fibrinolytic pathway that increase their risk of developing clots even in the absence of underlying predisposing factors. These conditions are termed congenital prothrombotic disorders (thrombophilias). They are:

- Protein C deficiency
- Protein S deficiency
- Antithrombin deficiency
- Factor V Leiden
- Prothrombin gene G20210A mutation.

Proteins C and S and antithrombin are natural anticoagulants and their deficiencies are inherited in an autosomal dominant manner. Heterozygotes are also predisposed to thrombosis, usually venous, during the second or third decade of life and only rarely in childhood. Homozygous deficiency of protein C and protein S are very uncommon and present with life-threatening thrombosis with widespread haemorrhage and purpura into the skin (known as 'purpura fulminans') in the neonatal period. Homozygous antithrombin deficiency is not seen, probably because it is lethal in the fetus.

Factor V Leiden is an inherited abnormality in the structure of the coagulation protein factor V, which makes it resistant to degradation by activated protein C as part of the body's normal anticoagulant mechanism. The prothrombin gene mutation is associated with high levels of plasma prothrombin.

Acquired disorders are:

- Catheter-related thrombosis
- DIC (disseminated intravascular coagulation)
- Hypernatraemia
- Polycythaemia (e.g. due to congenital heart disease)
- Malignancy
- SLE (systemic lupus erythematosus) and persistent antiphospholipid antibody syndrome.

Diagnosis

Although inherited thrombophilia is very uncommon, these disorders predispose to life-threatening thrombosis and so it is important not to miss the diagnosis in any child presenting with an unexplained thrombotic event. Therefore, screening tests for the presence of an inherited thrombophilia should be carried out in the following situations:

- Any child with unanticipated or extensive venous thrombosis, ischaemic skin lesions or neonatal purpura fulminans
- Any child with a positive family history of neonatal purpura fulminans.

The screening tests are assays for proteins C and S, antithrombin assay, polymerase chain reaction (PCR) for factor V Leiden and for the prothrombin gene mutation.

Mutations in factor V (factor V Leiden) and the prothrombin gene, respectively, are present in 5% and 2% of the northern European population. Children with protein C deficiency or factor V Leiden have 4–6 times higher risk of developing recurrent thromboses. The risk increases significantly if these conditions are inherited together. Therefore it is reasonable to screen children who develop thrombosis for all of these factors in order to plan the best management to prevent thrombosis. In the UK, current practice is not to screen asymptomatic children for genetic defects, which are not going to affect their medical management, e.g. on the basis of family history alone, until they are old enough to receive appropriate counselling and make decisions for themselves.

Summary

Thrombosis

All children with thrombosis should be screened for inherited or acquired predisposing disorders.

Further reading

Bailey S, **Skinner R**: *Paediatric Haematology and Oncology. Oxford Specialist Handbooks in Paediatrics.* Oxford, 2009, Oxford University Press.

Lilleyman JS, **Hann IM**, **Blanchette VS, editors:** *Pediatric Haematology*, ed 3, Edinburgh, 2005, Churchill Livingstone.

A single-volume, comprehensive textbook

Orkin SH, **Fisher DE**, **Look T**, **et al., editors:** *Nathan and Oski's Hematology of Infancy and Childhood*, ed 7, Philadelphia, PA, 2008, Saunders.

Comprehensive, two-volume textbook.

Websites (Accessed May 2011)

British Committee for Standards in Haematology guidelines: Available at: http://www.bcshguidelines. com.

Diamond–Blackfan syndrome: UK Diamond Blackfan Anaemia Support Group. Available at: http://www. diamondblackfan.org.uk.

Haemophilia: World Federation of Haemophilia. Available at: http://www.wfh.org/index.asp?lang=EN or The Haemophilia Society. Available at: http://www.haemophilia.org.uk.

Shwachman–Diamond syndrome: Shwachman–Diamond Support UK. Available at: http://sdsuk.org.

Sickle Cell Society: Available at: http:// www.sicklecellsociety.org.

UK Thalassaemia Society: Available at: http:// www.ukts.org.

Haematological disorders

23

Emotions and behaviour

Knowledge of children's emotions and behaviour is important in order to:

- know what constitutes the normal range
- understand common, normative and usually minor deviations and responses to stress, physical illness and injuries
- recognise and manage emotional and behavioural disorders.

Principles of normal development

Normal parenting

A child's behaviour, emotional responses and personality are the end result of interplay between genetic predisposition and environmental influences. The environment provides experience from which stems knowledge, learned behaviour or emotional responses and attitudes to oneself and the world. Interpersonal relationships are major environmental factors in promoting psychosocial development and the child's family is a principal source of these. Within the family, children should be protected, nurtured, educated and contained so that their development is supported optimally. Many societies are going through major demographic changes, including rising numbers of family breakdowns, lone-parent families and same gender parents. However, irrespective of the family structure, the essential elements of competent parenting or what is commonly referred to as 'good-enough parenting' are the same for all families (Box 23.1). Beyond this, the parents' attitude towards their children and how they handle their individual children help to determine how their personalities develop.

Normal early relationships

In the first 2 months of a baby's life, infants are not fussy about who responds to their needs. From 3 to 6 months they become more selective, demanding comfort from one or two caregivers. By 6–8 months they are particular about who responds to their needs or holds them, especially when distressed, and show tearful *separation anxiety* if their main caregiver, usually the mother, is not there. If tired, fearful, unhappy or in pain, they will cling to her and be comforted by her presence as an *attachment figure*. At this time, the child learns to crawl, and so is able to leave a primary caregiver and possibly encounter danger. The development of attachment behaviour allows the infant to keep track of their parent's whereabouts and resist separation. This close attachment relationship derives from social interaction and the mother's sensitive responsiveness to the baby's needs, not from any blood tie. It need not be with the biological mother, although it usually is. Its importance lies in it being:

- a particularly close relationship within which the child's development of trust, empathy, conscience and ideals is promoted, forming a prototype for future close relationships
- the child's primary source of comfort, providing the principal method of coping with stress (fear, anxiety, pain, etc.).

This underscores the importance of having a young child's parent 'rooming in' if admitted to hospital. Otherwise the child would be doubly distressed both by the absence of their attachment figure as well as by the threat of strange surroundings or procedures and by the stress of pain or illness.

If a young child is placed in strange, impersonal surroundings and separated from the mother for more than several hours, a *triphasic acute separation* reaction may set in (Fig. 23.1):

Box 23.1 Competent parents

- Are available physically and emotionally when needed
- Protect their children from harm
- Love their children – provide affection, support, comfort, food and shelter
- Exercise parental authority firmly, calmly and fairly, by setting clear and realistic limits for their children using rewards and praise to encourage compliance and non-physical sanctions to reduce non-compliance
- Respect their children's immature status and judge it accurately
- Keep adult business (sex, etc.) away from their children
- Model calm, positive and constructive problem-solving strategies for their children
- Have their own lives and do not live through their children
- Maintain their own self-esteem and personal development.

- Mounting anxiety about the fact that the child's mother fails to reappear produces distressed, irritable tearfulness (*protest*), which is hard to comfort
- After a day or two, this turns into a withdrawn state with no play, no interest in food and little speech or willingness for personal contact (*despair*)
- The child gradually cheers up from this but the close contact with the mother has been lost and the child is relatively indifferent to her when she reappears (*detachment*).

Recreating the original closeness can take weeks and is accompanied by a phase of irritability, misbehaviour and clinging. This can sometimes be seen when children who have been admitted to hospital as an emergency return home.

Children who have never had the opportunity for a close, secure attachment relationship in their early years are at risk of growing up as self-centred individuals who seek the affection and attention of others but have difficulty with close personal relationships and with learning to conform with social rules of conduct.

The selective clinging of early attachment behaviour diminishes over time so that in the second year of life children extend their emotional attachments to other family members and carers. By school age, they can tolerate separations from their parents for several hours. Children vary in their ability to do this depending on their temperament and social circumstances. For example, a child who is constitutionally apprehensive, who has an exceptionally anxious mother, or who has parents who threaten abandonment is likely to continue to cling to his/her mother for protection and comfort. A series of frightening events will tend to perpetuate clinging, which may persist well into middle childhood (age 5–12 years). This interferes with children's capacity to learn how to cope with anxiety on their own (Fig. 23.2).

The three stages of the acute separation response in children

Protest	Crying, distress Angry refusal to be comforted Asking for mummy

↓

Despair	Moping Not playing Not eating

↓

Detachment	Apparent cheering up and recovery Indifferent to parents on return to them

The above sequence develops over a period of days, but with considerable variation between children.

Figure 23.1 The three stages of the acute separation response in young children.

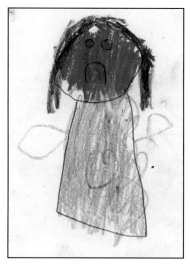

Figure 23.2 A 6-year-old with separation anxiety, showing what it feels like to leave her mother to go to school.

With entry into school, the importance of teachers and other children in shaping psychosocial development increases and their influence must be taken into account in understanding any schoolchild's development.

Summary

Early relationships:

Young children:

- develop a close attachment relationship with their mother (or main caregiver)
- if separated from their mother, may develop separation anxiety
- if admitted to hospital, should be able to have their parents stay with them.

Temperament

Children differ from each other in personality from birth, just as they do in physical appearance. This individuality in behavioural style or temperament is partly genetically determined. It is not fixed but changes slowly in the light of experience. It affects how other people deal with them.

A child born with a *difficult temperament* is prone to:

- predominantly negative moods – whinging, moaning, crying
- intense emotional reactions – screaming rather than whimpering, jumping for joy rather than smiling
- irregular biological functions – a lack of rhythm in sleeping, hunger or toileting
- negative initial responses to novel situations, e.g. pushing a new toy away
- protracted adjustment to new situations – taking weeks or months to settle into a new playgroup.

Such a pattern is a vulnerability factor for future emotional and behavioural problems. It may be hard for parents to maintain an affectionate relationship with a child who has a difficult temperament. Their self-confidence falters as they feel guilty that they have failed as parents. Such parents need support to maintain a positive, loving relationship with their child who will, if this can be done, soften and become easier to handle over a period of months. If parents lapse into irritable intolerance themselves, this is likely to maintain the child's grouchy and unsatisfied manner and may lead eventually to low self-esteem or the development of behavioural problems.

Self-esteem

Children develop views and make attributions about themselves. Most children experience praise and success in enough areas of their lives to develop a sense of inner self-confidence and self-worth. Those who do not are at increased risk of developing emotional and behavioural disorders which in turn may breed further shame and failure. A child who does not consider him/herself worthwhile and valued by others will play safe and not attempt new activities or explore new situations because of a fear of failure. This restricts the development of coping skills and knowledge of the world generally. It may also be a vulnerability factor for depression and anxiety disorders. Children who lack a belief in their own worth may adopt extraordinary and problematic behaviours in order to attract the attention and acclaim of others. For instance, one child took to openly eating dog faeces because it attracted a crowd of amazed children around her. Repeated failure, academically or socially, will undermine self-esteem, as will some disorders themselves (dyspraxia, enuresis and faecal soiling in particular). An important source of low self-esteem, however, is the child's parents, either because of their own low self-esteem or because of abuse (emotional, sexual or physical) and neglect.

Cognitive style

As children grow older, their thinking style evolves from one that is concrete to one that is able to cope with abstract thought. Below the age of about 5 years, thought is fundamentally egocentric, with the child being at the centre of his world (Box 23.2). During middle childhood, the dominant mode of thought is practical and orderly but tied to immediate circumstances and specific experiences rather than hypothetical possibilities or metaphors. Not until the mid-teens does the adult style of abstract thought begin to appear.

 Adjust the way you talk to children to be compatible with their thinking style.

Coping with chronic or serious illness or adversities in childhood

Children can respond to adversity, including illness, in a number of ways:

- *Cognitive response* – can lie anywhere along the spectrum of over-acceptance to denial, with fluctuation over time. In over-acceptance, the child may allow the illness to overtake their life resulting in more impairment than is expected for level of symptoms, and high levels of anxiety about the slightest symptom. With denial, symptoms and warning signs may be ignored and treatment poorly adhered to.
- *Emotional response* – to diagnosis of illness and at times of relapse, may have similarities to a bereavement reaction or reaction to loss, with shock, denial, anger, followed by acceptance and adjustment (Fig. 23.3). Such responses to a serious illness are normal as long as the child proceeds through the phases.
- *Behavioural response* – young children tend to regress when stressed and behave younger than they actually are. A toddler may become

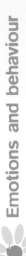

407

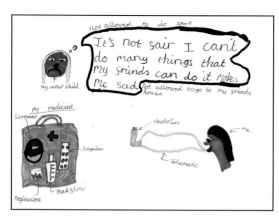

Figure 23.3 Drawing by a 10-year-old girl with asthma, showing how she felt about her illness. She was struggling to take her medicines and had multiple hospital admissions. Family therapy helped her to come to terms with her illness and take her medications.

overactive or clingy and display sleep and feeding difficulties. Regressive responses in older children predominantly manifest as problems with toileting, academic performance and peer relationships.

- *Somatic response* – can include expression of worry and distress through bodily symptoms such as recurrent abdominal pain.

Children suffering from chronic or serious illness are more vulnerable to mental health problems. This is related to:

- *Nature of illness* – this includes severity, chronicity, presence of constant discomfort and demands of treatment. Children with neurological disorders involving the brain, e.g. epilepsy, are at increased risk.
- *Stage of illness* – for example, diagnosis, deteriorations signalled by the need for new demanding treatments or by admissions to hospital.
- *Age of the child* – in infancy, illness may affect attachment and developmental milestones such as autonomy and mobility. Over 5 years of age there is a greater impact on educational progress, athletic activities and achievement. In adolescence, social adjustment, individual identity, independence from the family and poor adherence to treatment become more of an issue. Prolonged separation from parents resulting from illness will have a particularly negative impact between the age of 6 months and 3 years.
- *Temperament* – a child who is more adaptable to new situations will fare better. In contrast, a child who from early life has been difficult to soothe will fare worse
- *Intellectual capacity* – brighter children generally cope better.
- *Family factors* – the illness can have detrimental effects on the family and family difficulties can aggravate adaptation to illness.

Summary

Responses of children to illness or adversity include:

- Over-acceptance or refusal to accept the situation
- The sequence of shock, denial, anger, followed by acceptance and adjustment
- Regression of behaviour
- Somatic symptoms.

Adversities in the family

Family relationships are, for most children, the source of their most powerful emotions. Similarly, parents have more effect than anyone else on children's social learning and behaviour. The ecological model of child development indicates that families are generally the most potent environmental influence on a child's mental health. They are not all-powerful, since a predisposition to particular childhood emotional and behavioural problems can be inherited, but family influences interact with this so that overt disorder may or may not emerge. Not all disorders have their origin in family adversities: hyperkinetic disorder, tics and autism arise independently of them. Nevertheless, the non-genetic contribution of family interactions to emotional and behavioural disorders is often substantial and the mechanisms whereby they produce disorder are various. The following are some of the known risk factors:

- Angry discord between family members
- Parental mental ill health, especially maternal depression
- Divorce (Boxes 23.3 and 23.4) and bereavement
- Intrusive overprotection
- Lack of parental authority
- Physical and sexual abuse
- Emotional rejection or unremitting criticism
- Use of violence, terror, threats of abandonment or excessive guilt as disciplinary devices
- Taunting or belittlement of the child
- Inconsistent, unpredictable discipline
- Using the child to fulfil the unreasonable personal emotional needs of a parent
- Inappropriate responsibilities or expectations for the child's level of maturity.

Many of these risk factors can be aggravated by a difficult or unrewarding child whose behaviour or difficult temperament may make the adverse environment worse. While parents need to be made aware of changes required to improve the situation, it is unwise to blame them for causing their child's problem as it makes them less likely to engage in treatment.

Adversities may also arise outside the family. Experiences with other children are increasingly recognised as highly significant in psychosocial development. Bullying is a known adversity, as are instances of targeted peer rejection, and other forms of peer-mediated persecution. With widespread access to the internet, cyber bullying is becoming an increasing problem. Merely being left out of things by other children (as opposed to being driven away) is much less pernicious.

Summary

Regarding adversities

- The child's family is the most potent influence on the child's mental health
- Many but not all mental health problems originate from adversities in the family
- The child's temperament and adversities outside the family, e.g. bullying, may aggravate the situation.

Box 23.3 Reactions to parental divorce

Preschool
- Fear of further abandonment:
  - Intensified clinging at threatened separations
  - Sleep disturbances
  - Tearful, irritable and demanding
  - Disorganised play

Middle childhood
- Miserable at loss of parent, pining for restitution of family
- Self-blame in younger (age 6–8) age group
- Angry blaming of one parent for divorce in older (age 9–12) age group
- Loyalty conflicts
- Anxiety and jealousy at parents' new partners
- Educational underachievement

Adolescents
- Wide variation in response
- Various attempts to master the situation:
  - Detachment from family
  - Rapid maturation
  - Moral idealism
  - Critical of parents
- Educational underachievement
- Depression in some.

Box 23.4 Adjustment tasks facing children of divorced parents

- Acknowledgement of parental separation
- Regaining sense of direction in life activities
- Dealing with sense of loss and rejection
- Forgiving parents for break-up
- Accepting permanence of divorce, relinquishing wish for the previously intact family
- Feeling able to enter into new emotional relationships.

Conversely, having a number of steady, good-quality peer relationships is a marker for good prognosis in an emotional or behavioural problem which has resulted from environmental influences.

Problems of the preschool years

Meal refusal

A common scenario is a mother complaining that her child refuses to eat any or much of what she provides; mealtimes have become a battleground. Examination reveals a healthy, well-nourished child whose height and weight are securely within normal limits on a centile growth chart, or a small and thin child with faltering growth.

An account of what goes on at a typical mealtime may reveal:

- A past history of force-feeding
- Irregular meals so that the child is not predictably hungry
- Unsuitable meals
- Unreasonably large portions
- Multiple opportunities for distraction, e.g. TV.

Most importantly, how much does the child eat between meals? A well-nourished child is getting food from somewhere. Not all parents regard sweets and crisps as being food. Some mothers, while concerned about their child's apparently poor food intake, provide little variety in the child's diet. For strategies for dealing with meal refusal, see Box 23.5. Children with faltering growth may require specialist referral if they do not respond to this advice.

Sleep-related problems

Difficulty in settling to sleep at bedtime

This is a common problem in the toddler years. The child will not go to sleep unless the parent is present. Most instances are normal expressions of separation anxiety, but there may be other obvious reasons for it which can be explored in taking a history (Box 23.6), supplemented if necessary by the parents keeping a prospective sleep diary. Many cases will respond to simple advice:

- Creating a bedtime routine which cues the child to what is required
- Telling the child to lie quietly in bed until he/she falls asleep, recognising that children cannot fall asleep to order (although that is what everyone tells them to do).

If that advice does not resolve the problem, a more active intervention may be required. This involves parents imposing a graded pattern of lengthening periods between tucking their child up in bed and coming back after a few minutes to visit, but leaving the room before the child falls asleep, even if they are protesting. The object is to provide the opportunity for the child to learn how to fall sleep alone, a skill not yet

409

Mealtime history

What is the parent most concerned about?

- Nutrition?
  - Refer to growth chart
- Discipline and parenting?
  - Family history of eating problems
  - Parenting style
  - What do others say?
  - Is it part of a broader behavioural problem?

How much food is eaten between meals?

- Food diary to record child's intake over a number of days.

Advice

- As long as offered wholesome food with adequate range, children are remarkably good at eating a constant and appropriate quantity of food when allowed a reasonable choice.
- As it is impossible to force a child to eat, avoid confrontation at mealtimes.
- Develop a relaxed atmosphere.
- Use favourite foods as a reward. Introduce other rewards for compliance at mealtimes (e.g. additional privileges such as extra TV time).
- Reduce eating between meals if necessary, although many young children prefer small, frequent snacks.

developed. More refractory cases may require specialist referral.

Waking at night

This is normal, but some children cry because they cannot settle themselves back to sleep without their parent's presence. This is often associated with difficulty settling in the evenings, which should be treated first. Some children who can settle in the evening may be unable to settle when they wake in the night because the circumstances are different – it is quieter, darker, etc. The graded approach described above for evening settling can also be used in the middle of the night. Parents will find it helpful to take alternate nights on duty to share the burden.

Nightmares

These are bad dreams which can be recalled by the child. They are common, rarely requiring professional attention unless they occur frequently or are stereotyped in content, indicating a morbid preoccupation or symptomatic of a psychiatric disorder such as post-traumatic stress disorder. Unless a disorder is suspected, reassuring the child and his family will usually suffice.

Night (sleep) terrors

These are different from nightmares, occurring about 1.5 hours after settling. The parents find the child sitting up in bed, eyes open, seemingly awake but

- Too much sleep in the late afternoon
- Displaced sleep/wake cycle – not waking child in morning because did not settle until late on the previous night
- Separation anxiety
- Overstimulated or overwrought in the evening
- Kept awake by siblings or noisy neighbours or TV in the bedroom
- Erratic parental practices: no bedtime or routine to cue child into sleep readiness, sudden removal from play to go to bed without prior warning to wind down
- Use of bedroom as punishment
- Dislike of darkness and silence – night light and playing story tapes can be helpful
- Some chronic physical conditions may be associated with sleep problems, e.g. painful crisis in sickle cell disease.

obviously disorientated, confused and distressed and unresponsive to their questions and reassurances. The child settles back to sleep after a few minutes and has no recollection of the episode in the morning. A night terror is a *parasomnia*, a disturbance of the structure of sleep wherein a very rapid emergence from the first period of deep slow-wave sleep produces a state of high arousal and confusion. Sleepwalking has similar origins and the two may be combined. Most night terrors need little more than reassurance directed towards the parents. The most important intervention for sleepwalking is to make the environment safe to prevent injury to the child (e.g. not sleeping on the upper bunk of a double-bunk bed, putting gates before the staircase, locking the kitchen, etc.). Given that a common cause of night terrors and sleepwalking is a poor and erratic sleep schedule, a sleep routine can be helpful in preventing recurrence. Once parents have implemented the safety suggestions highlighted above, they can be reassured, as the natural course of these disorders is to decrease over time.

Disobedience, defiance and tantrums

Normal toddlers often go through a phase of refusing to comply with parents' demands, sometimes angrily ('the terrible 2s'). This is an understandable reaction to the discovery that the world is not organised around them. They also become confused and angered by the fact that the parent who provides them with comfort when they are distressed is also the person who is making them do things they do not wish to do. This seems exceptionally unfair to them. That is one reason why children play their parents up but may be fine with others. All this can exhaust and demoralise parents, not least because many people offer advice or criticism (everyone thinks themselves an expert in the area of children's development and behaviour). The points listed in Box 23.7 can be made.

Box 23.7 Managing toddler disobedience

- Ensure your demand is reasonable for the developmental stage of the child
- Tell the child what you want him/her to do rather than nagging about what you do not want him/her to do
- Praise for compliance, especially when it is spontaneous (catch doing the right thing)
- Use simple incentives to reward good behaviour
- Use instructions like 'If you (do this or that) … then we/I can do such and such' (not the other way round)
- Avoid threats that cannot be carried out
- Follow through with any consequences you indicated for non-compliance
- Ignore some episodes of defiance if they are not significant

Box 23.8 Analysing a tantrum

- **A**ntecedents – what happened in the minutes before the episode
- **B**ehaviour – exactly what did the episode consist of
- **C**onsequences – what happened as a result, including what you did and the outcome.

Box 23.9 Tantrums: management strategies

- Affection and attention before the tantrum
- Distraction
- Avoiding antecedents
- Ignoring:
  - Effective but can be difficult
  - No surrender (when parents give in, tantrums become harder to deal with over time)
- Time out from positive reinforcement:
  - Walk away, returning when quietens down
  - Separate from siblings
  - Put on a 'naughty chair' for a short time
- Holding firmly if the child is putting themselves or others in danger
- Star chart to prevent future episodes.

Temper tantrums are ordinary responses to frustration, especially at not being allowed to have or do something. They are common and normal in young preschool children. If asked for advice, a sensible first move is to take a history, analysing a couple of tantrums according to the ABC paradigm (Box 23.8). Next, examine the child to identify potential medical or psychological factors. Medical factors include global or language delay, hearing impairment (e.g. glue ear) and medication with bronchodilators or anticonvulsants. If none are present, there are management strategies that can be adopted, some of which are shown in Box 23.9.

The easiest course of action is to distract the child or, if this cannot be done, to let the tantrum burn itself out while the parent leaves the room, returning a few minutes later when things quieten down (provided it is safe to leave the child alone). Obviously this should be done in a calm, neutral manner and certainly not accompanied by threats of abandonment. Tantrums which are essentially coercive (when a child is demanding something from a parent) must be met by a refusal to give in. They can often be forestalled by the simple expedient of making rules which the child can be reminded of before the situation presents itself. An alternative course is to use 'time out', which is a form of structured ignoring. The child in a tantrum is placed somewhere such as the hallway, where no-one will talk to him for a short time, e.g. 1 min per year of age. During this period they are ignored completely. Parents

often expect this manoeuvre to produce a contrite child, complaining if it does not do so immediately. In fact, when used for tantrums, time out works according to different principles (not as a response to punishment but to the withdrawal of attention) and often takes several weeks to effect a gradual improvement. It may help to ask the mother to keep records to document this.

Disobedience can be dealt with by using a star chart to reward the child for complying with parental requests. The chart needs to be where the child can see it and it must be the case that the child knows what to do in order to get a star. It is wisest not to 'fine' the child by taking stars away once they have been earned. If the parent who is rewarding compliance by the child praises at the same time as giving the star, there may not be the need to tie stars with a material reward. However, if a tangible reward had been promised for a certain number of stars, it is important to follow through with this.

For temper tantrums

- **Analyse according to antecedents, behaviour and consequences**
- **Consider distraction, avoiding antecedents, ignoring and time out.**

Aggressive behaviour

Small children can be aggressive for a host of reasons, ranging from spite to exuberance. Much aggressive behaviour is learned, either by being rewarded (often inadvertently) or by copying parents, siblings or peers. For example, many instances of aggressive, demanding behaviour are provoked or intensified by a parent shouting at or hitting their child. In such cases, it is the parent's behaviour which needs to change. In most instances, the same principles as apply to tantrums are valid: make rules clear, stick to them, keep cool, do not give in and use time out if necessary. The latter can often be used on a 1–2–3 principle (Fig. 23.4). A tired or stressed child will be irritable and prone to

The 1–2–3 principle for tantrums or aggressive behaviour

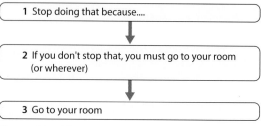

1 Stop doing that because....

2 If you don't stop that, you must go to your room (or wherever)

3 Go to your room

Figure 23.4 The 1–2–3 principle for tantrums or aggressive behaviour.

angry outbursts, as will children whose communication skills are compromised by deafness or a developmental language disorder so that they are frustrated and exasperated. Optimistic reassurance that the child will spontaneously grow out of a pattern of aggressive behaviour is mistaken; once established, an aggressive behavioural style is remarkably persistent over a period of years. Thus, aggressive behaviour in children needs to be proactively managed. There are several evidence-based parenting programmes that are effective for teaching parents to manage aggression in their children. Parents should be encouraged to attend such programmes.

Autism

This is considered in Chapter 4.

Problems of middle childhood

Nocturnal enuresis

Children can wet themselves by day or night, but in colloquial speech, 'enuresis' is synonymous with bedwetting. It is quite common: about 6% of 5-year-olds and 3% of 10-year-olds are not dry at night. Boys outnumber girls by nearly 2 to 1. There is a genetically determined delay in acquiring sphincter competence, with two-thirds of children with enuresis having an affected first-degree relative. There may also be interference in learning to become dry at night. Small children need reasonable freedom from stress and a measure of parental approval in order to learn night-time continence. It is well recognised that emotional stress can interfere and cause secondary enuresis (relapse after a period of dryness). Most children with enuresis are psychologically normal and the treatment of secondary enuresis still relies mainly on the symptomatic approach described below, although any underlying stress, emotional or physical disorder must be addressed.

Organic causes of enuresis are uncommon but include:

- Urinary tract infection
- Faecal retention severe enough to reduce bladder volume and cause bladder neck dysfunction
- Polyuria from osmotic diuresis, e.g. diabetes mellitus, or renal concentrating disorders, e.g. chronic renal failure.

A urine sample should always be tested for glucose and protein and checked for infection. Daytime and secondary enuresis are considered in Chapter 18.

The management of nocturnal enuresis is straightforward but needs to be painstaking to succeed. After the age of 4 years, enuresis resolves spontaneously in only 5% of affected children each year. In practice, treatment is rarely undertaken before 6 years of age.

Explanation

The first step is to explain to both child and parent that the problem is common and beyond conscious control. The parents should stop punitive procedures, as these are counterproductive.

Star chart

The child earns praise and a star each morning if the bed is dry. Wet beds are treated in a matter-of-fact way and the child is not blamed for them.

Enuresis alarm

If a child does not respond to a star chart, it may be supplemented with an enuresis alarm. This is a sensor, usually placed in the child's pants or under the child, which sounds an alarm when it becomes wet. In order to be effective, the alarm must wake the child, who gets out of bed, goes to pass urine, returns and helps to remake a wet bed before going back to sleep. It is not necessary to reset the alarm that night. Parental help can be enlisted in the night using a baby alarm to transmit the noise of the alarm to the parents' bedroom.

The alarm method takes several weeks to achieve dryness but is effective in most cases so long as the child is motivated and the procedure is followed fully. About one-third relapse after a few months, in which case repeat treatment with the alarm usually produces lasting dryness.

Desmopressin

Short-term relief from bedwetting, e.g. for holidays or sleepovers, can be achieved by the use of the synthetic analogue of antidiuretic hormone, desmopressin, taken as tablets or sublingually. This achieves a suppressant effect rather than a lasting cure.

Self-help groups

These provide advice and assistance to parents and health professionals, e.g. the Enuresis Resource and Information Centre (ERIC).

Summary

Nocturnal enuresis

- Common, males more than females
- Most affected children are psychologically and physically normal
- Treatment usually considered only at >6 years of age
- Management – explanation, star charts, enuresis alarm, sometimes desmopressin.

Faecal soiling

It is abnormal for a child to soil after the age of 4 years. Thereafter, children who soil fall into two broad groups: those with and those without a rectum loaded with faeces. Because of this, it is important to ascertain whether there is faecal retention by abdominal palpation. The reasons why a child's rectum becomes loaded are various, and commonly involve an interplay between constitutional factors and experience. Some children have a rectum that only empties occasionally, perhaps because of poor coordination with anal sphincter relaxation, and are thus more prone to developing retention. Superimposed upon this are a number of other factors:

- Constipation, possibly following dehydration during an illness
- Inhibition of defecation because of pain from a fissure
- Inhibition because of fear of punishment for incontinence
- Anxieties about using the toilet.

Once established, a huge bolus of hard faeces may be beyond the capacity of the child to shift. Furthermore, a rectum loaded with hard or soft faeces (both are found) dilates and habituates to distension so that the child becomes unaware of the need to empty it. The loaded rectum inhibits the anus via the rectoanal reflex and stool may seep out with spontaneous rectal contractions beyond the child's control. Soiling occurs in the child's pants, which may then be removed and hidden out of shame.

Any reasons for faecal retention, such as an anal fissure, should be identified and treated, but the most important thing is to empty the rectum as soon as possible. The child and parents need to understand that retention is present and how it leads to incontinence.

A stool softener (macrogol) is given for a couple of weeks, followed, if necessary, by a stimulant laxative (docusate, sodium picosulphate or senna) and an osmotic laxative (lactulose). Sometimes an enema is required. Once the rectum is disimpacted, maintenance laxative therapy is maintained (see Fig. 13.14 for details). The child can be encouraged to defecate regularly in the toilet, which earns stars on a star chart. Such retraining may take a number of weeks while the distended rectum shrinks to a normal size. Throughout this period a regular laxative is usually needed. The stars may therefore need to be cashed in for tangible rewards such as extra pocket money in order to maintain the incentive.

In some cases, repeated soiling will have been such a humiliating experience for the child that they psychologically deny there is a problem and cooperation is doubtful. Other children find that their involuntary soiling allows them a measure of control over parents and they are reluctant to surrender an apparently useful weapon. Such cases may need psychiatric referral.

Soiling may occur in conjunction with an empty rectum for various other uncommon reasons. Some children have an urgency of defecation for apparently constitutional reasons and can only postpone defecation for a few minutes; they can be taken by surprise. Some children have neuropathic bowel secondary to occult spinal abnormality, usually associated with urinary incontinence. Similarly, diarrhoea can overwhelm bowel control. The child may have a general learning disability with a mental age below 4 years, so that expectations of social bowel control need to be revised accordingly. Lastly, the child may defecate intentionally as a hostile act. Such children may be entrenched in distorted relationships with their parents and may have other behavioural problems requiring psychiatric referral.

> ## Summary
>
> ### Faecal retention
> - Present in most children who soil
> - May be due to constipation or reluctance to open the bowels because of pain or reluctance to use the toilet
> - When present, the rectum needs to be emptied, initially with a stool softener and laxative, followed by retraining.

Recurrent unexplained somatic symptoms/somatisation

Recurrent medically unexplained (functional somatic) symptoms are common in childhood and adolescence. In many cases, they are aggravated by stress but they can also be the expression of an anxiety or depressive disorder. Somatisation is the term used for the communication of emotional distress, troubled relationships and personal predicaments through bodily symptoms. The prepubertal child may experience affective distress as recurrent abdominal pain (this symptom peaking at age 9 years) and headaches (peaking at age 12 years). With increasing age, limb pain, aching muscles, fatigue and neurological symptoms become more prominent.

Recurrent central abdominal pain, often sharp and colicky, affects about 10% of school-age children. The causes are considered in Chapter 13. In the majority of cases, no organic cause can be objectively demonstrated, yet the child is obviously in pain. Some will have an emotional cause for their pain, but in many, no aetiology, medical or psychiatric, can be demonstrated.

The history must attend to possible sources of stress and the child should be interviewed about school, friends and family, noting the general level of anxiety and ability to communicate. This should be an integral part of the interview and not done as an afterthought when organic causes have been excluded. A thorough physical examination is important to reassure the child and family that there is no underlying organic cause. It also provides an opportunity to gain further information about the nature of the pain and the child's reaction to it. When examining the child, it is sensible to ask the child to point to where the pain is. In general, the further the pain is from the umbilicus, the more likely it is being caused by organic pathology (Apley's rule).

The pain may be limited to school days or coincide with upsetting events in the home, such as parental conflict, or other specific situations. A short interview with the child on their own can reveal sources of stress which may be otherwise unrecognised by parents or which the child is wary of mentioning in front of them. Problems at school, particularly bullying and teasing, or difficulties with a teacher or class work may only be known by the child. A report from the school may be helpful. A joint interview with both parents and the child is a good arena for explaining to the child and family how organic disease has been ruled out and, if appropriate, how tension can give rise to pain using familiar examples such as headache. It is often necessary to promote communication between family members to avoid any tendency for somatic symptoms to replace verbal communication of distress. Learning pain-coping skills, such as relaxation, may be helpful, especially for headaches. Referral to child and adolescent mental health services is indicated if any identified stressors cannot be relieved by straightforward means, if there is serious family dysfunction, or if the pain impairs the child's general functioning at home or school.

Summary

Somatic symptoms

- May be a means of communicating emotional distress
- Sources of stress should be identified, and ameliorated if possible
- In many children with unexplained recurrent abdominal pain or headaches, no significant sources of stress are identified.

Tics

A tic is a quick, sudden, coordinated movement, which is apparently purposeful and recurs in the same part of the child's body. It is not entirely involuntary in that it can be purposefully suppressed to some extent. About 1 in 10 children develop a tic at some stage, typically around the face and head – blinking, frowning, head-flicking, sniffing, throat clearing and grunting being the commonest. They are most likely to occur when the child is inactive (watching TV or on long car journeys) and often disappear when actively concentrating. They may worsen with anxiety but they are not themselves an emotional reaction. In most cases, there is a family history. These simple, *transient childhood tics* clear up over the next few months, although they may recur from time to time. They should be treated with reassurance in the first place.

Less commonly, the child has tics from which he/she is hardly ever free. They may be multiple, although there is fluctuation in the predominance of any particular tic and in overall severity. This is a chronic tic disorder which, if it includes both multiple motor tics and vocal tics such as hooting, yelping or swearing, is known as *Gilles de la Tourette's* syndrome. These conditions tend to be persistent in the medium term, requiring medication (such as clonidine or risperidone) under specialist supervision.

Hyperactivity

Young children are characteristically lively, some more than others, by virtue of their immaturity. When their level of motor activity exceeds that regarded as normal, they may be termed 'hyperactive' by their parents. This is a judgement that depends upon the parents' standards and expectations. The term can thus incorrectly be used as a complaint about a child who is normally active in overall terms but who can be cheeky and boisterous at times. Such a child is *not* hyperactive, but the parents need advice about how to handle unwanted behaviour.

In the true *hyperkinetic disorder* or *attention deficit hyperactivity disorder* (ADHD), the child is undoubtedly overactive in most situations and has impaired concentration with a short attention span or distractibility. Differences in diagnostic criteria and threshold mean that prevalence rates among prepubertal schoolchildren are variously estimated as between 10 and 50 per 1000 children, boys exceeding girls three-fold. There is a powerful genetic predisposition and the underlying problem is a dysfunction of brain neuron circuits that rely on dopamine as a neurotransmitter and which control self-monitoring and self-regulation.

Affected children are unable to sustain attention or persist with tasks. They cannot control their impulses – they manifest disorganised, poorly-regulated and excessive activity; have difficulty with taking turns; sharing; are socially disinhibited; and butt into other people's conversations and play. Their inattention and hyperactivity are worst in familiar or uninteresting situations. They also cannot regulate their activity according to the situation – they are fidgety; have excessive movements inappropriate to task completion; lose possessions; and are generally disorganised. Typically, they have short tempers and form poor relationships with other children, who find them exasperating.

The children do poorly in school and lose self-esteem. They may drift into antisocial activities for a variety of reasons, partly because their behaviour drives parents, teachers and peers to use coercion and punishment, which is ineffectual or breeds resentment.

In addition to child psychiatric or paediatric evaluation, the child will usually need to be assessed by an educational psychologist.

First-line management in preschool children and school-aged children with mild to moderately severe disorder is the active promotion of behavioural and educational progress by specific advice to parents and teachers to build concentration skills, encourage quiet self-occupation, increase self-esteem and moderate extreme behaviour. Behavioural interventions similar to those embedded in parenting programmes are helpful. These involve having clear rules and expectations, and consistent use of rewards to encourage adherence and where appropriate, consequences to discourage unacceptable behaviour.

For those children in whom this is insufficient, hyperactivity responds symptomatically to several types of medication, although this is usually reserved for children older than 6 years of age. Stimulants such as methylphenidate or dexamphetamine and non-stimulants, like atomoxetine, reduce excessive motor activity and improve attention on task, focused behaviour. The usual approach is not to put the child on medication until behavioural and educational progress is actively promoted by the specific measures mentioned above. However, in severe cases with high degrees of impairment, simultaneous psychosocial and medical treatment may be required. It may be necessary to continue medication for several years, sometimes into adulthood. Yearly trial off medication is recommended to evaluate the need for continuing treatment. Specialist supervision is mandatory. Close liaison with the school is required throughout the years of treatment.

The role of diet in the cause and management of hyperactivity is controversial. Current evidence indicates that the sort of diet which aims blindly to reduce sugar, artificial additives or colourants has no effect. A few children display an idiosyncratic behavioural reaction such as excitability or irritability to particular foods. If this seems likely, trying the child on an exclusion of that particular food may be useful. In general, food and drinks with caffeine are not advised. Overzealous dietary exclusion can lead to malnutrition, especially in a child on stimulant medication that may already have the side-effect of appetite reduction.

Summary

Attention deficit hyperactivity disorder (ADHD)

- Affects males more than females
- Clinical features: cannot sustain attention, excessively active, socially disinhibited, easily distracted and impulsive, may be poor at relationships, prone to temper tantrums, poor school performance
- Management: educational psychologist assessment, behavioural programmes in school, parenting intervention, medication if necessary.

Antisocial behaviour

Children steal, lie, disobey, light fires, destroy things and pick fights for various reasons:

- Failure to learn when to exercise social restraint
- Lack of social skills, such as the ability to negotiate a disagreement
- They may be responding to the challenges of their peers in spite of their parents' prohibitions
- They may be chronically angry and resentful
- They may find their own notions of good behaviour overwhelmed by emotion such as sadness or temptation.

When serious antisocial behaviour which infringes the rights of others is the dominant feature of the clinical picture and is so severe as to represent a handicap to general functioning, a diagnosis of *conduct disorder* is made. Children with conduct disorder may not have necessarily broken the law, although their behaviour excites strong social disapproval. They typically come from homes in which there are considerable discord, coercive relationships, limited boundaries that are inconsistently enforced, and poor supervision by adults. A milder form, characterised by angry, defiant behaviour to authority figures such as parents and teachers, is known as *oppositional-defiant disorder (ODD)*.

Treating conduct disorder can be difficult. Parent management training programmes (such as Webster–Stratton and Triple P) have an excellent evidence base and are highly recommended as primary interventions. However, poor parental cooperation and motivation can result in minimal benefit. Where parents are unwilling or unable to take up parenting programmes, affected children can be offered individual or group-based interventions focusing on problem-solving skills and anger management. Although these interventions show benefit in research settings, affected children do not often have the level of motivation required to benefit in routine clinic settings. In the absence of a coexisting psychiatric condition responsive to medication, it is not considered standard clinical practice to use medication for conduct disorder in the UK.

Summary

Antisocial behaviour

- It is important to exclude any coexisting psychiatric condition and treat this directly, e.g. ADHD or depression
- Parenting groups are an evidence-based treatment for these disorders, but require motivation.

Anxiety

Pathological anxiety exists in two forms: specific and general. In phobias there is fear of a specific object or situation that is excessive and handicapping and cannot be dealt with by reassurance. Most children have a number of irrational fears (the dark, ghosts, kidnappers, dogs, spiders, bats, snakes) which are common and do not usually handicap the child's ordinary life. Some of these persist into adulthood. If they are so severe that the child's ability to lead an ordinary life is affected, then treatment by cognitive behavioural therapy with graded exposure to the feared event may be indicated and is usually successful.

More diffuse general anxiety presents indirectly in childhood and it is uncommon for a child to complain directly about anxiety. Often, it is first manifest as physical complaints: nausea, headache or pain. It may take the form of health worries and the child repeatedly asks for reassurance that he is not going to die. Some children with generalised anxiety may develop unusual coping strategies that appear manipulative, in an attempt to gain control over their parents and the world in general. It may be a justifiable reaction to an event or situation, or be disproportionate. If the condition follows a recognisable precipitant such as a parental illness and the parents can be directed to provide comfort and support, prognosis is good. If it arises insidiously, specialist mental health referral is indicated.

 Children rarely say spontaneously that they are anxious – instead they tend to complain of aches and pains or behave in apparently manipulative ways to cope with or avoid the feared situation.

School refusal

During the years of compulsory school attendance, a child may be absent from school because of illness, because parents keep the child off school or because of truancy in which the child chooses to do something else rather than attend school. In truancy, a child leaves to go to school but never arrives or leaves early. It is often accompanied by other behavioural difficulties. A few non-attendees at school suffer from *school refusal*, an inability to attend school on account of overwhelming anxiety. Such children may not complain of anxiety but of its physical concomitants or the consequences of hyperventilation. Anxiety may present as complaints of nausea, headache or otherwise not being well, which are confined to weekday, term-time mornings, clearing up by midday. It may be rational, as when the child is being bullied or there is educational underachievement. If it is disproportionate to stresses at school, it is termed school refusal, an anxiety problem with two common causes – separation anxiety from parents persisting beyond the toddler years and anxiety provoked by some aspect of school, true school phobia. These can coexist.

School refusal based on separation anxiety is typical of children under the age of about 11 years. It may be provoked by an adverse life event such as illness, a death in the family or a move of house. The child is unable to tolerate separation from their attachment figure without whom the child cannot go anywhere, including school. Treatment is aimed at gently promoting increasing separations from the parents (e.g. staying overnight with relatives or friends), while arranging an early return to school. Some adolescents with school refusal have a depressive disorder, but more usually there is an interaction between an anxiety disorder and long-standing personality issues such as intolerance of uncertainty.

True school phobia is seen in slightly older, anxious children who are frequently uncommunicative and stubborn.

The management of school refusal is shown in Box 23.10.

Educational underachievement

Children who achieve less well in school than expected are sometimes brought to doctors. It is important to evaluate parents' and teachers' expectations and

Box 23.10 Treatment of school refusal

- Advise and support parents and school about the condition
- Treat any underlying emotional disorder
- Plan and facilitate an early and graded return to school at a pace tolerable for the child with all involved (child, family, teachers, educational psychologist and educational welfare officers)
- Help the parents make it more rewarding for the child to return to school than stay at home
- Address bullying or educational difficulties if present.

Box 23.11 Causes of underachievement at school

Long-standing problem

- Visual problems
- Hearing problems
- Dyslexia
- Generalised or specific learning problems
- Hyperactivity
- Anti-education family background
- Chaotic family background

Recent onset of problem

- Preoccupations (parental divorce, bullying, etc.)
- Fatigue
- Depression
- Rebellion against teacher, parents or 'swot' label
- Unsuspected poor attendance at school
- Sexual abuse
- Drug abuse
- Prodromal period of a psychotic illness (rare)
- Degenerative brain condition, rare but important.

ensure the child is actually able to rise to them. The services of an educational psychologist are indispensable. Core medical responsibilities include testing sight and hearing and attempting to elicit the cause of underachievement according to the list in Box 23.11. The topic is considered further in Chapter 4.

Adolescence

Although a popular image of adolescence is one of angry, rebellious teenagers, alienated from their parents and embroiled in emotional turmoil, studies show that most adolescents maintain good relationships with their parents. They do, however, tend to bicker with them about minor domestic matters and what they are allowed to do. Minor psychological symptoms such as moodiness or social sensitivity are quite common (as they are in adults), but serious psychiatric problems are no more prevalent than in adult life. Family relationships are often influenced by teenagers' negotiation of their own autonomy, the emergence of their own sense of themselves and the first moves towards a personal identity. At the same time, their parents may be experiencing mid-life crises of confidence in career, physical appearance or sexuality, so that parental and teenage preoccupations coincide, not always helpfully.

Cognitive style

The style of thought specifically associated with adolescence is formal operational (abstract) thought (Box 23.12), but this is acquired at various ages by different individuals during the teenage years, and a substantial minority do not develop it at all. Doctors are at a disadvantage here, as they have been selected by a series of examinations for excellence of their ability to manipulate abstractions and compare hypothetical predictions; they have often forgotten what it is like to think otherwise and communicate poorly with patients who still think concretely and practically (school-age children, about half of all teenagers and perhaps 1 in 5 adults). When interviewing adolescents, the skill is to avoid being patronising, while being sensitive as to whether abstract and reflective thought is solidly achieved. Using practical examples (not metaphors) and checking whether you have been understood will help to avoid the common problem of being faced with an adolescent who responds to questions with a sullen 'don't know'. This is considered further in Chapter 28.

Anorexia nervosa

Dieting to slim is endemic among teenage girls. Part of the reason for this is the contemporary equation between thinness and attractiveness, an assumption prevalent in advertising and fashion. Resonant with this is the finding that most teenage girls (but very few boys) overestimate their body width and depth, perceiving and judging themselves as fatter than they actually are.

Slimming through self-imposed calorie restriction is usually self-limiting because the goal is achieved or because the girl gives up; hunger wins through. In some girls, however, the slimming process takes over and there supervenes what has been called a 'relentless pursuit of thinness', typically with a phobic horror of normal body weight and shape. This is *anorexia nervosa*, and the features are:

- Self-induced weight loss resulting in a low body mass index (BMI); in children this needs to be plotted on a BMI centile chart, in older adolescents it is ≤17.5 kg/m^2
- A distorted perception of her body, which increases with weight loss
- A determined attempt to lose weight or avoid weight gain, by either restricting food intake, self-induced vomiting, laxative abuse, excessive exercising or using a combination of these methods
- When body weight falls below a critical point, pubertal development is halted and reversed so that menstruation ceases and the girl effectively becomes a prepubertal child. This may spare her some of the challenges of adolescence, particularly those related to sexuality
- The discovery by a girl who has felt powerless that through self-starvation she can control her shape and development and thus increase her sense of self-worth and self-effectiveness
- Preoccupations and dreams of food and cooking which come to dominate mental life as a response to starvation. There ensues a tremendous mental struggle not to give in and eat, which assumes prime importance in the girl's mental life
- The dramatic and visible effects of self-starvation on the girl, which can unite some parents in caring for their daughter and save a discordant marriage from divorce, something which she may fear is imminent.

An affected girl will often deny hunger, reassure everyone that she is in the peak of health, exercise to lose weight and disagree fervently that she is too thin. She will be careless of her own emaciation and seem unconcerned that she is starving herself to death. To the bewilderment of her parents, she may cook for others and read cookery books avidly. She may well be deceitful to anyone she perceives as thwarting her in her quest. Thus, she will conceal her poor eating by secretly disposing of her meals or lying about her weight. Both before and during her illness she will show obsessional, perfectionist character traits; without these she would not have the capacity to establish herself as a persistent dieter. Indeed, she is likely to be described as having been quiet, compliant and hard-working, 'the last person to develop anorexia nervosa'. Her parents will often present as nice people who avoid conflict.

As a result of starvation, her body develops a low metabolic rate with slow-to-relax tendon reflexes, reduced peripheral circulation, bradycardia and amenorrhea. Fine lanugo hair appears over her trunk and limbs. She does not lose pubic or axillary hair, although incompletely established puberty is delayed. Serum T$_3$ (triiodothyronine) may be low, giving rise to a false suspicion of hypothyroidism. Plasma proteins are sometimes low and ankle oedema not uncommon. Blood and urine levels of luteinising hormone and follicle-stimulating hormone are low and non-cyclical.

Some girls discover that self-restraint in carbohydrate intake can be bypassed by self-induced vomiting following repeated bouts of overeating and that further weight loss can be achieved by diuretics, and laxatives (in the belief that these will expedite food transit time and reduce absorption). This can cause wide fluctuations in weight and metabolic abnormalities such as hypokalaemia and alkalosis. This condition is *bulimia* which can occur at normal body weight or in association with low body weight as an ominous complication of anorexia nervosa. It tends to affect older rather than younger teenagers. Bulimia at normal body weight can be managed by encouraging a regular diet, monitoring this by a diary and providing individual or group cognitive behavioural therapy.

The prevalence rate among teenagers for anorexia nervosa is a little less than 1%, but the incidence rate may have increased over the last 50 years. The peak age of onset is 14 and girls outnumber boys by about 10:1. Bulimia is commoner, although prevalence rates vary widely, depending on the degree of severity. It also shows a markedly female preponderance and may also be becoming more frequent.

Management

Management is two-fold: medical and psychological. The initial management of anorexia nervosa is to restore near-normal body weight by refeeding. The emergence of physical complications may necessitate admission to hospital for refeeding, which may even involve nasogastric tube feeding in some instances. The cornerstone of treatment is family therapy. Individual psychological treatment is introduced to help the young person challenge the cognitions that drive anorexia and to acquire more constructive ways of confronting developmental demands, including handling conflict, maintaining self-esteem, personal autonomy and relationships.

Medical aspects

Anorexia has a high mortality rate compared with other psychiatric disorders. Some of the excess mortality arise from medical complications such as malnutrition, electrolyte imbalance and infection. This emphasises the importance of thorough physical examination, investigations and medical management. In the UK, NICE (National Institute for Health and Clinical Excellence) has produced a guideline for treatment of eating disorders including the physical management of anorexia nervosa.

Prognosis

The prognosis for children and adolescents is variable, with as many as 50% failing to make a full recovery. Factors predicting a poorer outcome include a low BMI and physical complications prior to treatment, bulimic symptoms, especially self-induced vomiting, as well as family disturbance, and interpersonal difficulties. Anorexia has the highest mortality of all psychiatric disorders. In addition to medical complications, the next important cause of mortality is suicide.

Chronic fatigue syndrome

Chronic fatigue syndrome (CFS) refers to persisting high levels of subjective fatigue, leading to rapid exhaustion on minimal physical or mental exertion. The term is broader and more neutral than the specific pathology or aetiology implied by myalgic encephalomyelitis (ME) or post-viral fatigue syndrome, which follows an apparently viral febrile illness. There is sometimes serological evidence of recent infection with coxsackie B or Epstein–Barr virus (EBV) or a hepatitis virus. Some cases have no history or evidence of a precipitating infection and there are no specific diagnostic tests. The clinical picture is somewhat diffuse and there are no pathognomonic symptoms. Myalgia, migratory arthralgia, headache, difficulty getting off to sleep, poor concentration and irritability are virtually universal. Stomach pains, scalp tenderness, eye pain and photophobia, and tender cervical lymphadenopathy are frequently encountered. Depressive symptoms are common and there is continuing debate as to how much of the clinical picture is physical and how much psychological. Usually parents insist on there being a physical cause and there is a risk that the doctor will carry out excessive unnecessary investigations. Most experienced doctors now regard the final clinical picture as resulting from both physical and psychological factors.

The majority of cases will remit spontaneously with time, but this takes months or sometimes years. Earlier recommendations of continuous rest have been shown to be unhelpful and can lead to secondary complications. The recommended treatment involves graded exercise therapy and/or cognitive behavioural therapy. Graded exercise therapy is usually provided by physiotherapists and aims to achieve gradual increase in exercise tolerance. If too much pressure is put upon the

Summary

In anorexia nervosa

- Female:male ratio is 10:1
- Peak age of onset – 14 years
- Affected girls have a distorted body image, so seldom agree that they are too thin and may deceive everyone by pretending to eat
- Features include: determined efforts to lose weight, arrest of puberty, cessation of periods
- May be accompanied by bulimia: overeating followed by self-induced vomiting
- Management is family therapy and individual therapy to restore body weight
- Some require hospitalisation; prognosis is variable, but has a mortality from suicide, malnutrition and infection.

Summary

In chronic fatigue syndrome

- There is exhaustion on minimal exertion
- There is thought to be a combination of physical and psychological factors
- Management is with graded exercise and/or cognitive behavioural therapy, but recovery may take months or years.

child, tantrums or mute withdrawal can occur. Argument about how much of the condition is physical and how much psychological is unhelpful. The parents and the child need continuing support to maintain as much of a normal life as possible, including school attendance. The mood of children with depressive symptoms may respond to antidepressant medication, but this is a treatment only for depressive symptoms and it is unlikely to result in alleviation of the fatigability. NICE guidelines are available.

Depression

Low mood can arise secondary to adverse circumstances or sometimes spontaneously. Depression as a clinical condition is more than sadness and misery; it extends to affect motivation, judgement, the ability to experience pleasure and provokes emotions of guilt and despair. It may disturb sleep, appetite and weight. It leads to social withdrawal, an important sign. Such a state is well recognised among adolescents, particularly girls, but occasionally affects prepubertal children. The general picture is comparable to depression in adults but there are differences (Box 23.13).

A diagnosis of depression depends crucially upon interviewing the adolescent on his own, as well as taking a history from the parents. Teenagers will, out of loyalty, often pretend to their parents that things are all right if interviewed in their presence. It is necessary to ask about feelings directly and to ask specifically about suicidal ideas and plans.

Treatment depends upon severity. Children with mild depression are managed initially in primary care and other non-specialist mental health settings. Many will recover spontaneously; hence a period of watchful waiting for up to 4 weeks may be appropriate. Alternatively, the child could be offered non-directive supportive therapy or guided self-help. However, if mild depression does not respond to these measures in 2–3 months, the child should be referred to specialist mental health services. Similarly, children with moderate and severe depression should be referred to specialist mental health services for more specific psychological intervention such as cognitive behavioural therapy, family therapy or interpersonal therapy. In all cases, any identified contributing factor such as bullying needs to be addressed. If psychological therapy for moderate or severe depression is insufficient after 6 weeks, then an SSRI (selective serotonin reuptake inhibitor antidepressant), fluoxetine, should be considered. Depressed young people who are suicidal may need admission to an adolescent psychiatric in-patient unit.

Self-harm

Like adults, young people who take overdoses do so for a variety of motives, of which suicide is the most serious one. For a high proportion, the overdose is a desperate gesture which may draw attention to a predicament perceived by them as irresolvable. Issues such as bullying or abuse should be considered. About half of teenagers who overdose are clinically depressed. Episodes of self-harm must be taken seriously as they carry significant risk of recurrence and suicide.

In those who have taken an overdose, a full psychiatric assessment is needed by a mental health professional. A useful adjunct in the assessment of suicide risk is the PATHOS score shown in Box 23.14; however, this needs to occur alongside a psychiatric assessment.

Drug misuse

Most teenagers are exposed to illicit drugs at some stage. A number will then experiment with them, some becoming habitual users. Usually, this is for recreational purposes, but a few use them to avoid unpleasant feelings or memories. A very small number become dependent, psychologically or physically. What is taken varies with culture and opportunity but alcohol and cannabis are common; solvents, LSD, ecstasy and amphetamine derivatives somewhat less so; and cocaine or heroin currently least prevalent, though their use is increasing. The addictive potential of the

---

Box 23.13 Features of depression in adolescents

More common than adults

- Apathy, boredom and an inability to enjoy oneself rather than depressed mood
- Separation anxiety which reappears, having resolved in earlier life
- Decline in school performance
- Social withdrawal
- Hypochondriacal ideas and complaints of pain in chest, abdomen and head
- Irritable mood or frankly antisocial behaviour

Less common than adults

- Loss of appetite and weight
- Loss of sleep
- Loss of libido
- Slowing of thought and movement
- Delusional ideas.

Box 23.14 PATHOS instrument to assess suicide risk after adolescent overdose

- **P:** Have you had **P**roblems for longer than a month?
- **A:** Were you **A**lone in the house at the time?
- **T:** Did you plan the overdose for longer than **T**hree hours?
- **HO:** Are you feeling **Ho**peless about the future?
- **S:** Were you feeling **S**ad for most of the time before the overdose?

Score 1 for Yes; 0 for No and add together. Child at high risk if score >2. However, the final judgement of suicide risk is a clinical and qualitative decision, not one based on a cut-off score.

Source: Kingsbury S. 1996. PATHOS: a screening instrument for adolescent overdose: a research note. *Journal of Child Psychology and Psychiatry* 37:609–611.

last two is the greatest and their dangers are well known.

Abuse implies heavy misuse. The signs vary with the agent but may include:

- Intoxication
- Unexplained absences from home or school
- Mixing with known users
- High rates of spending or stealing money
- Possession of the equipment required for drug use
- Medical complications associated with use.

Doctors may be approached by parents worried that their adolescent child may be abusing drugs. An assessment will involve interviewing the adolescent, possibly combined with taking a urine sample for drug screening. Most areas have specific services for adolescents with drug and/or alcohol problems. These services usually take self-referrals so that young people with these difficulties can access them directly. Medical involvement is predominantly focused on users who have other psychopathology including depression, or with the physical consequences of intoxication or injection when these threaten health. Solvent abuse (mainly glue and aerosol sniffing) is quite widespread as a group activity of young adolescents in some areas. It can occasionally give rise to cardiac dysrhythmias, bone marrow suppression or renal failure, and any of these can cause death, as may a fall or road traffic accident when intoxicated. Cannabis and LSD use may trigger anxiety or psychotic disorders. Ecstasy taken at dances or raves can cause dangerous hyperthermia, dehydration and death.

Doctors need to ensure that any adolescent known to them who is thought to be using drugs knows the specific risks to health. Dependence is rare among teenagers and most likely to involve alcohol. The few who are using illicit drugs for respite from psychological distress need referral to a psychiatrist.

Psychosis

Psychosis is a breakdown in the perception and understanding of reality and a lack of awareness that the person is unwell. This can affect ideas and beliefs, resulting in delusional thinking where abnormal beliefs are held with an unshakeable quality and lead to odd behaviour. The connectedness and coherence of thoughts may break down, so that speech is hard to follow, leading to thought disorder. Perceptual abnormalities lead to hallucinations, where a perception is experienced in the absence of a stimulus.

Psychotic disorders include:

- Schizophrenia, where no specific medical cause is identified and there is generally no major disturbance of mood other than blunting or flattening of affect
- Bipolar affective disorder, where the psychosis is associated with lowered mood as in depression or elevation in mood as in mania
- Organic psychosis occurs in delirium, substance-induced disorders and dementia.

Both schizophrenia and bipolar affective disorder are rare before puberty, but increase in frequency of presentation during adolescence. In these disorders the psychotic symptoms occur in clear consciousness.

Investigations should include a urine drug screen, exclusion of medication-induced psychosis (e.g. high-dose stimulants or anticholinergic drugs), exclusion of medical causes (i.e. infection, seizures, thyroid abnormalities and sleep disorders) and dementia.

Where schizophrenia and bipolar disorder is suspected, urgent referral to a psychiatrist is needed for comprehensive assessment and treatment with antipsychotic medication, psycho-education, family therapy and, where appropriate, individual therapy. In the case of an organic psychosis the underlying cause needs to be treated promptly by the paediatric team, with help from mental health professionals as appropriate.

Psychosis

- **May present during adolescence**
- **May be precipitated by or be a consequence of substance abuse.**

Management of emotional and behavioural problems

For most emotional and behavioural problems, there is an interplay between adversities in the family, peer group and school and strengths or vulnerabilities in the child. Sometimes, these are referred to as risk (predisposing) factors (things that do not in themselves produce a disorder but will do so when interacting with other adversities). Conversely, they are less likely to do so if there is a compensating strength (such as high intelligence, good self-esteem, secure attachment, good peer relations or an emotionally warm relationship with a parent). An environmental adversity may be acute (a life event) or chronic. It challenges the coping skills of the child, and emotional or behavioural problems result if these are overwhelmed. The problem may resolve spontaneously or persist.

With this in mind, it is possible to talk about the three **P**s of causation:

- **P**redisposition (vulnerability)
- **P**recipitation (usually an adverse life event)
- **P**erpetuation (usually chronic stresses).

In clinical practice, a precipitant is what many people call the 'cause', but it is often the factors that perpetuate or maintain the problem that one has to deal with.

Cultural considerations

Many developed countries are increasingly ethnically diverse in relation to language, religion and culture. This diversity has many important clinical implications for child mental health. The first implication relates to the need to recognise the subgroup of young people who are refugees or asylum seekers. These children and their families have often experienced major traumatic events before arriving in their host country. They remain highly vulnerable to mental and social-economic adversities due to past and ongoing stressful experiences.

The second implication relates to well-recognised ethnic differences in the epidemiology of some psychiatric disorders. For example, among people of African and Caribbean origin living in Western European countries, there is a clear increase in the incidence of schizophrenia but a lower incidence of anorexia nervosa compared with the indigenous Caucasian population.

Another implication of culture relates to the presentation of psychiatric symptoms. It is well recognised that the content of obsessions in children with obsessive compulsive disorder is sometimes shaped by the child's cultural and religious beliefs. This is also true of some delusions in young people with psychotic disorders. In these examples, understanding the child's religious and cultural background is essential for making an accurate diagnosis.

There are also important cultural differences about normative behaviour in children and thresholds for help-seeking. Differences in the level of stigma attached to mental illness across cultures also influence parent's help-seeking behaviour and access to child and adolescent mental health services.

The above implications suggest that cultural awareness and sensitivity are essential skills for all clinicians working or intending to work in ethnically diverse societies. The key message is that the presentation of psychiatric distress in children and young people may be coloured by their culture and language. It is therefore essential to avoid making assumptions about the significance of clinical information with cultural or religious meaning but instead to contextualise the information to the patient's culture, for example, through the use of trained interpreters.

Assessment

It is best to interview both parents if possible. While doing so, consider the quality of their relationship and the parents' mental state. Ask open questions where possible and feel able to ask directly about feelings. Assess the attitudes of the parents to the child. Obtain examples of the problem and estimate its frequency, severity, duration and the impact it has on both the child and family.

Interview the child and ask to see the older child alone as part of the assessment. Explain to the parents that you always like to have a few words with children on their own as they may have things they may feel too embarrassed to discuss with parents present. Assess the extent of the child's suffering (they may be somewhat brazen and minimise this). Keep your questions very simple and specific, making sure the child understands what it is you want to know. This also applies to teenagers. Ask about use of drugs and alcohol, experience of abuse, thoughts of self-harm and suicide. Consider whether reports from school or other involved agencies might help. In many instances, it is worth asking the parents to keep a prospective record of the problem by means of a diary or chart which you can inspect in a few days' time. Tell them what headings you want this under (such as 'antecedents, behaviour and consequences' for temper tantrums).

Treatment

Figure 23.5 shows an approach to managing a child displaying an emotional or behavioural problem. The process of making a referral to a child and adolescent mental health service (CAMHS) is most likely to succeed if the referrer has already taken some of the history and engaged the parents and child in an attempt to alleviate the problem. Many doctors, general practitioners and paediatricians in particular, are good generalists in child mental health issues and the mental health specialist should be seen as a specialist extension of their expertise, rather than a completely different sort of person.

In general, the management of children's emotional and behavioural problems:

- should be psychological rather than pharmacological
- does not need the child to be admitted to hospital (unless required as a place of safety for suicidal children or for child protection)
- involves parents as key participants
- may involve a variety of health and social service professionals.

Often more than one intervention is required and treatments are combined and several professionals become

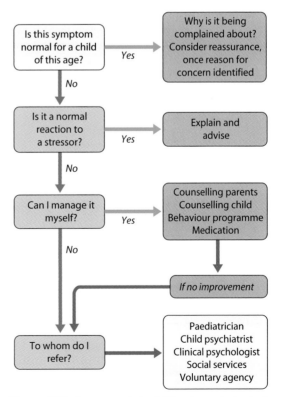

Figure 23.5 An approach to children's psychological problems.

Box 23.15 Main psychological treatment interventions employed for emotional and behavioural problems

Explanation and reassurance

Suitable for mild problems with a good prognosis arising in children from supportive families who can work out for themselves a sensible way of managing the problem until it subsides.

Counselling of child or parents

Used to provide non-directive, unstructured supportive therapy for children and families to aid coping with difficulties that are not severe enough to require specialist psychological interventions (e.g. bereavement counselling).

In parental counselling, the aim is to enhance parental coping not by telling the parent what to do but by helping them to find their own solutions, so increasing their confidence and effectiveness.

Parenting groups

Recently, parenting groups have become popular where a number of parents are seen together and given tools on how to play with their children and respond effectively to their challenging behaviour. Various approaches are rehearsed using role play and the facilitation of a therapist.

Behavioural therapy

A pragmatic approach to problems, which alters the environmental factors that trigger or maintain behaviours. It is particularly effective in the management of behavioural problems in young children.

Family therapy

Widely used by child mental health professionals. It uses a series of interviews with the entire household to alter dysfunctional patterns of relationships between family members on the basis that many children's problems are perpetuated by the ways in which family members live with and deal with each other.

Cognitive therapy

Used by specialists to explore the way thinking affects feelings and behaviour. It helps the young person to identify and challenge unhelpful thinking styles that perpetuate negative feelings and behaviour. Good evidence for efficacy in a range of disorders including depression.

Individual or group dynamic psychotherapy

More structured and intense extension of counselling, which can help children who, for example, have unconscious conflicts, which are manifest as relationship difficulties with a parent. Once the mainstay of child psychiatry, it is now less commonly used.

---

involved. The main treatment interventions employed are described in Box 23.15.

Medication plays a comparatively small role, although particular instances for which there is evidence for their efficacy are the use of stimulant and non-stimulant drugs in hyperkinetic disorder (ADHD), neuroleptics in psychosis and antidepressants for severely depressed adolescents. There is sometimes a temptation to sedate a child who is causing a problem but this is rarely effective and ethically questionable.

Further reading

Coghill D, Bonnar S, Duke S, et al: *Child and Adolescent Psychiatry*, Oxford Specialist Handbooks in Psychiatry, Oxford, 2009, Oxford University Press.

Goodman R, Scott S: *Child Psychiatry*, ed 2, Chichester, 2005, Wiley.

Lask B, Taylor S, Nunn K: *Practical Child Psychiatry*, London, 2003, BMJ Books.

Rutter M, Bishop D, Pine D, et al: *Rutter's Child and Adolescent Psychiatry*, Oxford, 2010, Blackwell.

24

Skin disorders

Features of skin disorders in children include:

- In the newborn, transient skin disorders are common but need to be distinguished from serious or permanent conditions
- Atopic eczema affects up to 20% of children
- Skin infections and infestations, especially viral warts and head lice, are common in school-aged children
- Acne is troublesome for many during adolescence.

The newborn

The skin at birth is covered with vernix caseosa. This chalky-white greasy coat, mainly composed of water, proteins and lipids, protects the skin in utero from the amniotic fluid. Shedding of vernix towards the end of gestation coincides with maturation of the transepidermal barrier. In the preterm infant, the skin is thin, poorly keratinised and lacks subcutaneous fat. Transepidermal water loss is markedly increased when compared with a term infant. The preterm infant is also unable to sweat until a few weeks old, whereas the term infant can sweat from birth.

Common naevi and rashes in the newborn period are described under the examination of the newborn infant (see Ch. 9). Some less common skin conditions presenting in the newborn period are described in this chapter.

Bullous impetigo

This is an uncommon but potentially serious blistering form of impetigo, the most superficial form of bacterial infection, seen particularly in the newborn (Fig. 24.1). It is most often caused by *Staphylococcus aureus*. Treatment is with systemic antibiotics, e.g. penicillinase-resistant penicillin (see also Ch. 14).

Melanocytic naevi (moles)

Congenital moles occur in up to 3% of neonates and any that are present are usually small. Congenital pigmented naevi involving extensive areas of skin (i.e. naevi >9 cm in diameter) are rare but disfiguring (Fig. 24.2) and carry a 4–6% lifetime risk of subsequent malignant melanoma. They require prompt referral to a paediatric dermatologist and plastic surgeon to assess the feasibility of removal.

Melanocytic naevi become increasingly common as children get older and the presence of large numbers

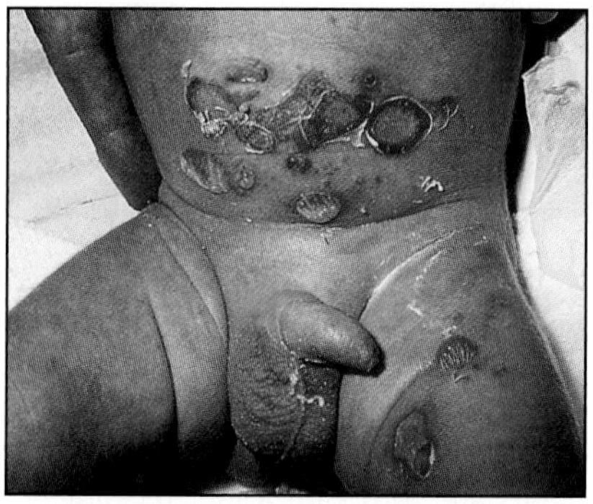

Figure 24.1 Bullous impetigo in a 2-week-old baby.

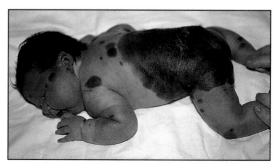

Figure 24.2 A large (giant) congenital pigmented hairy naevus. Other smaller naevi are also visible.

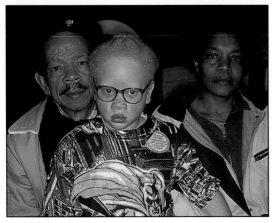

Figure 24.3 A child with oculocutaneous albinism, with her parents. The hair is silvery-white.

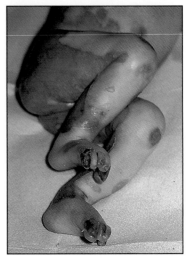

Figure 24.4 Severe, autosomal recessive form of epidermolysis bullosa. There is scarring following recurrent blistering.

in an adult may be indicative of childhood sun exposure. Prolonged exposure to sunlight should be avoided and sunscreen preparations with a sun protection factor exceeding 20 should be applied liberally to exposed skin in bright weather and reapplied every few hours.

Malignant melanoma is rare before puberty, except in giant naevi. However, in adults, the incidence of malignant melanoma has increased dramatically over the past 30 years. Risk factors for melanoma include a positive family history, having a large number of melanocytic naevi, fair skin, repeated episodes of sunburn and living in a hot climate with chronic skin exposure to the sun.

 Parents should prevent their children becoming sunburnt.

Albinism

This is due to a defect in biosynthesis and distribution of melanin. The albinism may be oculocutaneous, ocular or partial, depending on the distribution of depigmentation in the skin and eye (Fig. 24.3). The lack of pigment in the iris, retina, eyelids and eyebrows results in failure to develop a fixation reflex. There is pendular nystagmus and photophobia, which causes constant frowning. Correction of refractive errors and tinted lenses may be helpful. In a few children, the fitting of tinted contact lenses from early infancy allows the development of normal fixation. The disorder is an important cause of severe visual impairment. The pale skin is prone to sunburn and skin cancer. In sunlight, a hat should be worn and high factor barrier cream applied to the skin.

Epidermolysis bullosa

This is a rare group of genetic conditions with many types, characterised by blistering of the skin and mucous membranes. Autosomal dominant variants tend to be milder; autosomal recessive variants may be

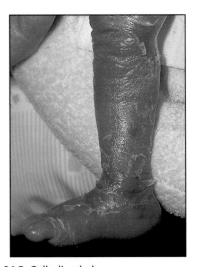

Figure 24.5 Collodion baby.

severe and even fatal. Blisters occur spontaneously or follow minor trauma (Fig. 24.4). They need to be differentiated from scalds. Management is directed to avoiding injury from even minor skin trauma and treating secondary infection. In the severe forms, the fingers and toes may become fused, and contractures of the limbs develop from repeated blistering and healing. Mucous membrane involvement may result in oral ulceration and stenosis from oesophageal erosions. Management, including maintenance of adequate nutrition, should be by a multidisciplinary team including a paediatric dermatologist, paediatrician, plastic surgeon and dietician.

Collodion baby

This is a rare manifestation of the inherited ichthyoses, a group of conditions in which the skin is dry and scaly. Infants are born with a taut parchment-like or collodion-like membrane (Fig. 24.5). Emollients are

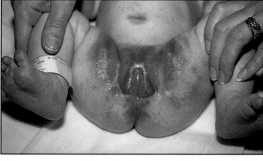

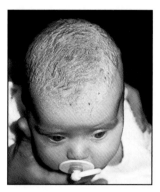

Figure 24.6 Napkin rash due to *Candida* infection. The skin flexures are involved and there are satellite pustules visible.

usually applied to moisturise and soften the skin. The membrane becomes fissured and separates within a few weeks, usually leaving either ichthyotic or less commonly, normal skin.

Rashes of infancy

Napkin rashes

Napkin rashes are common, although irritant reactions are much less of a problem with the widespread use of disposable nappies, as they are more absorbent. Some causes are listed in Box 24.1. Irritant dermatitis, the most common napkin rash, may occur if nappies are not changed frequently enough or if the infant has diarrhoea. However, irritant dermatitis can occur even when the napkin area is cleaned regularly. The rash is due to the irritant effect of urine on the skin of susceptible infants. Urea-splitting organisms in faeces increase the alkalinity and likelihood of a rash.

The irritant eruption affects the convex surfaces of the buttocks, perineal region, lower abdomen and top of thighs. Characteristically, the flexures are spared, which differentiates it from other causes of napkin rash. The rash is erythematous and may have a scalded appearance. More severe forms are associated with erosions and ulcer formation. Mild cases respond to the use of a protective emollient, whereas more severe cases may require mild topical corticosteroids. While leaving the child without a napkin will accelerate resolution, it is rarely practical at home.

Candida infection may cause and often complicates napkin rashes. The rash is erythematous, includes the skin flexures and there may be satellite lesions (Fig. 24.6). Treatment is with a topical antifungal agent.

Infantile seborrhoeic dermatitis

This eruption of unknown cause presents in the first 2 months of life. It starts on the scalp as an erythematous scaly eruption. The scales form a thick yellow adherent layer, commonly called cradle cap (Fig. 24.7a). The scaly rash may spread to the face, behind the ears and then extend to the flexures and napkin area (Fig. 24.7b). In contrast to atopic eczema, it is not itchy and the child is unperturbed by it. However, it is associated with an increased risk of subsequently developing

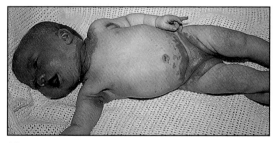

(a)

(b)

Figure 24.7 Infantile seborrhoeic dermatitis. **(a)** Cradle cap. **(b)** Involvement of face, axillae and napkin area.

atopic eczema. Mild cases will resolve with emollients. The scales on the scalp can be cleared with an ointment containing low-concentration sulphur and salicylic acid applied to the scalp daily for a few hours and then washed off. Widespread body eruption will clear with a mild topical corticosteroid, either alone or mixed with an antibacterial and antifungal agent if appropriate.

Atopic eczema (atopic dermatitis)

The prevalence of atopic eczema in children in the UK is about 20%. A genetic deficiency of skin barrier function is important in the pathogenesis of atopic eczema. Onset of atopic eczema is usually in the first year of life. It is, however, uncommon in the first 2 months, unlike infantile seborrhoeic dermatitis, which is relatively common at this age. There is often a family history of

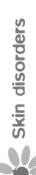

atopic disorders: eczema, asthma, allergic rhinitis (hay fever). Around one-third of children with atopic eczema will develop asthma. Exclusive breast-feeding may delay the onset of eczema in predisposed children but does not appear to have a significant impact on the prevalence of eczema during later childhood. Atopic eczema is mainly a disease of childhood, being most severe and troublesome in the first year of life and resolving in 50% by 12 years of age, and in 75% by 16 years.

Diagnosis

The diagnosis is made clinically. If tested, most affected children have an elevated total plasma IgE level. If there is a history to suggest a particular allergic cause, skin-prick and radioallergosorbent (RAST) tests may be helpful. This will also identify food and other allergens which may cause anaphylaxis. If the disease is unusually severe, atypical or associated with unusual infections or failure to thrive, an immune deficiency disorder should be excluded. Immunological changes in atopic disease are probably secondary to enhanced antigen penetration through a deficient epidermal barrier.

Clinical features

Rashes may itch in many conditions (Box 24.2), but in atopic eczema, itching (pruritus) is the main symptom at all ages and this results in scratching and exacerbation of the rash (Fig. 24.8). The excoriated areas become erythematous, weeping and crusted. Distribution of the eruption tends to change with age, as indicated in Figure 24.9.

Atopic skin is usually dry, and prolonged scratching and rubbing of the skin may lead to lichenification, in which there is accentuation of the normal skin markings (Fig. 24.10).

Complications

Causes of exacerbations of eczema are listed in Box 24.3. However, flare-ups are common, often for no obvious reason. Eczematous skin can readily become infected, usually with *Staphylococcus* or *Streptococcus* (Fig. 24.11). Inflammation increases the avidity of skin for *Staph. aureus* and reduces the expression of anti-microbial peptides, which are needed to control microbial infections. *Staph. aureus* thrives on atopic skin and releases superantigens which seem to maintain and worsen eczema. Herpes simplex virus infection, although less frequent, is potentially very serious as it can spread rapidly on atopic skin, causing an extensive vesicular reaction, eczema herpeticum (see Ch. 14). Regional lymphadenopathy is common and often marked in active eczema; it usually resolves when the skin improves.

Management

A number of treatment modalities are available.

Avoiding irritants and precipitants

It is advisable to avoid soap and biological detergents. Clothing next to the skin should be of pure cotton where possible, avoiding nylon and pure woollen garments. Nails need to be cut short to reduce skin damage from scratching, and mittens at night may be helpful in the very young. When an allergen such as cow's milk has been proven to be a precipitant, it should be avoided.

Emollients

These are the mainstay of management, moisturising and softening the skin. They should be applied liberally two or more times a day and after a bath. They include ointments such as one containing equal parts of white

---

Itching

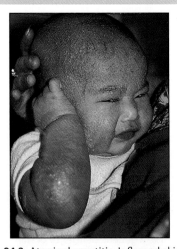

Figure 24.8 Atopic dermatitis. Inflamed skin worsened by rubbing/scratching. Itch is the key clinical feature in eczema at all ages, leading to an 'itch–scratch–itch' cycle.

Box 24.2 Some itchy rashes

- Atopic eczema
- Chickenpox
- Urticaria/allergic reactions
- Contact dermatitis
- Insect bites/papular urticaria
- Scabies
- Fungal infections
- Pityriasis rosea.

 No itch? – then it's not eczema

Eczema

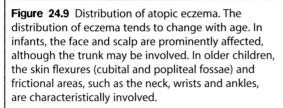

Infant >2 months old
(Predominantly face, also trunk)

Older child
(Predominantly flexor and friction surfaces)

Figure 24.9 Distribution of atopic eczema. The distribution of eczema tends to change with age. In infants, the face and scalp are prominently affected, although the trunk may be involved. In older children, the skin flexures (cubital and popliteal fossae) and frictional areas, such as the neck, wrists and ankles, are characteristically involved.

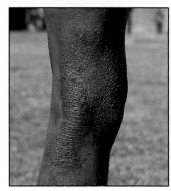

Figure 24.10 Lichenification.

Box 24.3 Causes of exacerbation of eczema

* Bacterial infection, e.g. *Staphylococcus*, *Streptococcus* spp.
* Viral infection, e.g. herpes simplex virus
* Ingestion of an allergen, e.g. egg
* Contact with an irritant or allergen
* Environment: heat, humidity
* Change or reduction in medication
* Psychological stress
* Unexplained.

Summary

Assessment of the child with eczema

Condition of the skin
Distribution of the eczema: is the skin excoriated, weeping, crusted, lichenified?
How troublesome is the itching?
Worse or better than usual?
What causes exacerbation – food or other allergens, irritants, medications, stress?
Does it disturb sleep?
Does it interfere with life?
Family knowledgeable about condition and its management?

Check:
* Any evidence of infection – bacterial or herpes simplex virus?
* Problems from other allergic disorders?
* Is growth normal?

Management
Avoiding soap, frequently using emollients?
Avoiding nylon and wool clothes?
Is there a need to give or change medications:
* Topical corticosteroids
* Immunomodulators
* Occlusive bandages
* Antibiotics or antiviral agents
* Antihistamines
Allergy test to egg +/- other foods – is it indicated to identify coexistent IgE – mediated food allergy?
On dietary elimination or is it indicated? If so, dietician supervision?
Need for psychosocial support?

Figure 24.11 Infected, excoriated atopic eczema.

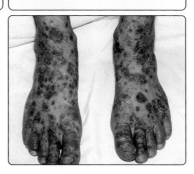

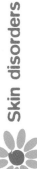

soft paraffin and liquid paraffin. Ointments are preferable to creams when the skin is very dry. A daily or alternate day bath using an emollient oil as a soap substitute is also beneficial.

Topical corticosteroids

These are an effective treatment for eczema, but must be used with care. Mildly potent corticosteroids, such as 1% hydrocortisone ointment, can be applied to the eczematous areas twice daily. Moderately potent topical steroids play a pivotal role in the management of acute exacerbations, but their use must be kept to a minimum. They should be applied thinly and their use on the face should be generally avoided. Excessive use of topical steroids may cause thinning of the skin as well as systemic side-effects. However, fear of these side-effects should not deter their use in controlling exacerbations.

Immunomodulators

In children over 2 years old, short-term topical use of tacrolimus or pimecrolimus may be indicated for eczema not controlled by topical corticosteroids and where there is a risk of important adverse effects from further topical steroid use.

Occlusive bandages

These are helpful over limbs when scratching and lichenification are a problem. They may be impregnated with zinc paste or zinc and tar paste. The bandages are worn overnight or for 2–3 days at a time until the skin has improved. For widespread itching in young children, short-term use of wet stockinette wraps may be helpful; diluted topical steroids mixed with emollient are applied to the skin and damp wraps fashioned for trunk and limbs are then applied with overlying dry wraps or clothes.

Antibiotics or antiviral agents

Antibiotics with hydrocortisone can be applied topically for mildly infected eczema. Systemic antibiotics are indicated for more widespread or severe infection. Eczema herpeticum is treated with systemic aciclovir.

Itch suppression is with an oral antihistamine. The newer second-generation antihistamines are not sedative. Antihistamines can be useful in raising the itching threshold so that scratching is reduced.

Dietary elimination

Food allergy may be present if the child reacted with immediate symptoms to a food, or in infants and young children with moderate or severe atopic eczema, particularly if associated with gut dysmotility (colic, vomiting, altered bowel habit) or failure to thrive. It may even occur in young infants with severe eczema who are exclusively breast-fed at the time. The most common food allergies are to egg, cow's milk and peanut. However, any food may be implicated in an eczema flare-up. Dietary elimination for 4–6 weeks is required to detect a response. A trial of an extensively hydrolysed protein formula or amino acid formula in place of cow's milk formula is also recommended for bottle-fed infants under 6 months old with severe atopic eczema

that has not been controlled by optimal treatment with emollients and mild topical corticosteroids. Dietary elimination should be carried out with the advice of a dietician to ensure complete avoidance of specific food constituents and that the diet remains nutritionally adequate. A food challenge is required to be fully objective. Children can usually tolerate the offending foods by the age of 3–4 years with the important exception of peanut allergy, which usually persists.

Psychosocial support

In most children, eczema is mild and can be controlled with emollients and mildly potent topical steroids, and additional psychological support is not required. However, eczema can be sufficiently severe to be disrupting both to the child and to the whole family. The parents and the child need considerable advice, help and support from health professionals, other affected families or fellow sufferers. In the UK, the National Eczema Society provides support and education about the disorder.

Infections and infestations

Bullous impetigo has been considered earlier in this chapter and acute bacterial and viral infections of the skin are considered in Chapter 14.

Viral infections

Viral warts

These are caused by the human papillomavirus, of which there are well over 100 types. Warts are common in children, usually on the fingers and soles (verrucae). Most disappear spontaneously over a few months or years and treatment is only indicated if the lesions are painful or are a cosmetic problem. They can be difficult to treat, but daily application of a proprietary salicylic acid and lactic acid paint or glutaraldehyde (10%) lotion can be used. Cryotherapy with liquid nitrogen is effective treatment but can be painful and often needs repeated application, and its use should be reserved for older children.

Molluscum contagiosum

This is caused by a poxvirus. The lesions are small, skin-coloured, pearly papules with central umbilication (Fig. 24.12). They may be single but are usually multiple. Lesions are often widespread but tend to disappear spontaneously within a year. If necessary, a topical antibacterial can be applied to prevent or treat secondary bacterial infection, and cryotherapy (2–3 s only) can be used in older children, away from the face, to hasten the disappearance of more chronic lesions.

Fungal infections

Ringworm

Dermatophyte fungi invade dead keratinous structures, such as the horny layer of skin, nails and hair. The term 'ringworm' is used because of the often ringed

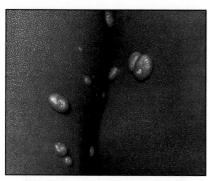

Figure 24.12 Molluscum contagiosum. Some of the pearly lesions show characteristic umbilication.

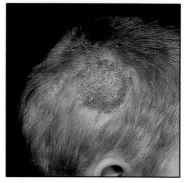

Figure 24.13 Ringworm of the scalp showing hair loss and kerion.

(annular) appearance of skin lesions. A severe inflammatory pustular ringworm patch is called a kerion (Fig. 24.13).

Tinea capitis (scalp ringworm), sometimes acquired from dogs and cats, causes scaling and patchy alopecia with broken hairs. Examination under filtered ultraviolet (Wood's) light may show bright greenish/yellow fluorescence of the infected hairs with some fungal species.

Rapid diagnosis can be made by microscopic examination of skin scrapings for fungal hyphae. Definitive identification of the fungus is by culture. Treatment of mild infections is with topical antifungal preparations, but more severe infections require systemic antifungal treatment for several weeks. Any animal source of infection also needs to be treated.

Summary

Tinea capitis (scalp ringworm)

- Annular scaling scalp lesion with patchy alopecia with broken hairs
- Fungal hyphae on skin scrapings
- Treated with topical or systemic antifungal
- Treat the dog or cat, if infected.

Parasitic infestations

Scabies

Scabies is caused by an infestation with the eight-legged mite *Sarcoptes scabiei*, which burrows down the epidermis along the stratum corneum. Severe itching occurs 2–6 weeks after infestation and is worse in warm conditions and at night.

In older children, burrows, papules and vesicles involve the skin between the fingers and toes, axillae, flexor aspects of the wrists, belt line and around the nipples, penis and buttocks. In infants and young children, the distribution often includes the palms (Fig. 24.14), soles and trunk. The presence of lesions on the soles can be helpful in making the diagnosis. The head, neck and face can be involved in babies but is uncommon.

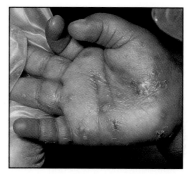

Figure 24.14 Scabies in a young child affecting the palm.

Diagnosis is made on clinical grounds with the history of itching and characteristic lesions. Although burrows are considered pathognomonic, they may be hard to identify because of secondary infection due to scratching. Itching in other family members is a helpful clinical indicator. Confirmation can be made by microscopic examination of skin scrapings from the lesions to identify mite, eggs and mite faeces.

Complications

The skin becomes excoriated due to scratching and there may be a secondary eczematous or urticarial reaction masking the true diagnosis. Secondary bacterial infection is common, giving crusted, pustular lesions. Sometimes slowly resolving nodular lesions are visible.

Treatment

As it is spread by close bodily contact, the child and whole family should be treated, whether or not they have evidence of infestation. Permethrin cream (5%) should be applied below the neck to all areas and washed off after 8–12 h. In babies, the face and scalp should be included, avoiding the eyes. Benzyl benzoate emulsion (25%) applied below the neck only, in diluted form according to age, and left on for 12 h, is also effective but smells and has an irritant action. Malathion lotion (0.5% aqueous) is another effective preparation applied below the neck and left on for 12 h.

 If a child and other members of the family are itching, suspect scabies.

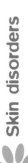

Summary

Scabies

- Very itchy burrows, papules and vesicles – distribution varies with age
- Scratching leads to excoriation, secondary eczematous or urticarial reaction often with secondary bacterial infection
- Not only the child but the whole family need treatment.

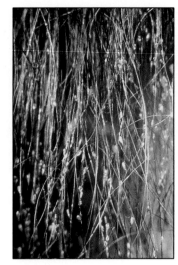

Figure 24.15 Head lice. Profuse nits (egg capsules) are visible on scalp hairs. Live lice were visible on the scalp.

Pediculosis

Pediculosis capitis (head lice infestation) is the most common form of lice infestation in children. It is widespread and troublesome among primary school children. Presentation may be itching of the scalp and nape or from identifying live lice on the scalp or nits (empty egg cases) on hairs (Fig. 24.15). Louse eggs are cemented to hair close to the scalp and the nits (small whitish oval capsules) remain attached to the hair shaft as the hair grows. There may be secondary bacterial infection, often over the nape of the neck, leading to a misdiagnosis of impetigo. Sub-occipital lymphadenopathy is common. Once infestation is confirmed by finding live lice, treatment is by applying a solution of 0.5% malathion to the hair and leaving it on overnight. The hair is then shampooed and the lice and nits removed with a fine-tooth comb. Treatment should be repeated a week later. Permethrin (1%) as a cream rinse would be an alternative application; it is left on for 10 min only. Flammability of alcohol-based lotions should be noted. Wet combing to remove live lice (bug-busting) every 3–4 days for at least 2 weeks is a useful and safe physical treatment, particularly when parents treat with enthusiasm.

Other childhood skin disorders

Psoriasis

This familial disorder rarely presents before the age of 2 years. The guttate type (Fig. 24.16) is common in children and often follows a streptococcal or viral sore throat or ear infection. Lesions are small, raindrop-like, round or oval erythematous scaly patches on the trunk and upper limbs, and an attack usually resolves over 3–4 months. However, most get a recurrence of psoriasis within the next 3–5 years. Chronic psoriasis with plaques or annular lesions is less common. Fine pitting of the nails may be seen in chronic disease but is unusual in children. Treatment for guttate psoriasis is with bland ointments. Coal tar preparations are useful for plaque psoriasis and scalp involvement. Dithranol preparations are very effective in resistant plaque psoriasis. Calcipotriol, a vitamin D analogue, which does not stain the skin, can also be useful for plaque psoriasis in those over 6 years old. Occasionally,

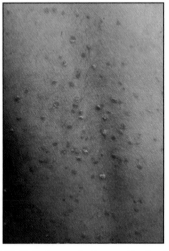

Figure 24.16 Guttate psoriasis over the back in a 5-year-old.

children with chronic psoriasis develop psoriatic arthritis. Chronic psoriasis may have a considerable effect on quality of life. The Psoriasis Association can be helpful in offering support and advice.

Pityriasis rosea

This acute, benign self-limiting condition is thought to be of viral origin. It usually begins with a single round or oval scaly macule, the herald patch, 2–5 cm in diameter, on the trunk, upper arm, neck or thigh. After a few days, numerous smaller dull pink macules develop on the trunk, upper arms and thighs. The rash tends to follow the line of the ribs posteriorly, described as the 'fir tree pattern'. Sometimes the lesions are itchy.

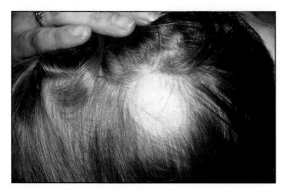

Figure 24.17 Alopecia areata. Smooth well-defined patch of non-inflamed hair fall.

No treatment is required and the rash resolves within 4–6 weeks.

Alopecia areata

This is a common form of hair loss in children and, understandably, a cause of much family distress. Hairless, single or multiple non-inflamed smooth areas of skin, usually over the scalp, are present (Fig. 24.17); remnants of broken-off hairs, visible as 'exclamation mark' hairs may be seen at the edge of active patches of hair fall. The more extensive the hair loss, the poorer the prognosis, but regrowth often occurs within 6–12 months in localised hair loss. Prognosis should be more guarded in children with atopic disorders.

Granuloma annulare

Lesions are typically ringed (annular) with a raised flesh-coloured non-scaling edge (unlike ringworm) (Fig. 24.18). They may occur anywhere but usually over bony prominences, especially over hands and feet.

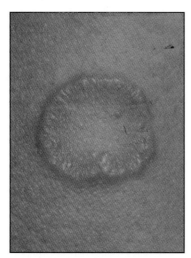

Figure 24.18 Granuloma annulare. Ringed lesion with a non-inflamed, non-scaling raised edge.

Lesions may be single or multiple, are usually 1–3 cm in diameter, and tend to disappear spontaneously but may take years to do so. There is also a subcutaneous form.

Acne vulgaris

Acne may begin 1–2 years before the onset of puberty following androgenic stimulation of the sebaceous glands and an increased sebum excretion rate. Obstruction to the flow of sebum in the sebaceous follicle initiates the process of acne. There are a variety of lesions, initially open comedones (blackheads) or closed comedones (whiteheads) progressing to papules, pustules, nodules and cysts. Lesions occur mainly on the face, back, chest and shoulders. The more severe cystic and nodular lesions often produce scarring. Menstruation and emotional stress may be associated with exacerbations. The condition usually resolves in the late teens, although it may persist.

Topical treatment is directed at encouraging the skin to peel using a keratolytic agent, such as benzoyl peroxide, applied once or twice daily after washing. Sunshine, in moderation, topical antibiotics or topical retinoids may be helpful. For more severe acne, oral antibiotic therapy with tetracyclines (only when over 12 years old, because they may discolour the teeth in younger children) or erythromycin is indicated. The oral retinoid isotretinoin is reserved for severe acne in teenagers unresponsive to other treatments.

Rashes and systemic disease

Skin rashes may be a sign of systemic disease. Examples are:

- Facial rash in systemic lupus erythematosus (SLE) or dermatomyositis
- Purpura over the buttocks, lower limbs and elbows in Henoch–Schönlein purpura
- Erythema nodosum (Fig. 24.19, Box 24.4) and erythema multiforme (Fig. 24.20, Box 24.5); both can be associated with a systemic disorder, but often no cause is identified
- Stevens–Johnson syndrome, a severe bullous form of erythema multiforme also involving the mucous membranes (Fig. 24.21). The eye involvement may include conjunctivitis, corneal ulceration and uveitis, and ophthalmological assessment is required. It may be caused by drug sensitivity or infection, with morbidity and sometimes even mortality from infection, toxaemia or renal damage
- Urticaria.

Urticaria

Urticaria (hives), characterised by flesh-coloured weals, is described in Chapter 15 and the management of anaphylaxis in Chapter 6.

Papular urticaria is a delayed hypersensitivity reaction most commonly seen on the legs, following a bite from a flea, bedbug, or animal or bird mite. Irritation,

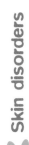

431

Erythema nodosum

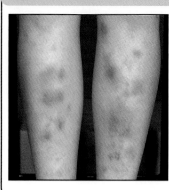

Figure 24.19 Erythema nodosum. There are tender nodules over the legs. She also had fever and arthralgia.

Box 24.4 Causes of erythema nodosum

- Streptococcal infection
- Primary tuberculosis
- Inflammatory bowel disease
- Drug reaction
- Idiopathic

(Sarcoidosis, a common association in adults, is rare in children)

Erythema multiforme

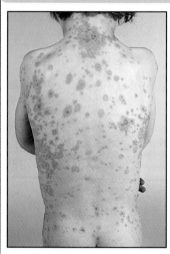

Box 24.5 Causes of erythema multiforme

- Herpes simplex infection
- *Mycoplasma pneumoniae* infection
- Other infections
- Drug reaction
- Idiopathic

Figure 24.20 There are target lesions with a central papule surrounded by an erythematous ring. Lesions may also be vesicular or bullous.

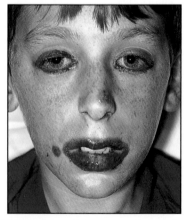

Figure 24.21 Stevens–Johnson syndrome showing severe conjunctivitis and ulceration of the mouth. (Courtesy of Dr Rob Primhak.)

vesicles, papules and weals appear and secondary infection due to scratching is common. It may last for weeks or months and may be recurrent.

Hereditary angioedema is a rare autosomal dominant disorder caused by a deficiency or dysfunction of C1-esterase inhibitor. There is no urticaria, but subcutaneous swellings occur, often accompanied by abdominal pain. The trigger is usually trauma. Angioedema may cause respiratory obstruction. Specific treatment of a severe acute attack is with a purified preparation of the inhibitor, but replacement therapy with fresh frozen plasma can be used as a short-term measure.

Further reading

Chiang NY, Verbov J: *Dermatology – A Handbook for Medical Students and Junior Doctors*, London, 2009, British Association of Dermatologists.

Available free from the British Association of Dermatologists, London

25

Endocrine and metabolic disorders

Points of note concerning endocrine and metabolic disorders in children are:

- The number of children developing diabetes mellitus is increasing
- The most common cause of hypothyroidism is congenital, which is detected on routine biochemical screening shortly after birth
- Inborn errors of metabolism are individually very rare and managed by a few specialist centres.

Diabetes mellitus

The incidence of diabetes in children has increased steadily over the last 20 years and now affects around 2 per 1000 children by 16 years of age. It has been estimated that the incidence of childhood diabetes will double by 2020 in developed countries. This is most likely to be a result of changes in environmental risk factors, although the exact causes remain obscure. There is considerable racial and geographical variation – the condition is more common in northern countries, with high incidences in Scotland and Finland. Almost all children have type 1 diabetes requiring insulin from the outset. Type 2 diabetes due to insulin resistance is starting to occur in childhood, as severe obesity becomes more common and in some ethnic groups. The other causes of diabetes are listed in Box 25.1.

Almost all children with diabetes have insulin-dependent (type 1) diabetes, although type 2 diabetes is increasingly common. In 2009, there were approximately 25 000 children and young people with type 1 diabetes and 200 with type 2 diabetes in the UK.

Aetiology of type 1 diabetes

Both genetic predisposition and environmental precipitants play a role. Inherited susceptibility is demonstrated by:

- An identical twin of a diabetic has a 30–40% chance of developing the disease

Box 25.1 Classification of diabetes according to aetiology

- **Type 1. Most childhood diabetes:**
  - Destruction of pancreatic β-cells by an autoimmune process
- **Type 2. Insulin resistance followed later by β-cell failure:**
  - Usually older children, obesity-related, positive family history, not as prone to ketosis, commoner in some ethnic groups (e.g. Indian subcontinent)
- **Type 3. Other specific types:**
  - Genetic defects in β-cell function (maturity-onset diabetes of the young, MODY) due to glucokinase or transcription factor mutations
  - Genetic defects in insulin action
  - Infections, e.g. congenital rubella
  - Drugs, e.g. corticosteroids
  - Pancreatic exocrine insufficiency, e.g. cystic fibrosis
  - Endocrine diseases, e.g. Cushing syndrome
  - Genetic/chromosomal syndromes, e.g. Down and Turner
  - Neonatal diabetes: transient and permanent
- **Type 4. Gestational diabetes (GDM).**

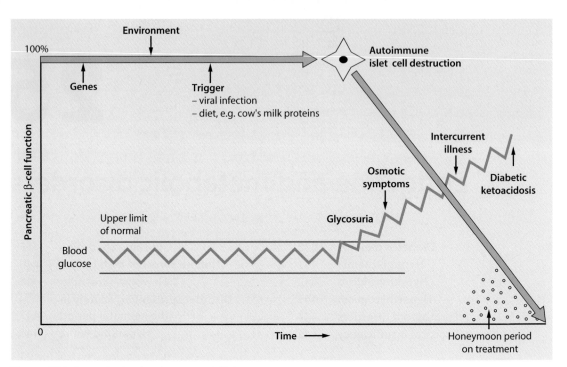

Figure 25.1 Stages in the development of diabetes.

- The increased risk of a child developing diabetes if a parent has insulin-dependent diabetes (1 in 20–40 if the father is affected, 1 in 40–80 if it is the mother – compared to about 1/400 in the population <16 years)
- The increased risk of diabetes among those who are HLA-DR3 or HLA-DR4 and a reduced risk with DR2 and DR5.

Molecular mimicry probably occurs between an environmental trigger and an antigen on the surface of β-cells of the pancreas. Triggers which may contribute are enteroviral infections, accounting for the more frequent presentation in spring and autumn, and diet, possibly cow's milk proteins (Fig. 25.1) and overnutrition. In genetically predisposed individuals, this results in an autoimmune process which damages the pancreatic β-cells and leads to increasing insulin deficiency. Markers of β-cell destruction include islet cell antibodies and antibodies to glutamic acid decarboxylase (GAD), the islet cells and insulin. There is an association with other autoimmune disorders such as hypothyroidism, Addison disease, coeliac disease and rheumatoid arthritis in the patient or family history.

Clinical features

There are two peaks of presentation of type 1 diabetes, preschool and teenagers. It is also commoner to present in spring and autumn months. In contrast to adults, children usually present with only a few weeks of polyuria, excessive thirst (polydipsia) and weight loss; young children may also develop secondary nocturnal enuresis. Most children are diagnosed at this early stage of the illness (Box 25.2). Advanced diabetic ketoacidosis has become an uncommon presentation

(<10% in some areas of the UK), but requires urgent recognition and treatment. Diabetic ketoacidosis may be misdiagnosed if the hyperventilation is mistaken for pneumonia or the abdominal pain for appendicitis or constipation.

Diagnosis

The diagnosis is usually confirmed in a symptomatic child by finding a markedly raised random blood

Box 25.2 Symptoms and signs of diabetes

Early

- *Most common – the 'classical triad':*
  - Excessive drinking (polydipsia)
  - Polyuria
  - Weight loss
- *Less common:*
  - Enuresis (secondary)
  - Skin sepsis
  - *Candida* and other infections

Late – diabetic ketoacidosis

- Smell of acetone on breath
- Vomiting
- Dehydration
- Abdominal pain
- Hyperventilation due to acidosis (Kussmaul breathing)
- Hypovolaemic shock
- Drowsiness
- Coma and death.

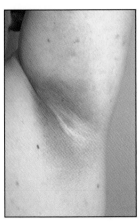

Figure 25.2 Acanthosis nigricans in axilla. A sign of insulin resistance.

glucose (>11.1 mmol/L by the current WHO definition), glycosuria and ketonuria. Where there is any doubt, a fasting blood glucose (>7 mmol/L) or a raised glycosylated haemoglobin (HbA_{1c}) are helpful. A diagnostic glucose tolerance test is rarely required in children.

Type 2 diabetes should be suspected if there is a family history, in children from the Indian subcontinent and in severely obese children with signs of insulin resistance (acanthosis nigricans – velvety dark skin on the neck or armpits (Fig. 25.2), skin tags or the polycystic ovary phenotype in teenage girls).

Initial management of type 1 diabetes

As type 1 diabetes in childhood is uncommon (1–2 children per large secondary school), much of the initial and routine care is delivered by specialist teams (Box 25.3).

The initial management will depend on the child's clinical condition. Those in advanced diabetic ketoacidosis require urgent hospital admission and treatment (see below). Most newly presenting children are alert and able to eat and drink and can be managed with subcutaneous insulin alone. Intravenous fluid is required if the child is vomiting or dehydrated. In most centres with sufficient resources, children newly presenting with diabetes who do not require intravenous therapy are not admitted to hospital but are managed entirely at home.

An intensive educational programme is needed for the parents and child, which covers:

- A basic understanding of the pathophysiology of diabetes
- Injection of insulin: technique and sites
- Diet: reduced refined carbohydrate; healthy diet with no more than 30% fat intake; 'carbohydrate counting', estimating the amount of carbohydrate in food to allow calculation of the insulin required for each meal or snack
- Adjustments of diet and insulin for exercise
- 'Sick-day rules' during illness to prevent ketoacidosis
- Blood glucose (finger prick) monitoring and blood ketones when unwell

- The recognition and staged treatment of hypoglycaemia
- Where to get advice 24 hours a day
- The help available from voluntary groups, e.g. local groups or 'Diabetes UK'
- The psychological impact of a lifelong condition with potentially serious short- and long-term complications.

A considerable period of time needs to be spent with the family to provide this information and psychological support. The information provided for the child must be appropriate for age, and updated regularly. The specialist nurse should liaise with the school (teachers, those who prepare school meals, physical education teachers) and the primary care team.

Insulin

Insulin is made chemically identical to human insulin by recombinant DNA technology or by chemical modification of pork insulin. All insulin that is used in the UK in children is human and in concentrations of 100 U/ml (U-100). The types of insulin include:

- Human insulin analogues. Rapid-acting insulin analogues, e.g. insulin lispro, insulin glulisine or insulin aspart (trade names Humalog, Apidra and NovoRapid, respectively) – with a much faster onset and shorter duration of action than soluble regular insulin. There are also very long-acting insulin analogues, e.g. insulin detemir (Levemir) or glargine (Lantus)
- 'Short-acting' soluble human regular insulin. Onset of action (30–60 min), peak 2–4 h, duration up to 8 h. Given 15–30 min before meals. Trade named examples are Actrapid and Humulin S
- Intermediate-acting insulin. Onset 1–2 h, peak 4–12 h. Isophane insulin is insulin with protamine, e.g. Insulatard and Humulin I
- Predetermined preparations of mixed short- and intermediate-acting insulins with 25% or 30% rapid-acting components.

Insulin can be given by continuous infusion of rapid-acting insulin from a pump or by injections using a variety of syringe and needle sizes, pen-like devices with insulin-containing cartridges, and jet injectors that inject insulin needle-free as a fine stream into the subcutaneous tissue.

Insulin may be injected into the subcutaneous tissue of the upper arm, the anterior and lateral aspects of the thigh, the buttocks and the abdomen. Rotation

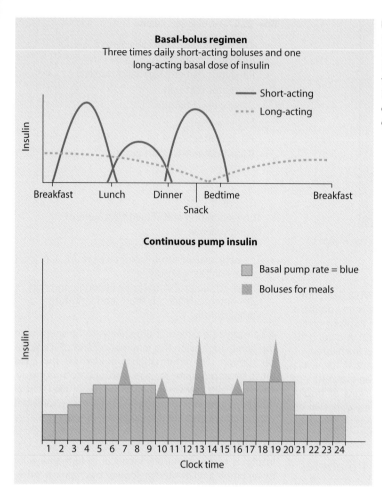

Figure 25.3 Basal-bolus insulin regimen and continuous pump insulin regimen, showing the basal levels of insulin programmed into the pump (blue bars) and the bolus insulin (red pulses) given before each meal/snack according to carbohydrate intake.

of the injection sites is essential to prevent lipohypertrophy or, more rarely, lipoatrophy. The skin should be pinched up and the insulin injected at a 45° angle. Using a long needle or an injection technique that is 'too vertical' causes a painful, bruised intramuscular injection. Shallow intradermal injections can also cause scarring and should be avoided.

Most children are started on an insulin pump or a 3–4 times/day injection regimen ('basal-bolus') with short-acting insulin (e.g. Lispro, Glulisine or Insulin Aspart) being given (bolus) before each meal and snack plus long-acting insulin (e.g. Glargine or Detemir) in the late evening and/or before breakfast to provide insulin background (basal). These treatments both allow greater flexibility by relating the insulin more closely to food intake and exercise (Fig. 25.3). Patients and families are also taught how to correct any sugar above 10 mmol/L between usual meal times by extra short-acting insulin injections. However, the input required by the teams to start these intensive regimens is high, as is the need for a supportive school environment, and some patients and families still rely on twice-daily treatment with premixed insulin.

Shortly after presentation, when some pancreatic function is preserved, insulin requirements often become minimal, the so-called 'honeymoon period'. Requirements subsequently increase to 0.5–1 U/kg or even up to 2 U/kg per day during puberty.

Diet

The diet and insulin regimen need to be matched (Fig. 25.4). The aim is to optimise metabolic control while maintaining normal growth. A healthy diet is recommended, with a high complex carbohydrate and relatively low fat content (<30% of total calories). The diet should be high in fibre, which will provide a sustained release of glucose, rather than refined carbohydrate, which causes rapid swings in glucose levels. 'Carbohydrate counting' allows patients to calculate their likely insulin requirements once their food choice for a meal is known, and taking into account their pre-meal sugar level and post-meal exercise pattern. Learning this balancing act requires a lot of educational input followed by refinement in the light of experience.

Blood glucose monitoring

Regular blood glucose profiles and blood glucose measurements, when a low or high level is suspected, are required to adjust the insulin regimen and learn how changes in lifestyle, food and exercise affect control. A record should be kept in a diary or transferred from the memory of the blood glucose meter. The aim is to maintain blood glucose as near to normal (4–6 mmol/L) as possible. In practice, in order also to avoid hypoglycaemic episodes, this means levels of 4–10 mmol/L in children and 4–8 mmol/L in

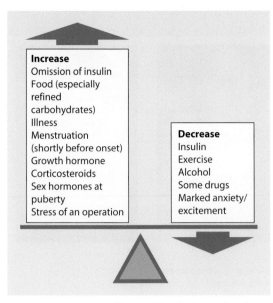

Increase
Omission of insulin
Food (especially refined carbohydrates)
Illness
Menstruation (shortly before onset)
Growth hormone
Corticosteroids
Sex hormones at puberty
Stress of an operation

Decrease
Insulin
Exercise
Alcohol
Some drugs
Marked anxiety/ excitement

Figure 25.4 Factors affecting blood glucose levels.

adolescents for as much of the time as possible. Realistic goals need to be agreed, with compromises reached about the frequency of monitoring and lifestyle issues, especially in teenagers. During changes in routine (e.g. holidays) or illness, it is not unreasonable to ask for four or more tests per day. In reality, many adolescents test less than once per week, if at all.

Continuous glucose monitoring sensors (CGMS), using subcutaneous or transcutaneous sensors to provide a continuous reading of blood glucose, are now widely available, and refinement is underway to allow these devices to help control the insulin delivered from a pump, or to suggest doses for a given meal composition and size. Continuous glucose monitoring sensors also allow the detection of unexpected asymptomatic episodes of nocturnal hypoglycaemia or times of poor control during the day. Blood ketone testing (often using the same meter as for blood glucose) is mandatory during infections or when control is poor to try to avoid severe ketoacidosis. Urine ketone testing is still used in some centres.

The measurement of glycosylated haemoglobin (HbA$_{1c}$) is particularly helpful as a guide of overall control over the previous 6–12 weeks and should be checked at least 3 times per year. The level is related to the risk of later complications in a non-linear fashion, such that the risk of complications increases more rapidly with higher levels, but may be misleading if the red blood cell lifespan is reduced, such as in sickle cell trait or if the HbA molecule is abnormal, as in thalassaemia. Since 2009, the units of HbA$_{1c}$ (originally expressed as a % figure) have been changed to an international reporting standard of mmol/mol. Until 2012, results will be reported in both old and new units to give everyone time to become familiar with the new units. A level of ≤58 mmol/mol (7.5%) is seen as an ideal target for patients, but in practice is only achieved in 50% or less of a clinic population in the UK.

Hypoglycaemia

Most children develop well-defined symptoms when their blood glucose falls below about 4 mmol/L. The symptoms are highly individual and change with age, but most complain of hunger, tummy ache, sweatiness, feeling faint or dizzy or of a 'wobbly feeling' in their legs. If unrecognised or untreated, hypoglycaemia may progress to seizures and coma. Parents can often detect hypoglycaemia in young children by their pallor and irritability, sometimes presenting as unreasonable behaviour. If there is any doubt, the blood glucose concentration should be checked or food given.

Treating a 'hypo' at an early stage requires the administration of easily absorbed glucose in the form of glucose tablets (e.g. Lucozade tablets or similar) or a non-diet sugary drink. Children should always have easy access to their hypo remedy, although young children quickly learn to complain of hypo-symptoms in order to leave class or obtain a sweet drink! Oral glucose gels (e.g. Glucogel) are easily and quickly absorbed from the buccal mucosa and so are helpful if the child is unwilling or unable to cooperate to eat. It can be administered by teachers or other helpers. Parents and school should be provided with a glucagon injection kit for the treatment of severe hypoglycaemia, and taught how to administer it intramuscularly to terminate severe hypos. After treatment of 'hypos', parents or carers should give the child some food (usually a biscuit or sandwich) to ensure the blood glucose does not drop again.

Severe hypoglycaemia can usually be predicted (or explained in retrospect – missed meal, heavy exercise). The aim is anticipation and prevention. Hypoglycaemia in an unconscious child brought to hospital is treated with glucose given intravenously.

Diabetic ketoacidosis

Presentation is described in Box 25.2, essential investigations in Box 25.4 and management in Figure 25.5.

Long-term management

The aims of long-term management are:

- Normal growth and development
- Maintaining as normal a home and school life as possible
- Good diabetic control through knowledge and good technique
- Encouraging children to become self-reliant, but with adult supervision until they are able to take responsibility
- Avoidance of hypoglycaemia
- The prevention of long-term complications and an HbA$_{1c}$ of 58 mmol/mol (7.5%) or less.

These aims are difficult to achieve in all patients at all stages of their condition.

Problems in diabetic control

Good blood glucose control is particularly difficult in the following circumstances:

- Eating too many sugary foods, such as sweets taken at odd times, at parties or on the way home from school

Endocrine and metabolic disorders

437

Diabetic ketoacidosis

Box 25.4 Essential early investigations

- Blood glucose (>11.1 mmol/L)
- Blood ketones (>3.0 mmol/L)
- Urea and electrolytes, creatinine (dehydration)
- Blood gas analysis (severe metabolic acidosis)
- Urinary glucose and ketones (both are present)
- Evidence of a precipitating cause, e.g. infection (blood and urine cultures performed)
- Cardiac monitor for T-wave changes of hypokalaemia
- Weight

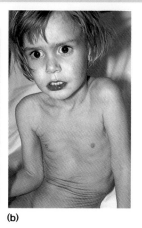
(b)

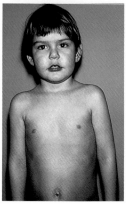
(c)

(a) Management priorities

This regimen is initiated if the child is vomiting or has a reduced level of consciousness. Otherwise, even if newly presenting, only subcutaneous insulin is required.

1. Fluids → If in shock, initial resuscitation is with normal saline. Dehydration should then be corrected gradually over 48–72 h (see Fig. 25.5b and c). Rapid rehydration should be avoided as it may lead to cerebral oedema. Initial rehydration fluids need to be taken into account in calculating fluid requirements. Monitor:
- fluid input and output
- electrolytes, creatinine and acid–base status regularly
- neurological state.
Insert central venous line (CVP) and urinary catheter if shocked.
A nasogastric tube is passed for acute gastric dilatation if there is vomiting or depressed consciousness.

2. Insulin → Insulin infusion (0.05–0.1 U/kg per h) is started after 1h, titrating the dose according to the blood glucose. Do not give a bolus. Monitor the blood glucose regularly. Aim for gradual reduction of blood glucose of about 2 mmol/h, as rapid reduction is dangerous. Change to 4% dextrose/ 0.18% saline after 24 h when the blood glucose has fallen to 14 mmol/L to avoid hypoglycaemia.

3. Potassium → Although the initial plasma potassium may be high, it will fall following treatment with insulin and rehydration. Potassium replacement must be instituted as soon as urine is passed. Continuous cardiac monitoring and regular plasma potassium measurements are indicated until the plasma potassium is stable.

4. Acidosis → Although a metabolic acidosis is present, bicarbonate should be avoided unless the child is shocked or not responding to therapy. The acidosis will self-correct with fluid and insulin therapy. Capillary ketones should be monitored.

5. Re-establish oral fluids, subcutaneous insulin and diet → Do not stop the intravenous insulin infusion until 1 h after subcutaneous insulin has been given.

6. Identification and treatment of an underlying cause → Ketoacidosis may be precipitated by an intercurrent infection. Diabetic ketoacidosis causes neutrophilia but not a fever. Antibiotics may be indicated. If the child was known to have diabetes, consider the reason for the ketoacidosis.

Figure 25.5 (a) Management priorities in diabetic ketoacidosis. **(b)** Severe dehydration and weight loss from diabetic ketoacidosis. **(c)** Four months later. (Courtesy of Dr Jill Challener.)

- Infrequent or unreliable blood glucose testing. 'Perfect' results are often invented and written down just before clinic to please the diabetes team
- Illness – viral illnesses are common in the young and although it is usually stated that infections cause insulin requirements to increase, in practice the insulin dose required is variable, partly because of reduced food intake. The dose of insulin should be adjusted according to regular blood glucose monitoring. Insulin *must* be continued during times of illness and the urine or blood tested for ketones. If ketosis is increasing along with a rising blood sugar, the family should know how to seek immediate advice to ensure that they increase the soluble insulin dose appropriately or seek medical help for possible intravenous therapy
- Exercise – vigorous or prolonged planned exercise (cross-country running, long-distance hiking, skiing) requires reduction of the insulin dose and increase in dietary intake. Late hypoglycaemia may occur during the night or even the next day, but may be avoided by taking an extra bedtime snack, including slow-acting carbohydrate such as cereal or bread. Less vigorous exercise such as sports lessons in school and spontaneous outdoor play can be managed with an extra snack or a reduction in short-acting insulin before the exercise
- Eating disorders, which are common in young females with diabetes.
- Family disturbance such as divorce or separation
- Inadequate family motivation, support or understanding. As children can never have a 'holiday' from their diabetes, they need a great deal of encouragement to continuously maintain good control. Educational programmes for children and families need to be arranged regularly and matched to their current level of education. Special courses and holiday camps are available; in the UK they are organised by Diabetes UK and local groups.

Management at school

An individualised care plan should be developed by the parents, diabetes team and the school to address the specific needs of the child. This will include the child's dietary needs, requirements to have snacks at specified times and what to do if the child becomes hypoglycaemic or loses consciousness. For younger children, support is needed to help calculate and give the pre-lunch insulin injection or bolus from the pump.

Puberty and adolescence

The rapid growth spurt in early puberty is governed by a complex interaction of hormonal changes, some of which involve insulin and insulin-like growth factors. Growth hormone, oestrogen and testosterone all antagonise insulin action and there is thus an increase in the insulin requirement from the usual 0.5–1.0 U/kg per day of early childhood up to ≥2 U/kg per day. The

increase may be especially marked first thing in the morning. The psychological changes accompanying adolescence may make this a time of rebellion where adherence to insulin and dietary regimens is minimal. Diabetic teenagers know that they will not become ill immediately if they cheat with their diet or miss an injection. Some will inevitably test the degree to which the rules can be broken, choosing to ignore the uncomfortable facts of diabetes provided that they 'feel OK'. This usually results in avoidance of blood testing and a tendency to work on the false assumption that feeling well equates with good control. Many teenage girls experiment with crash diets at some time, which are likely to cause major problems in diabetic control. They also learn that glycosuria can be used as an 'aid' to losing weight.

Battles with parents may concentrate on diabetic management instead of the more usual teenage concerns (Table 25.1). Conflict may also extend to involve the professionals of the diabetic team, because of intense anger against the disease which marks them out as different from their peers. Many parents are very protective at this time, whereas teenagers should be encouraged to take responsibility for their diabetes. Health education about smoking, alcohol and contraception may need to be provided. Liaison with a psychologist or child psychiatrist may be helpful. The professionals of the diabetic team may need to encourage diabetic teenagers to take better care of themselves. It is usually unhelpful to give lectures about the long-term risks to health, as these are likely to be seen as irrelevant by the teenagers. However, they may be helped if:

- There are clear short-term goals agreed by the patient
- Their efforts to improve their diabetic control, e.g. an improving or satisfactory HbA$_{1c}$ level, are communicated promptly and enthusiastically
- There is a united team approach, with agreement between professionals of the essentials they wish to promote and clear, unambiguous guidelines for health and diabetic management
- Peer group pressure is used to promote health. Activities such as holidays, etc., that allow teenagers to participate while learning about their diabetic management are encouraged. They may also benefit by being used as teachers of younger children.

Successful long-term diabetic management depends on education and increasing self-reliance and responsibility.

After many years in a children's clinic, it can be difficult for the patient and family to move to the adult care environment. This transition is helped by discussing and planning the move well ahead of the time, and by the provision of joint clinics with the adult diabetologists through to the early twenties or end of tertiary education. Special peri-conceptional clinics have been established in some centres to help achieve near-ideal control before conception in planned pregnancies. Conception of a fetus with a high HbA$_{1c}$ increases the risks of congenital abnormalities in the offspring.

Table 25.1 How diabetes interferes with normal adolescence

Normal adolescence	How diabetes interferes
Physical and sexual maturation	Delayed sexual maturation
	Invasion of privacy with frequent medical examinations
Conformity with peer group	Meals must be eaten on time
	Frequent injections and blood tests
Self-image	Hypoglycaemic attacks show that they are different
Self-esteem	Impaired body image
Independence from parents	Parental over-protection and reluctance to allow their child to be away from home
	Battles over diabetes
Economic independence	Loading of insurance premiums
	Discrimination by employers
	Statutory rules against becoming a pilot or driving heavy goods or public service vehicles

Summary

Regular assessment of the child with diabetes

Assessment of diabetic control:
- Any episodes of hypoglycaemia, diabetic ketoacidosis, hospital admission?
- Is there still awareness of hypoglycaemia?
- Absence from school? School supportive of diabetes care?
- Interference with normal life?
- HbA$_{1c}$ results – 58 mmol/mol (7.5%) or less?
- Diary of blood glucose results – if monitoring, is he reacting to results?
- Insulin regimen – appropriate? Correction bolus doses given?
- Lipohypertrophy or lipoatrophy (Fig. 25.6a and b) at injection sites?
- Diet – healthy diet, manipulating food intake and insulin to maintain good control?

General overview (periodic):
- Normal growth and pubertal development, avoiding obesity – measure each visit
- Blood pressure check for hypertension yearly (age-specific centiles)
- Renal disease – screening for microalbuminuria yearly from 12 years
- Eyes – photography for retinopathy or cataracts, yearly from 12 years
- Feet – maintaining good care – yearly
- Screening for coeliac and thyroid disease at diagnosis, thyroid screening yearly, coeliac again after 3 years or if weight gain poor.
- Annual reminder to have flu vaccination

Knowledge and psychosocial aspects:
- Good understanding of diabetes, would participation/holidays with other diabetic children be beneficial? Member of Diabetes UK?
- Becoming self-reliant, but appropriate supervision at home, school, diabetic team?
- Taking exercise, sport? Diabetes not interfering with it?
- Leading as normal life as possible?
- Smoking, alcohol?
- Is 'hypo' treatment readily available? Is stepped approach known?
- What are the main issues for the patient? Are there short-term goals to allow engagement with improving control?

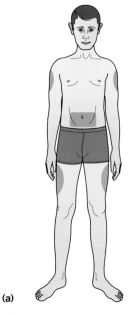

(a)

■ **Injection sites** – check for lipohypertrophy or lipoatrophy

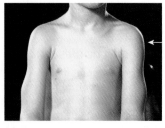

(b)

Figure 25.6 Lipohypertrophy from insulin injections. (a) Injection sites. (b) Lipohypertrophy (arrow) from insulin injections.

Prevention of long-term complications

It has been shown that meticulous diabetic control delays or prevents diabetic retinopathy and nephropathy and, if retinopathy occurs, it can slow the progression. There is also evidence that good early control reduces the risk of later complications, even if control deteriorates later in life. Levels of glycosylated haemoglobin above 58 mmol/mol (7.5%) are related to the risk of later complications in an almost exponential fashion, and so the ideal is to aim for below this level as much as possible.

Although long-term health problems are uncommon during childhood, there needs to be regular review for long-term complications and associated illnesses:

- *Growth and pubertal development.* Some delay in the onset of puberty may occur. Obesity is common, especially in females, if their insulin dose is not reduced towards the end of puberty. Intensive insulin regimens increase the risk of excessive weight gain and BMI should be plotted at each clinic visit
- *Blood pressure* – must be checked at least once a year for evidence of hypertension
- *Renal disease* – the detection of microalbuminuria is an early sign of nephropathy and should be screened annually in teenagers
- *Eyes* – retinopathy or cataracts requiring treatment are rare in children but should be monitored annually after 5 years of diabetes or from the onset of puberty, ideally with retinal photography
- *Feet* – children should be encouraged to take good care of their feet from an early age, to avoid tight shoes and treat any infections early
- *Other associated illnesses* – coeliac disease and thyroid disease are more common in type 1 diabetes and easily missed clinically, so screening for them is recommended at diagnosis and subsequently (thyroid function yearly post-diagnosis and coeliac screening by tissue transglutaminase levels after 3 years) or if suspected clinically. There should be a low threshold for investigating for other autoimmune disorders (rheumatoid, vitiligo, etc.).

Hypoglycaemia

Hypoglycaemia is a common problem in neonates during the first few days of life (see Chapter 10). Thereafter, it is uncommon in non-diabetics. It is often defined as a plasma glucose <2.6 mmol/L, although the development of clinical features will depend on whether other energy substrates can be utilised. Clinical features include:

- Sweating
- Pallor
- Central nervous system signs of irritability, headache, seizures and coma.

The neurological sequelae may be permanent if hypoglycaemia persists and include epilepsy, severe learning difficulties and microcephaly. This risk is

---

Box 25.5 Tests to perform when hypoglycaemia is present

Blood

- Confirm hypoglycaemia with laboratory blood glucose
- Growth hormone, IGF-1, cortisol, insulin, C-peptide, fatty acids, ketones (acetoacetate, 3-hydroxybutyrate), glycerol, branched-chain amino acids, acylcarnitine profile, lactate, pyruvate

First urine after hypoglycaemia

- Organic acids
- Consider saving blood and urine for toxicology, e.g. salicylate, sulphonylurea

---

greatest in early childhood during the period of most rapid brain growth.

Infants have high energy requirements and relatively poor reserves of glucose from gluconeogenesis and glycogenesis. They are at risk of hypoglycaemia with fasting. Infants should never be starved for more than 4 h, e.g. preoperatively. A blood glucose should be checked in any child who:

- becomes septicaemic or appears seriously ill. **ABC** then **DEFG** – '**D**on't **E**ver **F**orget **G**lucose'
- has a prolonged seizure
- develops an altered state of consciousness.

This is often done at the bedside, using glucose-sensitive strips, the accuracy of which is improved by use of a meter. However, the strips only indicate that the glucose is within a low range of values and any low reading must always be confirmed by laboratory measurement.

If the cause of the hypoglycaemia is unknown, *it is vital that blood is collected at the time of the hypoglycaemia* and the first available urine sent for analysis, so that a valuable opportunity for making the diagnosis is not missed (Box 25.5).

Causes

These are listed in Box 25.6.

Ketotic hypoglycaemia is a poorly-defined entity in which young children readily become hypoglycaemic following a short period of starvation, probably due to limited reserves for gluconeogenesis. The child is often short and thin and the insulin levels are low. Regular snacks and extra glucose drinks when ill will usually prevent hypoglycaemia. The condition resolves spontaneously in later life. A number of rare endocrine and metabolic disorders may present with hypoglycaemia at almost any age in childhood. Hepatomegaly would suggest the possibility of an inherited glycogen storage disorder, in which hypoglycaemia can be profound.

Transient neonatal hypoglycaemia in neonates may be due to exposure to high levels of insulin in utero if mothers are diabetic or glucose intolerant. In contrast, recurrent, severe neonatal hypoglycaemia may be

Box 25.6 Causes of hypoglycaemia beyond the immediate neonatal period

Fasting

- *Insulin excess*
  - Excess exogenous insulin, e.g. in diabetes mellitus/insulin given surreptitiously
  - β-cell tumours/disorders – persistent hypoglycaemic hyperinsulinism of infancy (PHHI, previously called nesidioblastosis), insulinoma
  - Drug-induced (sulphonylurea)
  - Autoimmune (insulin receptor antibodies)
  - Beckwith syndrome
- *Without hyperinsulinaemia*
  - Liver disease
  - Ketotic hypoglycaemia of childhood
  - Inborn errors of metabolism, e.g. glycogen storage disorders
  - Hormonal deficiency: GH↓, ACTH↓, Addison disease, congenital adrenal hyperplasia

Reactive/non-fasting

- Galactosaemia
- Leucine sensitivity
- Fructose intolerance
- Maternal diabetes
- Hormonal deficiency
- Aspirin/alcohol poisoning.

caused by persistent hypoglycaemic hyperinsulinism of infancy (PHHI, formerly called 'nesidioblastosis'). This is a rare disorder of infancy where there are gene mutations of various pathways leading to dysregulation of insulin release by the islet cells of the pancreas leading to profound non-ketotic hypoglycaemia. Treatment with high-concentration dextrose solutions and diazoxide (plus other medications) may be required to maintain safe blood sugar levels pending investigation. Special scans reveal that up to 40% of cases are caused by localised lesions in the pancreas amenable to partial resection, although the majority of cases either require long-term medication or total pancreatectomy with the attendant risk of diabetes and exocrine pancreatic insufficiency.

Treatment

Hypoglycaemia can usually be corrected with an intravenous infusion of glucose (2 ml/kg of 10% dextrose followed by 10% dextrose infusion). Care must be taken to avoid giving an excess volume as the solution is hypertonic and could cause cerebral oedema. If there is delay in establishing an infusion or failure to respond, glucagon is given intramuscularly (0.5–1 mg). If a higher concentration than a 10% solution is required in a neonate, the low sugar is highly likely to be secondary to hyperinsulinism.

Corticosteroids may also be used if there is a possibility of hypopituitarism or hypoadrenalism.

The correction of hypoglycaemia must always be documented with satisfactory laboratory glucose measurements.

Summary

Hypoglycaemia

- Should be excluded in any child with septicaemia, who is seriously ill, has a prolonged seizure or altered state of consciousness ('**D**on't **E**ver **F**orget **G**lucose')
- Low blood glucose on bedside testing must be confirmed by laboratory measurement
- If the cause is unknown, diagnostic blood and urine samples should, if possible, be taken at the time.

Hypothyroidism

There is only a small amount of thyroxine transfer from the mother to the fetus, although severe maternal hypothyroidism can affect the developing brain. The fetal thyroid predominantly produces 'reverse T_3', a derivative of T_3 which is largely inactive. After birth, there is a surge in the level of thyroid-stimulating hormone (TSH) which is accompanied by a marked rise in T_4 and T_3 levels. The TSH declines to the normal adult range within a week. Preterm infants may have very low levels of T_4 for the first few weeks of life, while the TSH is within the normal range; under these circumstances, additional thyroxine is not required.

Congenital hypothyroidism

Detection of congenital hypothyroidism is important, as it is:

- Relatively common, occurring in 1 in 4000 births
- One of the few preventable causes of severe learning difficulties.

Causes of congenital hypothyroidism are:

- *Maldescent of the thyroid and athyrosis* – the commonest cause of sporadic congenital hypothyroidism. In early fetal life, the thyroid migrates from a position at the base of the tongue (sublingual) to its normal site below the larynx. The thyroid may fail to develop completely or partially. In maldescent, the thyroid remains as a lingual mass or a unilobular small gland. The reason for this failure of formation or migration is not well understood
- *Dyshormonogenesis*, an inborn error of thyroid hormone synthesis, in about 5–10% of cases, although commoner in some ethnic groups with consanguineous marriage
- *Iodine deficiency*, the commonest cause of congenital hypothyroidism worldwide but rare in the UK. It can be prevented by iodination of salt in the diet

Box 25.7 Clinical features of hypothyroidism

Congenital	Acquired
Usually asymptomatic and picked up on screening. Otherwise:	Females > males
	Short stature/growth failure
Failure to thrive	Cold intolerance
Feeding problems	Dry skin
Prolonged jaundice	Cold peripheries
Constipation	Bradycardia
Pale, cold, mottled dry skin	Thin, dry hair
	Pale, puffy eyes with loss of eyebrows
Coarse facies	Goitre
Large tongue	Slow-relaxing reflexes
Hoarse cry	Constipation
Goitre (occasionally)	Delayed puberty
Umbilical hernia	Obesity
Delayed development	Slipped upper femoral epiphysis
	Deterioration in school work
	Learning difficulties

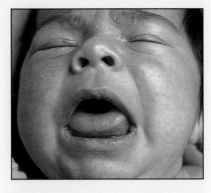

Figure 25.7 Untreated congenital hypothyroidism.

- Hypothyroidism due to *TSH deficiency* – isolated TSH deficiency is rare (<1% of cases) and is usually associated with panhypopituitarism, which usually manifests with growth hormone, gonadotrophin and ACTH deficiency leading to hypoglycaemia or micropenis and undescended testes in affected boys before the hypothyroidism becomes evident.

The clinical features (Box 25.7 and Fig. 25.7) are difficult to differentiate from normal in the first month of life, but become more prominent with age. There is a slight excess of other congenital abnormalities, especially heart defects.

Most infants with congenital hypothyroidism are detected on routine neonatal biochemical screening (Guthrie test), performed on all newborn infants, by identifying a raised TSH in the blood. However, thyroid dysfunction secondary to pituitary abnormalities may not be picked up at neonatal screening as they will have a low TSH. In some countries T_4 is also measured. Treatment with thyroxine is started at 2–3 weeks of age.

Early treatment of congenital hypothyroidism is essential to prevent learning difficulties. With neonatal screening, the results of long-term intellectual development have been satisfactory and intelligence should be in the normal range for the majority of children. Treatment is lifelong with oral replacement of thyroxine, titrating the dose to maintain normal growth, TSH and T_4 levels.

Juvenile hypothyroidism

This is usually caused by autoimmune thyroiditis. There is an increased risk in children with Down or Turner syndrome and of developing other autoimmune disorders, e.g. vitiligo, rheumatoid arthritis, diabetes mellitus. In some families, Addison disease may also occur.

The clinical features are listed in Box 25.7. It is commoner in females. There is growth failure accompanied by delayed bone age. Goitre is often present but this may also be physiological in pubertal girls. Treatment is with thyroxine.

> ### Summary
>
> **Congenital hypothyroidism**
>
> - Is identified on routine neonatal biochemical screening (Guthrie test)
> - Although present antenatally, treatment started soon after birth results in satisfactory intellectual development.

Hyperthyroidism

This usually results from Graves disease (autoimmune thyroiditis), secondary to the production of thyroid-stimulating immunoglobulins (TSIs). The clinical

443

Box 25.8 Clinical features of hyperthyroidism

Systemic	Eye signs (uncommon in children)
Anxiety, restlessness	Exophthalmos
Increased appetite	Ophthalmoplegia
Sweating	Lid retraction
Diarrhoea	Lid lag
Weight loss	
Rapid growth in height	
Advanced bone maturity	
Tremor	
Tachycardia, wide pulse pressure	
Warm, vasodilated peripheries	
Goitre (bruit)	
Learning difficulties/behaviour problems	
Psychosis	

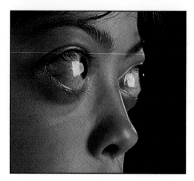

Figure 25.8 Exophthalmos in Graves disease.

features are similar to those in adults, although eye signs are less common (Box 25.8 and Fig. 25.8). It is most often seen in teenage girls. The levels of thyroxine (T_4) and/or tri-iodothyronine (T_3) are elevated and TSH levels are suppressed to very low levels. Antithyroid peroxisomal antibodies may also be present which may eventually result in spontaneous resolution of the thyrotoxicosis but subsequently cause hypothyroidism (so-called hashitoxicosis).

The first-line of treatment is medical, with drugs such as carbimazole or propylthiouracil that interfere with thyroid hormone synthesis. Initially, β-blockers can be added for symptomatic relief of anxiety, tremor and tachycardia. There is a risk of neutropenia from anti-thyroid medication and all families should be warned to seek urgent help and a blood count if sore throat and high fever occur on starting treatment. Medical treatment is given for about 2 years, which should control the thyrotoxicosis, but the eye signs may not resolve. When medical treatment is stopped, 40–75% relapse. A second course of drugs may then be given or surgery in the form of subtotal thyroidectomy will usually result in permanent remission. Radioiodine treatment is simple and is no longer considered to result in later neoplasia. Follow-up is always required as thyroxine replacement is often needed for subsequent hypothyroidism.

Neonatal hyperthyroidism may occur in infants of mothers with Graves disease from the transplacental transfer of TSIs. Treatment is required as it is potentially fatal, but it resolves spontaneously with time.

Parathyroid disorders

Parathyroid hormone (PTH) promotes bone formation via bone-forming cells (osteoblasts). However, when calcium levels are low, PTH promotes bone resorption via osteoclasts, increases renal uptake of calcium and activates metabolism of vitamin D to promote gut absorption of calcium. In hypoparathyroidism, which is rare in childhood, in addition to a low serum calcium, there is a raised serum phosphate and a normal alkaline phosphatase. The parathyroid hormone level is very low. Severe hypocalcaemia leads to muscle spasm, fits, stridor and diarrhoea. It is a common problem in premature infants, and increasingly seen as a presentation of severe rickets (see Ch. 12). Other causes are rare in childhood.

Hypoparathyroidism in infants is usually due to a congenital deficiency (DiGeorge syndrome), associated with thymic aplasia, defective immunity, cardiac defects and facial abnormalities. In older children, hypoparathyroidism is usually an autoimmune disorder associated with Addison disease.

In *pseudohypoparathyroidism* there is end-organ resistance to the action of parathyroid hormone caused by a mutation in a signalling molecule. Serum calcium and phosphate levels are abnormal but the parathyroid hormone levels are normal or high. Other abnormalities are short stature, obesity, subcutaneous nodules, short fourth metacarpals and learning difficulties. There may be teeth enamel hypoplasia and calcification of the basal ganglia. A related state, in which there are the physical characteristics of pseudohypoparathyroidism but the calcium, phosphate and PTH are all normal, is called *pseudopseudohypoparathyroidism*. There may be a positive family history of both disorders in the same kindred.

Treatment of acute symptomatic hypocalcaemia is with an intravenous infusion of calcium gluconate. The 10% solution of calcium gluconate must be diluted as extravasation of the infusion will result in severe skin damage. Chronic hypocalcaemia is treated with oral calcium and high doses of vitamin D analogues, adjusting the dose to maintain the plasma calcium concentration just below the normal range. Hypercalcuria is to be avoided as it may cause nephrocalcinosis and so the urinary calcium excretion should be monitored.

Hyperparathyroidism results in a high calcium level, which in turn produces constipation, anorexia, lethargy and behavioural effects, polyuria and polydipsia. Bony erosions of the phalanges may be seen on a wrist radiograph. In neonates and young children, it is associated with some rare genetic abnormalities (e.g. William syndrome), but in later childhood can be secondary to adenomas occurring spontaneously or as part of the multiple endocrine neoplasia (MEN) syndromes. Severe hypercalcaemia is treated with rehydration, diuretics and bisphosphonates.

Adrenal cortical insufficiency

Congenital adrenal hyperplasia is the commonest non-iatrogenic cause of insufficient cortisol and mineralocorticoid secretion (see Ch. 11).

Primary adrenal cortical insufficiency (Addison disease) is rare in children. It may result from:

- An autoimmune process, sometimes in association with other autoimmune endocrine disorders, e.g. diabetes mellitus, hypothyroidism, hypoparathyroidism
- Haemorrhage/infarction – neonatal, meningococcal septicaemia (usually fatal)
- X-linked adrenoleucodystrophy, a rare neurodegenerative metabolic disorder
- Tuberculosis, now rare.

Adrenal insufficiency may also be secondary to hypopituitarism from hypothalamic–pituitary disease or from hypothalamic–pituitary–adrenal suppression following long-term corticosteroid therapy.

Presentation

Infants present acutely (Box 25.9) with a salt-losing crisis, hypotension and/or hypoglycaemia. Dehydration may follow a gastroenteritis-like illness, from which the child recovers until the next episode. In older children, presentation is usually with chronic ill health and pigmentation (Fig. 25.9).

Diagnosis

This is made by finding hyponatraemia and hyperkalaemia, often associated with a metabolic acidosis and hypoglycaemia. The plasma cortisol is low and the plasma ACTH concentration high (except in hypopituitarism). With an ACTH (Synacthen) test, plasma cortisol concentrations remain low in both primary adrenal failure and in long-standing pituitary/hypothalamic Addison disease. A normal response excludes adrenal cortical insufficiency.

Management

An adrenal crisis requires urgent treatment with intravenous saline, glucose and hydrocortisone. Long-term treatment is with glucocorticoid and mineralocorticoid replacement. The dose of glucocorticoid needs to be increased by three times at times of illness or for an operation. Parents are taught how to inject intramuscular hydrocortisone in an emergency. All children at risk of an adrenal crisis should wear a MedicAlert bracelet.

Box 25.9 Features of adrenal cortical insufficiency

Acute	Chronic
Hyponatraemia	Vomiting
Hyperkalaemia	Lethargy
Hypoglycaemia	Brown pigmentation (gums, scars, skin creases)
Dehydration	
Hypotension	Growth failure
Circulatory collapse	

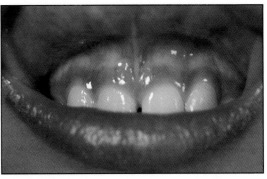

Figure 25.9 Buccal pigmentation in adrenal cortical insufficiency (Addison disease). This 9-year-old boy presented with salt craving and pigmentation. (Courtesy of Dr Steven Robinson.)

Summary

Adrenal cortical insufficiency

- Usually due to corticosteroid therapy, congenital adrenal hyperplasia or, rarely, Addison disease
- May result in an adrenal crisis requiring urgent treatment.

Cushing syndrome

Glucocorticoid excess in children is usually a side-effect of long-term glucocorticoid treatment (intravenous, oral or, more rarely, inhaled, nasal or topical) for conditions such as the nephrotic syndrome, asthma or, in the past, for severe bronchopulmonary dysplasia (Box 25.10 and Fig. 25.10). Corticosteroids are potent growth suppressors and prolonged use in high dosage will lead to reduced adult height and osteopenia. This unwanted side-effect of systemic corticosteroids is markedly reduced by taking corticosteroid medication in the morning on alternate days.

Other causes of glucocorticoid excess are rare. It may be ACTH-driven, from a pituitary adenoma, usually in older children, or from ectopic ACTH-producing tumours, but these almost never occur in children. ACTH-independent disease is usually from corticosteroid therapy, but may be from adrenocortical tumours

- Growth failure/short stature
- Face and trunk obesity
- Red cheeks
- Hirsutism
- Striae
- Hypertension
- Bruising
- Carbohydrate intolerance
- Muscle wasting and weakness
- Osteopenia
- Psychological problems.

(benign or malignant), when there may also be virilisation; these usually occur in young children. A diagnosis of Cushing syndrome is often questioned in obese children. Most obese children from dietary excess are of above-average height, in contrast to children with Cushing syndrome, who are short and have growth failure.

If Cushing syndrome is a possibility, then the normal diurnal variation of cortisol (high in the morning, low at midnight) may be shown to be lost – in Cushing syndrome the midnight concentration is also high. The 24-h urine free cortisol is also high. After the administration of dexamethasone, there is failure to suppress the plasma 09.00 h cortisol levels. Adrenal tumours are identified on CT or MRI scan of the abdomen and a pituitary adenoma on MRI brain scan. Adrenal tumours are usually unilateral and are treated by adrenalectomy and radiotherapy if indicated. Pituitary adenomas are best treated by trans-sphenoidal resection, but radiotherapy can be used.

Inborn errors of metabolism

Although individually rare, inborn errors of metabolism are an important cause of paediatric morbidity and mortality. The specialised nature of the diagnostic tests and subsequent management often means that these patients are managed in specialist centres. However, as the prognosis for most patients depends upon the speed of diagnosis, all doctors need to be familiar with their variable presentation and diagnosis. It is often assumed that a precise knowledge of a large number of biochemical pathways is necessary to make a diagnosis, but in fact a more than adequate diagnostic approach can be based on the correct use of only a few screening tests.

Presentation

An inborn error of metabolism may be suspected before birth from a positive family history or previous unexplained deaths in the family.

After birth, inborn errors of metabolism usually, but not invariably, present in one of five ways:

- As a result of newborn screening, e.g. phenylketonuria (PKU), or family screening, e.g. familial hypercholesterolaemia

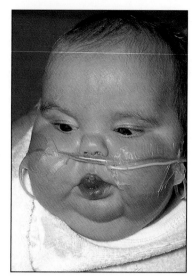

Figure 25.10 Facial obesity from prolonged course of high-dose corticosteroids for bronchopulmonary dysplasia in a preterm infant. Such prolonged courses are no longer used. Additional oxygen therapy is being given via nasal cannulae.

- After a short period of apparent normality, with a severe neonatal illness with poor feeding, vomiting, encephalopathy, acidosis, coma and death, e.g. organic acid or urea cycle disorders
- As an infant or older child with an illness similar to that described above but with hypoglycaemia as a prominent feature or as an ALTE (acute life-threatening episode) or near-miss 'cot death', e.g. a fat oxidation defect such as medium-chain acyl-CoA dehydrogenase deficiency (MCADD)
- In a subacute way, after a period of normal development, with regression, organomegaly and coarse facies, e.g. mucopolysaccharide disease or other lysosomal storage disorder or with enlargement of the liver and/or spleen alone, with or without accompanying biochemical upset such as hypoglycaemia, e.g. glycogen storage disease
- As a dysmorphic syndrome.

Newborn screening

The parents of all babies born in the UK are offered a screening test to detect hypothyroidism and phenylketonuria (PKU). The tests are done on a spot of blood from a heel-prick collected onto a filter paper. Although it is technically possible to screen for a much larger group of disorders, this has been resisted in the UK. However, the screening programme has been extended to include cystic fibrosis, haemoglobinopathies and the metabolic disorder MCADD.

Amino acid disorders

Phenylketonuria

This occurs in 1 in 10 000–15 000 live births in the UK. It is either due to a deficiency of the enzyme phenylalanine hydroxylase (classical PKU) or in the synthesis or recycling of the biopterin cofactor for this enzyme. Untreated, it usually presents with developmental delay at 6–12 months of age. There may be a musty odour due to the metabolite phenylacetic acid. Many affected children are fair-haired and blue-eyed and some develop eczema and seizures. Fortunately, most affected children are detected through the national biochemical screening programme (Guthrie test).

Treatment of classical PKU is with restriction of dietary phenylalanine, while ensuring there is sufficient for optimal physical and neurological growth. The blood plasma phenylalanine is monitored regularly. The current recommendation is to maintain the diet throughout life. This is particularly important during pregnancy, when high maternal phenylalanine levels may damage the fetus.

Cofactor defects, which have a much poorer prognosis than classical PKU, are treated with a diet low in phenylalanine and neurotransmitter precursors.

Homocystinuria

This is due to cystathionine synthetase deficiency. Presentation is with developmental delay and eventually subluxation of the ocular lens (ectopia lentis). There is progressive learning difficulty, psychiatric disorders and convulsions. Skeletal manifestations resemble Marfan syndrome. The complexion is usually fair with brittle hair. Thromboembolic episodes may occur at any age. Almost half respond to large doses of the coenzyme pyridoxine. Those who do not respond are treated with a low-methionine diet supplemented with cysteine and with the addition of the re-methylating agent betaine.

Tyrosinaemia

Tyrosinaemia (type 1) is a rare autosomal recessive disorder caused by a deficiency of fumarylacetoacetase. Accumulation of toxic metabolites results in damage to the liver (leading to liver failure) and renal tubules (resulting in Fanconi syndrome). Untreated the disorder is fatal, but effective therapy is now available with a drug called NTBC, which inhibits an enzyme required in the catabolism of tyrosine, together with a diet low in tyrosine and phenylalanine.

Disorders presenting acutely in the neonatal period

This group includes:

- Disorders of the catabolic pathways of several essential amino acids (the branched-chain amino acids, leucine, isoleucine and valine, and odd-chain amino acids, e.g. threonine) to cause maple syrup urine disease and other organic acid disorders
- Defects in the urea cycle
- A disorder of carbohydrate metabolism – classical galactosaemia.

In these disorders, the affected child is normal at birth and after several days develops non-specific signs and symptoms shared with other more common neonatal disorders, such as generalised infection. The most common patterns of illness are:

- Vomiting, acidosis and circulatory disturbance, followed by depressed consciousness and convulsions – suggestive of one of the organic acidaemias
- Neurological features of lethargy, refusal to feed, hypotonia, drowsiness, unconsciousness and apnoea – suggestive of primary defects of the urea cycle. Improvement when given intravenous fluids but relapse if milk feeds are restarted is characteristic of classical galactosaemia.

Diagnosis is with a 'metabolic screen' in addition to the standard investigations for unwell infants. The 'metabolic screen' varies between laboratories and should be discussed with the specialist laboratory before collecting samples. The urgency should also be indicated. Both blood and urine samples are likely to be required. A simple bedside test for ketones can be helpful as heavy ketosis and acidosis in an encephalopathic infant is strongly suggestive of an organic acid disorder. In patients with acidosis, calculation of the anion gap (the sum of serum concentrations of sodium and potassium minus the sum of the concentrations of chloride and bicarbonate) can be helpful. Values >25 mmol/L (normal 12–16 mmol/L) are usually secondary to an organic acidaemia. It is good practice to collect all urine passed by the infant for possible future analysis (or until a diagnosis is established), as well as collecting a sample of blood before any blood transfusion in case the latter interferes with the interpretation of laboratory tests. Both short-term and long-term management depend on the underlying diagnosis. In the immediate emergency situation, removal of toxic metabolites and limitation of catabolism have the highest priority. Transfer to a neonatal intensive care unit, mechanical ventilation and haemodialysis are often required. Long-term management involves skilled dietetic support as well as the use of specific medications depending on the underlying diagnosis.

Disorders of carbohydrate metabolism

Galactosaemia

This rare, recessively inherited disorder results from deficiency of the enzyme galactose-1-phosphate uridyltransferase, which is essential for galactose metabolism. When lactose-containing milk feeds such as breast or infant formula are introduced, affected infants feed poorly, vomit and develop jaundice and hepatomegaly and hepatic failure (see Ch. 20). Chronic liver disease, cataracts and developmental delay are inevitable if the condition is untreated. Management is with a lactose- and galactose-free diet for life. Even if treated early, there are usually moderate learning difficulties (adult IQ 60–80).

Glycogen storage disorders

These mostly recessively inherited disorders have specific enzyme defects which prevent mobilisation of glucose from glycogen, resulting in an abnormal

Table 25.2 Some of the glycogen storage disorders

Type	Enzyme defect	Onset	Liver	Muscle	Comments
Type I (von Gierke)	Glucose-6-phosphatase	Infant	+++	–	See Figure 25.11 Enlarged liver and kidneys Growth failure. Hypoglycaemia Good prognosis
Type II (Pompe)	Lysosomal α-glucosidase	Infant	++	+++	Hypotonia and cardiomegaly at several months. Enzyme replacement therapy (Myozyme). Death from heart failure
Type III (Cori)	Amylo-1,6-glucosidase	Infant	++	+	Milder features of type I, but muscles may be affected Good prognosis
Type V (McArdle)	Phosphorylase	Child	–	++	Temporary weakness and cramps muscles after exercise Myoglobinuria in later life

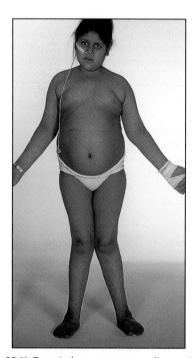

Figure 25.11 Type I glycogen storage disease in a 12-year-old girl. There is truncal obesity with a distended abdomen from an enlarged liver; short stature and hypotrophic muscles; 'doll' facies; nasogastric feeding to maintain blood glucose levels overnight.

storage of glycogen in liver and/or muscle. There are nine main enzyme defects, some of which are shown in Table 25.2. The disorder may predominantly affect muscle (e.g. types II, V), leading to skeletal muscle weakness. In type II (Pompe disease) there is generalised intralysosomal storage of glycogen. The heart is severely affected, leading to death from cardiomyopathy. In other types (e.g. I, III) the liver is the main organ of storage, and hepatomegaly and hypoglycaemia are prominent (Fig. 25.11). Long-term complications of type I include hyperlipidaemia, hyperuricaemia, the development of hepatic adenomas and cardiovascular disease.

Management is to maintain blood glucose by frequent feeds or by carbohydrate infusion via a gastrostomy or nasogastric tube in infancy. In older children, glucose levels can be maintained using slow-release oligosaccharides (corn starch). In type II (Pompe disease), treatment with enzyme replacement therapy (Myozyme) is now available. In type III disorder, a high-protein diet is recommended to prevent growth retardation and myopathy.

Hyperlipidaemia

Hyperlipidaemia is one of the main risk factors for coronary heart disease. Identification and treatment of hyperlipidaemia in childhood may delay the onset of cardiovascular disease in later life.

Children should be screened for hyperlipidaemia if they are at increased risk – if a parent or grandparent has a history of coronary heart disease before 55 years of age or if there is a family history of a lipid disorder. At present, screening all children is not thought justifiable in view of the many uncertainties about selecting who should be treated, what treatment should be given and its effect on outcome.

If the serum cholesterol is high (>5.3 mmol/L) on random testing, fasting serum cholesterol, triglyceride and low-density lipoprotein (LDL) and high-density lipoprotein (HDL) cholesterol are measured. Secondary causes of hypercholesterolaemia should be considered, such as obesity, hypothyroidism, diabetes mellitus, nephrotic syndrome and obstructive jaundice.

Familial hypercholesterolaemia (FH)

This autosomal dominant disorder of lipoprotein metabolism is due to a defect in the LDL receptor. About 1 in 500 of the population are affected. The serum LDL cholesterol concentration is markedly raised (>3.3 mmol/L). The condition is associated with premature coronary heart disease, which occurs in half by 50 years of age in males and by 60 years in females. Skin and tendon xanthomata (Fig. 25.12) may be present, but are uncommon in childhood. Drug therapy is considered in children aged 10 years and older and depends on how high the LDL cholesterol concentration is raised, if there is a family history of premature coronary heart disease (<55 years of age), if there is evidence of tissue lipid deposition (xanthomata or bruits) and other non-lipid risk factors, e.g. diabetes. The main drugs used are the non-systemically acting bile acid sequestrants and more recently the HMG-CoA reductase inhibitors, the statins. Although bile acid sequestrants are moderately effective, compliance remains a major problem with them. Statins have been shown to be effective in children, without adverse effects on growth, maturation or endocrine function. The fibrate drug fenofibrate has also been shown to reduce LDL cholesterol and to be well tolerated by children and adolescents.

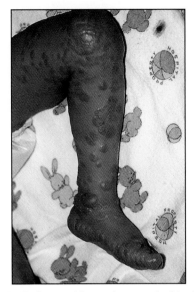

Figure 25.12 Severe skin xanthomata. In this child, it was secondary to liver failure and resolved within weeks of liver transplantation.

Homozygous disease is very rare and much more severe, causing xanthomata in childhood and clinical cardiovascular disease in the second decade. Affected children require referral to a specialist centre. Response to drugs is variable, depending on the gene mutation. Liver transplantation has been tried.

Further reading

Brook C, Clayton P, Brown R: *Brook's Paediatric Endocrinology*, ed 8, Oxford, 2009, Blackwell.

Sperling M: *Pediatric Endocrinology*, ed 3, Amsterdam, 2008, Elsevier.

Websites (Accessed April 2011)

International Society for Pediatric and Adolescent Diabetes: Available at http://www.ispad.org.

European Society for Paediatric Endocrinology: Available at http://www.eurospe.org.

Endotext.com Endocrine Source: Available at: http://www.endotext.org/pediatrics/index.htm. *Articles on endocrinology.*

Endocrine and metabolic disorders

Musculoskeletal disorders

Features of musculoskeletal disorders in children are:

- Although musculoskeletal presentations are common and often benign and self-limiting, they can be caused by a serious underlying condition such as infection, malignancy or non-accidental injury
- Many concerns of parents about their children's posture are variations of normal alignment in the growing skeleton
- Juvenile idiopathic arthritis (JIA) is the most common cause of chronic arthritis in children.

Assessment of the musculoskeletal system

This should, as a minimum, include the pGALS (paediatric Gait, Arms, Legs, Spine) screen (see p. 25) to identify and localise musculoskeletal problems; any suggestion of a musculoskeletal problem should be followed by more detailed regional musculoskeletal examination (called pREMS, see p. 26).

Variations of normal posture

Variations are common and may be noticed by parents or on routine developmental surveillance. Most resolve without any treatment but if severe, progressive, painful or asymmetrical, they should be referred for specialist opinion.

Bow legs (genu varum)

The normal toddler has a broad base gait. Many children evolve leg alignment with initially a degree of bowing of the tibiae, causing the knees to be wide apart – best observed while the child is standing with the feet together (Fig. 26.1). A pathological cause of bow legs is rickets; check for the presence of other clinical features (see Ch. 11). Severe progressive and often unilateral bow legs is a feature of Blount disease (infantile tibia vara), an uncommon condition predominantly seen in Afro-Caribbean children. Radiographs are characteristic with beaking of the proximal medial tibial epiphysis.

Knock-knees (genu valgum)

The feet are wide apart when standing with the knees held together (Fig. 26.2). It is seen in many young children and usually resolves spontaneously.

Flat feet (pes planus)

Toddlers learning to walk usually have flat feet due to flatness of the medial longitudinal arch and the presence of a fat pad which disappears as the child gets older (Fig. 26.3). An arch can usually be demonstrated on standing on tiptoe or by passively extending the big toe. Marked flat feet is common in hypermobility. A fixed flat foot, often painful, presenting in older children, may indicate a congenital tarsal coalition and requires an orthopaedic opinion. Symptomatic flat feet are often helped with footwear advice and, occasionally, an arch support may be required.

In-toeing and out-toeing

There are three main causes of in-toeing:

- *Metatarsus varus* (Fig. 26.4a) – an adduction deformity of a highly mobile forefoot

Variants of normal

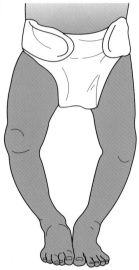

Figure 26.1 Bow legs.

Figure 26.2 Knock-knees.

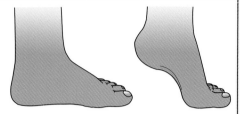

Figure 26.3 Pes planus showing the flat feet of toddlers. The medial longitudinal arch appears on standing on tiptoe.

In-toeing

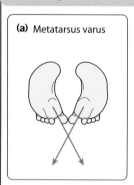

(a) Metatarsus varus

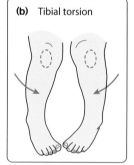

(b) Tibial torsion

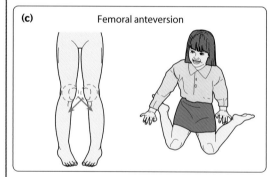

(c) Femoral anteversion

Figure 26.4 In-toeing **(a)** at the feet, **(b)** lower leg, **(c)** hip, with 'W' sitting.

Box 26.1 Clinical features of in-toeing in children

Metatarsus varus

- Occurs in infants
- Passively correctable
- Heel is held in the normal position
- No treatment required unless it persists beyond 5 years of age and is symptomatic

Medial tibial torsion

- Occurs in toddlers
- May be associated with bowing of the tibiae
- Self-corrects within about 5 years

Persistent anteversion of the femoral neck

- Presents in childhood
- Usually self-corrects by 8 years of age
- May be associated with hypermobility of the joints
- Children sit between their feet with the hips fully internally rotated ('W' sitting)
- Most do not require treatment but femoral osteotomy may be required for persistent anteversion.

- *Medial tibial torsion* (Fig. 26.4b) – at the lower leg, when the tibia is laterally rotated less than normal in relation to the femur
- *Persistent anteversion of the femoral neck* (Fig. 26.4c) – at the hip, when the femoral neck is twisted forward more than normal.

The clinical features are described in Box 26.1.

Out-toeing is uncommon but may occur in infants between 6 and 12 months of age.

When bilateral, it is often due to lateral rotation of the hips and resolves spontaneously.

Summary

Variations of musculoskeletal normality and differential diagnosis

Perceived disorder	Normal age range	Differential diagnoses to consider
Bow legs	1–3 years	Rickets osteogenesis imperfecta, Blount disease
Knock-knees	2–7 years	Juvenile idiopathic arthritis (JIA)
Flat feet	1–2 years	Hypermobility, congenital tarsal fusion
In-toeing	1–2 years	Tibial torsion, femoral anteversion
Out-toeing	6–12 months	Hypermobility, Ehlers–Danlos and Marfan syndromes
Toe walking	1–3 years	Spastic diplegia, muscular dystrophy, JIA

Toe walking

Common in young children and may become persistent, usually from habit; can walk normally on request. Needs to be distinguished from mild cerebral palsy or tightness of the Achilles tendons or inflammatory arthritis in the foot or ankle. In older boys, Duchenne muscular dystrophy should be excluded.

Abnormal posture

Talipes equinovarus (clubfoot)

Positional talipes from intrauterine compression is common. The foot is of normal size, the deformity is mild and can be corrected to the neutral position with passive manipulation. Often the baby's intrauterine posture can be recreated. If the positional deformity is marked, parents can be shown passive exercises by the physiotherapist.

Talipes equinovarus is a complex abnormality (Figs 26.5, 26.6). The entire foot is inverted and supinated, the forefoot adducted and the heel is rotated inwards and in plantar flexion. The affected foot is shorter and the calf muscles thinner than normal. The position of the foot is fixed, cannot be corrected completely and is often bilateral. The birth prevalence is 1 per 1000 live births, affects predominantly males (2 : 1), can be familial and is usually idiopathic. However, it may also be secondary to oligohydramnios during pregnancy, a feature of a malformation syndrome or of a neuromuscular disorder such as spina bifida. There is an association with developmental dysplasia of the hip (DDH).

Treatment is started promptly with plaster casting and bracing ('Ponsetti method'), which may be required for many months. It is usually successful unless the condition is very severe, when corrective surgery is required.

Vertical talus

Talipes equinovarus needs to be differentiated from the rare congenital vertical talus, where the foot is stiff and rocker-bottom in shape. Many of these infants

Talipes

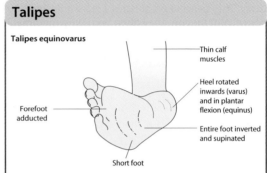

Talipes equinovarus

Thin calf muscles

Heel rotated inwards (varus) and in plantar flexion (equinus)

Forefoot adducted

Entire foot inverted and supinated

Short foot

Figure 26.5 Abnormalities in talipes equinovarus.

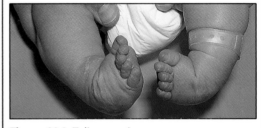

Figure 26.6 Talipes equinovarus.

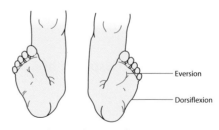

Talipes calcaneovalgus

Eversion

Dorsiflexion

Figure 26.7 Talipes calcaneovalgus.

have other malformations. The diagnosis can be confirmed on X-ray. Surgery is usually required.

Talipes calcaneovalgus

The foot is dorsiflexed and everted (Fig. 26.7). It usually results from intrauterine moulding and self-corrects. Passive foot exercises are sometimes advised.

Musculoskeletal disorders

453

There is an association with developmental dysplasia of the hip.

Flat feet

In older children and adolescents, a *rigid* flat foot is pathological. It is suggested by absence of a normal arch on tip toeing. It may be due to an associated tendo-Achilles contracture (ankle), or tarsal coalition (see below) or inflammatory arthropathy (juvenile idiopathic arthritis, JIA).

Tarsal coalition

Results from lack of segmentation between one or more bones of the foot, and coalitions that were fibrous or cartilaginous become symptomatic as they begin to ossify. They become progressively more rigid and limit normal foot motion. They often become symptomatic during the pre-adolescent years. Radiographs may be normal if the bars have not yet ossified. Corrective surgery may be required.

Pes cavus

In pes cavus, there is a high arched foot. When it presents in older children, it is often associated with neuromuscular disorders, e.g. Friedreich ataxia and type I hereditary motor sensory neuropathy (peroneal muscular atrophy). Treatment is required if the foot becomes stiff or painful.

Summary

Regarding talipes equinovarus
- Needs to be differentiated from positional talipes
- Check for neuromuscular disorder or spinal lesion and for developmental dysplasia of the hip (DDH).

Developmental dysplasia of the hip (DDH)

This is a spectrum of disorders ranging from dysplasia to subluxation through to frank dislocation of the hip. Early detection is important as it usually responds to conservative treatment; late diagnosis is usually associated with hip dysplasia, which requires complex treatment often including surgery. Neonatal screening is performed as part of the routine examination of the newborn (see Fig. 9.15), checking if the hip can be dislocated posteriorly out of the acetabulum (Barlow manoeuvre) or can be relocated back into the acetabulum on abduction (Ortolani manoeuvre). These tests are repeated at routine surveillance at 8 weeks of age. Thereafter, presentation of the condition is usually with

a limp or abnormal gait. It may be identified from asymmetry of skinfolds around the hip, limited abduction of the hip or shortening of the affected leg.

On neonatal screening, an abnormality of the hip is detected in about 6–10 per 1000 live births. Most will resolve spontaneously. The true birth prevalence of DDH is about 1.3 per 1000 live births. Clinical neonatal screening misses some cases. This may be because of inexperience of the examiner, but in some it is not possible to clinically detect dislocation at this stage, e.g. where there is only a mildly shallow acetabulum. To overcome these problems, some centres perform ultrasound screening on all newborn infants. It is highly specific in detecting DDH but is expensive and has a high rate of false positives, and is not recommended in the UK. It is performed in some centres in infants at increased risk (family history, of breech presentation).

If developmental dysplasia of the hip is suspected, a specialist orthopaedic opinion should be obtained. An ultrasound examination allows detailed assessment of the hip, quantifying the degree of dysplasia and whether there is subluxation or dislocation. If the initial ultrasound is abnormal, the infant may be placed in a splint or harness to keep the hip flexed and abducted for several months. Progress is monitored by ultrasound or X-ray. The splinting must be done expertly as necrosis of the femoral head is a potential complication.

In most instances, a satisfactory response is obtained. Surgery is required if conservative measures fail.

Scoliosis

Scoliosis is a lateral curvature in the frontal plane of the spine.

In structural scoliosis, there is rotation of the vertebral bodies which causes a prominence in the back from rib asymmetry. In most cases, the changes are mild, pain-free and primarily a cosmetic problem; however, in severe cases, the spinal curvature can lead to cardiorespiratory failure from distortion of the chest.

Causes of scoliosis are:

- *Idiopathic*. The most common, either early onset (<5 years old) or, most often, late onset, mainly girls 10–14 years of age during their pubertal growth spurt
- *Congenital*. From a congenital structural defect of the spine, e.g. hemivertebra, spina bifida, syndromes (e.g. VACTERL association – Vertebral, Anorectal, Cardiac, Tracheo-oEsophageal, Renal and Limb anomalies).
- *Secondary*. Related to other disorders such as neuromuscular imbalance (e.g. cerebral palsy, muscular dystrophy); disorders of bone such as neurofibromatosis or of connective tissues such as Marfan syndrome, or leg length discrepancy, e.g. due to arthritis of one knee in JIA.

Examination should start with inspection of the child's back while standing up straight. In mild scoliosis, there may be irregular skin creases and difference in shoulder

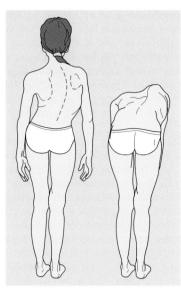

Figure 26.8 Structural scoliosis with vertebral rotation shown by rib rotation on bending forward.

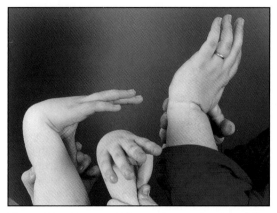

Figure 26.9 Hypermobility syndrome, showing ability to hyperextend the thumb onto the forearm of a mother and two of her children.

height. The scoliosis can be identified on examining the child's back when bent forward (Fig. 26.8). If the scoliosis disappears on forward bending, it is postural although leg lengths should be checked.

Mild scoliosis will resolve spontaneously, or progresses minimally. If more severe, the severity and progression of the curvature of the spine is determined by X-ray. Severe cases are managed in specialist spinal centres where the place of non-medical treatment such as bracing will be considered, with surgery indicated only if severe or there is coexisting pathology such as neuromuscular or respiratory disease.

Torticollis

The most common cause of torticollis (wry neck) in infants is a sternomastoid tumour (congenital muscular torticollis). They occur in the first few weeks of life and present with a mobile, non-tender nodule, which can be felt within the body of the sternocleidomastoid muscle. There may be restriction of head turning and tilting of the head. The condition usually resolves in 2–6 months. Passive stretching is advised, but its efficacy is unproven.

Torticollis presenting later in childhood may be due to muscular spasm or secondary to ENT infection, spinal tumour (such as osteoid osteoma), cervical spine arthritis or malformation or posterior fossa tumour.

The painful limb, knee and back

Growing pains

Episodes of generalised pain in the lower limbs, referred to as 'growing pains' or nocturnal idiopathic pain, are common in preschool and school-aged children. The pain often wakes the child from sleep and settles with

massage or comforting. The condition is poorly understood, but features to be fulfilled for this diagnosis are:

- Age range 3–12 years
- Pains symmetrical in lower limbs and not limited to joints
- Pains *never* present at the start of the day after waking
- Physical activities not limited; no limp
- Physical examination normal and otherwise well (with the exception of joint hypermobility in some).

Hypermobility

Older children or adolescents with hypermobility may complain of musculoskeletal pain mainly confined to the lower limbs, often worse after exercise. Joint swelling is usually absent or is transient. Hypermobility may be generalised or limited to peripheral joints (such as hands and feet). There is symmetrical hyperextension of the thumbs and fingers that can be hyperextended onto the forearms (Fig. 26.9), elbows and knees can be hyperextended beyond 10°, and palms can be placed flat on the floor with knees straight. Lower limb findings associated with hypermobility are hyperextensibility of the knee joint and flat feet with normal arches on tiptoe, which are over-pronated secondary to ankle hypermobility.

While mild degrees of hypermobility are a normal finding in younger female children, and many children with hypermobility are asymptomatic and find being very flexible an advantage in dancing and gymnastics, some experience recurrent mechanical joint and muscle pain, which is often activity related. These children require specialist assessment and may benefit from advice about footwear, exercises and occasionally orthotics. Hypermobility is also a feature of some chromosomal syndromes, e.g. Down syndrome and some inherited collagen disorders (e.g. Marfan and Ehlers–Danlos syndrome).

Complex regional pain syndromes

The most dramatic musculoskeletal pain is that encountered in complex regional pain syndromes (CRPS), formerly known as idiopathic pain syndromes, which may

Musculoskeletal disorders

455

be localised or generalised. They usually present in adolescent females.

Localised forms often present with foot and ankle involvement (typically unilateral); the pain can be extreme and incapacitating, often triggered by minor trauma or without a clear precipitant. Presentation to the clinic may be in a wheelchair. In addition to severe pain, there may be hyperaesthesia (increased sensitivity to stimuli), allodynia (pain from a stimulus that does not normally produce pain), and the affected part (often a foot or hand) may be cool to touch with swelling and mottling, held in flexion with minimal if any active movement, and bizarre posturing is not uncommon. Typically, with distraction, the normal range of passive movements is possible.

Diffuse forms are characterised by severe widespread pain with disturbed sleep patterns, feeling exhausted during the day, with extreme tenderness over soft tissues. The characteristic tender points that are found in adults with fibromyalgia may be absent or fewer in number in children.

The child or adolescent with complex regional pain is otherwise well and physical examination is otherwise normal.

Organic pathology needs to be excluded. The aetiology is unknown, but affected children often have significant associated stresses in their lives.

A multidisciplinary rehabilitation regimen is required, predominantly physical therapy-based, either community or inpatient.

Acute-onset limb pain

Limb pain of acute onset has a number of causes. Trauma is the most common, usually accidental from sports injuries or falls, but occasionally non-accidental. Osteomyelitis and bone tumours are uncommon, but need urgent treatment.

Osteomyelitis

In osteomyelitis, there is infection of the metaphysis of long bones. The most common sites are the distal femur and proximal tibia, but any bone may be affected (Fig. 26.10). It is usually due to haematogenous spread of the pathogen, but may arise by direct spread from an infected wound. The skin is swollen directly over the affected site. Where the joint capsule is inserted distal to the epiphyseal plate, as in the hip, osteomyelitis may spread to cause septic arthritis. Most infections are caused by *Staphylococcus aureus*, but other pathogens include *Streptococcus* and *Haemophilus influenzae* if not immunised. In sickle cell anaemia, there is an increased risk of staphylococcal and salmonella osteomyelitis. Infection may be from tuberculosis; although rare in the UK, it needs to be considered, especially in the immunodeficient child.

Presentation

This is usually with a markedly painful, immobile limb (pseudoparesis) in a child with an acute febrile illness. Directly over the infected site there is swelling and exquisite tenderness, and it may be erythematous and warm. Moving the limb causes severe pain. There may

be a sterile effusion of an adjacent joint. Presentation may be more insidious in infants, in whom swelling or reduced limb movement is the initial sign. Beyond infancy, presentation may be with back pain in a vertebral infection or with a limp or groin pain in infection of the pelvis. Occasionally, there are multiple foci (e.g. disseminated staphylococcal or *H. influenzae* infection).

Investigation

Blood cultures are usually positive and the white blood count and acute-phase reactants are raised. X-rays are initially normal, other than showing soft tissue swelling; it takes 7–10 days for subperiosteal new bone formation and localised bone rarefaction to become visible. Ultrasound may show periosteal elevation at presentation. MRI allows identification of infection in the bone (subperiosteal pus and purulent debris in the bone) and differentiation of bone from soft tissue infection. Radionuclide bone scan (Fig. 26.11) may be helpful if the site of infection is unclear. The X-ray changes of chronic osteomyelitis are shown in Figure 26.12.

Treatment

Prompt treatment with parenteral antibiotics is required for several weeks to prevent bone necrosis, chronic infection with a discharging sinus, limb deformity and amyloidosis. Antibiotics are given intravenously until there is clinical recovery and the acute-phase reactants have returned to normal, followed by oral therapy for several weeks. Aspiration or surgical decompression of the subperiosteal space may be performed if the presentation is atypical or in immunodeficient children. Surgical drainage is performed if the condition does not respond rapidly to antibiotic therapy. The affected limb is initially rested in a splint and subsequently mobilised.

> ### Summary
>
> **Osteomyelitis**
>
> - Presents with fever, a painful, immobile limb, swelling and extreme tenderness, especially on moving the limb
> - Blood cultures are usually positive
> - Parenteral antibiotics must be given immediately
> - Surgical drainage if unresponsive to antibiotic therapy.

Malignant disease

Acute lymphoblastic leukaemia may present with bone pain in children (sometimes primarily at night) and even frank arthritis. Neuroblastoma, usually in the young children, may present with systemic arthritis, or bone pain from metastases, which may be difficult to localise.

Bone tumours

Malignant bone tumours – osteogenic sarcoma and Ewing tumour – are rare. They present with pain or

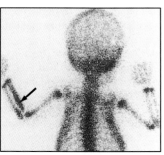

Epiphyseal plate

Joint

Epiphyseal centre

Septic arthritis

Capsular attachment below metaphysis as in the hip, shoulder and elbow

Infection of the metaphysis

Capsular attachment above metaphysis

Metaphysis

Subperiosteal abscess

Figure 26.10 Possible spread of osteomyelitis. In children, the epiphyseal growth plate limits the spread of metaphyseal infection. In infants, before there has been maturation of the growth plate, infection can spread directly to cause joint destruction and arrested growth.

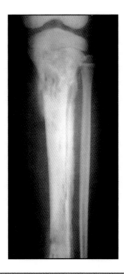

Figure 26.12 Chronic osteomyelitis, showing periosteal reaction along the lateral shaft of the tibia and multiple hypodense areas within the metaphyseal regions.

Figure 26.11 Bone scan of osteomyelitis with increased radionuclide uptake of the left radius. (Courtesy of Professor H. Carty.)

swelling, or occasionally with a pathological fracture. Further features are considered in Chapter 21.

Osteoid osteoma is a benign tumour affecting adolescents, especially boys, usually involving the femur or tibia or spine. The pain is more severe at night and improves with NSAID therapy. There may be some localised tenderness, soft tissue swelling, joint effusion if sited near a joint and scoliosis if in the spine. The X-ray is usually diagnostic, with a sharply demarcated radiolucent nidus of osteoid tissue surrounded by sclerotic bone. If the X-ray is normal, a CT or MRI scan is required. Treatment is by surgical removal.

The painful knee

When assessing a painful knee, the hip must always be examined, as hip pain is often referred to the knee.

Osgood–Schlatter disease

This is osteochondritis of the patellar tendon insertion at the knee, often affecting adolescent males who are physically active (particularly football or basketball). Usually presents with knee pain after exercise, localised tenderness and sometimes swelling over the tibial tuberosity. There is often hamstring tightness. It is bilateral in 25–50%. Most resolve with reduced activity and physiotherapy for quadriceps muscle strengthening, hamstring stretches and occasionally orthotics. A knee immobiliser splint may be helpful.

Chondromalacia patellae

There is softening of the articular cartilage of the patella. It most often affects adolescent females, causing pain when the patella is tightly apposed to the femoral condyles, as in standing up from sitting or on

457

walking up stairs. It is often associated with hypermobility and flat feet, suggesting a biomechanical component to the aetiology

Treatment is with rest and physiotherapy for quadriceps muscle strengthening.

Osteochondritis dissecans (segmental avascular necrosis of the subchondral bone)

This presents as persistent knee pain in the physically very active adolescent, with localised tenderness over the femoral condyles. Pain is caused by separation of bone and cartilage from the medial femoral condyle following avascular necrosis. Complete separation of articular fragments may result in loose body formation and symptoms of knee locking or giving way. Treatment is initially with rest and quadriceps exercises; sometimes arthroscopic surgery is required.

Subluxation and dislocation of the patella

Subluxation of the patella produces the feeling of instability or giving way of the knee. It is often associated with generalised hypermobility. Rarely, dislocation of the patella can occur, usually laterally, suddenly and with severe pain – reduction occurs spontaneously or on gentle extension of the knee. Treatment is with quadriceps exercises. Sometimes surgery is required to realign the pull of the quadriceps on the patellar tendon.

Injuries

Contact sports characteristically result in acute injuries to the knee, while non-contact sports with sustained activity tend to result in chronic injury and overuse syndromes. Sporting injuries to the menisci and ligaments are common in adolescents. MRI scans are helpful to determine the extent of damage. Management is usually conservative. In infants and young children, similar injuries are more likely to result in fractures, as their ligaments are relatively stronger than their bones.

Back pain

Back pain is a symptom of concern in the very young and pre-adolescent ages as, in contrast to adults, a cause can often be identified. The younger the child, the more likely there will be significant pathology. Red Flag clinical features are listed in Box 26.2.

Mechanical causes – there may be muscle spasm or soft tissue pain from injury, often sport-related or from poor posture or abnormal loading (such as carrying heavy school bags on one shoulder).

Tumours: benign or malignant – The spine is a common site for osteoid osteoma. It may also be the site of primary tumours or metastases.

Vertebral osteomyelitis or discitis – there is localised tenderness; in infants there is reluctance to walk or bear weight or pain on spine flexion along with fever and systemic upset. While plain X-rays may show abnormalities suggesting the diagnosis, further

Box 26.2 Red Flag clinical features of back pain

- Young age – pathology more likely
- High fever – infection
- Night waking, persistent pain – osteoid osteoma or tumours
- Painful scoliosis – infection or malignancy
- Focal neurological signs including nerve root irritation, loss of bowel/bladder control – nerve root/spinal cord compression
- Associated weight loss, systemic malaise – malignancy.

imaging (MRI) is often required. Treatment is with intravenous antibiotics.

Spinal cord or nerve root entrapment – from tumour or prolapsed intervertebral disc – often associated with trauma or heavy lifting,

Scheuermann disease – an osteochondrosis of the vertebral body; may present with a fixed thoracic kyphosis with or without back pain. The diagnosis is usually made on X-ray. In many cases, the radiographic changes are a coincidental finding and the patient is asymptomatic.

Spondylolysis/spondylolisthesis – stress fracture of the pars interarticularis of the vertebra. Increased risk with certain sporting activities, e.g. bowling in cricket or gymnastics. If bilateral, can result in spondylolisthesis, forward slip of the vertebral body and potential cord or nerve root compression. There is pain on spine extension and localised tenderness. Change may be apparent on X-ray but often further imaging (CT scan) is required.

Complex regional pain syndrome (CRPS) – diagnosed when no physical cause is found; may be exacerbated by psychological stress.

Limp

Limp can be divided into acute painful limp and chronic or intermittent limp, where pain may or may not be the presenting feature, and by age (Table 26.1).

Transient synovitis ('irritable hip')

This is the most common cause of acute hip pain in children. It occurs in children aged 2–12 years old. It often follows or is accompanied by a viral infection. Presentation is with sudden onset of pain in the hip or a limp. There is no pain at rest, but there is decreased range of movement, particularly internal rotation. The pain may be referred to the knee. The child is afebrile or has a mild fever and does not appear ill.

It can be difficult to differentiate transient synovitis from early septic arthritis of the hip joint (Table 26.2), and if there is any suspicion of septic arthritis, joint aspiration and blood cultures are mandatory.

In a small proportion of children, transient synovitis precedes the development of Perthes disease. Management of transient synovitis is with bed rest

Table 26.1 Causes of limp

	Acute painful limp	Chronic and intermittent limp
1–3 years	Infection – septic arthritis, osteomyelitis of hip or spine	Developmental dysplasia of the hip (DDH), talipes
	Transient synovitis	
	Trauma – accidental/non-accidental	Neuromuscular, e.g. cerebral palsy
	Malignant disease – leukaemia, neuroblastoma	Juvenile idiopathic arthritis (JIA)
3–10 years	Transient synovitis	Perthes disease (chronic)
	Septic arthritis/osteomyelitis	Neuromuscular disorders, e.g. Duchenne muscular dystrophy
	Trauma and overuse injuries	
	Perthes disease (acute)	Juvenile idiopathic arthritis (JIA)
	Juvenile idiopathic arthritis (JIA)	Tarsal coalition
	Malignant disease, e.g. leukaemia	
	Complex regional pain syndrome	
11–16 years	Mechanical – trauma, overuse injuries, sport injuries	Slipped capital femoral epiphysis (chronic)
	Slipped capital femoral epiphysis (acute)	Juvenile idiopathic arthritis (JIA)
	Avascular necrosis of the femoral head	
	Reactive arthritis	Tarsal coalition
	Juvenile idiopathic arthritis (JIA)	
	Septic arthritis/osteomyelitis	
	Osteochondritis dissecans of the knee	
	Bone tumours and malignancy	
	Complex regional pain syndrome	

Table 26.2 Contrast in clinical features of transient synovitis and septic arthritis of the hip

	Transient synovitis	Septic arthritis
Onset	Acute limp, non-weight bearing	Acute onset, non-weight bearing
Fever	Mild/absent	Moderate/high
Child's appearance	Child often looks well	Child looks ill
Hip movement	Comfortable at rest, limited internal rotation and pain on movement	Hip held flexed; severe pain at rest and worse on any attempt to move joint
White cell count	Normal	Normal/high
Acute-phase reactant/ESR	Slight increase/normal	Raised
Ultrasound	Fluid in joint	Fluid in joint
Radiograph	Normal	Normal/widened joint space
Management	Rest, analgesia	Joint aspiration, usually under ultrasound guidance
		Prolonged antibiotics, rest and analgesia
Course	Resolves <1 week, approx 3% develop Perthes disease	Progressive and severe joint damage if not treated

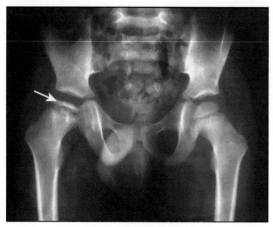

Figure 26.13 Perthes disease, showing flattening with sclerosis and fragmentation of the right femoral capital epiphysis; the left hip is normal.

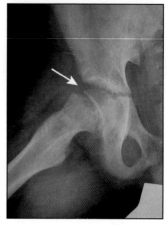

Figure 26.14 Slipped capital femoral epiphysis of the right hip.

and, rarely, skin traction. It usually improves within a few days.

Perthes disease

This is an avascular necrosis of the capital femoral epiphysis of the femoral head due to interruption of the blood supply, followed by revascularisation and reossification over 18–36 months. It mainly affects boys (male:female ratio of 5:1) of 5–10 years of age. Presentation is insidious, with the onset of a limp, or hip or knee pain. The condition may initially be mistaken for transient synovitis. It is bilateral in 10–20%. If suspected, X-ray of both hips (including frog views) should be requested; early signs of Perthes include increased density in the femoral head, which subsequently becomes fragmented and irregular (Fig. 26.13).

Even if the initial X-ray is normal, a repeat may be required if clinical symptoms persist. A bone scan and MRI scan can be helpful in making the diagnosis.

Prognosis is dependent on early diagnosis; if identified early and less than half the femoral head is affected, only bed rest and traction may be required. In more severe disease or late presentations, the femoral head needs to be covered by the acetabulum to act as a mould for the re-ossifying epiphysis and is achieved by maintaining the hip in abduction with plaster or calipers, or by performing femoral or pelvic osteotomy.

In most children, the prognosis is good, particularly in those below 6 years of age with less than half the epiphysis involved. In older children or with more extensive involvement of the epiphysis, deformity of the femoral head and metaphyseal damage are more likely, with potential for subsequent degenerative arthritis in adult life.

Slipped capital femoral epiphysis (SCFE)

Results in displacement of the epiphysis of the femoral head postero-inferiorly requiring prompt treatment in order to prevent avascular necrosis. It is most common

at 10–15 years of age during the adolescent growth spurt, particularly in obese boys and is bilateral in 20%. There is an association with metabolic endocrine abnormalities, e.g. hypothyroidism and hypogonadism. Presentation is with a limp or hip pain, which may be referred to the knee. The onset may be acute, following minor trauma or insidious. Examination shows restricted abduction and internal rotation of the hip. Diagnosis is confirmed on X-ray (Fig. 26.14), and a frog lateral view should also be requested. Management is surgical, usually with pin fixation in situ.

Summary

Regarding hip disorders

- Developmental dysplasia of the hip – identified on screening at birth or 8 weeks, detection of asymmetry of skinfolds around the hip, limited abduction of the hip, shortening of the affected leg or a limp or abnormal gait
- Transient synovitis – most common cause of acute hip pain or a limp; must be differentiated from septic arthritis
- Perthes disease – usually school-aged children with hip pain or limp
- Slipped capital femoral epiphysis – adolescent with a limp or hip pain.

Arthritis

Acute arthritis presents with pain, swelling, heat, redness and restricted movement in a joint. In a monoarthritis of acute onset, the child is also likely to be systemically unwell with fever; if septic arthritis or osteomyelitis is the cause, urgent diagnosis and treatment is required. With infection, more than one joint can be affected, although a single joint is more common.

The causes of polyarthritis are listed in Table 26.3.

Table 26.3 Causes of polyarthritis

Infection	Bacterial – septicaemia/septic arthritis, TB
	Viral – rubella, mumps, adenovirus, coxsackie B, herpes, hepatitis, parvovirus
	Other – *Mycoplasma*, Lyme disease, rickettsia
	Reactive – gastrointestinal infection, streptococcal infection
	Rheumatic fever
Inflammatory bowel disease	Crohn disease, ulcerative colitis
Vasculitis	Henoch–Schönlein purpura, Kawasaki disease
Haematological disorders	Haemophilia, sickle cell disease
Malignant disorders	Leukaemia, neuroblastoma
Connective tissue disorders	Juvenile idiopathic arthritis (JIA), systemic lupus erythematosus (SLE), dermatomyositis, mixed connective tissue disease (MCTD), polyarteritis nodosa (PAN)
Other	Cystic fibrosis

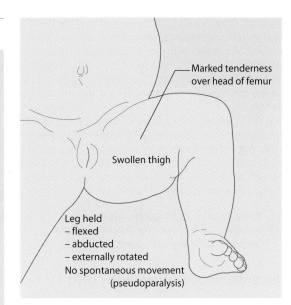

Figure 26.15 Septic arthritis of the hip in infants, showing the characteristic posture to reduce intracapsular pressure. Any leg movement is painful and is resisted.

Reactive arthritis

Reactive arthritis is the most common form of arthritis in childhood. It is characterised by transient joint swelling (usually <6 weeks) often of the ankles or knees. It usually follows (or rarely accompanies) evidence of extra-articular infection. The enteric bacteria (*Salmonella*, *Shigella*, *Campylobacter* and *Yersinia*) are often the cause in children, but viral infections, sexually transmitted infections in adolescents (chlamydia, gonococcus), *Mycoplasma* and *Borrelia burgdorferi* (Lyme disease) are other causes. Rheumatic fever and post-streptococcal reactive arthritis are rare in developed countries but are frequent in many developing countries.

Fever is low grade. Acute-phase reactants are normal or mildly elevated and X-rays are normal. No treatment or only NSAIDs are required and complete recovery can be anticipated.

Septic arthritis

This is a serious infection of the joint space, as it can lead to bone destruction. It is most common in children <2 years old. It usually results from haematogenous spread, but may also occur following a puncture wound or infected skin lesions, e.g. chickenpox. In young children, it may result from spread from adjacent osteomyelitis into joints where the capsule inserts below the epiphyseal growth plate. Usually only one joint is affected, with the hip being a particular concern in infants and young children. Beyond the neonatal period, the most common organism is *Staphylococcus aureus*, and usually only one joint is affected. *H. influenzae* was an important cause in young children prior to Hib immunisation and often affected multiple sites. Underlying and predisposing illnesses such as immunodeficiency and sickle cell disease should be considered.

Presentation

This is usually with an erythematous, warm, acutely tender joint, with a reduced range of movement, in an acutely unwell, febrile child. Infants often hold the limb still (pseudoparesis, pseudoparalysis) and cry if it is moved. A joint effusion may be detectable in peripheral joints. In osteomyelitis, although a sympathetic joint effusion may be present, the tenderness is over the bone, but in up to 15% there is coexistent septic arthritis. The diagnosis of septic arthritis of the hip can be particularly difficult in toddlers, as the joint is well covered by subcutaneous fat (Fig. 26.15). Initial presentation may be with a limp or pain referred to the knee.

Investigation

There is an increased white cell count and acute-phase reactants. Blood cultures must be taken. Ultrasound of deep joints, such as the hip, is helpful to identify an effusion. X-rays are used to exclude trauma and other bony lesions. However, in septic arthritis, the X-rays are initially normal, apart from widening of the joint space

Musculoskeletal disorders

461

and soft tissue swelling. A bone scan may be helpful and an MRI scan may demonstrate an adjacent osteomyelitis. Aspiration of the joint space under ultrasound guidance for organisms and culture is the definitive investigation. Ideally, this is performed immediately, unless this would cause a significant delay in giving antibiotics. A prolonged course of antibiotics is required, initially intravenously. Washing out of the joint or surgical drainage may be required if resolution does not occur rapidly or if the joint is deep-seated, such as the hip. The joint is initially immobilised in a functional position, but subsequently must be mobilised to prevent permanent deformity.

 Early treatment of septic arthritis is essential to prevent destruction of the articular cartilage and bone.

Juvenile idiopathic arthritis (JIA)

This is the commonest chronic inflammatory joint disease in children and adolescents in the UK. It is defined as persistent joint swelling (of >6 weeks duration) presenting before 16 years of age in the absence of infection or any other defined cause. Ninety-five per cent of children have a disease that is clinically and immunogenetically distinct from rheumatoid arthritis in adults. It has a prevalence of approximately 1 in 1000 children, (i.e. similar to epilepsy), with over 12 000 affected children in the UK.

There are at least seven different subtypes of JIA. Its classification is clinical and based on the number of joints affected in the first 6 months, as polyarthritis (more than four joints) (Fig. 26.16) and oligoarthritis (up to and including four joints) or systemic (with fever and rash). Psoriatic arthritis and enthesitis are further subtypes. Subtyping is further classified according to the presence of rheumatoid factor and HLA B27 tissue type. The subtypes and their clinical features are shown in Table 26.4.

Features in the history are gelling (stiffness after periods of rest, such as long car rides), morning joint stiffness and pain. In the young child, it may present with intermittent limp or deterioration in behaviour or mood or avoidance of previously enjoyed activities, rather than complaining of pain.

Initially, there may be only minimal evidence of joint swelling, but subsequently there may be swelling of the joint due to fluid within it, inflammation and, in chronic arthritis, proliferation (thickening) of the synovium and swelling of the periarticular soft tissues.

Long term, with uncontrolled disease activity, there may be bone expansion from overgrowth, which in the knee may cause leg lengthening or valgus deformity, in the hands, discrepancy in digit length, and in the wrist, advancement of bone age.

If systemic features are present, sepsis and malignancy must always be considered.

Complications

Chronic anterior uveitis

This is common but asymptomatic and can lead to severe visual impairment. Regular ophthalmological

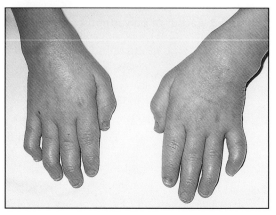

Figure 26.16 Polyarticular juvenile idiopathic arthritis, showing swelling of the wrists, metacarpal and interphalangeal joints and early swan-neck deformities of the fingers.

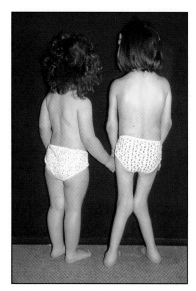

Figure 26.17 Growth failure and marked genu valgum (knock-knees) in an 8-year-old girl with juvenile idiopathic arthritis. For comparison, her sister on the left is 4 years old.

screening using a slit lamp is indicated, especially for children with oligoarticular disease.

Flexion contractures of the joints

These occur when the joint is held in the most comfortable position, thereby minimising intra-articular pressure. Chronic untreated disease can lead to joint destruction and the need for joint replacement.

Growth failure

This may be generalised from anorexia, chronic disease and systemic corticosteroid therapy (Fig. 26.17). May also be localised overgrowth such as leg length discrepancy due to prolonged active knee synovitis and undergrowth, such as micrognathia, usually seen in

Table 26.4 Classification and clinical features of JIA (juvenile idiopathic arthritis)

JIA subtype (approximate %)	Onset age	Sex ratio (F:M)	Articular pattern	Extra-articular features	Laboratory abnormalities
Oligoarthritis (persistent) (49%)	1–6 years	5:1	1–4 (max) joints involved; knee, ankle or wrist most common	Chronic anterior uveitis in 20%, leg length discrepancy Prognosis excellent	ANA+/−
Oligoarthritis (extended) (8%)	1–6 years	5:1	>4 joints involved after first 6 months. Asymmetrical distribution of large and small joints	Chronic anterior uveitis 20%, asymmetrical growth Prognosis moderate	ANA+/−
Polyarthritis (RF negative) (16%)	1–6 years	5:1	Symmetrical large and small joint arthritis, often with marked finger involvement Cervical spine and temporomandibular joint may be involved	Low-grade fever, chronic anterior uveitis 5%, late reduction of growth rate Prognosis moderate	
Polyarthritis (RF) positive (3%)	10–16 years	5:1	Symmetrical large and small joint arthritis, often with marked finger involvement	Rheumatoid nodules 10% Similar to adult rheumatoid arthritis Prognosis poor	RF+ (long term)
Systemic arthritis (9%)	1–10 years	1:1	Oligoarthritis or polyarthritis. May have aches and pains in joints and muscles (arthralgia/myalgia) but initially no arthritis	Acute illness, malaise, high daily fever initially, with salmon-pink, macular rash, lymphadenopathy, hepatosplenomegaly, serositis Prognosis variable to poor	Anaemia, raised neutrophils and platelets, high acute-phase reactants (see Case History 26.1)
Psoriatic arthritis (7%)	1–16 years	1:1	Usually asymmetrical distribution of large and small joints, dactylitis	Psoriasis, nail pitting or dystrophy, chronic anterior uveitis 20% Prognosis moderate	
Enthesitis-related arthritis (7%)	6–16 years	1:4	Lower limb, large joint arthritis initially, mild lumbar spine or sacroiliac involvement later on	Enthesitis – localised inflammation at insertion of tendons or ligaments into bone, often in feet, Achilles insertion Occasional acute uveitis Prognosis moderate	HLAB27+
Undifferentiated arthritis (1%)	1–16 years	2:1 (variable)	Overlapping articular and extra-articular patterns between ≥2 subtypes or insufficient criteria for sub-classification	Prognosis variable	

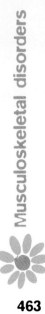

Musculoskeletal disorders

463

Case History

26.1 Systemic-onset juvenile idiopathic arthritis

A 2-year-old boy presented with a high fever (Fig. 26.18a) and malaise. A salmon-coloured rash was present at times of fever (Fig. 26.18b). Investigation showed markedly raised acute-phase reactants. Shortly afterwards, he developed severe polyarthritic joint disease. A diagnosis of systemic-onset juvenile idiopathic arthritis was made on the basis of the clinical presentation and exclusion of other disorders (Table 26.3).

He was treated with high-dose intravenous corticosteroids with rapid improvement, started on oral corticosteroids and weekly methotrexate given by subcutaneous injection. His mother was taught by the nurse specialist how to give the injections to him at home and a daily exercise programme to improve his mobility was provided. A year later he remained on weekly methotrexate. He had persistent problems with his hips, with joint damage on X-ray and may ultimately require hip replacements in his adult years. He is shorter than his peers. He is now at university studying economics and drives his own car.

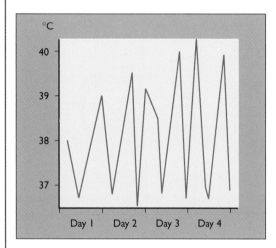

Figure 26.18a Temperature chart.

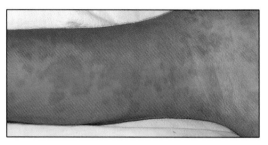

Figure 26.18b Salmon-pink rash.

---

long-standing or suboptimally treated arthritis due to premature fusion of epiphyses.

Constitutional problems

Anaemia of chronic disease, delayed puberty.

Osteoporosis

Multifactorial aetiology, including diet, reduced weight bearing, systemic corticosteroids and delayed menarche. Reduce risk by dietary supplements of calcium and vitamin D; regular weight-bearing exercise; and minimise oral corticosteroids use and sometimes bisphosphonates.

Amyloidosis

Very rare now, causes proteinuria and subsequent renal failure and has a high mortality.

Management

The management of JIA has radically changed in the last decade and improvement in outcome is evident as long as children access appropriate care. Deformity and disability are much less common with current treatment approaches. The overall management aim is to induce remission as soon as possible.

All children suspected of having JIA should be managed by specialist paediatric rheumatology multidisciplinary teams, often working in shared care with local hospitals; such teams have specific paediatric expertise in the use and monitoring of immunosuppressive treatments that are now routinely used. There is need for education and support for the child and family, physical therapy to maintain joint function, and links to other specialities including ophthalmology, dentistry and orthopaedics. The team work closely with school, social services and primary healthcare providers. The child is encouraged to take part in all activities except contact sports during active flares. With optimal care, most children are managed as outpatients.

Medical management includes:

- *NSAIDs (non-steroidal anti-inflammatory drugs) and analgesics* – do not modify disease but help relieve symptoms during flares
- *Joint injections, increasingly under ultrasound guidance* – effective, first-line treatment for oligoarticular JIA; in polyarticular disease multiple joint injections are used as bridging agent when starting methotrexate. Often requires sedation or inhaled anaesthesia (Entonox)
- *Methotrexate* – early use reduces joint damage. Effective in approximately 70% with polyarthritis, less effective in systemic features of JIA. It is given as weekly dose (tablet, liquid or injection) and regular blood monitoring is required (for abnormal liver function and bone-marrow suppression). Nausea is common.

- *Systemic corticosteroids* – avoided if possible, to minimise risk of growth suppression and osteoporosis. Pulsed intravenous methylprednisolone often used for severe polyarthritis as an induction agent. May be life-saving for severe systemic arthritis or macrophage activation syndrome.
- *Cytokine modulators ('biologics') and other immunotherapies* – Many agents (e.g. anti-TNF alpha, IL-1, CTLA-4 or IL-6) now available and useful in severe disease refractory to methotrexate. Costly and given under strict national guidance with registries for long-term surveillance. T-cell depletion coupled with autologous haematopoetic stem cell rescue (bone marrow transplant) is an option for refractory disease.

Prognosis

Long-term outcome studies have shown that at least one in three children will have ongoing active disease into adult years, with significant morbidity from previous inflammation, such as joint damage requiring joint replacement surgery, visual impairment from uveitis, or fractures from osteoporosis. There is also significant psychosocial morbidity. However, with current management approaches it is anticipated that long-term outcomes will improve.

Transitional care programmes are increasingly provided to facilitate the changes through adolescence and young adulthood and to help young people learn how to manage their chronic disease independently.

Henoch–Schönlein purpura

This is the most common vasculitis of childhood and presents with a purpuric rash over the lower legs and buttocks, usually associated with arthritis of the ankles or knees. Other features are abdominal pain, haematuria and proteinuria (see Ch. 18).

Systemic lupus erythematosus

Systemic lupus erythematosus is rare in children, but may present in adolescent females typically with

---

Summary

Diagnostic clues regarding musculoskeletal disorders

'Typical' symptom combinations	Pivotal clinical features	Possible diagnoses
Nocturnal wakening with leg pain	Normal child	'Growing pains'
		Osteoid osteoma
	Anaemia, bruising, irritability, infections	Leukaemia, lymphoma, neuroblastoma (young child)
'Clunk' on hip movement on screening, limp in an older infant	Asymmetrical upper leg skin folds, limited hip abduction	Developmental dysplasia of the hip (DDH)
Febrile, toxic-looking infant, irritability with nappy changing	Restricted joint range (especially hip)	Septic arthritis
		Osteomyelitis
Sudden limp in a otherwise well young child	Unilateral restricted hip movement	Transient synovitis of the hip
		Perthes disease
Fever, erythematous rash, red eyes, irritability in infant or young child	Erythema/oedema of hands and feet, oral mucositis, cervical lymphadenopathy	Kawasaki disease
Irritability, fever, reluctance to move in an infant or young child	Stiff back, 'tripod' sitting	Discitis
		Vertebral osteomyelitis
Joint pain, stiffness and restriction **Loss of joint function**	Persistent joint swelling Loss of joint range	Juvenile idiopathic arthritis
Hip pain in an obese adolescent boy	Unilateral hip restriction	Slipped capital femoral epiphysis
Lethargy, unwilling to do physical activities, irritability, rash	Eyelid erythema Proximal muscle weakness	Juvenile dermatomyositis
Constitutional symptoms, lethargy, arthralgia in an adolescent female	Multi-system abnormalities, haematuria, facial erythema	Systemic lupus erythematosus

malaise, arthralgia and malar rash (often photosensitive). Organ involvement (kidneys, lung or CNS) are serious complications.

Juvenile dermatomyositis

Juvenile dermatomyositis (JDMS) is rare. It usually begins insidiously with malaise, progressive weakness (often difficulty climbing stairs) and facial rash with erythema over the bridge of the nose and malar areas and a violaceous (heliotropic) discoloration of the eyelids (see Fig. 27.10). The skin over the metacarpal and proximal interphalangeal joints may be hypertrophic and pink, and the nailfold capillaries may be dilated and tortuous. Muscle pain is a common, if non-specific, symptom and arthritis is present in 30%. Respiratory failure and aspiration pneumonia may be life-threatening. The condition is described further in Chapter 27.

Genetic skeletal conditions

These are inherited abnormalities resulting in generalised developmental disorders of the bone, of which there are several hundred types. They usually result in reduced growth and abnormality of bone shape rather than impaired strength, except for osteogenesis imperfecta. The bones of the limbs and spine are often affected, resulting in short stature. Intelligence is usually normal. Improved knowledge of the molecular basis of collagen and its disorders is allowing better understanding and delineation of some of these disorders.

Achondroplasia

Inheritance is autosomal dominant, but about 50% are new mutations. Clinical features are short stature from marked shortening of the limbs, a large head, frontal bossing and depression of the nasal bridge (see Fig. 11.10). The hands are short and broad. A marked lumbar lordosis develops. Hydrocephalus sometimes occurs.

Thanatophoric dysplasia

This results in stillbirth. The infants have a large head, extremely short limbs and a small chest. The appearance of the bones on X-ray is characteristic. The importance of the correct diagnosis of this disorder is that, in contrast to achondroplasia, its inheritance is sporadic. It may be identified on antenatal ultrasound.

Cleidocranial dysostosis

In this autosomal dominant disorder, there is absence of part or all of the clavicles and delay in closure of the anterior fontanelle and of ossification of the skull. The child is often able to bring the shoulders together in front of the chest to touch each other as a 'party trick'. Short stature is usually present. Intelligence is normal.

Arthrogryposis

This is a heterogeneous group of congenital disorders in which there is stiffness and contracture of joints. The cause is usually unknown, but there may be an association with oligohydramnios, widespread congenital anomalies or chromosomal disorders. It is usually sporadic. Marked flexion contractures of the knees, elbows and wrists, dislocation of the hips and other joints, talipes equinovarus and scoliosis are common, but the disorder may be localised to the upper or lower limbs. The skin is thin, subcutaneous tissue is reduced and there is marked muscle atrophy around the affected joints. Intelligence is usually unaffected. Management is with physiotherapy and correction of deformities, where possible, by splints, plaster casts or surgery. Walking is impaired in the more severe forms of the disorder.

Osteogenesis imperfecta (brittle bone disease)

This is a group of disorders of collagen metabolism causing bone fragility, with bowing and frequent fractures.

In the most common form (type I), which is autosomal dominant, there are fractures during childhood (Fig. 26.19a) and a blue appearance to the sclerae (Fig. 26.19b) and some develop hearing loss. Treatment with bisphosphonates reduces fracture rates. The prognosis is variable. Fractures require splinting to minimise joint deformity.

There is a severe, lethal form (type II) with multiple fractures already present before birth (Fig. 26.20). Many affected infants are stillborn. Inheritance is variable but mostly autosomal dominant or due to new mutations. In other types, scleral discoloration may be minimal.

Osteopetrosis (marble bone disease)

In this rare disorder, the bones are dense but brittle. The severe autosomal recessive disorder presents with failure to thrive, recurrent infection, hypocalcaemia, anaemia and thrombocytopenia. Prognosis is poor, but bone marrow transplantation can be curative. A less severe autosomal dominant form may present during childhood with fractures.

Marfan syndrome

This is an autosomal dominant disorder of connective tissue associated with tall stature, long thin digits (arachnodactyly), hyperextensible joints, a high arched palate, dislocation (usually upwards) of the lenses of the eyes and severe myopia. The body proportions

Osteogenesis imperfecta

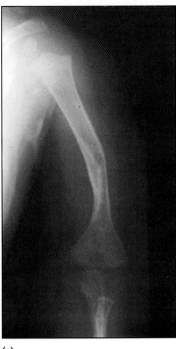

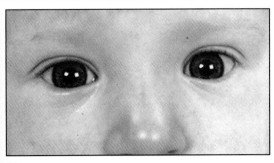

(b)

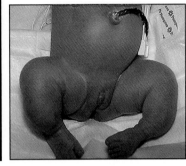

Figure 26.20 Osteogenesis imperfecta (type II) showing shortened, deformed lower limbs from gross deformity of the bones with multiple fractures.

(a)

Figure 26.19 Osteogenesis imperfecta type I, showing **(a)** fracture of the humerus and osteoporotic bones, **(b)** blue sclerae.

 Osteogenesis imperfecta is often considered in the evaluation of unexplained fractures in suspected child abuse.

are altered, with long, thin limbs resulting in a greater distance between the pubis and soles (lower segment) than from the crown to the pubis (upper segment). The arm span, measured from the extended fingers, is greater than the height. There may be chest deformity and scoliosis. The major problems are cardiovascu- lar, due to degeneration of the media of vessel walls resulting in a dilated, incompetent aortic root with valvular incompetence and mitral valve prolapse and regurgitation. Aneurysms of the aorta may dissect or rupture. Monitoring by echocardiography is required.

Further reading

Cassidy J, Petty RE, Laxer R et al: *Textbook of Pediatric Rheumatology*, ed 5, Edinburgh, 2005, Elsevier Saunders.

Foster HE, Brogan P: *Oxford Handbook of Paediatric Rheumatology*, Oxford, 2011, Oxford University Press.

Szer IS, Kimura Y, Malleson PN et al, editors: *Arthritis in Children and Adolescents: Juvenile Idiopathic Arthritis*, Oxford, 2006, Oxford University Press.

Woo P, Laxer RM, Sherry DD: *Pediatric Rheumatology in Clinical Practice*, New York, 2007, Springer.

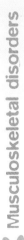

Musculoskeletal disorders

Websites (Accessed May 2011)

Arthritis Research UK: Free educational materials for medical students including pGALS. Available at: http://www.arthritisresearchuk.org/arthritis_information/information_for_medical_profes/medical_student_handbook.aspx.

Arthritis Research UK: Information about arthritis for health professionals. Available at: http://www.arthritisresearchuk.org/.

British Society for Paediatric and Adolescent Rheumatology: Information about clinical guidelines and protocols. Available at: http://www.bspar.org.uk/pages/bspar_home.asp.

Neurological disorders

The central nervous system comprises 100 000 million neurones and when it malfunctions it has the potential to generate a wide spectrum of clinical problems. The site of the dysfunctional neurones determines the nature of the problem, which may involve impaired movement, vision, hearing, sensory perception, memory or consciousness. Classifying this wide range of symptom complexes can be problematic.

Headache

Headache is a frequent reason for older children and adolescents to consult a doctor. The International Headache Society (IHS) has devised a classification, as shown in Box 27.1, which defines:

- Primary headaches: four main groups, comprising migraine, tension-type headache, cluster headache (and other trigeminal autonomic cephalalgias); and other primary headaches (such as cough or exertional headache). They are thought to be due to a primary malfunction of neurones.
- Secondary headaches: symptomatic of some underlying pathology, e.g. from raised intracranial pressure and space-occupying lesions
- Trigeminal and other cranial neuralgias, and other headaches including root pain from herpes zoster.

Primary headaches

Tension-type headache

This is a symmetrical headache of gradual onset, often described as tightness, a band or pressure. There are usually no other symptoms.

Migraine without aura

This accounts for 90% of migraine. In children, episodes may last 1–72 h; the headache is commonly bilateral but may be unilateral. Characteristically pulsatile, over temporal or frontal area, it is often accompanied by unpleasant gastrointestinal disturbance such as nausea, vomiting and abdominal pain and photophobia or phonophobia (sensitivity to sounds). Aggravated by physical activity.

Migraine with aura

Accounts for 10% of migraine. The headache is preceded by an aura (visual, sensory or motor), although the aura may occur without a headache. Features are the absence of problems between episodes and the frequent presence of premonitory symptoms (tiredness, difficulty concentrating, autonomic features, etc.).

The most common aura comprises visual disturbance, which may include:

- Negative phenomena, such as hemianopia (loss of half the visual field) or scotoma (small areas of visual loss)
- Positive phenomena such as fortification spectra (seeing zigzag lines).

Rarely, there are unilateral sensory or motor symptoms.

Episodes usually last for a few hours, during which time children often prefer to lie down in a quiet, dark place. Sleep often relieves the bout.

Symptoms of *tension-type headache* or a *migraine* often overlap. They are probably part of the same pathophysiological continuum, with evidence that both result from primary neuronal dysfunction,

Box 27.1 The classification of headache disorders

Primary headaches	Secondary headaches	Cranial neuralgias, central and primary facial pain and other headaches
• Migraine • Tension-type headache • Cluster headache and other trigeminal autonomic cephalalgias • Other primary headaches	Headache attributed to: • Head and/or neck trauma • Cranial or cervical vascular disorder – vascular malformation or intracranial haemorrhage • Non-vascular intracranial disorder – raised intracranial pressure, idiopathic intracranial hypertension • A substance or its withdrawal – alcohol, solvent or drug abuse • Infection – meningitis or encephalitis • Disorder of homeostasis – hypercapnia or hypertension • Disorder of facial or cranial structures – acute sinusitis • Psychiatric disorder	• Trigeminal and other cranial neuralgias and central causes of facial pain • Other headaches.

including channelopathies, with vascular phenomena as secondary events. There is a genetic predisposition, with first- and second-degree relatives often also affected. Bouts are often triggered by a disturbance of inherent biorhythms, such as late nights or early rises, stress, or winding down after stress at home or school. Certain foods, e.g. cheese, chocolate and caffeine, are only rarely a reliable trigger. In girls, headaches can be related to menstruation and the oral contraceptive pill.

Uncommon forms of migraine

These include:

- *Familial* – linked to a calcium channel defect, dominantly inherited
- *Sporadic hemiplegic migraine*
- *Basilar-type migraine* – vomiting with nystagmus and/or cerebellar signs
- *Periodic syndromes* – often precursors of migraine and include:
  - *Cyclical vomiting* – recurrent stereotyped episodes of vomiting and intense nausea associated with pallor and lethargy. The child is well in between.
  - *Abdominal migraine* – an idiopathic recurrent disorder characterised by episodic midline abdominal pain in bouts lasting 1–72 h. Pain is moderate to severe in intensity and associated with vasomotor symptoms, nausea and vomiting. The child is well in between episodes.
  - *Benign paroxysmal vertigo* of childhood – a heterogeneous disorder characterised by recurrent brief episodes of vertigo occurring without warning and resolving spontaneously in otherwise healthy children. Between episodes, neurological examination,

audiometric and vestibular function tests are normal.

Secondary headaches

Raised intracranial pressure and space-occupying lesions

Headaches often raise the fear of brain tumours; it may well be the reason for parents to consult a doctor. Headaches due to a space-occupying lesion are worse when lying down and morning vomiting is characteristic. The headaches may also cause night-time waking. There is often a change in mood, personality or educational performance. Other features suggestive of a space-occupying lesion are:

- Visual field defects – from lesions pressing on the optic pathways, e.g. craniopharyngioma (a pituitary tumour)
- Cranial nerve abnormalities causing diplopia, new-onset squint or facial nerve palsy. The VIth (abducens) cranial nerve has a long intracranial course and is often affected when there is raised pressure, resulting in a squint with diplopia and inability to abduct the eye beyond the midline. It is a false localising sign. Other nerves are affected depending on the site of lesion, e.g. pontine lesions may affect the VIIth (facial) cranial nerve and cause a facial nerve palsy
- Abnormal gait
- Torticollis (tilting of the head)
- Growth failure, e.g. craniopharyngioma or hypothalamic lesion
- Papilloedema – a late feature
- Cranial bruits – may be heard in arteriovenous malformations but these lesions are rare.

Other causes

These are listed in Box 27.1.

Management

The mainstay of management is a thorough history and examination with detailed explanation and advice. Imaging is unnecessary in the absence of any Red Flag features.

Children and parents should be informed that recurrent headaches are common. For most there are good and bad spells, with periods of months or even years in between the bad spells, and that they cause no long-term harm. Written child-friendly information for the family to take home is helpful. Children should be advised on how to live with and control the headaches, rather than allowing the headaches to dominate their lives. There is nothing medicine can do to cure this problem but there is much it can offer to make the bad spells more bearable.

Rescue treatments

- Analgesia – paracetamol and non-steroidal anti-inflammatory drugs (NSAIDs), taken as early as possible in an individual troublesome episode
- Anti-emetics – prochlorperazine and metoclopramide
- Serotonin (5-HT$_1$) agonists, e.g. sumatriptan. A nasal preparation of this is licensed for use in children over 12 years of age.

Summary

History
Premonitory symptoms, aura, character, position, radiation, frequency, duration, triggers, relieving and exacerbating factors?   *Special consideration:*   Triggers – stress, relaxation, food, menstruation?   Emotional or behavioural problems at home or school?   Vision checked – refractive error?   Head trauma?   Alcohol, solvent, or drug abuse?   Analgesia over-use?

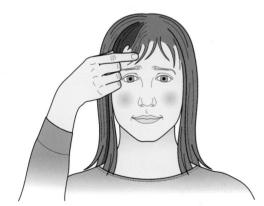

Investigations
Only consider these if Red Flag features

Headache type
Tension-type headache – constriction band.   **Migraine without aura** – bilateral or unilateral, pulsatile, gastrointestinal disturbance, e.g. nausea, vomiting, abdominal pain, photophobia. Lies in quiet, dark place. Relieved by sleep   **Migraine with aura** – preceded by aura (visual, sensory or motor), premonitory symptoms   **Mixed-type headaches** – common

Red flag symptoms – space-occupying lesion
Headache – worse lying down or with coughing and straining   Headache – wakes up child (different from headache on awakening, not uncommon in migraine)   Associated confusion, and/or morning or persistent nausea or vomiting   Recent change in personality, behaviour or educational performance

Red flag physical signs – space-occupying lesion
• Growth failure   • Visual field defects – craniopharyngioma   • Squint   • Cranial nerve abnormality   • Torticollis   • Abnormal coordination – for cerebellar lesions   • Gait – upper motor neurone or cerebellar signs   • Fundi – papilloedema   • Bradycardia   • Cranial bruits – arteriovenous malformation

Other physical signs
Visual acuity – for refractive errors   **Sinus tenderness** – for sinusitis   **Pain on chewing** – temporomandibular joint malocclusion   **Blood pressure** – for hypertension

Neurological disorders

Prophylactic agents

Where headaches are frequent and intrusive:

- Pizotifen (5-HT antagonist) – can cause weight gain and sleepiness
- Beta-blockers – propranolol; contraindicated in asthma.
- Sodium channel blockers – valproate or topiramate.

Psychosocial support

- Psychological support – is it required to ameliorate a particular stressor, e.g. bullying, anxiety over exams or illness in friends or family?
- Relaxation and other self-regulating techniques.

Systematic reviews highlight the need for further evidence on which to base headache management.

Seizures

A seizure is a clinical event in which there is a sudden disturbance of neurological function caused by an abnormal or excessive neuronal discharge. Seizures may be epileptic or non-epileptic.

The causes of seizures are listed in Box 27.2.

Febrile seizures

A febrile seizure is a seizure accompanied by a fever in the absence of intracranial infection due to bacterial meningitis or viral encephalitis. These occur in 3% of children, between the ages of 6 months and 5 years. There is a genetic predisposition, with a 10% risk if the child has a first-degree relative with febrile seizures. The seizure usually occurs early in a viral infection when the temperature is rising rapidly. The seizures are usually brief, and are generalised tonic-clonic seizures. About 30–40% will have further febrile seizures. This is more likely the younger the child, the shorter the duration of illness before the seizure, the lower the temperature at the time of seizure and if there is a positive family history.

Simple febrile seizures do not cause brain damage; the child's subsequent intellectual performance is the same as in children who do not experience a febrile seizure. There is a 1–2% chance of developing epilepsy, similar to the risk for all children.

However, complex febrile seizures; i.e. those which are focal, prolonged, or repeated in the same illness, have an increased risk of 4–12% of subsequent epilepsy.

The acute management of seizures is described in Chapter 6. Examination should focus on the cause of the fever, which is usually a viral illness, but a bacterial infection including meningitis should always be considered. The classical features of meningitis such as neck stiffness and photophobia may not be as apparent in children <18 months of age, so an infection screen (including blood cultures, urine culture and lumbar puncture for CSF) may be necessary. If the child is unconscious or has cardiovascular instability, lumbar puncture is contraindicated and antibiotics should be started immediately.

Parents need reassurance and information. Advice sheets are usually given to parents. Antipyretics have not been shown to prevent febrile seizures and tepid sponging is no longer recommended. The family should be taught the first aid management of seizures. If there is a history of prolonged seizures (>5 min), rescue therapy with rectal diazepam or buccal midazolam can be supplied. Oral prophylactic anti-epileptic drugs are not used as they do not reduce the recurrence rate of seizures or the risk of epilepsy. An EEG is not indicated as it does not serve as a guide for treatment; nor does it predict seizure recurrence.

Box 27.2 Causes of seizures

Epilepsy

- Idiopathic (70–80%) – cause unknown but presumed genetic
- Secondary
  - Cerebral dysgenesis/malformation
  - Cerebral vascular occlusion
  - Cerebral damage, e.g. congenital infection, hypoxic-ischaemic encephalopathy, intraventricular haemorrhage/ischaemia
- Cerebral tumour
- Neurodegenerative disorders
- Neurocutaneous syndromes

Non-epileptic

- Febrile seizures
- Metabolic
  - Hypoglycaemia
  - Hypocalcaemia/hypomagnesaemia
  - Hypo/hypernatraemia
- Head trauma
- Meningitis/encephalitis
- Poisons/toxins.

Summary

Febrile seizures

- Affect 3% of children; have a genetic predisposition
- Occur between 6 months and 6 years of age
- Are usually brief, generalised tonic-clonic seizures occurring with a rapid rise in fever
- If a bacterial infection, especially meningitis, is present, it needs to be identified and treated
- Advise family about management of seizures, consider rescue therapy
- If simple – does not affect intellectual performance or risk of developing epilepsy
- If complex, 4–12% risk of subsequent epilepsy.

Paroxysmal disorders

There is a broad differential diagnosis for children with paroxysmal disorders ('funny turns'). Epilepsy is a clinical diagnosis based on the history from eyewitnesses and the child's own account. If available, videos of the seizures or suspected seizures can be of great help. The diagnostic question is whether the paroxysmal events are that of an epilepsy of childhood or one of the many conditions which mimic it (Fig. 27.1). The most common pitfall is that of syncope leading to an anoxic (non-epileptic) tonic-clonic seizure.

The key to the diagnosis lies in a detailed history, which, together with clinical examination, will determine the need for an EEG or other investigations.

Causes of funny turns

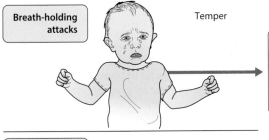

Breath-holding attacks	Temper

Occur in some toddlers when they are upset. The child cries, holds his breath and goes blue. Sometimes children will briefly lose consciousness but rapidly recover fully. Drug therapy is unhelpful. Attacks resolve spontaneously, but behaviour modification therapy, with distraction, may help.

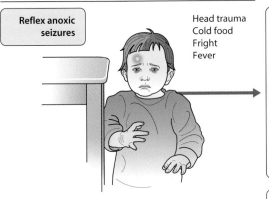

Reflex anoxic seizures	Head trauma Cold food Fright Fever

Occur in infants or toddlers. Many have a first-degree relative with a history of faints. Commonest triggers are pain or discomfort, particularly from minor head trauma, cold food (such as ice-cream or cold drinks), fright or fever. Some children with febrile seizures may have experienced this phenomenon. After the triggering event, the child becomes very pale and falls to the floor. The hypoxia may induce a generalised tonic–clonic seizure. The episodes are due to cardiac asystole from vagal inhibition. The seizure is brief and the child rapidly recovers. Ocular compression under controlled conditions often leads to asystole and paroxysmal slow-wave discharge on the EEG.

Syncope

Children may faint if in a hot and stuffy environment, on standing for long periods, or from fear. Clonic movements may occur.

Migraine

May sometimes lead to paroxysmal headache involving unsteadiness or light-headedness as well as the more common visual or gastrointestinal disturbance. In some young people these episodes occur without headache.

Benign paroxysmal vertigo

This is characterised by recurrent episodes of vertigo, lasting from one to several minutes, associated with nystagmus, unsteadiness or even falling. It is a primary headache disorder of childhood occasionally due to a viral labyrinthitis.

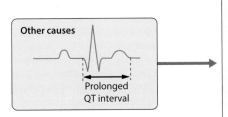

Other causes

Prolonged QT interval

Cardiac arrhythmia – prolonged QT interval may rarely cause collapse or cardiac syncope which may be related to exercise
Tics, daydreaming, night terrors
Self-gratification – young children may stimulate their genitalia in order to achieve a feeling of comfort rather than sexual gratification
Non-epileptic attack disorder (NEAD)
Pseudoseizures – when children feign seizures
Fabricated – seizures are fabricated by parent
Induced illness (non-accidental injury) – e.g. seizures, from hypoglycaemia from an adult deliberately injecting insulin
Paroxysmal movement disorders – well-circumscribed episodes, genetically determined, no loss of consciousness.

Figure 27.1 Causes of 'funny turns'.

Summary

Breath-holding and reflex anoxic seizures

In toddlers:

- Breath-holding episodes – toddler, precipitated by anger, holds breath, goes blue, then limp, rapid recovery
- Reflex anoxic seizures – toddler, precipitated by pain, stops breathing, goes pale, brief seizure sometimes, rapid recovery
- Other non-epileptic paroxysmal disorders: see Fig. 27.1.

Epilepsies of childhood

Epilepsy has an incidence of about 0.05% (after the first year of life when it is even more common) and a prevalence of 0.5%. This means that most large secondary schools will have about six children with an epilepsy. Epilepsy is a chronic neurological disorder characterised by recurrent unprovoked seizures, consisting of transient signs and/or symptoms associated with abnormal, excessive or synchronous neuronal activity in the brain. Most epilepsy is idiopathic but other causes of seizures are listed in Box 27.2.

An international classification of epilepsy is used, which has recently been revised (International League Against Epilepsy (ILAE) 2010 Classifications). This broadly classifies seizures as either:

- *Generalised* – discharge arises from both hemispheres. They may be – absence, myoclonic, tonic, tonic-clonic and atonic
- *Focal* – where seizures arise from one or part of one hemisphere.

Focal seizure manifestations will depend on the part of the brain where the discharge originates:

- *Frontal* seizures – involve the motor or premotor cortex. May lead to clonic movements, which may travel proximally (Jacksonian march). Asymmetrical tonic seizures can be seen, which may be bizarre and hyperkinetic and can be mistakenly dismissed as non-epileptic events. Atonic seizures may arise from mesial frontal discharge.
- *Temporal lobe* seizures, the most common of all the epilepsies – may result in strange warning feelings or aura with smell and taste abnormalities and distortions of sound and shape. Lip-smacking, plucking at one's clothing and walking in a non-purposeful manner (automatisms) may be seen, following spread to the pre-motor cortex. Déjà-vu and jamais-vu are described (intense feelings of having been, or never having been, in the same situation before). Consciousness can be impaired and the length of event is longer than a typical absence.
- *Occipital* seizures – cause distortion of vision.
- *Parietal lobe* seizures – cause contralateral dysaesthesias (altered sensation), or distorted body image.

In focal seizures, the level of consciousness may be retained, consciousness may be lost, or the seizure may be followed by generalised tonic-clonic seizure. In the new classification, the terms simple or complex or discognitive are no longer used and the impairment of consciousness is not classified but described.

In many children, especially under 5 years old, it may be unclear whether a seizure is generalised or focal.

The main seizure types are summarised in Figure 27.2 and the epilepsy syndromes in Table 27.1.

Diagnosis

The diagnosis of epilepsy is primarily based on a detailed history from the child and eyewitnesses, substantiated by a video if available. This is increasingly available on mobile phones. Particular attention is focussed on any specific triggers and if the child has any impairments, as there may be educational, psychological or social problems. Clinical examination should include checking for skin markers for a neurocutaneous syndrome or neurological abnormalities. Although epilepsy is usually idiopathic, it may be the presentation or a complication of an underlying neurological disorder.

Investigation of seizures

EEG

An EEG is indicated whenever epilepsy is suspected. It is interpreted to identify a background that is abnormal for the child's age; asymmetry or slowing that might suggest underlying structural abnormalities; or evidence of neuronal hyperexcitability such as sharp waves or spike-wave complexes. Many children with epilepsy have a normal initial EEG; and many children who will never have epilepsy have EEG abnormalities. Unless a seizure is actually captured, an EEG does no more than add supportive evidence (or not) for the diagnosis. If the standard EEG is normal, a sleep or sleep-deprived record can be helpful. Additional techniques are 24-h ambulatory EEG or, ideally, video-telemetry. For assessment prior to surgery, more invasive techniques such as subdural electrodes can be used.

Imaging

- *Structural*. MRI and CT brain scans are not required routinely for childhood generalised epilepsies. They are indicated if there are neurological signs between seizures, or if seizures are focal, in order to identify a tumour, vascular lesion, or area of sclerosis which could be treatable. MRI FLAIR (fluid-attenuated inversion recovery) sequences better detect mesial temporal sclerosis in temporal lobe epilepsy.
- *Functional scans*. While it is not always possible to see structural lesions, techniques have advanced to allow functional imaging to detect areas of abnormal metabolism suggestive of seizure foci. These include PET (positron emission tomography) and SPECT (single positron emission computed tomography), which use isotopes and ligands, injected and taken up by metabolically active cells. Both can be used between seizures to detect areas of hypometabolism in epileptogenic lesions. SPECT

Epilepsy seizure types

Generalised seizures

Onset in both hemisphere

In generalised seizure disorders, there is:
- always a loss of consciousness
- no warning
- symmetrical seizure
- bilaterally synchronous seizure discharge on EEG or varying asymmetry

Absence seizures → Transient loss of consciousness, with an abrupt onset and termination, unaccompanied by motor phenomena except for some flickering of the eyelids and minor alteration in muscle tone. Absences may be typical (petit mal) or atypical and can often be precipitated by hyperventilation

Myoclonic seizures → Brief, often repetitive, jerking movements of the limbs, neck or trunk
Non-epileptic myoclonic movements are also seen physiologically in hiccoughs (myoclonus of the diaphragm) or on passing through stage II sleep (sleep myoclonus)

Tonic seizures → Generalised increase in tone

Tonic–clonic seizures → Rhythmical contraction of muscle groups following the tonic phase.
In the rigid tonic phase, children may fall to the ground, sometimes injuring themselves. They do not breathe and become cyanosed. This is followed by the clonic phase, with jerking of the limbs. Breathing is irregular, cyanosis persists and saliva may accumulate in the mouth. There may be biting of the tongue and incontinence of urine. The seizure usually lasts from a few seconds to minutes, followed by unconsciousness or deep sleep for up to several hours

Atonic seizures → Often combined with a myoclonic jerk, followed by a transient loss of muscle tone causing a sudden fall to the floor or drop of the head

Focal seizures

Onset in neural network limited to one cerebral hemisphere

Parietal
Frontal
Temporal
Occipital

Focal seizures:
- begin in a relatively small group of dysfunctional neurones in one of the cerebral hemispheres
- may be heralded by an aura which reflects the site of origin
- may or may not be associated with change in consciousness or more generalised tonic-clonic seizure

Focal seizures → Frontal seizures – motor phenomena
Temporal lobe seizures – auditory or sensory (smell or taste) phenomena
Occipital – positive or negative visual phenomena
Parietal lobe seizures – contralateral altered sensation (dysaesthesia)

Figure 27.2 Epilepsy seizure types.

can also be used to capture seizures and areas of hypermetabolism. Functional MRI can be used alongside psychological testing –including memory assessment – to minimise the risk of postoperative impairment.

Other investigations

Metabolic investigations may be warranted when there is developmental regression or seizures are related to feeds or fasting. Genetic studies will become increasingly helpful as certain epilepsy syndromes are now known to be due to genetic deletions causing abnormalities of sodium and other ion channels (e.g. SCN1A mutations in severe myoclonic epilepsy of infancy).

Management

Management begins with explanation and advice to help adjustment to the condition. A specialist epilepsy nurse may assist families by providing education and continuing advice on lifestyle issues. The decision whether to treat or not is related to the level of inconvenience seizures are bringing into the young person's life. It is common practice not to institute treatment after a single unprovoked seizure.

Anti-epileptic drug (AED) therapy

Principles governing use are:

- Not all seizures require AED therapy. This decision should be based on the seizure type, frequency

Neurological disorders

Table 27.1 Some epilepsy syndromes – arranged by age of onset

Name	Age	Seizure pattern	Comments
West syndrome	4–6 months	Violent flexor spasms of the head, trunk and limbs followed by extension of the arms (so-called 'salaam spasms'). Flexor spasms last 1–2 s, often multiple bursts of 20–30 spasms, often on waking, but may occur many times a day. May be misinterpreted as colic. Social interaction often deteriorates – a useful marker in the history	Many causes; two-thirds have underlying neurological cause. The EEG shows hypsarrhythmia, a chaotic pattern of high-voltage slow waves, and multi-focal sharp wave discharges (Fig. 27.3). Treatment is with vigabatrin or corticosteroids; good response in 30–40%, but unwanted effects are common. Most will subsequently lose skills and develop learning disability or epilepsy
Lennox–Gastaut syndrome	1–3 years	Multiple seizure types, but mostly drop attacks (astatic seizures), tonic seizures and atypical absences. Also neurodevelopmental arrest or regression and behaviour disorder	Often other complex neurological problems or history of infantile spasms. Prognosis is poor
Childhood absence epilepsy	4–12 years	Stare momentarily and stop moving, may twitch their eyelids or a hand minimally. Lasts only a few seconds and certainly not longer than 30 s. Child has no recall except realises they have missed something and may look puzzled or say 'pardon' on regaining consciousness. Developmentally normal but can interfere with schooling. Accounts for only 2% of childhood epilepsy	Two-thirds are female. The episodes can be induced by hyperventilation, the child being asked to blow on a piece of paper or windmill for 2–3 min, a useful test in the outpatient clinic. The EEG shows generalised 3/second spike and wave discharge, which is bilaterally synchronous during and sometimes between episodes (Fig. 27.4). Prognosis is good, with 95% remission in adolescence; 5–10% may develop tonic-clonic seizures in adult life
Benign* epilepsy, with centrotemporal spikes (BECTS)	4–10 years	Tonic-clonic seizures in sleep, or simple focal seizures with awareness of abnormal feelings in the tongue and distortion of the face (supplied by the Rolandic area of the brain)	Comprises 15% of all childhood epilepsies. EEG shows focal sharp waves from the Rolandic or centrotemporal area. Important to recognise as it is benign and does not always require treatment. Almost all remit in adolescence
Early-onset benign* childhood occipital epilepsy (Panayiotopoulos type)	1–14 years	Younger children – periods of unresponsiveness, eye deviation, vomiting and autonomic features. Older children – headache and visual disturbance including distortion of images and hallucinations	Uncommon. EEG shows occipital discharges. Remit in childhood
Juvenile myoclonic epilepsy	Adolescence-adulthood	Myoclonic seizures, but generalised tonic-clonic seizures and absences may occur, mostly shortly after waking. A typical history is throwing drinks or cornflakes about in the morning as myoclonus occurs at this time. Learning is unimpaired	Characteristic EEG. Response to treatment is usually good but lifelong. A genetic linkage has been identified. Remission unlikely

*Although called benign, may be specific learning difficulties in some children.

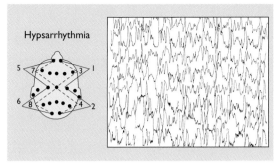

Figure 27.3 EEG of hypsarrhythmia in West syndrome. There is a chaotic background of slow-wave activity with sharp multi-focal components.

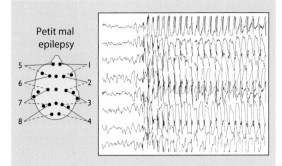

Figure 27.4 EEG in a typical absence seizure in childhood absence epilepsy. There is three per second spike and wave discharge which is bilaterally synchronous during, and sometimes between, attacks.

and the social and educational consequences of the seizures set against the possibility of unwanted effects of the drugs.

- Choose the appropriate drug for the seizure. Inappropriate AEDs may be detrimental, e.g. carbamazepine can make absence and myoclonic seizures worse.
- Monotherapy at the minimum dosage is the desired goal, although in practice more then one drug may be required.
- All AEDs have potential unwanted effects and these should be discussed with the child and parent.
- Drug levels are not measured routinely, but may be useful to check for adherence to advice or with some drugs with erratic pharmacokinetics, e.g. phenytoin.
- Children with prolonged seizures are given rescue therapy to keep with them. This is usually a benzodiazepine, e.g. rectal diazepam or buccal midazolam.
- AED therapy can usually be discontinued after 2 years free of seizures.

Guidance regarding treatment options for different seizure types are shown in Table 27.2. Common unwanted effects of AEDs are shown in Table 27.3.

Other treatment options

In children with intractable seizures, there are a number of radical treatment options.

- *Ketogenic (fat-based) diets* may be helpful in some children. Its mechanism of action is poorly understood.
- *Vagal nerve stimulation*, delivered using externally programmable stimulation of a wire implanted around the vagal nerve, may possibly be useful; trials are being conducted.
- *Surgery*. Cessation of seizures and drug therapy may be achieved in some children whose clinical seizures are well-localised as demonstrated by good concordance between EEG, MRI and functional imaging findings. The main procedure is temporal lobectomy for mesial temporal sclerosis, but other procedures include hemispherectomy or hemispherotomy (isolation of hemisphere which is not removed so as avoid post-operative shifts in space) and other focal resections. Detailed assessment is required to ensure that the benefits outweigh the risks.

Advice and prognosis

The aim is to promote independence and confidence. Some children with epilepsy and their families need psychological help to adjust to the condition. The school needs to be aware of the child's problem and teachers advised on the management of seizures. Unrecognised absences may interfere with learning, which is an indication for being vigilant about 'odd

Table 27.2 Choice of anti-epileptic drugs (NICE 2004)

Seizure type	First-line	Second-line
Generalised seizures		
Tonic-clonic	Valproate, carbamazepine	Lamotrigine, topiramate
Absence	Valproate, ethosuximide	Lamotrigine
Myoclonic	Valproate	Lamotrigine
Focal seizures	Carbamazepine, valproate	Topiramate, levetiracetam, oxcarbazepine, gabapentin, tiagabine, vigabatrin
	Lamotrigine shown since to be most effective – but slow titration	

Table 27.3 Common or important unwanted effects of anti-epileptic drugs

Drug	Side-effects
Valproate	Weight gain, hair loss
	Rare idiosyncratic liver failure
Carbamazepine/oxcarbazepine	Rash, neutropenia, hyponatraemia, ataxia
	Liver enzyme induction, can interfere with other medication
Vigabatrin	Restriction of visual fields, which has limited its use
	Sedation
Lamotrigine	Rash
Ethosuximide	Nausea and vomiting
Topiramate	Drowsiness, withdrawal and weight loss
Gabapentin	Insomnia
Levetiracetam	Sedation – rare
Benzodiazepines – clobazam, clonazepam, diazepam, nitrazepam	Sedation, tolerance to effect, increased secretions

All the above may cause drowsiness and occasional skin rashes.

episodes' which may represent seizures. Relatively few restrictions are required, but situations where having a seizure could lead to injury or be fatal should be avoided. This includes avoiding deep baths (showers are preferable) and not swimming alone in deep water. Those with photosensitivity should sit at a distance from televisions, can cover one eye, and check that TVs and VDUs in use are acceptable (Epilepsy Action consider most modern TVs and VDUs to be suitable and can provide advice).

For adolescents, there may be issues to discuss around driving (only after 1 year free of seizures), contraception and pregnancy. There may also be issues with adherence and precipitation of seizures by alcohol and poor sleep routines.

Sudden unexpected death in epilepsy, SUDEP, may be discussed, and its low risks emphasised. Information is available from self-help groups and organisations such as Epilepsy Action.

Children with epilepsy do less well educationally, with social outcomes and with future employment than those with other chronic illnesses such as diabetes.

Two-thirds of children with epilepsy go to a mainstream school, but some require educational help for associated learning difficulties. One-third attend a special school, but they often have multiple disabilities and their epilepsy is part of a severe brain disorder. A few children require residential schooling where there are facilities and expertise in monitoring and treating intractable seizures.

Status epilepticus

Status epilepticus, a seizure lasting 30 min or repeated seizures for 30 min without recovery of consciousness is described in Chapter 6.

Summary

Epilepsy

- Affects 1 in 200 children
- Classified according to seizure type; the identification of a syndrome, where possible; and underlying aetiology
- If suspected, an EEG is indicated
- Anti-epileptic drug therapy should be considered where the seizures are intrusive, selected according to seizure type, monotherapy if possible and with the least potential for unwanted effects
- Requires liaison with the school about the management of seizures and avoiding situations which could lead to injury.

Motor disorders

Movement is governed by three main cerebral control centres. Patterns of information, modulated by afferent sensory information (joint position, crude touch, visual, auditory and vestibular), pass down the brainstem and spinal cord, through synapses in the anterior horns and along peripheral nerves to the target muscles. In clinical practice the first question to ask when seeing a child with a motor disorder is whether this is a central or a peripheral nervous system disorder. The pattern of movement usually gives the answer.

Table 27.4 Causes of movement disorders

Corticospinal (pyramidal) tract disorders	Basal ganglia disorders	Cerebellar disorders
Cerebral dysgenesis, e.g. neuronal migration problem	Acquired brain injury:	Acute – medication and drugs, including alcohol and solvent abuse
Global hypoxia-ischaemia	– Acute and profound hypoxia-ischaemia	Post-viral – particularly varicella infection
Arterial ischaemic stroke	– Carbon monoxide poisoning	Posterior fossa lesions or tumours, e.g. medulloblastoma
Cerebral tumour	– Post cardiopulmonary bypass chorea	Genetic and degenerative disorders, e.g. ataxic cerebral palsy, Friedreich ataxia and ataxia-telangiectasia
Acute disseminated encephalomyelitis	Post-streptococcal chorea (rheumatic fever)	
Post-ictal paresis	Mitochondrial cytopathies	
Hemiplegic migraine	Wilson disease	
	Huntington disease	

Central motor disorders

The three central movement control centres are:

- *Motor cortex*, lying along the pre-central gyrus (the homunculus reflects the body upside down, legs superiorly and face inferiorly, just above the Sylvian fissure; with large areas to govern fine movements of the tongue, fingers and thumb). Information from here passes down the corticospinal (pyramidal) tracts to link with the basal ganglia.
- *Basal ganglia*, deep grey matter structures, store patterns of movement so that we need not put conscious effort into every movement we make.
- *Cerebellum*, acting as the 'air-traffic controller'; receiving feedback on joint position nanosecond by nanosecond to keep us on course as we execute movements.

Disorders of these central movement control centres are:

- *Corticospinal (pyramidal) tract disorders* – there is weakness with a pattern of adduction at the shoulder, flexion at the elbow and pronation of the forearm; adduction and internal rotation at the hip, flexion at hip, knee and plantar flexion at the ankle with brisk hyper-reflexia and extensor plantars. Fine finger movement will be lost.
- *Basal ganglia disorders* – will lead either to difficulty initiating movement, with fluctuating (largely increased) tone – a 'dystonia', or a 'dyskinesia', where packets of movement information are released to give jerky movement (chorea) or writhing movement (athetosis).
- *Cerebellar disorders* – will lead to difficulty holding a posture (particularly with eyes closed); past-pointing (dysmetria); poor alternating movements (dysdiadochokinesis); and a characteristic scanning dysarthria. Posterior sensory pathway problems may give a similar clinical picture but are much

rarer in childhood. The gait is wide-based. Associated nystagmus may be seen. Causes of these disorders are listed in Table 27.4.

Cerebral palsy

This is described in Chapter 4.

Peripheral motor disorders: the neuromuscular disorders

Any part of the lower motor pathway can be affected in a neuromuscular disorder, so that anterior horn cell disorders, peripheral neuropathies, disorders of neuromuscular transmission and primary muscle diseases can all occur. The causes of neuromuscular disorders are shown in Figure 27.5. The key clinical feature of a neuromuscular disorder is weakness, which may be progressive or static. Affected children may present with:

- Floppiness
- Delayed motor milestones
- Muscle weakness
- Unsteady/abnormal gait
- Fatiguability
- Muscle cramps (suggesting a metabolic myopathy).

History and examination may provide useful clues. Children with myopathy often show a waddling gait or positive Gowers sign suggestive of proximal muscle weakness. Gowers sign is the need to turn prone to rise to a standing from a supine position. This is normal until the age of 3 years. It is only when children have become very weak that they 'climb up the legs with the hands' to gain the standing position (Fig. 27.6). A pattern of more distal wasting and weakness, particularly in the presence of pes cavus, suggests an

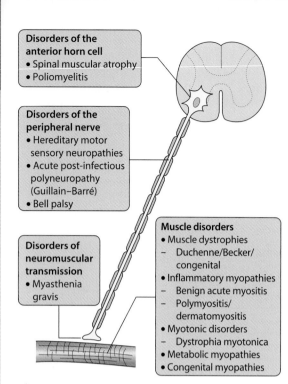

Disorders of the anterior horn cell
• Spinal muscular atrophy
• Poliomyelitis

Disorders of the peripheral nerve
• Hereditary motor sensory neuropathies
• Acute post-infectious polyneuropathy (Guillain–Barré)
• Bell palsy

Disorders of neuromuscular transmission
• Myasthenia gravis

Muscle disorders
• Muscle dystrophies
   – Duchenne/Becker/ congenital
• Inflammatory myopathies
   – Benign acute myositis
   – Polymyositis/ dermatomyositis
• Myotonic disorders
   – Dystrophia myotonica
• Metabolic myopathies
• Congenital myopathies

Figure 27.5 Neuromuscular disorders.

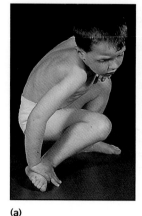
(a)

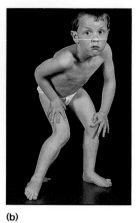
(b)

Figure 27.6 (a,b) Gowers sign. The child needs to turn prone to rise (the key, early feature of Gowers sign), then uses his hands to climb up on his knees before standing (late feature), because of poor hip girdle fixation and/or proximal muscle weakness. Any child continuing to turn prone to rise after 3 years of age is likely to have a neuromuscular condition.

hereditary motor sensory neuropathy. Increasing fatiguability through the day, often with ophthalmoplegia and ptosis, would be more consistent with depletion at the motor end-plate and a diagnosis of myasthenia gravis.

It is usually difficult to differentiate a myopathy from a neuropathy on clinical grounds but there are some broad points to look for:

• Anterior horn cell – there are signs of denervation: weakness, loss of reflexes, fasciculation and wasting as the nerve supply to the muscle fails.
• Neuropathy – often distal nerves affected. Motor neuropathy will give weakness, sensory neuropathy will give impaired perception of pain and temperature, or touch, with a loss of reflexes in either.
• Myopathy – there is weakness (often proximal), wasting, gait disturbance.
• Neuromuscular junction – as end-plate acetylcholine stores become depleted, there is diurnal worsening through the day, leading to fatiguability.

Investigations

Myopathy:

• Serum creatine phosphokinase – markedly elevated in Duchenne and Becker muscular dystrophy and inflammatory myopathies
• Muscle biopsy, needle or open – modern histochemical techniques often enable a definitive diagnosis
• DNA testing – to identify abnormal genes
• Ultrasound and MRI of muscles – used in specialist centres to diagnose and monitor progress.

Neuropathy:

• Nerve conduction studies – to identify delayed motor and sensory nerve conduction velocities seen in neuropathy
• DNA testing – for abnormal genes
• Nerve biopsy – rarely performed
• EMG (electromyography) helps in differentiating myopathic from neuropathic disorders, e.g. fatiguability on repetitive nerve stimulation in myasthenia. However, it should be used selectively in children, as the nerve conduction studies cause a tingling sensation and electromyography requires insertion of fine needle electrodes.

Diagnosis of neuromuscular disorders has been made easier by the advances made in confirmatory DNA tests for many of them, e.g. spinal muscular atrophy (SMA), Duchenne muscular dystrophy, myotonic dystrophy, the congenital muscular dystrophies and hereditary neuropathies. This also allows antenatal testing and genetic counselling and often obviates the need for the discomfort of peripheral neurophysiology.

Disorders of the anterior horn cell

Presentation is with weakness, wasting and absent reflexes. The features of poliomyelitis are described in Chapter 14.

Spinal muscular atrophy

This is an autosomal recessive degeneration of the anterior horn cells, leading to progressive weakness and wasting of skeletal muscles due to mutations in the survival motor neurone (SMN) gene. This is the second most common cause of neuromuscular disease in the UK after Duchenne muscular dystrophy. A number of phenotypes are recognised.

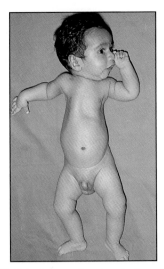

Figure 27.7 Spinal muscular atrophy type 1 (Werdnig–Hoffmann disease) showing proximal muscle wasting, chest deformity from weakness of the intercostal muscles and thighs held abducted because of hypotonia.

Spinal muscular atrophy type 1 (Werdnig–Hoffmann disease)

A very severe progressive disorder presenting in early infancy (Fig. 27.7). Diminished fetal movements are often noticed during pregnancy and there may be arthrogryposis (positional deformities of the limbs with contractures of at least two joints) at birth. Typical signs include:

- Lack of antigravity power in hip flexors
- Absent deep tendon reflexes
- Intercostal recession
- Fasciculation of the tongue.

These children never sit unaided. Death is from respiratory failure within about 12 months. There are milder forms of the disorder with a later onset. Children with type 2 spinal muscular atrophy can sit, but never walk independently. Those with type 3 (Kugelberg–Welander) do walk and can present later in life.

Peripheral neuropathies

The hereditary motor sensory neuropathies (HMSN)

This group of disorders typically leads to symmetrical, slowly progressive muscular wasting, which is distal rather than proximal. Type I, formerly known as peroneal muscular atrophy (Charcot–Marie–Tooth disease), is usually dominantly inherited and the most common. Affected nerves may be hypertrophic due to demyelination followed by attempts at remyelination. Nerve biopsy typically shows 'onion bulb formation' due to these two processes. Onset is in the first decade with distal atrophy and pes cavus, the legs being affected more than the arms. Rarely, there may be distal sensory loss and the reflexes are diminished. The disease is

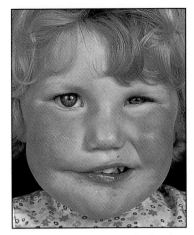

Figure 27.8 Bell palsy. There is right facial weakness of both the upper and lower face.

chronic and only rarely do those affected lose the ability to walk. The initial presentation of Friedreich ataxia can be similar.

Acute post-infectious polyneuropathy (Guillain–Barré syndrome)

Presentation is typically 2–3 weeks after an upper respiratory tract infection or campylobacter gastroenteritis. There may be fleeting abnormal sensory symptoms in the legs, but the prominent feature is an ascending symmetrical weakness with loss of reflexes and autonomic involvement. Sensory symptoms, usually in the distal limbs, are less striking than the paresis but can be unpleasant. Involvement of bulbar muscles leads to difficulty with chewing and swallowing and the risk of aspiration. Respiratory depression may require artificial ventilation. The maximum muscle weakness may occur only 2–4 weeks after the onset of illness. Although full recovery may be expected in 95% of cases, this may take up to 2 years. ①

The CSF protein is characteristically markedly raised, but this may not be seen until the second week of illness. The CSF white cell count is not raised. Nerve conduction velocities are reduced. ②

Management of post-infectious polyneuropathy is supportive, particularly of respiration. The disorder is probably due to the formation of antibody attaching itself to protein components of myelin. Corticosteroids have no beneficial effect and may delay recovery. Controlled trials indicate the ventilator-dependent period can be significantly reduced by immunoglobulin infusion. If this is not successful, plasma exchange may be effective.

Bell palsy and facial nerve palsies

Bell palsy is an isolated lower motor neurone paresis of the VIIth cranial nerve leading to facial weakness (Fig. 27.8). Although the aetiology is unclear, it is probably post-infectious with an association with herpes simplex virus in adults. Corticosteroids may be of value in reducing oedema in the facial canal during the first week; no benefit from aciclovir has been

CSF
Protein ↑↑
WBC –
Glucose –

Neurological disorders

Neurological disorders

481

7+8 → Compressive lesion at cerebellopontine angle

demonstrated. Recovery is complete in the majority of cases but may take several months. The main complication is conjunctival infection due to incomplete eye closure on blinking. This may require the eye to be protected with a patch or even tarsorrhaphy.

There is an important differential diagnosis. If symptoms of an VIIIth nerve paresis are also present then the most likely diagnosis is a compressive lesion in the cerebellopontine angle. The herpes virus may invade the geniculate ganglion and give painful vesicles on the tonsillar fauces and external ear, along with a facial nerve paresis. Treatment for this is with aciclovir.

Ramsay Hunt

Hypertension should be excluded, as there is an association between Bell palsy and coarctation of the aorta. If the facial weakness is bilateral, sarcoidosis should be suspected, and this is also seen in Lyme disease.

Disorders of neuromuscular transmission

Myasthenia gravis

This presents as abnormal muscle fatiguability which improves with rest or anticholinesterase drugs.

Transient neonatal myasthenia

This is described in Chapter 9.

Juvenile myasthenia

This is similar to adult autoimmune myasthenia and is due to binding of antibody to acetylcholine receptors on the post-junctional synaptic membrane. This gives a reduction of the number of functional receptors. Presentation is usually after 10 years of age with ophthalmoplegia and ptosis, loss of facial expression and difficulty chewing (Fig. 27.9). Generalised, especially proximal, weakness may be seen.

Diagnosis is made by observing improvement following the administration of intravenous edrophonium and can be further confirmed by testing for acetylcholine receptor antibodies (seen in 60–80%) or, more rarely, anti-muscle-specific kinase (anti-MuSK) antibodies. Treatment is with the anti-muscarinic drugs neostigmine or pyridostigmine. In the longer term, immunosuppressive therapy with prednisolone or azathioprine is of value. Plasma exchange is used for crises. Thymectomy is considered if a thymoma is present or if the response to medical therapy is unsatisfactory. About a quarter will show remission post thymectomy and up to half show some improvement.

Muscle disorders

The muscular dystrophies

This is a group of inherited disorders with muscle degeneration, often progressive.

Duchenne muscular dystrophy

Duchenne muscular dystrophy is the most common phenotype, affecting 1 in 4000 male infants. It is inherited as an X-linked recessive disorder, although about a third have new mutations. It results from a deletion on the short arm of the X chromosome (at the Xp21 site). This site codes for a protein called dystrophin, which connects the cytoskeleton of a muscle fibre to the surrounding extracellular matrix through the cell membrane. Where it is deficient, there are several aberrant intracellular signalling pathways associated with an influx of calcium ions, a breakdown of the calcium calmodulin complex and an excess of free radicals, ultimately leading to myofibre necrosis. The serum creatine phosphokinase (CPK) is markedly elevated. Some countries, e.g. Wales, have introduced neonatal screening for Duchenne dystrophy; affected children are detected in the neonatal screening test by an elevated CPK.

Children present with a waddling gait and/or language delay; they have to mount stairs one by one and run slowly compared to their peers. Although the average age of diagnosis remains 5.5 years, children often become symptomatic much earlier. They will show Gowers sign (the need to turn prone to rise). There is pseudohypertrophy of the calves because of replacement of muscle fibres by fat and fibrous tissue.

In the early school years, affected boys tend to be slower and clumsier than their peers. The progressive muscle atrophy and weakness means that they are no longer ambulant by the age of about 10–14 years. Life expectancy is reduced to the late twenties from respiratory failure or the associated cardiomyopathy. About one-third of affected children have learning difficulties. Scoliosis is a common complication.

Management – Appropriate exercise helps to maintain muscle power and mobility and delays the onset of scoliosis. Contractures, particularly at the ankles, should be prevented by passive stretching and the provision of night splints. Walking can be prolonged with the provision of orthoses, in particular those which allow ambulation by leaning from side to side. Lengthening of the Achilles tendon may be required to facilitate ambulation. Attention to maintaining a good sitting posture helps to minimise the risk of scoliosis. Scoliosis is managed with a truncal brace, a moulded seat and ultimately surgical insertion of a metal spinal rod. Later in the condition, episodes of nocturnal hypoxia secondary to weakness of the intercostal muscles may present with lassitude or irritability. Respiratory aids, particularly overnight CPAP (continuous

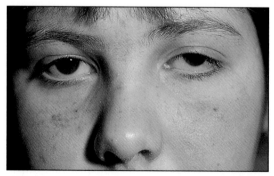

Figure 27.9 Myasthenia gravis showing ptosis from ocular muscle fatigue which improved with edrophonium.

positive airway pressure) or non-invasive positive pressure ventilation (NIPPV), may be provided to improve the quality of life. As with all chronic disabling conditions, parent self-help groups are a useful continuing source of information and support for families. Affected children should be reviewed periodically at a specialist regional centre. Ambulant children with Duchenne dystrophy are increasingly treated with corticosteroids (prednisolone for 10 days each month) to preserve mobility and prevent scoliosis. The precise mechanism by which glucocorticoids may help is not known.

It may be possible to identify female carriers if they have a mildly raised CPK or if the gene deletion can be detected on DNA analysis. Antenatal diagnosis is then possible.

Becker muscular dystrophy

In Becker dystrophy some functional dystrophin is produced. The features are similar to those of Duchenne dystrophy but clinically the disease progresses more slowly. The average age of onset is 11 years, inability to walk in the late twenties, with life expectancy being from the late forties to normal.

Congenital muscular dystrophies

This is a heterogeneous group of disorders, most with recessive inheritance, which present at birth or early infancy with weakness, hypotonia or contractures. Typically the proximal weakness is slowly progressive with a tendency to contracture when the ability to walk is lost. Some may run a more static course. Biopsy shows dystrophic features with a reduction of one of the extracellular matrix proteins such as laminin (most common); or one of several glycosyltransferases. These dystrophies may be linked with central nervous abnormalities, which may result in learning difficulties.

Congenital myopathies

These present at birth or in infancy with generalised hypotonia and muscle weakness. They are static or slowly progressive. They are named according to the changes seen on muscle biopsy or electron microscopy. Creatine phosphokinase levels are normal or only mildly elevated.

Metabolic myopathies

Metabolic conditions can affect muscles, due either to the deposition of storage material or to energy-depleting enzyme deficiencies. Presentation is as a floppy infant or, in older children, with muscle weakness or cramps on exercise. The main causes are:

- Glycogen storage disorders (see Ch. 25).
- Disorders of lipid metabolism. Fatty acids are important muscle fuel. Fatty acid oxidation occurs in the mitochondria and defects in this pathway can result in weakness. Carnitine is essential to supply long-chain fatty acids to the mitochondria for breakdown, and carnitine deficiency causes weakness.
- Mitochondrial cytopathies. Rare disorders which are coded as maternally inherited mitochondrial DNA. Myopathy may be the major manifestation or

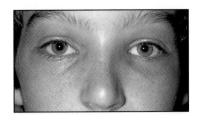

Figure 27.10 Heliotrope rash in dermatomyositis.

the disorder may be multisystem, with lactic acidosis and encephalopathy. Mitochondrial DNA testing is available.

The inflammatory myopathies

Benign acute myositis

This is assumed to be a post-viral phenomenon, as it often follows an upper respiratory tract infection and runs a self-limiting course. Pain and weakness occur in affected muscles. CPK is usually raised.

Dermatomyositis

This is a systemic illness, probably due to an angiopathy. Usual onset is between 5 and 10 years. This can be acute, but more typically is insidious with fever, misery, and eventually symmetrical muscle weakness, which is mainly proximal. Sometimes pharyngeal muscle involvement affects swallowing. There is also a characteristic violaceous (heliotrope) rash to the eyelids, and periorbital oedema (Fig. 27.10). The rash may also affect the extensor surfaces of joints, e.g. elbow, and with time subcutaneous calcification can appear. Inflammatory markers (CRP, ESR) can be raised but not invariably. Muscle biopsy shows an inflammatory cell infiltrate and atrophy. Physiotherapy is needed to prevent contractures. Corticosteroids are the standard treatment, and continue at a tailored dose for 2 years. Other immunosuppressants, e.g. methotrexate, ciclosporin, may be needed. Mortality is 5–10%.

Myotonic disorders

Myotonia is delayed relaxation after sustained muscle contraction. It can be identified clinically and on electromyography.

Dystrophia myotonica

This relatively common illness is dominantly inherited and caused by a nucleotide triplet repeat expansion, so this means there can be anticipation through generations, especially when maternally transmitted (see Ch. 8). Newborns can present with hypotonia and feeding and respiratory difficulties due to muscle weakness. It is then useful to examine the mother for myotonia. This manifests as slow release of handshake or difficulty releasing the tightly clasped fist. This may be mild and not have been appreciated. Sensitivity is required as diagnosis in the neonate may have repercussions for the family. Older children can present with myopathic facies (Fig. 27.11), learning difficulties and myotonia. Adults develop cataracts and males develop baldness and testicular atrophy. Death is usually due to cardiomyopathy.

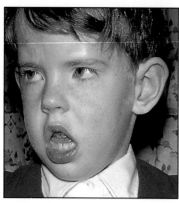

Figure 27.11 Dystrophia myotonica in an 8-year-old who has marked facial weakness and moderately severe learning difficulties.

The 'floppy infant'

Persisting hypotonia in infants can be readily felt on picking up the infant, who tends to slip through the fingers or hang like a rag doll when suspended prone. There will be marked head lag when the head is lifted by the arms from supine. The causes are listed in Box 27.3. The clinical examination may help determine the site of the lesion, whether cortical or neuromuscular. Central hypotonia is associated with poor truncal tone but preserved limb tone. Dysmorphic features suggest a genetic cause. Lower motor neurone lesions are suggested by a frog-like posture (Fig. 27.7), poor antigravity movements and absent reflexes.

Summary

Neuromuscular disorders

- Present with muscle weakness, which may manifest with floppiness, delayed motor milestones, unsteady gait or muscle fatiguability
- Anterior horn cell – *spinal muscular atrophy*: progressive weakness and wasting of skeletal muscles; tongue fasciculation may aid diagnosis
- Peripheral nerve
  - *Hereditary motor sensory neuropathies* (HMSN): symmetrical wasting of the distal muscles
  - *Acute post-infectious polyneuropathy* (Guillain–Barré syndrome): ascending symmetrical weakness; may be bulbar palsy and respiratory depression
- Neuromuscular transmission – *juvenile myasthenia*: >10 years old, ophthalmoplegia and ptosis, loss of facial expression and difficulty chewing
- Muscle – *Duchenne muscular dystrophy*: X-linked recessive, presents with waddling gait and difficulty climbing stairs

Box 27.3 Causes of the floppy (hypotonic) infant

Central
Cortical
- Hypoxic-ischaemic encephalopathy
- Cortical malformations

Genetic
- Down syndrome
- Prader–Willi syndrome

Metabolic
- Hypothyroidism
- Hypocalcaemia

Peripheral
Neuromuscular
- Spinal muscular atrophy
- Myopathy
- Myotonia
- Congenital myasthenia.

Ataxia

Friedreich ataxia

This is an autosomal recessive condition. The gene mutation (Frataxin) is an example of a trinucleotide repeat disorder. It presents with worsening ataxia, distal wasting in the legs, absent lower limb reflexes but extensor plantar responses because of pyramidal involvement, pes cavus and dysarthria. This is similar to the hereditary motor sensory neuropathies, but in Friedreich ataxia, there is impairment of joint position and vibration sense, extensor plantars and there is often optic atrophy. The cerebellar component becomes more apparent with age. Evolving kyphoscoliosis and cardiomyopathy can cause cardiorespiratory compromise and death at 40–50 years.

Ataxia telangiectasia

This disorder of DNA repair is an autosomal recessive condition. The gene (ATM) has been identified. There may be mild delay in motor development in infancy and oculomotor problems with incoordination and delay in ocular pursuit of objects (oculomotor dyspraxia), with difficulty with balance and coordination becoming evident at school age. There is subsequent deterioration, with a mixture of dystonia and cerebellar signs. Many children require a wheelchair for mobility in early adolescence. Telangiectasia develops in the conjunctiva (Fig. 27.12), neck and shoulders from about 4 years of age. These children:

- Have an increased susceptibility to infection, principally from an IgA surface antibody defect
- Develop malignant disorders, principally acute lymphoblastic leukaemia (about 10%)
- Have a raised serum alpha-fetoprotein

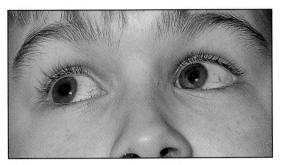

Figure 27.12 Telangiectasia of the conjunctiva are present from about 4 years of age in ataxia telangiectasia.

- Have an increased white cell sensitivity to irradiation, which can be used diagnostically, but the ATM gene test is now mostly used.

Other hereditary cerebellar ataxias

There is a growing number of these, largely dominantly inherited (genotypes identified), with a relatively benign course in childhood.

Summary

Cerebellar ataxia

- Causes – medication and drugs, varicella infection, posterior fossa lesions or tumours, genetic and degenerative disorders, e.g. ataxic cerebral palsy, Friedreich ataxia and ataxia telangiectasia.

Cerebrovascular disease

Intracranial haemorrhage

Extradural haemorrhage

This usually follows direct head trauma, often associated with skull fracture (tearing of middle meningeal artery as it passes through the foramen spinosum of the sphenoid bone). It results from arterial or venous bleeding into the extradural space. There is often a lucid interval until the conscious level deteriorates, with seizures, secondary to increasing size of the haematoma. There may be focal neurological signs with dilatation of the ipsilateral pupil, paresis of the contralateral limbs and a false localising uni- or bilateral VIth nerve paresis. In young children, initial presentation may be with anaemia and shock. The diagnosis is confirmed with a CT scan. Management is to correct hypovolaemia, urgent evacuation of the haematoma and arrest of the bleeding.

Subdural haematoma

This results from tearing of the veins as they cross the subdural space. It is a characteristic lesion in non-accidental injury caused by shaking or direct trauma in infants or toddlers. Retinal haemorrhages are usually present. There has been recent controversy surrounding the relative contributions of direct trauma, shearing injury and hypoxia. Subdural haematomas are occasionally seen following a fall from a considerable height.

Subarachnoid haemorrhage

This is much more common in adults. Presentation is usually with acute onset of head pain, neck stiffness and occasionally fever. Retinal haemorrhage is usually present. Seizures and coma may develop. A CT scan of the head usually identifies blood in the CSF. A lumbar puncture in the acute situation is best avoided as haemorrhage may extend following the release of intracranial pressure. The cause is often an aneurysm or arteriovenous malformation (AVM). It can be identified on MR angiography (MRA), CT or conventional angiography. Treatment can be neurosurgical or with interventional radiography.

Summary

Cerebral haemorrhage

- History of significant head injury – remember that an extradural haemorrhage may be present even if lucid afterwards
- Subdural haematoma and retinal haemorrhages in an infant – consider non-accidental injury caused by shaking or direct trauma.

Stroke

Infantile stroke is dealt with in Chapter 10. Childhood stroke may be due to vascular, thromboembolic or haemorrhagic disease. The clinical presentation is determined by the vascular territory involved. There is compromise of the anterior circulation (internal carotid, anterior and middle cerebral arteries), which leads to hemiparesis with or without speech disturbance. Less common is compromise of the posterior circulation (vertebrobasilar arteries) with associated visual or cerebellar signs.

Causes include:

- Cardiac: congenital cyanotic heart disease, e.g. Fallot tetralogy, endocarditis
- Haematological: sickle cell disease; deficiencies of anti-thrombotic factors, e.g. protein S
- Post-infective: following varicella or other viral infection
- Inflammatory: damage to vessels in autoimmune disease, e.g. SLE (systemic lupus erythematosus)
- Metabolic/genetic: homocystinuria, mitochondrial disorders, e.g. MELAS (**m**yoclonic **e**pilepsy, **l**actic **a**cidosis and **s**troke); CADASIL (**c**erebral **a**utosomal **d**ominant **a**rteriopathy with **s**ubcortical **i**nfarcts

and leukoencephalopathy), the most common form of hereditary stroke disorder

- Vascular malformations: moyamoya disease. These children have abnormal vasculature. Moyamoya comes from the Japanese for 'puff of smoke', similar to the blurred appearance seen on angiography.

Investigations should include an assessment of cerebral vasculature with MRI and MRA and carotid Doppler studies to rule out dissection of the carotid arteries (formal angiography may be required later); echocardiography to detect a source of embolism, along with a thrombophilia and vasculitis screen, and metabolic tests for homocysteine and mitochondrial cytopathy. Often no cause can be identified. Rehabilitation requires the involvement of the remedial therapy team. Aspirin prophylaxis is recommended but further evidence is needed on the advisability of anti-thrombolytic agents.

Summary

Strokes

- Occur in infants and children
- Occur in the antenatal or perinatal period, and may present in late infancy with a hemiplegia or at the time with seizures
- Are most often seen in association with cardiac or sickle cell disease, but varicella infection is another cause.

Neural tube defects and hydrocephalus

Neural tube defects

Neural tube defects result from failure of normal fusion of the neural plate to form the neural tube during the first 28 days following conception. Their birth prevalence in the UK has fallen dramatically from 4 per 1000 live births in the 1970s to 0.15 per 1000 live births in 1998 and to 0.11 per 1000 live births in 2005 (Fig. 27.13). This is mainly because of a natural decline, as well as antenatal screening.

The reason for the natural decline is uncertain, but may be associated with improved maternal nutrition. Mothers of a fetus with a neural tube defect have a 10-fold increase in risk of having a second affected fetus. Folic acid supplementation reduces this risk. High doses are now recommended periconceptually for women with a previously affected infant planning a further pregnancy. Low-dose periconceptual folic acid supplementation is recommended for all pregnancies. In some countries e.g. United States, folic acid is added to flour for bread.

Anencephaly

This is failure of development of most of the cranium and brain. Affected infants are stillborn or die shortly after birth. It is detected on antenatal ultrasound screening and termination of pregnancy is usually performed.

Encephalocele

There is extrusion of brain and meninges through a midline skull defect, which can be corrected surgically. However, there are often underlying associated cerebral malformations.

Spina bifida occulta

This failure of fusion of the vertebral arch (Fig. 27.14a) is often an incidental finding on X-ray, but there may be an associated overlying skin lesion such as a tuft of hair, lipoma, birth mark or small dermal sinus, usually in the lumbar region. There may be underlying tethering of the cord (diastematomyelia), which, with growth, may cause neurological deficits of bladder function and lower limbs. The extent of the underlying lesion can be delineated using ultrasound and/or MRI scans. Neurosurgical relief of tethering is usually indicated.

Meningocele and myelomeningocele

Meningoceles (Fig. 27.14b) usually have a good prognosis following surgical repair.

Myelomeningoceles (Figs 27.14c, 27.15) may be associated with:

- Variable paralysis of the legs
- Muscle imbalance, which may cause dislocation of the hip and talipes
- Sensory loss
- Bladder denervation (neuropathic bladder)
- Bowel denervation (neuropathic bowel)
- Scoliosis
- Hydrocephalus from the Chiari malformation (herniation of the cerebellar tonsils and brainstem tissue through the foramen magnum), leading to disruption of CSF flow.

Management – The back lesion is usually closed soon after birth.

Paralysis and muscle imbalance – physiotherapy helps prevent joint contractures. Walking aids or a wheelchair help mobility.

For sensory loss – skin care is required to avoid the development of skin damage and ulcers.

Neuropathic bladder – an indwelling catheter may be required for a neurogenic bladder, or intermittent

Summary

Neural tube defects

- Include anencephaly, encephalocele, spina bifida occulta, meningocele and myelomeningocele
- The birth prevalence in the UK has fallen dramatically, mainly owing to a natural decline but also to antenatal screening
- The birth prevalence is reduced by periconceptual folic acid
- Myelomeningoceles can cause paralysis of the legs, dislocation of the hip and talipes, sensory loss, neuropathic bladder and bowel, scoliosis and hydrocephalus from the Chiari malformation.

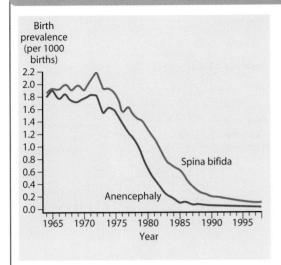

Figure 27.13 The decline in the number of babies born with neural tube defects. This has resulted from a natural decrease together with antenatal diagnosis and termination of pregnancy.

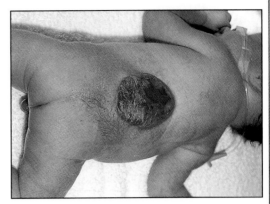

Figure 27.15 Myelomeningocele showing the exposed neural tissue and the patulous anus from neuropathic bowel.

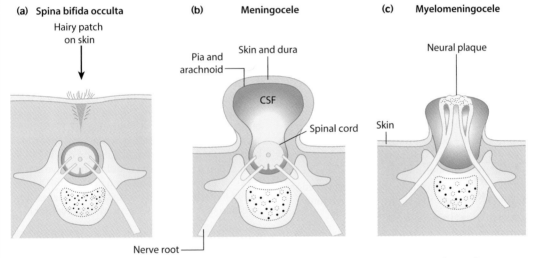

Figure 27.14 Neural tube defects: **(a)** spina bifida occulta; **(b)** meningocele; **(c)** myelomeningocele.

urinary catheterisation may be performed by parents or by older children themselves. There should be regular checks for hypertension, renal function and urinary infection. Prophylactic antibiotics may be necessary. Medication (such as ephedrine or oxybutynin) may improve bladder function and improve urinary dribbling.

Bowel denervation – requires regular toileting, and laxatives and suppositories are likely to be necessary with a low roughage diet for lesions above L3.

Scoliosis – is monitored and may require surgical treatment. Ventricular dilatation associated with a Chiari malformation – often present at birth and 80% of affected infants require a shunt for progressive hydrocephalus during the first few weeks of life.

The most severely disabled have a spinal lesion above L3 at birth. They are unable to walk, have a scoliosis, neuropathic bladder, hydronephrosis and frequently develop hydrocephalus.

Modern medical care has improved the quality of life for severely affected children. Their care is best managed by a specialist multidisciplinary team.

Hydrocephalus

In hydrocephalus, there is obstruction to the flow of cerebrospinal fluid, leading to dilatation of the ventricular system proximal to the site of obstruction. The obstruction may be within the ventricular system or aqueduct (non-communicating or obstructive hydrocephalus), or at the arachnoid villi, the site of absorption of CSF (communicating hydrocephalus) (Box 27.4).

Hydrocephalus

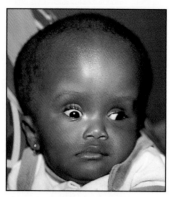

Figure 27.16 Grossly enlarged head and downward deviation of the eyes (setting-sun sign) from untreated hydrocephalus.

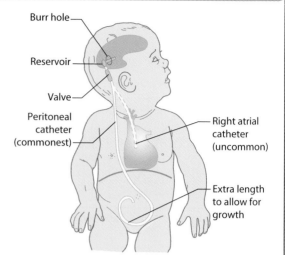

Burr hole
Reservoir
Valve
Peritoneal catheter (commonest)
Right atrial catheter (uncommon)
Extra length to allow for growth

Figure 27.17 Ventriculoperitoneal shunt for drainage of symptomatic hydrocephalus. A sufficient length of shunt tubing is left in the peritoneal cavity to allow for the child's growth. Right atrial catheters require revision with growth.

Box 27.4 Causes of hydrocephalus

Non-communicating (obstruction in the ventricular system)

Congenital malformation
- Aqueduct stenosis
- Atresia of the outflow foramina of the fourth ventricle (Dandy–Walker malformation)
- Chiari malformation

Posterior fossa neoplasm or vascular malformation
Intraventricular haemorrhage in preterm infant

Communicating (failure to reabsorb CSF)

Subarachnoid haemorrhage
Meningitis, e.g. pneumococcal, tuberculous

Some can cause both non-communicating and communicating hydrocephalus.

Clinical features

In infants with hydrocephalus, as their skull sutures have not fused, the head circumference may be disproportionately large or show an excessive rate of growth. The skull sutures separate, the anterior fontanelle bulges and the scalp veins become distended. An advanced sign is fixed downward gaze or sun setting of the eyes (Fig. 27.16). Older children will develop signs and symptoms of raised intracranial pressure.

Hydrocephalus may be diagnosed on antenatal ultrasound screening or in preterm infants on routine cranial ultrasound scanning. For suspected hydrocephalus, initial assessment is with cranial ultrasound (in infants) or imaging with CT or MRI. Head circumference should be monitored over time on centile charts.

Treatment is required for symptomatic relief of raised intracranial pressure and to minimise the risk of neurological damage. The mainstay is the insertion of a ventriculoperitoneal shunt (Fig. 27.17), but endoscopic treatment to create a ventriculostomy can now be performed. Shunts can malfunction due to blockage or infection (usually with coagulase-negative staphylococci). They then need replacing or revising. Overdrainage of fluid can cause low-pressure headaches but the insertion of regulatory valves can help avoid this.

Summary

Hydrocephalus

- In infants, presents with excessive increase in head circumference, separation of skull sutures, bulging of the anterior fontanelle, distension of scalp veins and sun setting of the eyes
- Older children present with raised intracranial pressure
- Treatment is usually with a ventriculoperitoneal shunt.

The neurocutaneous syndromes

The nervous system and the skin have a common ectodermal origin. Embryological disruption causes syndromes involving abnormalities to both systems – the neurocutaneous syndromes.

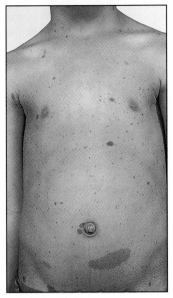

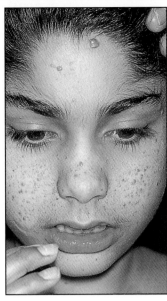

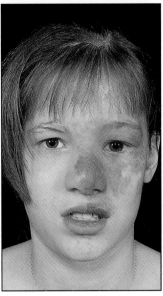

Figure 27.18 Café-au-lait patches and axillary freckling in neurofibromatosis.

Figure 27.19 Adenoma sebaceum in tuberous sclerosis.

Figure 27.20 Sturge–Weber syndrome. There is a port-wine stain in the distribution of the trigeminal nerve.

Neurofibromatosis type 1 (NF1)

This affects 1 in 3000 live births. It is an autosomal dominant, highly penetrant condition. One-third have new mutations. The gene has been identified.

In order to make the diagnosis, two or more of these criteria need to be present:

- Six or more café-au-lait spots >5 mm in size before puberty, >15 mm after puberty (Fig. 27.18)
- More than one neurofibroma, an unsightly firm nodular overgrowth of any nerve
- Axillary freckles (Fig. 27.18)
- Optic glioma which may cause visual impairment
- One Lisch nodule, a hamartoma of the iris seen on slit-lamp examination
- Bony lesions from sphenoid dysplasia, which can cause eye protrusion
- A first-degree relative with NF1.

The cutaneous features tend to become more evident after puberty, and there is a wide spectrum of involvement from mild to severe. Neurofibromata appear in the course of any peripheral nerve, including cranial nerves. They may look unsightly or cause neurological signs if they occur at a site where a peripheral nerve passes through a bony foramen. Visual or auditory impairment may result if there is compression of the IInd or VIIIth cranial nerve. Megalencephaly with learning difficulties and epilepsy are sometimes seen.

Neurofibromatosis type 2 (NF2; bilateral, acoustic or central) is less common and presents in adolescence. Bilateral acoustic neuromata are the predominant feature and present with deafness and sometimes a cerebellopontine angle syndrome with a facial (VIIth) nerve paresis and cerebellar ataxia.

There may be an overlap between the features of NF1 and NF2. Both NF1 and NF2 can be associated with endocrinological disorders, the multiple endocrine neoplasia (MEN) syndromes.

Other associations are phaeochromocytoma, pulmonary hypertension, renal artery stenosis with hypertension, and gliomatous change, particularly in central nervous system lesions. Rarely, the benign tumours undergo sarcomatous change. However, most people with the disorder carry no features other than the cutaneous stigmata.

Tuberous sclerosis

This disorder is a dominantly inherited disorder, but up to 70% are new mutations. Prevalence is 1 in 9000 live births.

The cutaneous features consist of:

- Depigmented 'ash leaf'-shaped patches which fluoresce under ultraviolet light (Wood's light)
- Roughened patches of skin (shagreen patches) usually over the lumbar spine
- Adenoma sebaceum (angiofibromata) in a butterfly distribution over the bridge of the nose and cheeks, which are unusual before the age of 3 years (Fig. 27.19).

Neurological features are:

- Infantile spasms and developmental delay
- Epilepsy – often focal
- Intellectual impairment.

Neurological disorders

489

These children have severe learning difficulties and often have autistic features to their behaviour when older. Other features are:

- Fibromata beneath the nails (subungual fibromata)
- Dense white areas on the retina (phakomata) from local degeneration
- Rhabdomyomata of the heart which are identifiable in the early weeks on echocardiography but usually resolve in infancy
- Polycystic kidneys.

As with neurofibromatosis, gliomatous change can occur in the brain lesions. Many people who carry the gene have no stigmata other than the cutaneous features and no associated neurological features.

CT scans will detect the calcified subependymal nodules and tubers from the second year of life. MRI is more sensitive and more clearly identifies other tubers and lesions.

Sturge–Weber syndrome

This is a sporadic disorder with a haemangiomatous facial lesion (a port-wine stain) in the distribution of the trigeminal nerve associated with a similar lesion intracranially. The ophthalmic division of the trigeminal nerve is always involved (Fig. 27.20). Calcification of the gyri used to show characteristic 'rail-road track' calcification on skull X-ray, but MRI is the imaging modality of choice nowadays. In the most severe form, it may present with epilepsy, learning disability and hemiplegia. Children presenting with intractable epilepsy in early infancy may benefit from hemispherectomy. For children who are less severely affected, deterioration is unusual after the age of 5 years, although there may still be seizures and learning difficulties. There is a high risk of glaucoma, which should be assessed in the neonatal period.

Summary

The neurocutaneous syndromes

Include neurofibromatosis, tuberous sclerosis and Sturge–Weber syndrome.

Neurodegenerative disorders

These are disorders that cause a deterioration in motor and intellectual function. Abnormal neurological features develop, including seizures, spasticity, abnormal

Table 27.5 Lipid storage disorders

Disorder	Enzyme defect	Clinical features
Tay–Sachs disease	Hexosaminidase A	Autosomal recessive disorder
		Most common among Ashkenazi Jews
		Developmental regression in late infancy, exaggerated startle response to noise, visual inattention and social unresponsiveness
		Severe hypotonia, enlarging head
		Cherry red spot at the macula
		Death by 2–5 years
		Diagnosis – measurement of the specific enzyme activity
		Carrier detection of high-risk couples is practised
		Prenatal detection is possible
Gaucher disease	Beta-glucosidase	Occurs in 1 in 500 Ashkenazi Jews
		Chronic childhood form – splenomegaly, bone marrow suppression, bone involvement, normal IQ
		Splenectomy may alleviate hypersplenism
		Enzyme replacement therapy is available, but is expensive
		Acute infantile form – splenomegaly, neurological degeneration with seizures
		Carrier detection and prenatal diagnosis are possible
Niemann–Pick disease	Sphingomyelinase	At 3–4 months, feeding difficulties and failure to thrive, hepatosplenomegaly, developmental delay, hypotonia and deterioration of hearing and vision
		Cherry red spot in macula affects 50%
		Death by 4 years

head circumference (macro- or microcephaly), involuntary movement disorders, visual and hearing loss and behaviour change. While individually rare, they are numerous and include:

- Lysosomal storage disorders, e.g. lipid storage disorders and mucopolysaccharidoses, in which absence of an enzyme leads to accumulation of a harmful metabolite
- Peroxisomal enzyme defects, e.g. X-linked adrenoleucodystrophy. Peroxisomes are catalase- and oxidase-containing organelles involved in long-chain fatty acid oxidation. Enzyme deficiencies can lead to accumulation of very long-chain fatty acids (VLCFAs)
- Heredodegenerative disorders, e.g. Huntington disease, which presents with progressive dystonia, dementia, seizures and corticospinal tract signs

- Wilson disease, from the accumulation of copper, may cause changes in behaviour and additional involuntary movements or a mixture of neurological and hepatic symptoms
- Subacute sclerosing panencephalitis (SSPE), a delayed response in adolescence to previous measles infection causing neurological regression with a characteristic EEG, but has become rare since measles immunisation.

Lysosomal storage disorders

In metachromatic leucodystrophy, a sulfatidosis, an accumulation of sulphatides causes a destruction of myelin and is diagnosed on testing white cell enzymes.

In lipid storage disorders (Table 27.5), which are sphingolipidoses, there is an accumulation of

Mucopolysaccharidoses

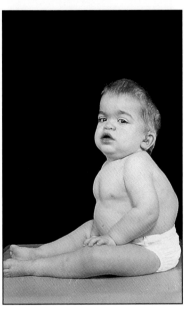

Figure 27.21 Hurler syndrome showing the characteristic facies and skeletal dysplasia.

Table 27.6 Clinical features of mucopolysaccharidoses

Eyes	Corneal clouding
	Retinal degeneration
	Glaucoma
Skin	Thickened skin
	Coarse facies
Heart	Valvular lesions
	Cardiac failure
Neurology	Developmental regression
Skeletal	Thickened skull
	Broad ribs
	Claw hand
	Thoracic kyphosis
	Lumbar lordosis
Other	Hepatosplenomegaly
	Carpal tunnel syndrome
	Conductive deafness
	Umbilical and inguinal hernias

Table 27.7 Types of mucopolysaccharidoses

Type	Inheritance	Cornea	Heart	Brain	Skeletal
MPS I (Hurler)	AR	+++	++	+++	++
MPS II (Hunter)	X-linked	–	+	++	+
MPS III (Sanfilippo)	AR	±	–	+	+
MPS IV (Morquio)	AR	+	+	–	+++
MPS VI (Maroteaux–Lamy)	AR	+++	++	–	++

AR, autosomal recessive.

sphingolipids, essential components of CNS membranes. They are diagnosed on testing white cell enzymes.

The mucopolysaccharidoses are progressive multisystem disorders which may affect the neurological, ocular, cardiac and skeletal systems (Table 27.6). Hepatosplenomegaly is usually present. Most children present with developmental delay following a period of essentially normal growth and development up to 6–12 months of age. Developmental attainment then slows and children may show some loss of skills. It is only in the second 6 months of life that the characteristic facies begin to emerge, with coarsening of the facial features and prominent forehead due to frontal bossing (Fig. 27.21).

The characteristics of five of the varieties are shown in Table 27.7. The diagnosis is made by identifying the enzyme defect and the excretion in the urine of the major storage substances, the glycosaminoglycans (GAGs). Treatment is supportive according to the child's needs. Successful enzyme replacement by bone marrow transplantation has been performed but cannot reverse any established neurological abnormality.

Summary

In neurodegenerative disorders

There is developmental regression with the evolution of abnormal neurological signs.

Further reading

Forsyth R, Newton R: *Paediatric Neurology. Oxford Specialist Handbook in Paediatrics*, Oxford, 2007, Oxford University Press.

Newton RW: *Colour Atlas of Pediatric Neurology*, London, 1995, Mosby-Wolfe.
A well-illustrated textbook.

Websites (Accessed May 2011)

British Paediatric Neurology Association: Available at: http://www.bpna.org.uk.

Child Neurology: Available at: http://www.familyvillage.wisc.edu/.
Provides 'family village' library with information on many neurological diagnoses.

International Headache Society classification: Available at: http://ihs-classification.org/en.

International League Against Epilepsy (ILAE): Available at: http://www.ilae.org.

Neuromuscular Disease Center: (Washington University School of Medicine, St Louis, MO). Available at: http://neuromuscular.wustl.edu.

Systematic reviews of migraine treatment in children, epilepsy, steroids for facial palsy and treatment of Guillain–Barré syndrome can be found in the Cochrane Library. Available via: http://www.thecochranelibrary.com.

Adolescent medicine

Adolescence is the transition from childhood to adulthood. There is no clearly defined age range, but it is usually considered to be from puberty until 18 years of age. There are 7.8 million adolescents in the UK, 12–13% of the population, with increased proportions observed in ethnic minority groups.

The transition from being a child to an adult involves many biological, psychological and social changes (Table 28.1). Pubertal development is considered in Chapter 11. Difficulties may arise if the pubertal changes are early or delayed.

Table 28.1 Developmental changes of adolescence

	Biological	Psychological	Social
Early adolescence	Early puberty: Females – breast bud, pubic hair development, start of growth spurt Males – testicular enlargement, start of genital growth	Concrete thinking (Fig. 28.1a), but begin to develop moral concepts and awareness of their sexual identity	The early emotional separation from parents, start of a strong peer identification, early exploratory behaviours, e.g. may start smoking
Mid-adolescence	Females – end of growth spurt, menarche, change in body shape Males – sperm production, voice breaks, start of growth spurt Acne Blushing Need for more sleep	Abstract thinking, but still seen as 'bulletproof', increasing verbal dexterity, may develop a fervent ideology (religious, political)	Continuing emotional separation from parents, heterosexual peer interest, early vocational plans
Late adolescence	Males – end of puberty, continued growth in height, strength and body hair	Complex abstract thinking (Fig. 28.1b), identification of difference between law and morality, increased impulse control, further development of personal identity, further development or rejection of ideologies	Social autonomy, may develop intimate relationships, further education or employment, may begin or develop financial independence

Adapted from Adolescent development. In: Viner R, ed. 2005. *ABC of Adolescence*. Blackwell, Oxford.

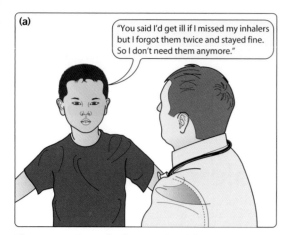

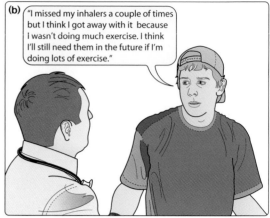

Figure 28.1 Example showing the difference between **(a)** concrete and **(b)** abstract thinking in the management of asthma in an older child and an adolescent.

While general practitioners will see all adolescent medical problems, difficulties may arise when obtaining specialist medical care. Those less than 16 years old are generally looked after by paediatricians; over 16 years old, by either paediatricians or more often by adult physicians and surgeons. However, paediatric facilities, e.g. children's wards, are often geared to the needs of young children rather than adolescents, whilst older adolescents may be overwhelmed by the medical conditions encountered on adult wards and the independence expected of them. Adolescent females with gynaecological problems are often cared for by gynaecologists, usually in adult facilities. Some paediatricians in the UK are now specialising in adolescent medicine in a similar way to North America and Australia.

Communicating with adolescents

The adolescent consultation differs from the paediatric consultation for young children, in that the adolescent has a greater active role in the consultation.

As well as seeing adolescents with their parents, an integral component of adolescent healthcare is offering young people the opportunity to be seen independently of their parents for at least part of the visit The principle is that the parents should not be seen alone after the adolescent has spent time with the doctor, so that the adolescent can trust that whatever confidences have been disclosed to the doctor have been kept.

Some practical points about communicating and working with adolescents are:

- Make the adolescent the central person in the consultation.
- Be yourself. When establishing rapport, it may be appropriate to engage the adolescent by talking about their interests, e.g. football, clothes or music, but do not try to be cool, false or patronising; your relationship should be as their doctor, not their friend.

- Consider the family dynamics. Is the mother or father answering for the adolescent? Does the adolescent seem to want this or resent being interrupted?
- Avoid being judgemental or lecturing. Avoid 'You ....' statements and use 'I ....' statements in preference, e.g. 'I am concerned that you ....'. A frank and direct approach works best. Your role should be that of a knowledgeable, trusted adult from whom they can get advice if they so choose.
- An authoritarian approach is likely to result in a rebellious stance. Working things out together in a practical way has the best chance of success.
- Frame difficult questions so they are less threatening and judgemental, e.g. 'Lots of teenagers drink alcohol, do any of your friends drink? How much do they drink in a week? Do you drink alcohol – how much do you drink compared to them?' Likewise, when asking sensitive questions on, e.g. sexual health, always give young people warning and explain the rationale of why such questions need to be asked.
- Confidentiality is particularly important to this age group and must be respected. Explain that you will keep everything you are told confidential, unless they or somebody else is at risk of serious harm. Always assess their understanding of confidentiality and correct any misunderstanding.
- Bear in mind proxy presentations, e.g. abdominal pain, when the real reason is anxiety about the possibility of pregnancy, or sexually transmitted infection or the result of recreational drug use.
- A full adolescent psychosocial history is useful to engage the young person, to assess the level of risk as well as provide information which will aid the formulation of effective interventions. The HEADS acronym may be helpful in this regard (Table 28.2), although questions must always be tailored to stage of development and the right of the young person to not answer should be respected.

Table 28.2 HEADS acronym for psychosocial history taking in adolescents

H	**Home life**	Relationships, social support, household chores
E	**Education**	School, exams, work experience, career, university, financial issues
A	**Activities**	Exercise, sport, other leisure activities
		Social relationships, friends, peers, who can they rely on?
D	**Driving**	Aged 16 if has high rate mobility component of the Disability Living Allowance (DLA)
	Drugs	Drug use, cigarettes, alcohol. How much? How often?
	Diet	Weight, caffeine (diet drinks), binges/vomits
S	**Sex**	Concerns, periods, contraception (and in relation to medication)
	Sleep	How much? Hard to get to sleep? Wake often?
	Suicide/affect	Early waking? Depression, self-harm, body image

- Communicate and explain concepts appropriate to their cognitive development. For young adolescents, use concrete examples ('here and now') rather than abstract concepts ('if … then') .
- History-taking should avoid making the assumption of heterosexuality with questions about romantic and sexual partners asked in a gender neutral way.
- If they need to have a physical examination, consider their privacy and personal integrity – Who do they want present? As with any age, young people have the right to a chaperone but it should not be assumed the young person will want this to be their parent. Also, find out if they would prefer a doctor of the same sex, if this is an option.

> **Summary**
>
> **Talking and listening with young people**
> - Always give them the opportunity to be seen independently of their parents
> - Explain and assure confidentiality
> - Psychosocial screening is useful to:
>   - Engage young people
>   - Assess risk
>   - Assist formulation of interventions.

Consent and confidentiality

Consent

In the UK, young people can give consent if they are sufficiently informed and either over 16 years old or under 16 years and competent to make decisions for themselves. Conflict rarely arises about a treatment, as usually the adolescent, their parents and doctors agree that it is necessary. Handling of disagreement over consent is considered in Chapter 5.

Confidentiality

Confidentiality is regarded by adolescents as of crucial importance in their medical care. They want to know that information they have disclosed to their doctor is not revealed to others, whether parents, school or police, without their permission. In most circumstances, their confidentiality should be kept unless there is a risk of serious harm, either to themselves from physical or sexual abuse or from suicidal thoughts or to others from homicidal intent. Difficulties relating to confidentiality for adolescents are usually about contraception, abortion, sexually transmitted infections, substance abuse or mental health. It is usually desirable for the parents to be informed and involved in the management of these situations and the adolescent should be encouraged to tell them or allow the doctor to do so. However, if the young person is competent to make these decisions for himself/herself, the courts have supported medical management of these situations without parental knowledge or consent.

Range of health problems

Adolescence is considered a healthy stage of life compared with early childhood or old age. In spite of this, the majority of young people will consult their general practitioner more than once in a year and 13% of adolescents report a chronic illness. The range of health problems affecting adolescents include:

- Common acute illnesses: respiratory disorders, skin conditions, musculoskeletal problems including sports injuries and somatic complaints. Acute serious illness has become rare, with mortality predominantly from trauma
- Chronic illness and disability: e.g. asthma, epilepsy, diabetes, cerebral palsy, juvenile idiopathic arthritis, sickle cell disease. The prevalence of some of the common chronic disorders in adolescence is shown in Table 28.3. There is also a range of uncommon disorders with serious chronic morbidity such as malignant disease and connective tissue disorders. In addition, children

Adolescent medicine

Table 28.3 Prevalence of some chronic illnesses per 1000 adolescents (12–18 years old)

Disease	Prevalence per 1000 adolescents
Musculoskeletal conditions	41
Skin conditions	32
Significant mental health problems	120
Diabetes	
Type 1	2
Type 2	1–2
Respiratory conditions	150
Asthma	100
Cystic fibrosis	0.1
Epilepsy	4
Hearing problems	18
Cerebral palsy	1.5

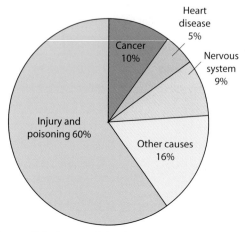

Figure 28.3 Causes of death, 15–19 years of age, in England and Wales, 2008. (Source: ONS, 2010.)

with many congenital disorders which often used to be fatal in childhood now survive into adolescence or adult life, e.g. cystic fibrosis, Duchenne muscular dystrophy, complex congenital heart disease, metabolic disorders, etc.
- High prevalence of somatic symptoms: fatigue, headaches, backache, etc.
- Mental health problems including suicide and deliberate self-harm
- Eating disorders and weight problems
- Those associated with health-risk behaviours, such as smoking, drinking, drug abuse and sexual health, contraception and teenage pregnancy.

Mortality

The dramatic improvement in the mortality of young children seen since the 1960s has not been matched in adolescents, who now have a higher mortality rate than that of 1–4-year-olds (Fig. 28.2). Although deaths in adolescents from communicable diseases have declined markedly, this has not been matched by mortality from road traffic accidents, other injuries and suicide, and these now predominate (Fig. 28.3). Alcohol is thought to be a contributing factor in one-third of these deaths.

Impact of chronic conditions

Chronic illness may disrupt biological, psychological and social development. In addition, these developmental changes may affect the control and management of the disorder (Table 28.4). The impact of chronic illness on children, young people and their families is considered in Chapter 23.

Adherence

Poor adherence is a problem for many people, including adolescents as they are beginning to take over management of their illness, wish to avoid parental supervision and may give the management of their illness a lower priority than social and recreational activities. They may not believe that taking the

Figure 28.2 Mortality by age group in England and Wales 1960–2008, showing that the mortality rate is now greater at 15–19 years than at 1–4 years. (Source: ONS, 2010.)

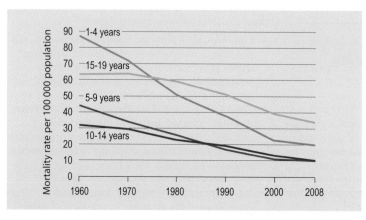

Table 28.4 Some of the ways in which chronic illness and development interact with each other

	Effect of chronic illness on development	Effect of development on chronic illness
Biological	Delayed puberty Short stature Reduced bone mass accretion Malnutrition secondary to inadequate intake due to increased caloric requirement of disease or anorexia Localised growth abnormalities in inflammatory joint disease, e.g. premature fusion of epiphyses	Pubertal hormones may impact on disease, e.g. growth hormone worsens diabetes and increases insulin requirements; females with cystic fibrosis may have deterioration in lung function; corticosteroid toxicity worse in peripubertal phase Increased caloric requirement may worsen disease control or result in undernutrition – may need dietary supplements or overnight feeding with nasogastric tube or gastrostomy Growth may cause scoliosis
Psychological	Regression to less mature behaviour Adopt sick role Impaired development of sense of attractive/sexual self Parental stress, depression, financial problems in providing care; siblings may suffer	Deny that their health may suffer from their actions Poor adherence and disease control Reject medics like parents
Social	Reduced independence when should be separating Failure of peer relationships Social isolation – unable to participate in sports or social events School absence and decline in school performance, may lower self-esteem Vocational failure	Risk behaviour may adversely affect disease, e.g. smoking and asthma or cystic fibrosis, alcohol and diabetic control, sleep deprivation and epilepsy Chaotic eating habits lead to malnutrition or obesity

medication really matters, especially if it is preventative or of long-term rather than short-term benefit.

Peer relationships and self-image are very important when considering adherence. For example, it may be more important for an adolescent with diabetes to lunch promptly, so he can sit with his friends rather than go to the school nurse first for his insulin injection. Side-effects are also important, particularly those that affect well-being or appearance. They may assess risk differently from adults, so that the risk of not being one of their crowd because of having to adhere to a certain treatment may appear to be more important than the risks attached to not taking any medication.

Adherence may be influenced by lack of knowledge and/or poor recall of previous disease education. The disorder may have presented when the child was much younger, so that the original consultation will have taken place primarily between the doctor and parents. If this communication has not been updated with increasing age, the adolescent's knowledge may be poor, with little understanding about his/her illness, what medications he/she is taking and why. As the responsibility for management moves to the young

person, information needs to be provided about medications and treatment appropriate for his/her development. Other ways to maximise adherence are summarised in Table 28.5.

The implications of their condition on the rest of their health needs to be considered. This may include sexual health, future vocational development, including the need for disclosure and their rights under the Disability Discrimination Act. Similarly, the implications of other health-risk behaviours such as substance use, tattoos and piercing may need to be discussed.

Transition to adult services

The young person with a chronic condition must eventually leave paediatric and adolescent services for adult services. This often involves changing from a treatment model based around close contact between the adolescent and healthcare professionals (unlimited telephone advice from clinical nurse specialists, possibly home visits, frequent appointments) and involvement with parents and other family members, to one where they are likely to be seen infrequently in a busy adult

Adolescent medicine

497

Table 28.5 Ways to maximise adherence

Assess the size of the problem and be non-judgemental	Ask: 'Most people have trouble taking their medication. When was the last time you forgot?'
Take time to explore practicalities	Try to put yourself in the adolescent's shoes and think through the detail of their regimen with them. Make regimen as simple as possible. Don't forget practical issues – poor adherence may be as simple as not having anywhere private at school to take the treatment
Explore beliefs	May harbour strange or incorrect beliefs about medications, e.g. falsely attribute a side-effect and therefore refuse to take the medication
Use daily routines to 'anchor' adherence	Find daily activities to anchor taking the medication, e.g. brushing teeth, or 'with breakfast and dinner' instead of 'twice a day'. Find the least chaotic time of day: may be morning or evening! Let the suggestions come from the adolescent
Motivation	Negotiate short-term treatment goals. Search for factors that motivate the young person
Involve and contract	Plan the regimen with the adolescent. Some may respond to a written contract that both sides agree to stick to
Written instructions	Most of what is said has been shown to be forgotten once they leave the room!
Take time to explain	Check level of knowledge on each occasion
Solution-focused approach	Find out what has been going well and why. Use this information, e.g. 'How have you managed to remain out of hospital for 3 weeks this month?'

clinic where parental involvement may be minimal or discouraged.

Young people and their parents need both information about the transfer process and time to prepare. Transitional care encompasses this preparation which, by definition, addresses the medical, psychosocial and educational/vocational needs as a young person moves from child- to adult-centred services. Parents are often concerned that the adult team will not address their teenager's healthcare needs. It is helpful if an identified healthcare professional, often a nurse specialist, is responsible for coordinating transition arrangements.

Whereas transitional care starts in early adolescence, some flexibility in age of transfer is desirable, so that it can occur when the young person is developmentally ready and has the necessary maturity to cope with adult services.

Transfer may be via an adolescent or young adult service with clinics run by both adolescent and adult teams together. Such bridging arrangements have many advantages, but require a sufficient number of patients and medical staff able and willing to provide this service. These clinics are usually for specialist conditions, e.g. diabetes, juvenile idiopathic arthritis, cystic fibrosis or congenital heart disease. Alternatively, transfer may be successfully accomplished if there is good communication between teams, although it usually involves a radical change in ethos for the adolescent and family. The general practitioner may be a source of continuity between changing specialty practitioners.

> ### Summary
>
> **Chronic conditions during adolescence**
> - Chronic illness and/or disability may disrupt adolescent development
> - Consideration should be made of the impact of the chronic condition on the rest of health (including sexual and reproductive health) as well as education and leisure
> - Transitional care aims to address medical, psychosocial and educational/vocational issues as young people move from child- to adult-centred services.

Fatigue, headache and other somatic symptoms

Fatigue, headache, abdominal pain, backache and dizziness are common in adolescence. International surveys of adolescents in Europe reveal that two-thirds report morning fatigue more than once a week, 25% have a headache and 15% stomach ache, backache or sleep problems more than once a week. In many, these symptoms appear to be a feature of adolescence, although organic disease must be excluded by history, examination and, occasionally, investigation. For a minority, they may be a physical manifestation of

Table 28.6 Main mental health problems and disorders in adolescents

Problem or disorder	Prevalence (%)
Depression	3–5
Anxiety	4–6
Attention deficit hyperactivity disorder	2–4
Eating disorders	1–2
Conduct disorder	4–6
Substance misuse disorder	2–3

Source: Michaud P-A, Fombonne E. 2005. Common mental health problems. In: Viner R, ed. 2005. *ABC of Adolescence*. Blackwell, Oxford.

psychological problems, and are precipitated by or maintained by factors such as bullying or parental discord.

Occasionally, the symptoms are so severe and persistent that they considerably affect quality of life, with impairment of school attendance, academic results and peer relationships. This may be from chronic fatigue syndrome or chronic idiopathic pain syndromes. Further investigation and assessment will be required and multidisciplinary rehabilitation and cognitive behavioural therapy within the family may be beneficial. The management of somatic symptoms and chronic fatigue syndrome are considered further in Chapter 23.

Mental health problems

The prevalence of mental health problems in adolescents is estimated to be about 11%. The main problems are listed in Table 28.6.

Deliberate self-harm varies from little actual harm, where there is a wish to communicate distress or escape from an interpersonal crisis, to suicide. About 7–14% of adolescents will self-harm, depending on its definition.

Eating disorders are common during adolescence. About 40% of females and 25% of males begin dieting in adolescence because of dissatisfaction with their body. In anorexia nervosa and bulimia, there is a morbid preoccupation with weight and body shape. This is discussed in more detail in Chapter 23.

Health-risk behaviour

During adolescence, young people begin to explore 'adult' behaviours, including smoking, drinking, drug use and sex. These behaviours, often referred to as 'risk-taking' behaviours, may reflect the adolescent's search for pleasure and excitement by participating in new and enjoyable experiences, as well as exerting independence from parents or rebelling against parents' wishes and lifestyle. There is also considerable pressure to fit in with peers.

Adolescents do not always understand the risks involved and may behave as if they are immune from harm. Participating in these activities may also deflect attention away from themselves to mask shyness or anxiety. Unfortunately, health-risk behaviours started in adolescence tend to continue into adult life.

Sexual health

The average age for first sexual intercourse in the UK is 16 years, with one-fifth of 14-year-olds having had intercourse. Having sexual intercourse at an early age is often associated with unsafe sex. This may be because of a lack of knowledge, lack of access to contraception, inability to negotiate obtaining contraception, being drunk or high on drugs or unable to resist being pressurised by their partner.

Risk-taking behaviour in adolescents can result in sexually transmitted infections (STIs) or unplanned pregnancy. STIs may present with urethral or vaginal discharge, urinary symptoms, pain on micturition, abdominal or loin pain, or post-coital vaginal bleeding. Chlamydia is asymptomatic in 50% of cases and can lead to later infertility. In young teenagers, it is more likely to present with a vaginal discharge. Studies have shown that up to one-third of sexually active teenage girls have a sexually transmitted infection. They are also at risk of HIV infection.

Management of sexually transmitted infections

Taking a sexual history from an adolescent should be approached sensitively, in a developmentally appropriate manner, giving the young person warning of the topic, as well as why the questions are being asked. Relevant questions include those related to the risk of STIs: number of partners; any partners during travel abroad; contraception used; whether vaginal, oral or anal sex; any discharge, lower abdominal pain, urinary symptoms; last menstrual period. However, many sexually transmitted infections are asymptomatic, especially in younger teenagers, male and female.

If indicated, swabs should be taken for virology and microbiology (to look for human papillomavirus (HPV), herpes simplex virus (HSV), chlamydia and gonorrhoea). HIV testing may be indicated. In England, in response to the high rates of chlamydia in the under-25-year-old age group, there is a national chlamydia screening programme enabling them to test themselves with easy-to-use kits.

Treatment regimens vary, depending on prevalent antibiotic resistance. Chlamydia can be treated with azithromycin or doxycycline, gonorrhoea with a cephalosporin. Metronidazole can be added for pelvic inflammatory disease. It is advisable to inform and treat partners.

Contraception

Most adolescents who are sexually active *are* using contraception, albeit sometimes haphazardly. In the UK, contraception is used by only half at first intercourse. Condoms, followed by the oral contraceptive pill, are the commonest forms of contraception used. As teenagers have a relatively high failure rate in their ability to use condoms correctly and with the oral contraceptive pill having irregular use, the 'double Dutch' method of condom and oral contraception is advocated to protect against both sexually transmitted infections and pregnancy.

Adolescents with chronic disease, e.g. diabetes, even without microvascular complications, are generally started on lower doses of the contraceptive pill. Some medications prescribed in adolescents are potentially teratogenic (e.g. retinoids for acne, methotrexate for juvenile idiopathic arthritis or other disorders) and may therefore need to be combined with an oral contraceptive pill or depot hormonal implant. Discussions, however, must also reinforce condom use to prevent STIs.

Emergency contraception

Emergency contraception (in the past misleadingly known as the 'morning after pill') can provide significant protection from pregnancy for up to 72 h after unprotected intercourse. Emergency contraception is available from a pharmacist without prescription for those 16 years and over, and on prescription for those under 16 years. If taken within 72 h, it has a 2% failure rate. Side-effects include nausea and lethargy. However, knowledge of emergency contraception is poor among many young people.

Teenage pregnancy

The UK has the highest rate of teenage pregnancy in Western Europe. Teenage girls may present with complaints such as abdominal pain, fatigue, breast tenderness or appetite changes rather than late or missed menstrual period.

Becoming a teenage mother can be a positive life choice and is influenced by culture. There may be considerable support from the extended family, and this may work well. However, in those where the pregnancy was unintended or who are emotionally deprived themselves or unsupported and live in poverty, there may be many adverse consequences for the mother and child. Children of teenage mothers have a higher infant mortality, a higher rate of childhood accidents, illness and admission to hospital, being taken into care, low educational achievement, sexual abuse and mental health problems. Deprivation, from the mother's lack of financial and emotional support and the paucity of her own education and life experiences, is the strongest risk factor. Protective factors are having a supportive family, religious belief and a stable, long-term relationship with the partner.

Health promotion

The reasons to undertake health promotion in adolescents are:

- It is the period for starting health-risk behaviours (smoking, alcohol, drug misuse, unsafe sexual activity)
- Health-risk behaviours started in adolescence often continue into adult life
- Health behaviours may have a direct effect on their lives, e.g. teenage pregnancy, road traffic accidents
- Increasing morbidity, e.g. obesity and diabetes.

The main areas for health promotion are:

- Health-risk behaviours
- Mental health
- Violent behaviour
- Physical activity, nutrition and obesity
- Parent–adolescent communication.

There are a number of approaches to health promotion for adolescents:

- Provide suitable information in a user-friendly way for young people. An example is the website: Teenage Health Freak (Fig. 28.4).
- Health promotion by society as a whole, e.g. banning cigarette advertising, making emergency contraception available in pharmacies. These can be very effective. However, there is increasing evidence that improving the socioeconomic circumstances of young people would be the most effective intervention for health promotion. Also, as adolescents often embark on more than one risk behaviour, tackling the underlying problem may reduce other risk-taking behaviours: e.g. a programme to reduce bullying in a whole school may also reduce other behaviour such as drug misuse.
- Training programmes to improve adolescents' ability to accept or reject certain courses of behaviour can be effective for the individual, but is time-consuming and expensive.

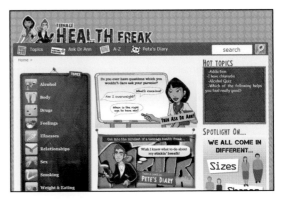

Figure 28.4 The website Teenage Health Freak promotes health in a user-friendly way to teenagers. Available at: http://www.teenagehealthfreak.org (Accessed May 2011). (Reproduced with permission.)

Summary

The main health problems of adolescents

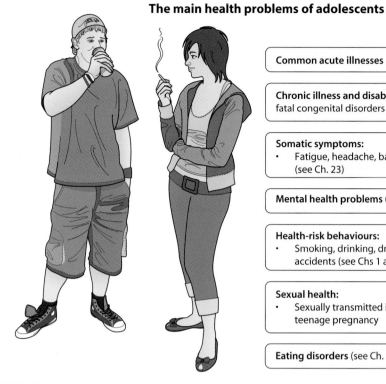

Common acute illnesses

Chronic illness and disability, including previously fatal congenital disorders

Somatic symptoms:
* Fatigue, headache, backache and abdominal pain (see Ch. 23)

Mental health problems (see Ch. 23)

Health-risk behaviours:
* Smoking, drinking, drug abuse, road traffic accidents (see Chs 1 and 23)

Sexual health:
* Sexually transmitted infections, contraception, teenage pregnancy

Eating disorders (see Ch. 23) **and obesity** (see Ch. 12)

* Health promotion by professionals. Exhorting adolescents not to smoke, to eat a balanced diet, use contraception, etc., has not been found to be effective, and may be counter-productive. Health professionals do have a role in health promotion at an individual level. It is likely to be most effective if targeted at those who are receptive or contemplating change in their health-risk behaviour. However, motivational interviewing techniques (which do not assume that they are ready to change their behaviour, but aim to increase their intrinsic motivation to change) have also been shown to be useful with this age group.

Further reading

Not Just a Phase: A Guide to the Participation of Children and Young People in Health Services, London, 2010, Royal College of Paediatrics and Child Health (RCPCH).

Viner R: *ABC of Adolescence*, London, 2005, BMJ Books.

Websites (Accessed May 2011)

Teenage Health Freak: Available at: http://www.teenagehealthfreak.org.

Youth Health Talk: Available at: http://www.youthhealthtalk.org.

Adolescent medicine

Appendix

Growth charts

Examples of growth charts used in the UK for:

- low birthweight males (A.1a) and females (A.1b)
- 0–1 years, boys (A.1c) and girls (A.1d)
- 1–4 years, boys (A.1e) and girls (A.1f)
- Birth–20 years, boys (A.1g).

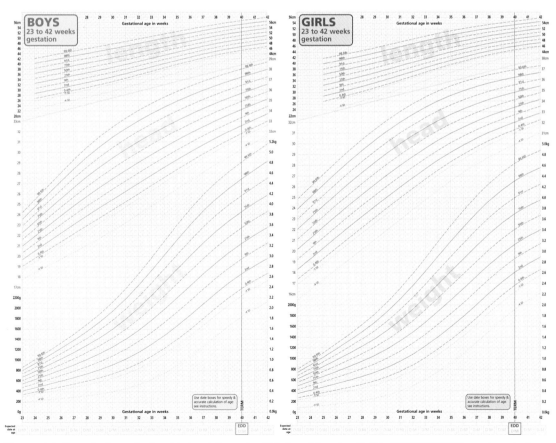

Figure A.1 Growth charts for low birthweight males (A.1a) and females (A.1b). (RCPCH/WHO/Department of Health. ©2009 Department of Health).

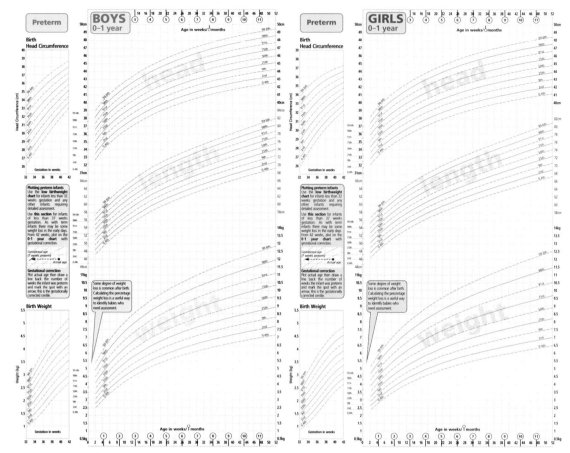

Figure A.1, cont'd Growth charts 0–1 year Boys (A.1c) Girls (A.1d). (RCPCH/WHO/Department of Health. ©2009 Department of Health).

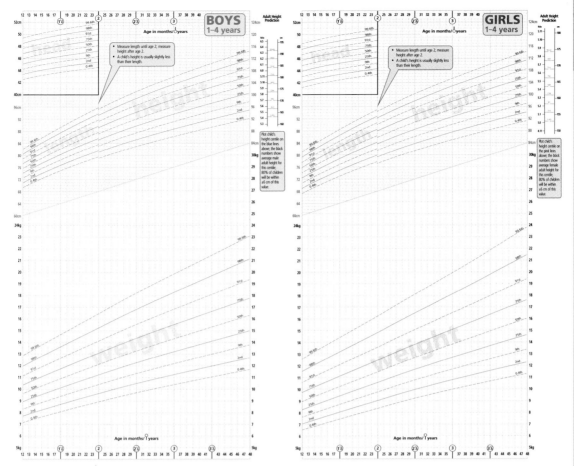

Figure A.1, cont'd Growth charts 1-4 years Boys (A.1e) Girls (A.1f). (RCPCH/WHO/Department of Health. ©2009 Department of Health.)

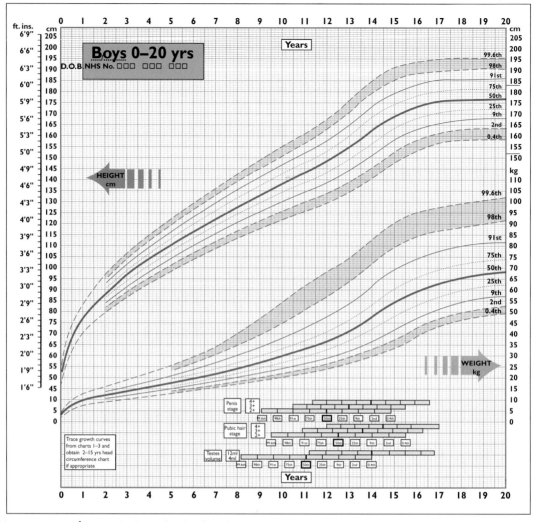

Figure A.1, cont'd Growth chart of males from birth to 20 years using the nine centile UK chart (A.1g). The interval between each pair of centile lines is the same (²⁄₃ standard deviation). It shows the 0.4 and 99.6 centile lines, which are 2²⁄₃ standard deviations below and above the median respectively. It also shows the timing of the stages of puberty. (Chart ©Child Growth Foundation.)

Gestational age assessment of newborn infants

Neuromuscular maturity

	−1	0	1	2	3	4	5
Posture							
Square window (wrist)	>90°	90°	60°	45°	35°	0°	
Arm recoil		180°	140°–180°	110°–140°	90°–110°	<90°	
Popliteal angle	180°	160°	140°	120°	100°	90°	<90°
Scarf sign							
Heel to ear							

Physical maturity

Skin	Sticky, friable, transparent	Gelatinous, red, translucent	Smooth pink, visible veins	Superficial peeling and/or rash, few veins	Cracking pale areas rare veins	Parchment, deep cracking, no vessels	Leathery, cracked, wrinkled
Lanugo	None	Sparse	Abundant	Thinning	Bald areas	Mostly bald	
Plantar surface	Heel-toe 40–50 mm: −1 < 40 mm: −2	>50 mm no crease	Faint red marks	Anterior transverse crease only	Creases ant. 2/3	Creases over entire sole	
Breast	Imperceptible	Barely perceptible	Flat areola, no bud	Stippled areola 1–2 mm bud	Raised areola 3–4 mm bud	Full areola 5–10 mm bud	
Eye/ear	Lids fused loosely: −1 tightly −2	Lids open Pinna flat, stays folded	Sl. curved pinna; soft; slow recoil	Well-curved pinna; soft but ready recoil	Formed and firm, instant recoil	Thick cartilage, ear stiff	
Genitalia male	Scrotum flat, smooth	Scrotum empty, faint rugae	Testes in upper canal, rare rugae	Testes decending, few rugae	Testes down, good rugae	Testes pendulous, deep rugae	
Genitalia female	Clitoris prominent, labia flat	Prominent clitoris, small labia minora	Prominent clitoris, enlarging minora	Majora and minora equally prominent	Majora large, minora small	Majora cover clitoris and minora	

(c) Maturity rating

Score	Weeks
−10	20
−5	22
0	24
5	26
10	28
15	30
20	32
25	34
30	36
35	38
40	40
45	42
50	44

Figure A.2 Scoring system for assessment of gestational age in newborn infants (Ballard score). This is a method of assessing gestational age according to neuromuscular and physical maturity. The infant's gestation or age (±2 weeks) is determined from the total score using the conversion chart. (Adapted from: Ballard JL, Khoury JC, Wedig K , et al. 1991. New Ballard score, expanded to include extremely premature infants. *Journal of Pediatrics* 119:417–423.)

Management plan for asthma

Green zone – GO

Your asthma is under control if:
- your breathing feels good
- you do not have a cough or wheeze
- you can take part in normal activities and play games / sport.
- your are sleeping through the night
- you are not missing school because of your asthma

Peak Flows are between:

....

....

Green zone action –
Your normal medicines are:
Preventer

....

....

Other Medicines

....

....

Reliever

....
as required.
Remember: If necessary take this before exercise or if you have cold-like symptoms. Take 2–4 puffs every 4 hours if you need it.
If there is no improvement, move to the Amber zone.

Amber zone – WARNING

Your asthma is getting worse if you:
- wake at night with asthma symptoms
- have a cough, wheeze or 'tight' chest
- need to use the reliever inhaler once a day, more than usual or it is not lasting for four hours.

Peak Flows are between:

....

....

Amber zone action –
Take all medicines as normal.

Take 4–10 puffs of reliever – one puff at a time as taught. Use a spacer if you have one and shake the MDI in between puffs. Take every four hours if needed.

- If no improvement – make an appointment to see your doctor for that day.
- If you have a Symptom/Peak Flow Diary – start filling it in and take it with you to the doctor.

Or
Start your home prednisolone ....mgs daily, if you have it. See your doctor if you are not better after 12 hours.

Remember: If no better after 10 puffs of reliever, move to Red zone.

Red zone – DANGER

Your asthma is severe if after taking 10 puffs of reliever you:
- are still breathing hard and fast
- can't talk or feed easily
- are exhausted
- are frightened and look anxious
- are very pale/grey/blue in colour

Peak Flow reading (if able) below:

....

....

Red zone action –
   Call an ambulance now

- Keep taking one puff of reliever every 20–30 seconds or 4 slow breaths or, if you have one, nebulized reliever with oxygen until the ambulance arrives.
- Take a dose of oral steroids if not already taken.
- Don't move about
- Keep calm

Figure A.3 Example of patient management plan for asthma.

Blood pressure chart

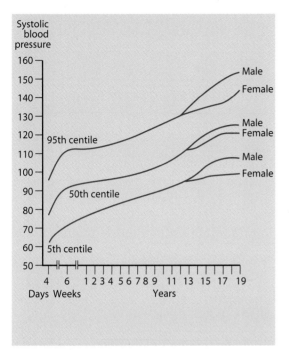

Figure A.4 Systolic blood pressure according to age. Blood pressure charts are also available according to height. (Data from: de Swiet M, Fayers P, Shinebourne EA. 1980. Blood pressure in a population of infants in the first year of life: the Brompton Study. *Pediatrics* 65:1028–1035 and de Man SA, Andre JL, Bachmann H et al. 1991. Blood pressure in childhood: pooled findings of six European studies. *Journal of Hypertension* 9:109–114.)

Peak flow chart

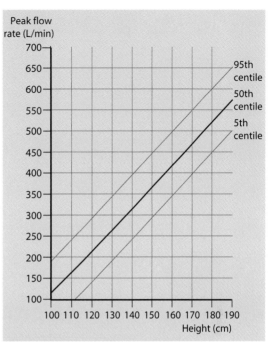

Figure A.5 The normal range of peak flow measurements according to height. (Reproduced with permission from: Godfrey S, Kamburoff PL, Nairn JR. 1970. Spirometry, lung volumes and airway resistance in normal children aged 5 to 18 years. *British Journal of Diseases of the Chest* 64:15–24.)

Normal ranges: haematology

Age	Hb (g/dl)	MCV (fL)	WBC (×10⁹/L)	Platelets (×10⁹/L)
Birth	14.5–21.5	100–135	10–26	150–450 at all ages
2 weeks	13.4–19.8	88–120	6–21	
2 months	9.4–13.0	84–105	6–18	
1 year	11.3–14.1	71–85	6–17.5	
2–6 years	11.5–13.5	75–87	5–17	
6–12 years	11.5–15.5	77–95	4.5–14.5	
12–18 years:				
Male	13.0–16.0	78–95	4.5–13	
Female	12.0–16.0	78–95	4.5–13	

Index

Nutrition, 201–218
    assessment of status, 209–212
    Crohn disease, 236
    in cystic fibrosis patients, 297
    demands for growth, 201
    dental caries, 217–218
    in diabetes, 436
    dietary elimination, atopic eczema, 428
    enteral, 164, 210–211
    failure to thrive see Failure to thrive
    gastroenteritis, 232
    infantile growth, 181
    intensive support, role, 210–211
    and kidney disease, 344
    and liver disease, 363
    long-term outcome of deficiency, 202
    low stores, in infants and children, 201–202
    malnutrition, 201–202, 209–212, 212b, 257
    and neuronal development, 201–202
    and obesity, 6, 181, 215–217
    parenteral, 160, 211
    during pregnancy, 134
    in pre-term infants, 164
    seizures, 477
    and short stature, 187
    in very low birthweight infants, 167f
    vitamin deficiency see Vitamin A deficiency;
        Vitamin D deficiency
    vulnerability of infants and children, 201–202
Nystagmus, 23–24

O

Obesity, 6, 215–217, 218b
    complications, 216b
    definitions, 216–217
    endogenous causes, 217
    and low birthweight, 181
    management of, 217
    prevention, 217
    reduced, in breast-feeding, 203
Obstructive sleep apnoea (OSA), 279, 298
Occipital plagiocephaly, 192
Occipital seizures, 474
Occlusive bandages, 428
Oedema, pulmonary, 88
Oesophageal atresia, 177
Oesophageal varices, 362–363
Oesophagitis, acid-related, 222
Omalizumab, 289
Omeprazole, 222, 228
Omphalocele, 178–179
Ophthalmoscopy, 24–27
Opiates, maternal drug abuse with, 140
Oral allergy syndrome, 273
Orchidopexy, 349–350
Orchitis, 257
Orlistat, 217
Ortolani manoeuvre, 152f
Osgood-Schlatter disease, 457
Osteochondritis dissecans, 458
Osteogenesis imperfecta, 112, 122, 466, 467f
Osteomalacia, 213
Osteomyelitis, 456, 456b
Osteopaenia of prematurity, 167f
Osteopetrosis, 466
Osteoporosis, 464
Otitis media (OM), 59, 80
    acute, 278–279

Otitis media with effusion (OME), 279
    recurrent, 279
Otosclerosis, 122
Outflow obstruction
    in sick child, 301, 318–320
    in well child, 301, 315–318, 318b
Oxygen dissocation curve, 382f
Oxygen therapy, pre-term infants, 162
Oxytocin, 140

P

Pain, 71, 71f
    acute, 71
    assessing, 71f
    back, 458
    chest, 321
    chronic, 71
    limbs, 456–457
    management of, 71
Palliative care, 378
Palpation
    abdominal examination, 20
    cardiovascular system examination, 19
    respiratory system examination, 17
Pancreatic exocrine insufficiency, in CF,
        296
Parainfluenza viruses, 280
Paralytic squints, 61
Paraphimosis, 353
Parasitic infestations, 429–430
Parathyroid disorders, 444–445
Parathyroid hormone, 213
Paravertebral tumours, 374
Parental chromosomal analysis, 117, 129
Parental employment, 3
Parenteral nutrition, 160, 211
Parenting, normal, 405
Parenting styles, 3
Parietal lobe seizures, 474
Paroxysmal disorders, 473
Partially sighted children, 62
Participation rights of child, 6
Parvovirus B19, 255, 385
Patau syndrome (trisomy 13), 118, 119b
Patent ductus arteriosus, pre-term infants, 163
Peak expiratory flow rate (PEFR), 288–289
Pectus carinatum (pigeon chest), 17
Pectus excavatum (hollow chest), 17
Pedestrian road traffic accidents, 98
Pediculosis capitis, 430
Peer groups, 4
Pelvic kidney, 329
Pelviureteric junction (PUJ) obstruction, 228
D-penicillamine, 105–106
Penicillin resistance, 245
Penis, 351–353
    circumcision, 352–353
    hypospadias, 198, 351, 352f
    paraphimosis, 353
Peptic ulceration, 228
Percussion
    cardiovascular system examination, 19
    masses, abnormal, 21
    respiratory system examination, 17
Performance IQ (PIQ), 41–42
Periarticular oedema, 339
Pericarditis, 255
Perinatal isoimmune thrombocytopenia, 136

surfactant therapy in, 80, 159, 162f
temperature control, 163
very low birthweight, 167f, 168
see also Infants; Jaundice; Neonates
Prevenar vaccine, 284
Preventers (inhaled corticosteroids), 289
Primary care, 67
Primitive reflexes, 34t, 54
Primordial dwarfism, 187
Progressive familial intrahepatic cholestasis (PFIC), 358
Prop-feeding, discouraging, 218
Prostaglandin F2, 140
Protease inhibitor (Pi), 356
Protection rights of child, 6
Protein
importance in obese children, 217
requirements, reference values, 202t
transient intolerances, 234
Proteinuria, 336–338
Proteus infection, 331
Proton pump inhibitors, 222, 228
Prune-belly syndrome, 329
Pruritis
eczema, 426
liver disease, 364
Pseudohepatomegaly, 20
Pseudohypoparathyroidism, 444
Pseudomembranous croup (bacterial tracheitis), 281
Pseudomonas, 174
Pseudomonas aeruginosa, 295–296
Pseudopseudohypoparathyroidism, 444
Psoriasis, 430
Psychosis, 420
Psychosocial deprivation, and short stature, 181, 187
Psychosocial support
atopic eczema, 428
headache, 472
hospital care, 70
malignant disease, 368
Puberty, 183–186
in both sexes, 185
delayed, 195–196
constitutional delay, 186, 196
diabetes management, 439
in females, 183, 184f
growth spurt, 181
in males, 184
precocious, 193–194
Tanner stages, 184f
timing of, 185f
see also Adolescents
Public health issues, 6
Pulmonary hypertension, 323–324
in newborn, 173
Pulmonary hypoplasia, 173
Pulmonary interstitial emphysema (PIE), 162
Pulmonary oedema, 88
Pulmonary stenosis, 316–317
Pulse oximetry, 280
Pulses
examining, 18–19
normal resting, in children, 19t
Pupillary signs, in coma, 90f
Purified protein derivative (PPD), 260
Purpura fulminans, 252
P-wave, 320
Pyelonephritis, 330, 334
Pyloric stenosis, 222, 222b–223b
Pyloromyotomy, 222

Pyramidal tract dysfunction, 22–23
Pyrazinamide, 260
Pyridoxine, 260

Q

QRS complex, 320
Quadriplegia, 54

R

Radiological investigation
kidneys and urinary tract disorders, 326t
malignant disease, 366
Radiotherapy, 367, 371, 377
Rashes, 425–428
chickenpox, 252–253
in febrile child, 243, 251t
German measles, 133, 140–141, 257
Langerhans cell histiocytosis, 378f
measles, 256–257
nephritis, 339
and systemic disease, 431–432
systems review, 15
see also Meningitis
RAST test, 426
allergies, 274
RB gene, 366
Reactive arthritis, 461
Reconstituted families, 3
Rectal atresia, 178
Rectal examination, 21–22
Recurrent abdominal pain (RAP), 227–228
Red cell aplasia, 385–386
Red cells
abnormally shaped, 386f
increased destruction in haemolytic anaemia, 386–394
reduced production in newborn, 392
Reflexes
absent, 23
corneal light reflex test, 61
neurological examination, 23
postural, 34t
primitive, 34t, 54
Refractive errors, 62
Refugees, 3
Regurgitation, 219–220
Relievers (short-acting β_2-agonists), 289
Remission induction, in leukaemia, 369–370
Renal acidosis, 344–345
Renal agenesis, 325
Renal calculi, 341
Renal failure, 343
acute, 343b–344b
chronic, 187, 325, 345b
and liver disease, 363
postrenal, 343
prerenal, 343
see also Kidneys and urinary tract disorders;
Urinary tract infection (UTIs)
Renal function, assessment in children, 326t
Renal masses, 341
Renal osteodystrophy, prevention, 344
Renal scarring, 335
Renal tubular disorders, 341–342
Research in paediatrics, ethics of, 75–76
Respiratory depression, 146

testicular torsion, 350
undescended testes, 349
Umbilical infection, 175
Umbilical venous catheter, 160
Unconsciousness
near-drowning, 101
see also Coma
Undescended testes, 348–350
bilateral, 198, 348–349
examination, 349
retractile testis, 349
unilateral, 348–349
Undressing children, for examination, 16
Uniparental disomy, 125, 126f
United Nations Convention on the Rights of the Child,
6b, 66, 106
Upper respiratory tract infection (URTI), 243, 278–279
Urease, 228
Urinalysis, 22
Urinary tract infection (UTIs), 330–335
acute abdominal pain, 224
acute scrotum, 350–351
bacterial and host factors, predisposing to, 331–332
case histories, 333, 335
circumcision, 352–353
clinical features, 330
dipstick testing, 331, 331t
first, 333f, 334b
haematuria, 338
incomplete bladder emptying, 332
infecting organism, 331
investigations, 332–334
management of, 334
presentation in infancy/childhood, 330b
prevention, medical measures, 334–335
recurrent, follow-up, 335
sample collection, 330–331, 335
see also Kidneys and urinary tract disorders
Urinary tract obstruction, 328b, 329
Urticaria, 275, 276b, 431–432
neonatal, 150f
Utility, 74
Uveitis, 462

V

VACTERL association, 128, 177
Vagal nerve stimulation, 477
Vaginal discharge, 354
Varicella zoster, 141, 253
Varicocele, 350
Vasculitis, 245
Kawasaki disease, 258, 258b–259b, 323
kidney disorder, 340
Venous lines, 160
Ventilation
long-term, in cystic fibrosis, 299–300
neonatal resuscitation, 143
Ventricular septal defect (VSD), 305, 308–309, 309f
Ventricular tap, 164
Verbal IQ (VIQ), 41–42
Vernix caseosa, 423
Vertical talus, 453
Vesicoureteric reflux (VUR), 332
Vincristine, 368
Viral infections, 250–257
hepatitis, 358–360
see also Hepatitis
meningitis, 245–246, 257
molluscum contagiosum, 428

uncommon, 256–257
warts, 428
see also Respiratory infections
Vision
abnormalities, 61–62, 116
development, 34–40, 36f, 39f, 44–47
severe impairment, 62
Vision testing, 47
Visual reinforcement audiometry, 44, 46f
Vitamin deficiency
vitamin A, 205–206, 215, 257, 363
vitamin D, 205–206, 213–215, 364
vitamin E, 363
vitamin K, 356–358, 363
Vitamin K therapy, 152
Vitamins, fat-soluble, 363–364
VLBW (very low birthweight infants), 167f, 168
Vomiting, 219–222
in allergic conditions, 273
cancer treatment, 368
causes, 220f
cyclical, 470
investigation, 221–222
'red flag' clinical features, 219b, 220
Von Willebrand disease (vWD), 396t, 398
Vulvovaginitis, 354

W

Walking, 33
late, 33f, 52
Warfarin, 133
War/natural disasters, 6, 6b
Warts, 428
Wealth, 5
Weaning, 206
Wegener granulomatosis, 340
Werdnig-Hoffmann disease, 481
Wheezing, 18
persistent and recurrent, 287
transient early, 285–287
Whooping cough (pertussis), 166, 266, 282
Williams syndrome, 120, 128f
Wilms' tumour, 20, 375, 375b
Wilson disease, 361–362
Wiskott-Aldrich syndrome, 400
Wolff-Parkinson-White (WPW) syndrome, 320
Wong Baker Faces scale, pain assessment, 71f
World Health Organization (WHO)
on breast-feeding, 203
Child Growth Standards, 182–183
Wound management
burns and scalds, 99–101
dog bites, 101
Wrist, X-rays, 185f

X

Xerophthalmia, 215
X-linked dominant inheritance, 123
X-linked recessive inheritance, 122b, 124b, 124f

Y

Y-linked inheritance, 123

Z

Zinc deficiency, 232